Molecular Pharmacology

From DNA to Drug Discovery

Molecular Pharmacology

From DNA to Drug Discovery

John Dickenson, Fiona Freeman, Chris Lloyd Mills,
Shiva Sivasubramaniam and Christian Thode
Nottingham Trent University

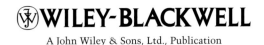

A John Wiley & Sons, Ltd., Publication

Registered office: John Wiley & Sons, Ltd, The Atrium, Southern Gate, Chichester, West Sussex, PO19 8SQ, UK

Editorial offices: 9600 Garsington Road, Oxford, OX4 2DQ, UK

The Atrium, Southern Gate, Chichester, West Sussex, PO19 8SQ, UK

111 River Street, Hoboken, NJ 07030-5774, USA

For details of our global editorial offices, for customer services and for information about how to apply for permission to reuse the copyright material in this book please see our website at www.wiley.com/wiley-blackwell.

Library of Congress Cataloging-in-Publication Data

Molecular pharmacology : from DNA to drug discovery / John Dickenson . . . [et al.].
    p. ; cm.
  Includes index.
  ISBN 978-0-470-68444-3 (cloth) – ISBN 978-0-470-68443-6 (pbk.)
  I. Dickenson, John.
  [DNLM: 1. Molecular Targeted Therapy. 2. Pharmacogenetics–methods.
3. Drug Delivery Systems. 4. Drug Discovery. QV 38.5]
  615.1′9–dc23

                                                2012034772

A catalogue record for this book is available from the British Library.

Wiley also publishes its books in a variety of electronic formats. Some content that appears in print may not be available in electronic books.

Typeset in 9.25/11.5pt Minion by Laserwords Private Limited, Chennai, India.
Printed and bound in Singapore by Markono Print Media Pte Ltd.

First Impression 2013

Contents

Preface

Nottingham Trent University offers a suite of successful MSc courses in the Biosciences field that are delivered by full-time, part-time and distance (e-learning) teaching. The authors are members of the Pharmacology team at Nottingham Trent University and teach extensively on the MSc Pharmacology and Neuropharmacology courses. The content of this book was inspired by these courses as there is no comparable postgraduate textbook on molecular pharmacology and it is a rapidly expanding subject. The primary aim of this text was to provide a platform to complement our courses and enhance the student experience. Given the breadth and depth of this volume it will be of use to students from other institutions as a teaching aid as well as an invaluable source of background information for post-graduate researchers. The value of this book is enhanced by the research portfolio of the Bioscience Department and individual authors who have research careers spanning over 25 years.

This textbook illustrates how genes can influence our physiology and hence our pharmacological response to drugs used to treat pathological conditions. Tailoring of therapeutic drugs is the future of drug design as it enables physicians to prescribe personalised medical treatments based on an individual's genome. The book utilises a drug target-based approach rather than the traditional organ/system-based viewpoint and reflects the current advances and research trends towards *in silico* drug design based on gene and derived protein structure.

The authors would like to thank Prof Mark Darlison (Napier University, Edinburgh, UK) for providing the initial impetus, inspiration and belief that a book of such magnitude was possible. We would also like to acknowledge the unflagging encouragement and support of the Wiley-Blackwell team (Nicky, Fiona and Clara) during the preparation of this work. Finally thanks should also be given to the helpful, constructive and positive comments provided by the reviewers. We hope that you enjoy this book as much as we enjoyed writing it.

John Dickenson, Fiona Freeman, Chris Lloyd Mills, Shiva Sivasubramaniam and Christian Thode.

Abbreviations

$[Ca^{2+}]_i$	intracellular free ionised calcium concentration	**ARC channels**	arachidonic acid regulated Ca^{2+} channels
$[Ca^{2+}]_n$	nuclear free ionised calcium concentration	**Arg**	arginine (R)
$[Ca^{2+}]_o$	extracellular free ionised calcium concentration	**ASIC**	acid sensing ion channels
		ASL	airways surface liquid
2-APB	2-aminoethoxydiphenyl borate	**Asn**	asparagine (N)
4EFmut DREAM	4th EF hand mutant DREAM	**Asp**	aspartic acid (D)
5F-BAPTA	1,2-bis(2-amino-5,6-diflurophenoxy) ethane-N,N,N′,N′-tetracacetic acid	**ATF1**	activation transcription factor 1
		ATP	adenosine triphosphate
		AV	adenovirus
5-HT	5-hydroxytyrptamine / serotonin	**Aβ**	amyloid β peptide
AAV	adeno-associated virus	**BAC**	bacterial artificial chromosome
ABC	ATP-binding cassette (transporter)	**BBB**	blood brain barrier
AC	adenylyl cyclase	**BCRP**	breast cancer resistant protein
ACC	mitochondrial ADP/ATP carrier (transporter)	**BDNF**	brain-derived neurotrophic factor
		BK_{Ca}	big conductance Ca^{2+}-activated K^+ channels
ACh	acetylcholine		
ACS	anion-cation subfamily	**BLAST**	Basic Local Alignment Search Tool
AD	Alzheimer's disease	**bp**	base pairs
ADAR	adenosine deaminase acting on RNA (1, 2 or 3)	**BRET**	bioluminescence resonance energy transfer
ADCC	antibody-dependent cellular cytotoxicity	**Brm/brg1**	mammalian helicase like proteins
		BTF	basal transcription factors
ADEPT	antibody-directed enzyme pro-drug therapy	**BZ**	benzodiazepine
		Ca-CaM	Ca^{2+}-calmodulin
ADHD	attention deficit hyperactivity disorder	**CaCC**	calcium activated chloride channel
AF1/2	transcriptional activating function (1 or 2)	**cADPr**	cyclic adenosine diphosphoribose
		CaM	calmodulin
Ala	alanine (A)	**CaMK**	calcium-dependent calmodulin kinase
AM	acetoxylmethyl	**cAMP**	cyclic adenosine 3′,5′ monophsophate
AMPA	α-amino-3-hydroxy-5-methylis oxazole 4-propionic acid	**CaRE**	calcium responsive element
		catSper	cation channels in sperm
Apo-	apolipoproteins (A, B or C)	Ca_V	voltage-gated Ca^{2+} channels
APP	amyloid precursor protein	**CBAVD**	congenital bilateral absence of the vas deferens
AQP	aquaporins		

CBP	CREB binding protein
CCCP	carbonyl cyanide *m*-chlorophenylhydrazone
CCK	cholecystokinin
CDAR	cytosine deaminase acting on RNA
cDNA	complementary DNA
CDR	complementarily-determining region
CF	cystic fibrosis
CFP	cyan fluorescent protein
CFS	colony stimulating factors
CFTR	cystic fibrosis transmembrane conductance regulator
cGMP	cyclic guanosine $3',5'$ monophosphate
CHF	congestive heart failure
CHO	Chinese hamster ovary cell line
CICR	calcium induced calcium release
CIF	calcium influx factor
ClC	chloride channel
CMV	cytomegalovirus
CNG	cyclic nucleotide-gated channel
CNS	central nervous system
CNT	concentrative nucleoside transporter
COS	CV-1 cell line from Simian kidney cells immortalised with SV40 viral genome
COX	cyclooxygenases (1, 2 or 3)
CPA	monovalent cation/proton antiporter super family
CpG	cytosine-phosphate-guanine regions in DNA
CPP	cell penetrating peptide (transporter)
CRE	cAMP responsive element
CREB	cAMP responsive element binding protein
CREM	CRE modulator
CRF	corticotropin-releasing factor
CRM	chromatin remodelling complex
CRTC	cAMP-regulated transcriptional co-activator family
CSF	cerebral spinal fluid
CTD	C terminal domain
CTL	cytotoxic T lymphocyte
CYP	cytochrome P_{450}
Cys	cysteine (C)
DAG	diacylglycerol
DAX1	dosage-sensitive sex reversal gene/TF
DBD	DNA-binding domain
DC	dicarboxylate
DHA	drug:H^+ antiporter family (transporter)

Dlg1	drosophila disc large tumour suppressor
DNA	deoxyribonucleic acid
DOPA	dihydroxyphenylalanine
DPE	downstream promoter element
DRE	downstream regulatory element
DREAM	DRE antagonist modulator
dsRNA	double-stranded RNA
EBV	Epstein Barr virus
EGF	epidermal growth factor
EGFR	epidermal growth factor receptor
EGTA	ethylene glycol tetraacetic acid
ELISA	enzyme linked immunosorbent assay
ENaC	epithelial sodium channel
EPO	erythropoietin
ER	endoplasmic reticulum
ERK	extracellular-signal-regulated kinases
eRNA	enhancer RNA
ERTF	oestrogen receptor transcription factor
ES cells	embryonic stem cells
ESE	exon splicing enhancer
ESS	exon splicing silencer
EST	expressed sequence tag
Fab	antibody binding domain
FACS	fluorescent-activated cell sorting
Fc	constant fragment of the monoclonal antibodies
FEV_1	forced expiratory volume in 1 second
FGF-9	fibroblast growth factor
FIH	factor inhibiting HIF
FISH	fluorescence *in situ* hybridisation
FOXL2	fork-head box protein
FRET	fluorescence resonance energy transfer
FXS	fragile-X syndrome
G3P	glucose-3-phosphate
GABA	gamma-aminobutyric acid
GAT	GABA transporters
GC	guanylyl cyclase
GFP	green fluorescent protein
GIRK	G-protein-gated inwardly rectify K^+ channel
Gln	glutamine (Q)
GlpT	sn-glycerol-3-phosphate/phosphate antiporter
GltPh	Pyrococcus horikoshii glutamate transporters
Glu	glutamic acid (E)
GLUT	glucose transporters
Gly	glycine (G)
GLYT	glycine transporters

GMP	guanosine monophosphate
GPCR	G protein coupled receptor
GPN	glycyl-L-phenylalanine-2-napthylamide
GRK	G-protein coupled receptor kinase
GST	Glutathione S-transferase
H^+	hydrogen ion; proton
HAD	histone deacetylases
HAMA	human anti-murine antibodies
HAT	histone acetyltransferases
HCF	host cell factor
HCN	hyperpolarisation-activated cyclic nucleotide-gated channels
HDL	high density lipoprotein
HIF	hypoxia inducible factor
His	histidine (H)
HMG	high mobility group
HMIT	H^+/myo-inositol transporter
hnRNP	nuclear ribonucleoproteins
HOX	homeobox
HPLC	high-performance liquid chromatography
HRE	hypoxia response elements
Hsp70	heat shock protein of the 70 kilodalton family
HSV	herpes simplex virus
HSV-tk	herpes simplex virus thymidine kinase
HTS	high-throughput screening
Htt	Huntingtin
IBMX	3-isobutyl-1-methylxanthine
I_{crac}	calcium release activated Ca^{2+} channel
ICSI	intra-cytoplasmic sperm injection
Ifs	interferons
Ig	immunoglobulins
IGF-1	insulin-like growth factor-I
iGluR	ionotropic glutamate receptor
IHD	ischaemic heart disease
IL-10	interleukin-10
Ile	isoleucine (I)
INN	international non-proprietary names
INR	initiator element
INSL3	insulin-like factor 3
IP_3	inositol 1,4,5-triphosphate
IP_3R	IP_3 receptor
$iPLA_2\beta$	β isoform of Ca^{2+} independent phospholipase A_2
IRT	immunoreactive trypsinogen
I_{sc}	short circuit current
ISE	introns splicing enhancer
ISS	introns splicing silencer
K_{2P}	two-pore potassium channels

K3K4 HMT	histone methyl transferase
K_{ATP}	ATP-sensitive K^+ channels
kb	kilobase
K_{Ca}	Ca^{2+}-activated K^+ channels
KCC	K^+-Cl^- co-transporter
KChIP	K^+ channel interacting protein
KCO	K^+ channel openers
Kd	Ca^{2+} dissociation constant
K_G	G-protein gated K^+ channels
KID	kinase-inducible domain
K_{ir}	inwardly rectifying K^+ channels
K_V	voltage-gated K^+ channel
LacY	lactose:H^+ symporter
LBD	ligand binding domains
LDL	low density lipoprotein
Leu	leucine (L)
LeuTAa	Aquifex aeolicus leucine transporter
LGIC	ligand-gated ion channel
lncRNA	long non-coding RNA
LPS	lipopolysaccharide
lys	lysine (K)
Mab	monoclonal antibodies
MAC	membrane attack complex
MAPK	mitogen-activated protein kinase
MATE	multidrug and toxic compound extrusion superfamily (transporter)
Mb	megabase
MCT	mono carboxylate transporters
MCU	mitochondrial Ca^{2+} uniporter
MDR	multidrug resistance (transporter)
MDR1	multidrug resistant transporter 1
Met	methionine (M)
MFP	periplasmic membrane fusion protein family (transporter)
MFS	major facilitator superfamily (transporter)
MHC	histocompatibility complex
miRNA	microRNA
mPTP	mitochondrial permeability transition pore
mRNA	messenger RNA
MSD	membrane spanning domain
MTF	modulatory transcription factors
Myc	myc oncogene
NAADP	nicotinic acid adenine dinucleotide phosphate
nAChR	nicotinic acetylcholine receptors
NAD^+	nicotinamide adenine dinucleotide
$NADP^+$	nicotinamide adenine dinucleotide phosphate

NALCN	sodium leak channel non-selective protein channel	PGE$_2$	prostaglandin E$_2$
NAT	natural antisense transcript	P-gp	permeability glycoprotein (transporter)
Na$_V$	voltage-gated Na$^+$ channels	Phe	phenylalanine (F)
NBD	nucleotide binding domain	Pi	inorganic phosphate
ncRNA	non-coding RNA	PI3	phosphatidylinositol 3-kinases
neoR	neomycin resistance	PIP$_2$	phosphatidylinositol 4,5-bisphosphate
NES	nuclear endoplasmic space	PKA	protein kinase A
NFAT	nuclear factor of activated T cells	PKC	protein kinase C
NFκB	nuclear factor kappa of activated B cells	PLC	phospholipase C
		PLCβ	β isoform of phospholipase C
NHA	Na$^+$/H$^+$ antiporters	pLGICs	pentameric ligand-gated ion channels
NhaA	Escherichia coli Na$^+$/H$^+$ antiporter	PM	plasma membrane
NHE	Na$^+$/H$^+$ exchanger	PMCA	plasma membrane Ca^{2+} ATPase
NKCC	sodium potassium 2 chloride cotransporter	PP1	protein phosphatase 1
NM	nuclear membrane	PPAR	peroxisome proliferator-activated receptors (α, β, δ, or γ)
NMDA	N-methyl-D-aspartate		
NMR	nuclear magnetic reasonance	PPRE	PPAR response element
NO	nitric oxide	pRB	retinoblastoma protein
NPA	Asn-Pro-Ala motif	Pro	proline (P)
NPC	nuclear pore complex	PSD$_{95}$	post synaptic density protein-95
NR	nucleoplasmic reticulum	Q1/Q2	glutamine-rich domains (1 or 2)
NR-HSP	nuclear receptor-heat shock protein complex	RaM	rapid mode uptake
		RAMP	receptor-activity modifying protein
NRSE	neuron restrictive silencer element	Ras	rat sarcoma (causing factor)
NSS	neurotransmitter sodium symporter (transporter)	RBC	red blood cell
		REST	repressor element-1 transcription factor
nt	nucleotide		
NTD	N- terminal domain	RFLP	restriction fragment length polymorphism
NVGDS	non viral gene delivery systems		
OA-	organic anion	rhDNase	recombinant human DNase
OAT	organic anion transporters	RICs	radio-immunoconjugates
OCT	organic cation transporters	RIP	receptor-interacting protein
Oct/OAP	octomer/octomer associated proteins	RISC	RNA-induced silencing complex
OMF	outer membrane factor family (transporter)	RLF	relaxin-like factor
		RNA pol	RNA polymerases
ORCC	outwardly rectifying chloride channel	RNA	ribonucleic acid
ORF	open-reading frame	RNAi	RNA interference
OSN	olfactory sensory neurons	RND	resistance-nodulation-cell division (transporter)
OxlT	oxalate:formate antiporter		
Pax	paired box gene/TF	ROS	reactive oxygen species
pCa	-log$_{10}$ of the Ca^{2+} concentration	rRNA	ribosomal RNA
PCR	polymerase chain reaction	RSPO1	R-spondin-1
PD	potential difference	RT-PCR	reverse-transcription polymerase chain reaction
PDE	phosphodiesterase		
PDZ	PSD$_{95}$-Dlg1-zo-1 (protein motif)	RXR	retinoic acid receptor
PEPT	dipeptide transporters	RyR	ryanodine receptors
PG	prostaglandins	SAM	intraluminal sterile α motif
PGC-1α	peroxisome proliferator-activated receptor α, co-activator 1α	SBP	substrate binding protein
		Ser	serine (S)

SERCA	sarco/endoplasmic reticulum Ca^{2+} ATPase	TIF-1	transcription intermediary factor
Shh	sonic hedgehog homolog gene/TF	TIRF	total internal reflection fluorescence imaging
siRNA	short interfering RNA	TMAO	trimethylamine N-oxide
SK$_{Ca}$	small conductance Ca^{2+}-activated K$^+$ channels	TMD	transmembrane domain
SLC	solute carrier superfamily (transporter)	TMS	transmembrane segments
		TNFs	tumour necrosis factors
SMN	survival of motor neurons protein	TPC	two pore calcium channels
SMR	small multidrug resistance superfamily (transporter)	TPEN	N,N,N′,N′-tetrakis(2-pyridylmethyl)ethylenediamine
snoRNA	small nucleolar RNA	Trk	tyrosine kinase receptor (A, B or C)
SNP	single nucleotide polymorphism	tRNA	transfer RNA
snRNA	spliceosomal small nuclear RNA	TRP	transient receptor potential channels
SOC	store operated Ca^{2+} channel	Trp	tryptophan (W)
Sox9	SRY-related HMG box-9 gene/factor	TTX	tetrodotoxin
SR	sarcoplasmic reticulum	Tyr	tyrosine (Y)
SRC-1	steroid receptor co-activator-1.	TZD	thiazolidinedione
SREBP	sterol regulatory element-binding proteins	Ubi	ubiquitination
		UTR	untranslated region
SRY	sex-determining region Y	Val	valine (V)
SSS	solute sodium symporter (transporter)	VDAC	voltage dependent anion channel
STAT	signal transducer and activator of transcription (1, 2 or 3)	VEGF	vasculoendothelial growth facto
		VFT	venus flytrap
STIM	stromal interaction molecule	vGLUT	vesicular glutamate transporter
SUG-1	suppressor of gal4D lesions −1	VHL	von Hippel-Lindau protein
SUMO	small ubiquitin like modifier	VIP	vasoactive intestinal peptide
SUR	sulfonylureas receptor	VLDL	very low density lipoprotein
SW1/SNF	switching mating type/sucrose non-fermenting proteins	V$_m$	membrane potential
		VOCC	voltage-operated calcium channels
TAD	transactivation domain	WNT4	wingless-type mouse mammary tumour virus integration site
TAP	transporters associated with antigen processing		
		YAC	yeast artificial chromosome
TCA	tricarboxlyic acid	YFP	yellow fluorescent protein
TCR	T cell receptor	YORK	yeast outward rectifying K$^+$ channel
TDF	testis-determining factor	ZAC	zinc-activated channel
TEAD	TEA domain proteins	Zo-1	zonula occludens-1 protein
TEF	transcription enhancer factor		
TESCO	testis-specific enhancer of Sox9		
TGF	transforming growth factor		
TGN	trans-Golgi network		
TH	tyrosine hydroxylase		
Thr	threonine (T)		

POST-FIXes

Chimeric antibodies – *xiMabs*

Human antibodies – *muMbs*

Humanised antibodies – *zumab*

Monoclonal antibodies – *oMabs*

1

Introduction to Drug Targets and Molecular Pharmacology

1.1 Introduction to molecular pharmacology

During the past 30 years there have been significant advances and developments in the discipline of molecular pharmacology – an area of pharmacology that is concerned with the study of drugs and their targets at the molecular or chemical level. Major landmarks during this time include the cloning of the first G-protein coupled receptor (GPCR) namely the β_2-adrenergic receptor in 1986 (Dixon et al., 1986). This was quickly followed by the cloning of additional adrenergic receptor family genes and ultimately other GPCRs. The molecular biology explosion during the 1980s also resulted in the cloning of genes encoding ion channel subunits (e.g. the nicotinic acetylcholine receptor and voltage-gated Na^+ channel) and nuclear receptors. The cloning of numerous drug targets continued at a pace during the 1990s but it was not until the completion of the human genome project in 2001 that the numbers of genes for each major drug target family could be determined and fully appreciated. As would be expected, the cloning of the human genome also resulted in the identification of many potentially new drug targets. The completion of genome projects for widely used model organisms such as mouse (2002) and rat (2004) has also been of great benefit to the drug discovery process.

The capacity to clone and express genes opened up access to a wealth of information that was simply not available from traditional pharmacology-based approaches using isolated animal tissue preparations. In the case of GPCRs detailed expression pattern analysis could be performed using a range of molecular biology techniques such as *in situ* hybridisation, RT-PCR (reverse transcriptase-polymerase chain reaction) and Northern blotting. Furthermore having a cloned GPCR gene in a simple DNA plasmid made it possible for the first time to transfect and express GPCRs in cultured cell lines. This permitted detailed pharmacological and functional analysis (e.g. second messenger pathways) of specific receptor subtypes in cells not expressing related subtypes, which was often a problem when using tissue preparations. Techniques such as site-directed mutagenesis enable pharmacologists to investigate complex structure-function relationships aimed at understanding, for example, which amino acid residues are crucial for ligand binding to the receptor. As cloning and expression techniques developed further it became possible to manipulate gene expression *in vivo*. It is now common practice to explore the consequences of deleting a

Molecular Pharmacology: From DNA to Drug Discovery, First Edition. John Dickenson, Fiona Freeman, Chris Lloyd Mills, Shiva Sivasubramaniam and Christian Thode.
© 2013 John Wiley & Sons, Ltd. Published 2013 by John Wiley & Sons, Ltd.

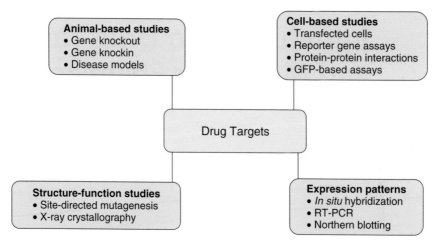

Figure 1.1 Molecular pharmacology-based methods used to interrogate drug targets.

specific gene either from an entire genome (knockout) or from a specific tissue/organ (conditional knockout). It is also possible to insert mutated forms of genes into an organism's genome using knockin technology. These transgenic approaches allow molecular pharmacologists to study developmental and physiological aspects of gene function *in vivo* and in the case of gene knockin techniques to develop disease models.

The molecular biology revolution also enabled the development of novel approaches for studying the complex signal transduction characteristics of pharmacologically important proteins such as receptors and ion channels. These include reporter gene assays, green fluorescent protein (GFP) based techniques for visualising proteins in living cells and yeast two hybrid-based assays for exploring protein-protein interactions. You will find detailed explanations of these and other current molecular-based techniques throughout this textbook. Another major breakthrough in the 2000s was the development of methods that allowed high resolution structural images of membrane-associated proteins to be obtained from X-ray crystallography. During this time the first X-ray structures of GPCRs and ion channels were reported enabling scientists to understand how such proteins function at the molecular level. Indeed crystallography is an important tool in the drug discovery process since crystal structures can be used for *in silico* drug design. More recently researchers have used NMR spectroscopy to obtain a high-resolution structural information of the β_2-adrenergic receptor (Bokoch et al., 2010). A distinct advantage of NMR-based structural

studies, which are already used for structural studies of other drug targets such as kinases, would be the ability to obtain GPCR dynamics and ligand activation data which is not possible using X-ray based methods. Some of the molecular pharmacology based approaches used to interrogate drug targets are outlined in Figure 1.1.

Despite this increased knowledge of drug targets obtained during the molecular biology revolution, there has been a clear slowdown in the number of new drugs reaching the market (Betz, 2005). However, since it takes approximately 15 years to bring a new drug to market it may be too early to assess the impact of the human genome project on drug discovery. In 2009 the global pharmaceutical market was worth an estimated $815 billion. However during the next few years a major problem facing the pharmaceutical industry is the loss of drug patents on key blockbusters. The hope for the future is that the advances in molecular pharmacology witnessed during the last decade or so will start to deliver new blockbuster therapeutics for the twenty-first century.

1.2 Scope of this textbook

As briefly detailed above there have been numerous exciting developments in the field of molecular pharmacology. The scope of this textbook is to explore aspects of molecular pharmacology in greater depth than covered in traditional pharmacology textbooks (summarised in Figure 1.2). Recent advances and developments in the four major human drug target families (GPCRs, ion channels, nuclear receptors and transporters) are

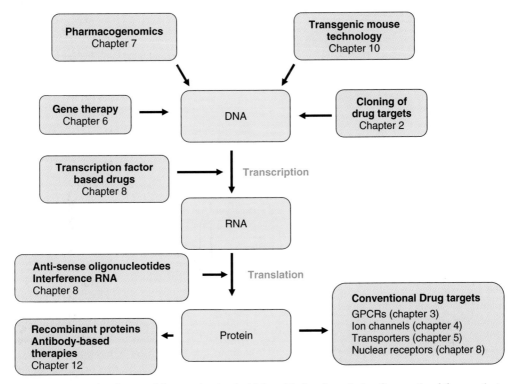

Figure 1.2 Drug targets within the central dogma of molecular biology. To date the majority of conventional therapeutics target a relatively small group of protein families that include G-protein coupled receptors, ion channels, and transporters. Novel therapeutic strategies include blocking translation of mRNA into protein using anti-sense oligonucleotide and/or RNA interference technology. Gene transcription can also be targeted via the activation/inhibition of nuclear receptor function. The chapters covering these topics are indicated.

covered in separate chapters (Chapters 3–5 and 8). The molecular targets of anti-infective drugs (anti-bacterial and anti-viral) whilst of great importance are not covered in this book. Other chapters deal with the cloning of drug targets (Chapter 2) and transgenic animal technology (Chapter 10). The concept of gene therapy is explored in a case study-based chapter which looks at current and possible future treatment strategies for cystic fibrosis, the commonest lethal genetic disease of Caucasians (Chapter 6). Another major development in molecular pharmacology has been the discipline of pharmacogenomics: the study of how an individual's genetic makeup influences their response to therapeutic drugs (Chapter 7). These naturally occurring variations in the human genome are caused predominantly by single nucleotide polymorphisms (DNA variation involving a change in a single nucleotide) and there is a major research consortium aimed at documenting all the common variants of the human genome (The International HapMap project).

The information from the project, which is freely available on the internet, will enable scientists to understand how genetic variations contribute to risk of disease and drug response. Finally, we take an in depth look at the role of calcium in the cell, looking at techniques used to measure this important second messenger (Chapter 9).

1.3 The nature of drug targets

How many potential drug targets are there in the human genome? This is an important question often asked by the pharmaceutical industry since they are faced with the task of developing novel therapeutics for the future. When the draft sequence of the human genome was completed in 2001 it was estimated to contain approximately 31,000 protein-coding genes. However since its completion the number of human protein-coding genes has been continually revised with current estimates ranging

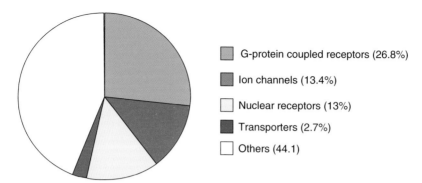

G-protein coupled receptors (26.8%)

Ion channels (13.4%)

Nuclear receptors (13%)

Transporters (2.7%)

Others (44.1)

Figure 1.3 The molecular targets of prescribed drugs. The data is expressed as a percentage of all FDA approved drugs as of December 2005. Drugs that target ligand-gated ion channels and voltage-gated ion channels have been grouped together as ion channels. Drug targets grouped together as others encompass 120 different specific targets many of which are enzymes. Data taken from Overington et al. (2006).

between 20,000 and 25,000. Of these it is predicted that about 3000 are feasible protein drug targets. In 2005 it was calculated that about 100 drug targets account for all prescription drugs. On this basis there is obviously considerable scope for the development and discovery of novel drug targets to treat disease. At present the classical drug targets include GPCRs (Chapter 3), ion channels (Chapter 4), nuclear receptors (Chapter 8), transporters (Chapter 5) and enzymes. These important classical drug targets, whilst briefly covered in this Introduction, are extensively covered in later chapters. The distribution of drug targets expressed as a percentage of total products approved by the Food and Drug Administration (FDA; agency in the USA responsible for approving drugs for therapeutic use) is illustrated in Figure 1.3.

G-protein coupled receptors (GPCRs)

GPCRs represent the largest single family of pharmaceutical drug target accounting for approximately 30% of the current market. Their primary function is to detect extracellular signals and through heterotrimeric G-protein activation trigger intracellular signal transduction cascades that promote cellular responses (Figure 1.4). Whilst their share of the overall drug market is likely to fall in the future they still represent 'hot' targets for drug discovery programmes. GPCRs are conventionally targeted using small molecules (typically less than 500 Da) that are classified as agonists (receptor activating) or antagonists (inhibit receptor function by blocking the effect of an agonist). Some key examples of drugs that target GPCRs are listed in Table 1.1. Chapter 3 will explain in detail many of the recent developments in GPCR structure, function, pharmacology and signal transduction

including GPCR dimerisation. Many of these exciting advances have revealed new pharmaceutical approaches for targeting GPCRs such as inverse agonists, allosteric modulators, biased agonists and bivalent ligands that target GPCR heterodimers. Since the completion of the human genome project it has emerged that the total number of human GPCRs may be as high as 865, which would account for approximately 3.4% of total predicted protein-coding genes (assuming a total of 25,000). For many cloned GPCRs the endogenous ligand(s) are unknown (so called 'orphan' GPCRs) and the identification of these orphan receptor ligands is the focus of drug discovery programmes within the pharmaceutical industry. The process of GPCR de-orphanisation is addressed in Chapter 2. In Chapter 11 the concept that GPCRs interact with a host of accessory proteins that are important in modulating many aspects in the life of a GPCR including the formation of signalling complexes will be explored. Indeed, targeting such GPCR signalling complexes with drugs that disrupt proteinprotein interactions is another exciting avenue for future drug development not only in the field of GPCRs but also in other areas of signal transduction.

Ion channels

Ion channels represent important drug targets since they are involved in regulating a wide range of fundamental physiological processes. Indeed, at present they are the second largest class of drug target after GPCRs. They operate the rapid transport of ions across membranes (down their electrochemical gradients) and in doing so trigger plasma and organelle membrane hyperpolarisation or depolarisation. They are also potential drug

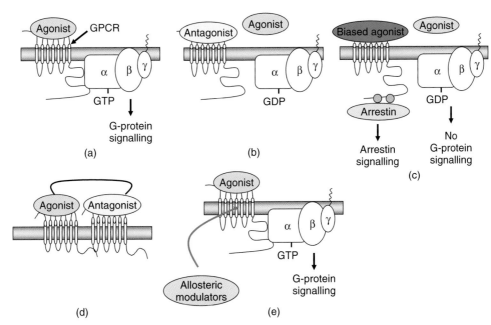

Figure 1.4 G-protein coupled receptors as drug targets. (a) GPCRs can be targeted using selective synthetic agonists which trigger receptor activation thus enabling G-protein coupling and subsequent cell signalling responses. (b) antagonists can be used to block the binding of an endogenous agonist thus preventing receptor activation. (c) GPCRs can also trigger G-protein independent cell signalling pathways which are dependent on arrestin binding to the activated receptor. Biased agonists are being developed that specifically promote the activation of arrestin-dependent signalling pathways. (d) bivalent ligands targeting specific GPCR heterodimers. (e) GPCRs can also be targeted using allosteric modulators which bind to sites on the receptor that are distinct from the agonist (orthosteric) binding site.

Table 1.1 G-protein coupled receptors as drug targets.

GPCR	Drug (brand name)	Agonist/Antagonist	Condition/use
Histamine H_2 receptor	Famotidine (Pepcidine)	Antagonist	Stomach ulcers
α_1-adrenergic receptor	Doxazosin (Cardura)	Antagonist	Hypertension
$GnRH_1$ receptor	Leuprorelin (Lupron)	Agonist	Prostate cancer
$5\text{-}HT_{1D}$ receptor	Sumatriptan (Imigran)	Agonist	Migraine
μ-opioid receptor	Fentanyl (Sublimaze)	Agonist	Analgesic

Abbreviations: GnRH, gonadotropin-releasing hormone.

targets for the treatment of rare monogenic hereditary disorders caused by mutations in genes that encode ion channel subunits. Such conditions termed 'ion channelopathies' include mutations in sodium, chloride and calcium channels that cause alterations in skeletal muscle excitability. The understanding of ion channel diversity and complexity increased significantly following the completion of the human genome project which identified over 400 genes encoding ion channel subunits. Given this number of genes it has been suggested that ion

channels may rival GPCRs as drug targets in the future (Jiang et al., 2008). Other major developments include the first 3D resolution of ion channel structure by X-ray crystallography, which was reported for the voltage-gated potassium channel in 2003 (MacKinnon et al., 2003). Despite these important advances in the understanding of ion channel diversity and structure very few new ion channel drugs have reached the market during the last decade. Some key examples of ion channels as drug targets are shown in Table 1.2.

Table 1.2 Ion channels as drug targets.

Ion channel	Drug (brand name)	Condition/use
Voltage-gated Ca^{2+} channel	Amlodipine (Norvasc)	Hypertension and angina
Voltage-gated Na^+ channel	Phenytoin (Dilantin)	Epilepsy
ATP-sensitive K^+ channel	Glibenclamide (Glimepride)	Type II diabetes
$GABA_A$ receptor	Benzodiazepines (Diazepam)	Anxiety
$5\text{-}HT_3$ receptor	Ondansetron (Zofran)	Nausea and vomiting

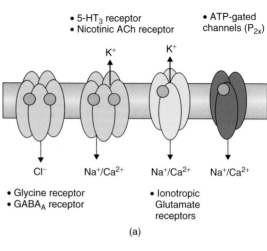

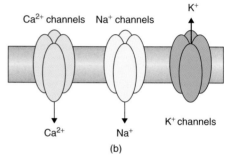

Figure 1.5 Ion channel classification. (a) Ligand-gated ion channels comprise a family of multi-subunit transmembrane proteins that are activated by a diverse set of ligands (indicated by the orange circle) that include amino acids (glycine, glutamate and GABA), 5-hydroxytryptamine (5-HT), acetylcholine (ACh), and ATP. (b) voltage-gated channel channels, which are also multi-subunit proteins, open in response to local changes in membrane potential.

Ion channels are broadly classified into two main groups (Figure 1.5). Firstly there are ligand-gated ion channels or ionotropic receptors which open when activated by an agonist binding to a specific ion channel subunit. Examples of this class include the nicotinic acetylcholine receptor, $GABA_A$ receptor, glycine receptor, $5\text{-}HT_3$ receptor, ionotropic glutamate receptors, and ATP-gated channels. The second group which includes voltage-gated or voltage-operated ion channels are opened by other mechanisms including changes in plasma membrane potential. Examples include voltage-gated Ca^{2+}, Na^+, and K^+ channels. The molecular structure and classification of ion channels together with their use as drug targets will be explored in detail in Chapter 4.

Nuclear receptors

Nuclear receptors are a large family of transcription factors that play a pivotal role in endocrine function. In contrast to other families of transcription factor the activity of nuclear receptors (as their name suggests) is specifically regulated by the binding of ligands (Figure 1.6). Such ligands, which are small and lipophilic, include steroid hormones (glucocorticoids, mineralo-corticoids, androgens, oestrogens and progestogens), thyroid hormones (T_3 and T_4), fat soluble vitamins D and A (retinoic acid) and various fatty acid derivatives. Since the completion of the human genome sequencing project 48 members of the human nuclear receptor family have been identified. However, for many nuclear receptors the identity of the ligand is unknown. These 'orphan' nuclear receptors are of significant interest to the pharmaceutical industry since they may lead to the discovery of novel endocrine systems with potential therapeutic use. Whilst the total number of nuclear

receptors is small in comparison to GPCRs they are the target of approximately 13% of all prescribed drugs. For example, the chronic inflammation associated with asthma can be suppressed by inhaled glucocorticoids and oestrogen-sensitive breast cancer responds to treatment with the oestrogen receptor antagonist tamoxifen. The structure, classification, signal transduction mechanisms and therapeutic uses of nuclear receptor targeting drugs will be explored in detail in Chapter 8.

Neurotransmitter transporters

The concentration of some neurotransmitters within the synaptic cleft is tightly regulated by specific plasma membrane-bound transporter proteins. These transporters, which belong to the solute carrier

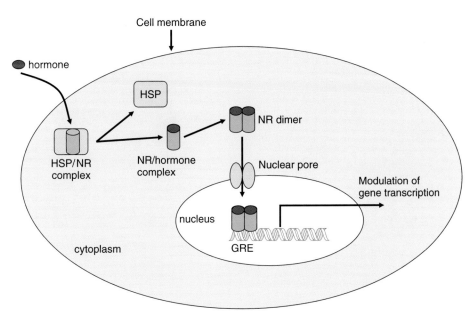

Figure 1.6 Type I nuclear receptor-mediated signal transduction. In the absence of hormone (e.g. glucocorticoid) the nuclear receptor (NR) is located in the cytoplasm bound to a heat shock protein (HSP). Hormone binding triggers dissociation of the HSP from the NR/HSP complex, dimerisation of the NR and translocation to the nucleus. Once in the nucleus the NR dimer binds to a specific DNA sequence known as glucocorticoid response element (GRE) and modulates gene transcription.

(SLC) transporter family, facilitate the movement of neurotransmitter either back into the pre-synaptic neuron or in some cases into surrounding glial cells. There are two major subclasses of plasma-membrane bound neurotransmitter transporter: the SLC1 family which transports glutamate and the larger SLC6 family which transports dopamine, 5-HT, noradrenaline, GABA and glycine (Figure 1.7). Both SLC1 and SLC6 families facilitate neurotransmitter movement across the plasma membrane by secondary active transport using extracellular Na^+ ion concentration as the driving force. As might be expected drugs that target neurotransmitter transporters have a wide range of therapeutic applications such as treatment for depression, anxiety and epilepsy. Indeed, neurotransmitter transporters are the target for approximately one-third of all psychoactive drugs (see Table 1.3). The molecular structure and classification of neurotransmitter transporters and their value as important current and future drug targets will be discussed in detail in Chapter 5.

1.4 Future drug targets

At present more than 50% of drugs target only four major gene families, namely GPCRs, nuclear receptors,

ligand-gated ion channels and voltage-gated ion channels (Figure 1.3). It is likely that the market share of these classical drug targets will shrink as new drug targets and approaches are developed in the future.

Protein kinases

It is predicted that protein kinases (and lipid kinases), one of the largest gene families in eukaryotes, will become major drug targets of the twenty-first century. Protein phosphorylation is reversible and is one of the most common ways of post-translationally modifying protein function. It regulates numerous cellular functions including cell proliferation, cell death, cell survival, cell cycle progression, and cell differentiation. The enzymes that catalyse protein phosphorylation are known as protein kinases, whereas the enzymes that carry out the reverse dephosphorylation reaction are referred to as phosphatases (Figure 1.8a). The human genome encodes for 518 protein kinases and approximately 20 lipid kinases. The predominant sites of protein phosphorylation are the hydroxyl groups ($-OH$) in the side chains of the amino acids serine, threonine and tyrosine (Figure 1.8b). When a phosphate group is attached to a protein it introduces a strong negative charge which can alter protein conformation and thus function.

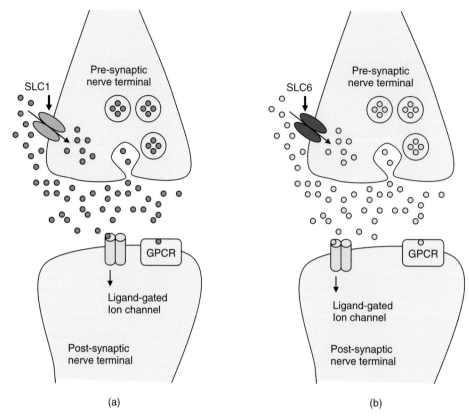

(a)   (b)

Figure 1.7 Neurotransmitter transporter classification. (a) Glutamate released into the synaptic cleft activates both ion channels (ionotropic glutamate receptors) and GPCRs (metabotropic glutamate receptors) located on the post-synaptic membrane. Released glutamate is subsequently removed from the extracellular space by SLC1 transporters located on pre-synaptic membranes. (b) Dopamine, 5-hydroxytryptamine (5-HT), γ-aminobutyric acid (GABA), noradrenaline and glycine released into the synaptic cleft activate specific ligand-gated ion channels and/or GPCRs located on the post-synaptic membrane. These released neurotransmitters are subsequently transported back into the pre-synaptic nerve terminal via SLC6 transporters. For clarity specific vesicular transporters responsible for transporting neurotransmitters from the cytoplasm into synaptic vesicles have been omitted. Figure adapted from Gether et al. (2006). Trends in Pharmacological Sciences 27: 375–383.

Table 1.3 Transporters as drug targets.

Transporter	Drug (brand name)	Condition/ use
5-HT transporter (SERT)	Sertraline (Zoloft)	Antidepressant
Dopamine transporter (DAT)	Cocaine	Drug of abuse
Noradrenaline transporter (NET)	Bupropion[a] (Welbrutin)	Antidepressant
GAT-1 (GABA)	Tiagabine	Epilepsy

[a] Affinity for DAT as well

Enzymes

Enzymes are the drug target for approximately 50% of all prescribed drugs. Some key examples are listed in Table 1.4. However, because of their diverse nature they will not be the focus of a specific chapter in this book. It is also important to remember that many prescribed drugs target bacterial and viral enzymes for the treatment of infectious disease and HIV. Also many enzymes, whilst not direct drug targets, play important roles in drug metabolism for example cytochrome P450 enzymes.

Protein kinases are classified according to the amino acid they phosphorylate and are grouped into two main types: serine/threonine kinases and tyrosine kinases. In

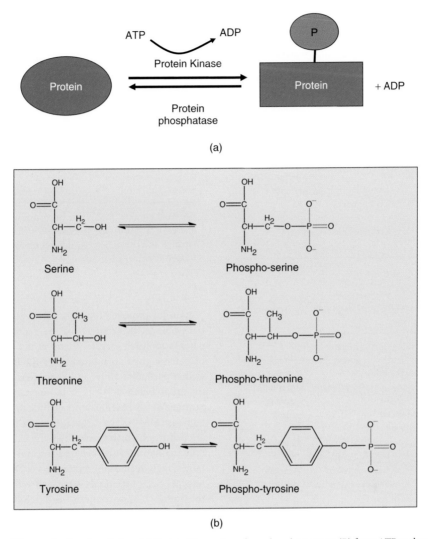

Figure 1.8 Reversible protein phosphorylation. (a) Protein kinases transfer a phosphate group (P) from ATP to the target protein altering its biological activity. The removal of phosphate from a phosphorylated protein is catalysed by protein phosphatases. (b) Phosphate groups are transferred to the amino acids serine, threonine and tyrosine.

both cases ATP supplies the phosphate group with the third phosphoryl group (γ; gamma phosphate) being transferred to the hydroxyl group of the acceptor amino acid. Examples of serine/threonine kinases include protein kinase A (PKA; activated by the second messenger cyclic AMP) and protein kinase C (PKC; activated by the second messenger diacylglycerol). Examples of tyrosine kinases include tyrosine kinase linked receptors for insulin and epidermal growth factor and non-receptor tyrosine kinases such as Src and JAK (Janus-associated kinase). Given the prominent role of protein phosphorylation in

regulating many aspects of cell physiology it is not surprising that dysfunction in the control of protein kinase signalling is associated with major diseases such as cancer, diabetes and rheumatoid arthritis. These alterations in protein kinase and in some cases lipid kinase function arise from over-activity either due to genetic mutations or over-expression of the protein. It is estimated that up to 30% of all protein targets currently under investigation by the pharmaceutical industry are protein or lipid kinases. Indeed, there are approximately 150 protein kinase inhibitors in various stages of clinical development,

Table 1.4 Enzymes as drug targets.

Enzyme	Drug (brand name)	Condition/use
HMG-CoA reductase	Statins	Used to lower blood cholesterol levels
Phosphodiesterase type V	Sildenafil (Viagra)	Erectile dysfunction and hypertension
Cyclo-oxygenase	Aspirin	Analgesic and anti-inflammatory
Angiotensin-converting enzyme	Captopril (Capoten)	Hypertension
Dihydrofolate reductase	Methotrexate	Cancer

Table 1.6 Small-molecule protein kinase inhibitors approved for clinical use.

Drug (brand name)	Targets	Use
Imatinib (Gleevec®)	c-Abl-kinase, c-Kit	Chronic myeloid leukaemia
Gefitinib (Iressa®)	EGFR	Various cancers
Sunitinib (Sutent®)	PDGFR, VEGFR	Renal cell carcinoma
Dasatinib (Sprycel®)	c-Abl-kinase, Src	Various cancers
Everolimus (Afinitor®)	mTOR[a]	Various cancers

[a]Serine/threonine kinase. Abbreviations: EGFR, epidermal growth factor receptor; mTOR, mammalian target of rapamycin; PDGFR, platelet-derived growth factor receptor; VEGFR, vascular endothelial growth factor receptor.

Table 1.5 Selected small-molecule protein kinase inhibitors in clinical development.

Drug	Protein kinase target	Use
AZD 1152	Aurora B Kinase	Various cancers
NP-12	Glycogen synthase kinase 3 (GSK3)	Alzheimer's disease
Bay 613606	Spleen tyrosine kinase (Syk)	Asthma
INCB-28050	Janus-associated kinase 1/2 (JAK1/2)	Rheumatoid arthritis
BMS-582949	p38 mitogen-activated protein kinase (p38 MAPK)	Rheumatoid arthritis

some of which are highlighted in Table 1.5. Whilst protein kinases are important new human drug targets they are also present in bacteria and viruses and thus represent potential targets for infectious disease treatment.

Since the launch of imatinib in 2001 several other small-molecule protein kinase inhibitors have successfully made it to the market place as novel anti-cancer treatments (Table 1.6). The majority of these drugs are tyrosine kinase inhibitors and in some cases function as multi-kinase inhibitors (e.g. sunitinib) targeting PDGFR (proliferation) and VEGFR (angiogenesis) dependent signalling responses. Monoclonal antibodies are also used to block the increased tyrosine kinase linked receptor activity that is associated with many forms of cancer and these will be discussed in Chapter 12.

A useful approach for assessing the therapeutic potential of novel drug targets is the number of approved patents for each target (Zheng et al., 2006). The level of patents gives an indication of the degree of interest in that particular target and hence likelihood of successful drugs being developed. Future targets with a high number of US-based patents include matrix metalloproteinases (MMPs) as a target for cancer treatment. MMPs are proteases which break down the extracellular matrix thus facilitating cancer cell invasion and metastasis. Other targets include phosphodiesterase 4 (PDE4), caspases and integrin receptors. Only time will tell whether any of these novel targets result in the development of effective therapeutics. For further reading on the identification and characteristics of future drug targets see the review by Zheng et al. (2006).

Therapeutic oligonucleotides

In addition to the development of small-molecule-based drugs there are several other approaches to treat human disease including the exciting prospect of therapeutic oligonucleotides (anti-sense and RNA interference based) as tools for gene silencing and the continued quest for gene therapy-based techniques. These molecular biology-based strategies for combating human disease will be addressed later in Chapter 8.

Another new class of drugs are short single-stranded oligonucleotides (DNA or RNA based) that have been selectively engineered to target specific intracellular proteins (Dausse et al., 2009). These oligonucleotides which fold into defined three-dimensional structures are known as aptamers or 'chemical antibodies'. They are generated and repeatedly selected through a method known as SELEX (Systematic Evolution of Ligands by Exponential Enrichment). Essentially the process begins with the synthesis of a large oligonucleotide library, containing randomly generated sequences of fixed length, which is screened for binding to the target protein usually by affinity chromatography. Those that bind are repeatedly selected using stringent elution conditions that ultimately result in the identification of the tightest binding sequences. These high affinity sequences can be chemically modified to increase their affinity and effectiveness as potential therapeutic oligonucleotides. The first aptamer-based drug approved by the US Food and Drug Administration (FDA) targets the VEGFR and is used to treat age-related macular degeneration. Several other aptamer oligonucleotides are also undergoing clinical trials.

1.5 Molecular pharmacology and drug discovery

The process of drug discovery is a long and costly process with new drugs taking up to 12 years to reach the clinic. Many novel molecular pharmacology-based techniques play important roles in the process of drug discovery and development. A problem faced by many pharmaceutical companies is the huge task of screening their vast chemical libraries (in some cases this can exceed one million compounds) against an increasing number of possible drug targets. The development, in the early 1990s, of high-throughput screening (HTS) technology using 96-well microtiter plates enabled the drug screening process to be miniaturised and automated. Using such methodology it became possible to screen up to 10,000 compounds per day. However during the last decade 384-well microtiter plates and more recently 1536-well microtiter plate-based assays have been developed that allow for screening of up to 200,000 compounds a day (ultra-high-throughput screening). Since the screening of large chemical libraries is expensive several alternative strategies to increase the chances of success have been introduced in recent years. One such approach has been the introduction of fragment-based screening (FBS) or fragment-based lead discovery (FBLD). This involves screening the biological target with small libraries of chemical fragments (molecular weights around 200 Da) with the aim of identifying scaffolds or 'chemical backbones' that can be developed into lead compounds. This

approach may also be combined with computer-based 'virtual screening' approaches. For example structure-based virtual screening involves the use of 3D protein structures, many of which are now widely available via public databases, to assess whether a ligand can interact or dock with the protein of interest. This can be linked with ligand-based virtual screening which involves *in silico* screening of chemical libraries for compounds that display similar structural features associated with the binding of the ligand to the target. As indicated above structure-based virtual screenings rely on the availability of accurate 3D structures of the drug target. The discipline of structural biology uses a range of biophysical techniques including X-ray crystallography, NMR spectroscopy and electron cryo-microscopy to determine protein structure. The latter is an emerging technique that can be used to determine the 3D structure of macromolecular complexes that are too large to be studied using X-ray crystallography and/or NMR spectroscopy. So far in this section we have briefly covered some of the up-and-coming techniques that can used to interrogate drug target structure and screen drug targets for lead compounds. There is also a drive towards the development novel cell-based and animal-based models that are more representative of human physiology and hence more suitable for drug screening. For example, 3D 'organotypic' cell microarrays are currently being developed that will allow drug screening in a system that is close to the *in vivo* environment of cells. In summary, we

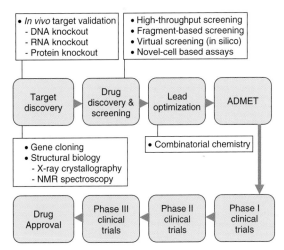

Figure 1.9 Schematic representation of the drug discovery process. ADMET (**A**dsorption, **D**istribution, **M**etabolism, **E**xcretion and **T**oxicity studies).

are witnessing exciting times in the process of drug discovery with the continued development of *in silico* and nanotechnology-based methods and the introduction of novel cell-based screening models. Has there ever been a better time to be a molecular pharmacologist? A schematic representation of the drug discovery process is shown in Figure 1.9.

References

Betz UAK (2005). How many genomics targets can a portfolio support? Drug Discovery Today 10: 1057–1063.

Bokoch MP, Zou Y, Rasmussen SGF, Liu CW, Nygaard R, Rosenbaum DM, Fung JJ, Choi H-J, Thian FS, Kobilka TS, Puglisi JD, Weis WI, Pardo L, Prosser RS, Mueller L and Kobilka BK (2010). Ligand-specific regulation of the extracellular surface of a G protein coupled receptor. Nature 463: 108–112.

Dausse E, Da Rocha Gomes S and Toulme J-J (2009). Aptamers: a new class of oligonucleotides in the drug discovery pipeline. Current Opinion in Pharmacology 9: 602–607.

Dixon RA, Kobilka BK, Strader DJ, Benovic JL, Dohlman HG, Frielle T, Bolanowski MA, Bennett CD, Rands E, Diehl RE, Munford RA, Slater EE, Sigal IS, Caron MG, Lefkowitz RJ and Strader CD (1986). Cloning of the gene and cDNA for mammalian beta-adrenergic receptor and homology with rhodopsin. Nature 321: 75–79.

Gether U, Andersen PH, Larsson OM and Schousboe A (2006). Neurotransmitter transporters: molecular function of important drug targets. Trends in Pharmacological Sciences 27: 375–383.

Jiang Y, Lee A, Chen J, Ruta V, Cadene M, Chait BT and MacKinnon R (2003). X-ray structure of a voltage-dependent K^+ channel. Nature 423: 33–41.

Kaczorowski GJ, McManus OB, Priest BT and Garcia ML (2008). Ion channels as drug targets: the next GPCRs. Journal General Physiology 131: 399–405.

Overington JP, Al-Lazikani B and Hopkins AL (2006). How many drug targets are there? Nature Reviews 5: 993–996.

Zheng CJ, Han LY, Yap CW, Ji ZL, Cao ZW and Chen YZ (2006). Therapeutic targets: progress of their exploration and investigation of their characteristics. Pharmacological Reviews 58: 259–279.

2 Molecular Cloning of Drug Targets

2.1 Introduction to molecular cloning – from DNA to drug discovery

Over four decades ago, the discovery and characterisation of molecular tools, in the form of DNA ligases (Zimmerman et al., 1967), restriction endonucleases (Linn and Arber, 1968; Smith and Wilcox, 1970; Danna and Nathans, 1971) and reverse transcriptases (Baltimore, 1970; Temin and Mizutani, 1970) provided the platform for the emerging recombinant DNA technology (Cohen et al., 1972, 1973; Jackson et al., 1972), an array of applications used to cut, join, amplify, modify and express DNA fragments. Molecular cloning, in this context, refers to the process that introduces an isolated piece of DNA into a vector (recombination) and generates multiple copies (clones) of it. (It should not be confused with cloning of animals or cells!)

Recombinant DNA technology quickly transformed the field of pharmacology, as it overcame several technical limitations faced with traditional pharmacology at that time: Supported by Sanger's rapid DNA sequencing method (Sanger et al., 1977), it offered a range of novel approaches for pharmacological studies, sufficient biological material – and data of previously unknown quantity and quality. DNA as a starting material was the new focal point that led to the molecular cloning of targets for endogenous ligands as well as therapeutic drugs, and thus facilitated drug discovery (see 2.3 below). The technical possibilities seemed infinite.

Consequently, molecular cloning sparked a global race amongst scientists for the identification of DNAs of major drug targets, the molecular nature of which was often unknown back then! This work revealed a surprising diversity of drug targets and complexity of intracellular signalling cascades. It was frequently accompanied by the realisation that a single 'known' drug target indeed existed in a multitude of subtypes, which traditional investigations failed to distinguish. And it highlighted the necessity to develop subtype-specific drugs. However, the initial DNA cloning process could now be complemented

Molecular Pharmacology: From DNA to Drug Discovery, First Edition. John Dickenson, Fiona Freeman, Chris Lloyd Mills, Shiva Sivasubramaniam and Christian Thode.
© 2013 John Wiley & Sons, Ltd. Published 2013 by John Wiley & Sons, Ltd.

by expression studies in host cells, where previously-identified or potential novel drug targets could be functionally and pharmacologically characterised *in vitro*. It also marked the beginning of reverse pharmacology.

The chapter *Molecular Cloning of Drug Targets* starts with a brief overview of traditional pharmacology, followed by technical insights into the main methods, which nowadays are used routinely in molecular cloning. It concludes with a particular example, where molecular cloning enabled the identification of a natural endogenous ligand for a receptor. (The interested reader is referred to Sambrook and Russel's (2001) *Molecular Cloning: A Laboratory Manual*, (3rd ed) CSH Press, for detailed protocols).

2.2 'Traditional' pharmacology

'Traditional' pharmacology refers here to the characterisation of 'native' drug targets, that is, proteins in their natural molecular environment, such as in cells, tissues and organs. Typically employed techniques include:

- electrophysiological recordings from cells; these permit the study of ion fluxes across the plasma membrane (see Chapter 4), for example in response to the exposure to ligands.
- radioligand binding to tissue extracts and isolated membranes; a radiolabelled molecule, whether the natural ligand or another compound, can be used to determine the binding affinity of a drug for a particular target in its native state.
- receptor autoradiography; the incubation of thin tissue sections with a radiolabelled ligand is used to obtain signals (autoradiographs) on X-ray films; their pattern and intensity reveals qualitative (location) and quantitative information (amount) about a drug target *in situ*.
- 'classical' preparations; for example, isolated tissue strips (such as muscle fibres) can be maintained in tissue baths for the purpose of measuring a drug-induced response (e.g. contraction).
- enzyme assays; the activity of a particular enzyme is recorded in response to different drug concentrations.

Despite the negative connotation that the word 'traditional' may hold for some, this approach still offers an important means of investigation, frequently supplementing the data from molecular cloning. However, prior to the advent of molecular cloning studies, 'traditional' pharmacology on its own had several disadvantages. For example, cells, tissues, and organs may contain more than one target for any given compound that lacks selectivity.

Thus, an observed response could be due to the activation of more than one protein, such as a receptor (a so-called mixed response), and this might go undetected. It might be possible to detect the presence of multiple targets if the experimenter had access to one or more selective antagonists. However, a given antagonist might inhibit a response that was due to the activity of multiple proteins, but blocking all of them. Famous examples, where 'traditional' pharmacology has erroneously postulated the existence of too few subtypes exist among G-protein coupled receptors (GPCRs; i.e. muscarinic acetylcholine receptors and dopamine receptors) and ligand-gated ion channels (LGICs; i.e. $GABA_A$ receptors; see section 2.5 for details). Conversely, a single GPCR could give rise to different responses, depending on the cell type and the intracellular signalling pathways that it coupled to via different guanine nucleotide binding proteins (G-proteins).

2.3 The relevance of recombinant DNA technology to pharmacology/drug discovery

The acquisition and successive use of sequence information plays a central role in recombinant DNA technology. Although the first – perhaps explorative – experiments are often limited to the isolation, cloning and identification of a relatively short DNA fragment, they can set the foundation for a number of more elaborate studies, such as genetic engineering (see Chapter 10), with access to physiological information of a different quality. The initially-obtained cloned nucleotide sequence, though, can already provide the deduced primary amino-acid sequence of a drug target, a map of recognition sites for restriction endonucleases, or some limited structural information. For instance (see 2.5), many drug targets (e.g. LGICs or GPCRs) are membrane-bound, and the results of molecular cloning can reveal the number of their membrane-spanning domains or indicate their topology (i.e. whether the amino- and carboxy-termini are intracellular or extracellular). This information is important because we do not currently have the ability to purify them in sufficient amounts for crystallographic studies.

By searching appropriate databases (e.g. http://blast.ncbi.nlm.nih.gov/Blast.cgi, http://www.ebi.ac.uk/embl) with a cloned sequence, it is also possible to find homologous sequences, either in the same or a different species. These sequence comparisons may indicate the full length of the open-reading frame of a partially-cloned fragment or even help to identify protein families.

Indeed, the increasing availability of genomic data from a range of diverse organisms has facilitated this process considerably. *In silico* analysis – also known as 'clone by phone' among senior scientists – can frequently replace the necessity to carry out molecular cloning. In combination with the polymerase chain reaction (PCR), it has accelerated the discovery and subsequent cloning of a large number of 'orphan' GPCRs (see 2.7). Such receptors potentially represent novel drug targets, and the challenge now is to identify their natural, endogenous agonists and their *in vivo* physiological functions.

In addition, as a result of DNA cloning, specific probes can be developed, to determine the sites of gene expression and the location of the encoded product, through Northern blotting and *in situ* hybridisation (i.e. detection of mRNA), or Western blotting and immunocytochemistry (protein detection), respectively.

However, perhaps the most significant advance over 'traditional' pharmacological approaches is the ability to express the corresponding complementary DNA (cDNA) of a 'cloned' drug target *in vitro*, such as in mammalian cells. (NB: Proteins cannot be 'cloned', only the encoding nucleic acids). The expression permits the detailed functional and pharmacological characterisation of the encoded protein 'in isolation' – an advantage exploited by the pharmaceutical industry in high-throughput screens for new therapeutic compounds. It is not uncommon to over-express a cloned cDNA, with the help of appropriate promoters, because high levels of the protein of interest are likely to produce strong signals in the functional tests.

Finally, the effect of mutation or single-nucleotide polymorphisms (via the use of *in vitro* mutagenesis) on function and pharmacology can be investigated (see Chapter 7). This can give insights into binding sites for natural ligands and drugs, or confirm a hypothesised link between a disease and naturally-occurring gene mutation.

2.4 The 'cloning' of drug targets

Four main methods have been used to 'clone' drug targets. These involve the use of:
- peptide sequences that derive from the target of interest; this requires protein purification and sequencing, oligonucleotide synthesis and a cDNA library.
- specific antibodies; this requires an expression library (e.g. in the bacteriophage vector λgt11) in which the different polypeptides that are encoded by the various cDNAs in the library, are produced as fusion proteins.

- functional assays; this requires a cDNA expression library, an appropriate expression system (e.g. *Xenopus laevis* oocytes or mammalian cells) and some activity that can be measured (e.g. ion flux or radioligand binding).
- the polymerase chain reaction; this technique amplifies a specific DNA fragment with the help of oligonucleotide primers, a heat-resistant DNA polymerase and repeated cycles of alternating temperature conditions.

Cloning using peptide sequence(s)

This method is carried out in several stages, in which the initial aim is to obtain one or more peptide sequences, from the target of interest, that allow conclusions about the underlying DNA sequence to be drawn. Thus, the first necessary step is to purify the drug target. This is often not easy and usually laborious, since numerous drug targets are membrane-bound and have to be solubilised from the membrane prior to the purification. It also requires some kind of assay to monitor the purification process, such as a (radiolabelled) ligand that specifically binds to the target to allow its enrichment in a protein fraction. The nicotinic acetylcholine receptor, for instance, was the first membrane-bound receptor to be isolated in this way (Olsen et al., 1972) – and later the first one to be cloned (Noda et al., 1982). The success was based on the earlier discovery that certain snake α-neurotoxins (e.g. α-bungarotoxin) bind with high affinity to this pentameric complex in the electric organ of the electric eel (*Electrophorus electricus*), which has a high density of cholinergic synapses. However, assays to purify LGICs, voltage-gated ion channels and transporters cannot rely on activity, as this is lost, together with the native conformation, when the proteins are stripped from the membrane.

Design of oligonucleotide probes

Once the drug target has been purified (e.g. using affinity chromatography), its amino-terminus can be sequenced by Edman degradation, or the protein can be digested by proteases and the resulting peptide fragments sequenced. Oligonucleotides that are based on the deduced peptide sequence(s) can then be designed using the genetic code (Figure 2.1). In the method's final stage, these short and single-stranded DNA fragments act as probes, which recognise the corresponding cDNA of the protein of interest.

Depending on the peptide's unveiled amino-acid sequence, the oligonucleotide(s) that is/are designed can be either a 'best-guess', with one defined DNA sequence, or degenerate (Figure 2.2), that is, a mixture

		second base in codon								
		T		**C**		**A**		**G**		
	T	TTT	Phe	TCT	Ser	TAT	Tyr	TGT	Cys	**T**
		TTC	Phe	TCC	Ser	TAC	Tyr	TGC	Cys	**C**
		TTA	Leu	TCA	Ser	TAA	*Stop*	TGA	*Stop*	**A**
		TTG	Leu	TCG	Ser	TAG	*Stop*	TGG	Trp	**G**
first base in codon	**C**	CTT	Leu	CCT	Pro	CAT	His	CGT	Arg	**T**
		CTC	Leu	CCC	Pro	CAC	His	CGC	Arg	**C**
		CTA	Leu	CCA	Pro	CAA	Gln	CGA	Arg	**A**
		CTG	Leu	CCG	Pro	CAG	Gln	CGG	Arg	**G**
	A	ATT	Ile	ACT	Thr	AAT	Asn	AGT	Ser	**T**
		ATC	Ile	ACC	Thr	AAC	Asn	AGC	Ser	**C**
		ATA	Ile	ACA	Thr	AAA	Lys	AGA	Arg	**A**
		ATG	Met	ACG	Thr	AAG	Lys	AGG	Arg	**G**
	G	GTT	Val	GCT	Ala	GAT	Asp	GGT	Gly	**T**
		GTC	Val	GCC	Ala	GAC	Asp	GGC	Gly	**C**
		GTA	Val	GCA	Ala	GAA	Glu	GGA	Gly	**A**
		GTG	Val	GCG	Ala	GAG	Glu	GGG	Gly	**G**

(right-hand axis label: third base in codon)

Figure 2.1 The genetic code, showing the 64 possible triplets, the 20 encoded amino acids (three-letter code) and the stop codons, respectively. Note that RNA contains uracil instead of thymine (DNA).

peptide sequence	NH$_2$	Met	Pro	Asp	Glu	Trp	Gly	Cys	COOH
	5'	ATG	CCT	GAT	GAA	TGG	GGT	TGT	3'
possible codons			CCC	GAC	GAG		GGC	TGC	
			CCA				GGA		
			CCG				GGG		
no. of different codons		1	4	2	2	1	4	2	

Figure 2.2 This example demonstrates the design of a 'degenerate' oligonucleotide of 21 nucleotides in length (i.e. a 21 mer). Due to the different triplet combinations, all of which can encode the peptide sequence shown above, the oligonucleotide yields a degeneracy of: $1 \times 4 \times 2 \times 2 \times 1 \times 4 \times 2 = 128$; it therefore is a mixture of 128 different 21 mers. (A similar approach may be chosen for the design of the primers in certain PCR applications; see 2.7, below).

of different sequences that contain all of the possible codons encoding the peptide. The latter approach takes into account that the genetic code is degenerate, whereby most amino acids are specified by more than one codon (also called a triplet; see Figure 2.1). Thus, valine (Val) is encoded by GTT, GTC, GTA and GTG, and leucine (Leu) is encoded by TTA, TTG, CTT, CTC, CTA and CTG. Only the amino acids methionine (Met; ATG) and tryptophan (Trp; TGG) are encoded by single triplets.

'Best guess' oligonucleotides are designed based on the fact that codon usage is not random. Interestingly, although the majority of amino acids are specified by several codons, they are not all used with equal frequency. For example, as codon usage tables (e.g. http://www.kazusa.or.jp/codon) illustrate, for the amino acid valine in rat, GTG is the most commonly used codon, while GTA is used the least; the other two triplets GTT and GTC are used at intermediate frequencies.

Following the design and synthesis, the oligonucleotide is radiolabelled, using the enzyme T4 polynucleotide kinase, which adds a (radioactive) phosphate group to the 5'-end of the probe, and used to screen a cDNA library. Two important examples from the early days of molecular cloning of receptors, in which this approach has been applied, include the human epidermal growth factor receptor (Ullrich et al., 1984) and two subunits of the GABA$_A$ receptor (Schofield et al., 1987).

Synthesis of cDNA and construction of a cDNA library

A cDNA library is a collection of cloned cDNA fragments, which can be synthesised enzymatically from mRNA in two stages (see Figure 2.3). Firstly, total RNA is isolated from the tissue known to contain the protein of interest. The corresponding mRNA is subsequently purified from this with the help of oligonucleotides, such as oligo(dT).

These comprise a string of thymine bases, enabling the binding (hybridisation) to the poly(A) tail of mRNA. First-strand cDNA is synthesised from mRNA using the enzyme reverse transcriptase (Baltimore, 1970; Temin and Mizutani, 1970).

To initiate synthesis, it requires a partially double-stranded template, which is provided by the oligo(dT)/poly(A) hybrid. The second strand of the cDNA is then synthesised using DNA polymerase I. Also this enzyme requires a partially double-stranded DNA template, which can be generated in a number of ways (for details, see Sambrook and Russel's (2001) *Molecular Cloning: A Laboratory Manual*, (3rd ed) CSH Press); in Figure 2.3 it is achieved through random hexamer primers. Finally, the mixed population of double-stranded cDNA molecules is joined (ligated) to a linearised cloning vector (either a plasmid or a bacteriophage), using the enzyme T4 DNA ligase.

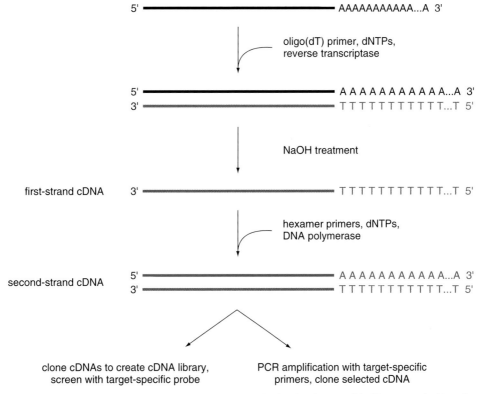

Figure 2.3 Synthesis of double-stranded cDNA. In the first step, the polyadenylated mRNA (black) is transcribed into first-strand cDNA (blue) and an mRNA/DNA hybrid is generated. Following the removal of the mRNA through alkali treatment, a partially double-stranded template is provided for the DNA polymerase by the inclusion of a mixture of random 6 mers (hexamers), which anneal to the first-strand cDNA. Apart from the preparation of a cDNA library, the cDNA may serve as substrate for PCR amplifications of selected clones.

These recombinant vectors, that is, the library of several million independent 'cDNA clones', are then introduced into suitable strains of bacteria (e.g. *Escherichia coli*) and can be immediately screened for a clone of interest or stored for several years.

Screening a cDNA library

To screen a cDNA library, the bacteria carrying it are plated out, at high density, on Petri dishes and incubated (Figure 2.4). This yields either colonies, if the cDNA library is based on plasmid vectors, or plaques on the bacterial layer in the case of bacteriophage vectors. Circular nitrocellulose filters, having the same diameter as the Petri dish, are then overlaid to produce replica of the colonies/plaques, that is, traces of the recombinant cDNAs are transferred and later immobilised onto the filters. In the next step, the filters are first treated with alkali to denature the cDNAs (i.e. to

separate the DNA strands), neutralised and eventually incubated, usually overnight, with the single-stranded and radiolabelled oligonucleotide, which anneals (hybridises) to a complementary DNA sequence. The excess, unbound or loosely-bound probe is washed away the following day, and the filters are exposed to X-ray film.

Colonies/plaques that give a signal on the X-ray film can be identified by comparing the film with the original Petri dish; these positive 'individual' colonies or plaques are picked. However, they need to be re-plated at a lower density, to avoid any overlap of adjacent cDNA clones, and re-screened. Once again, the radiolabelled oligonucleotide probe is utilised until a single, pure recombinant clone is obtained. This is achieved when all colonies/plaques in the Petri dish produce a positive signal on the X-ray film. The cDNA insert of the selected clone is then subjected to DNA sequencing to reveal its identity (see Figure 2.4).

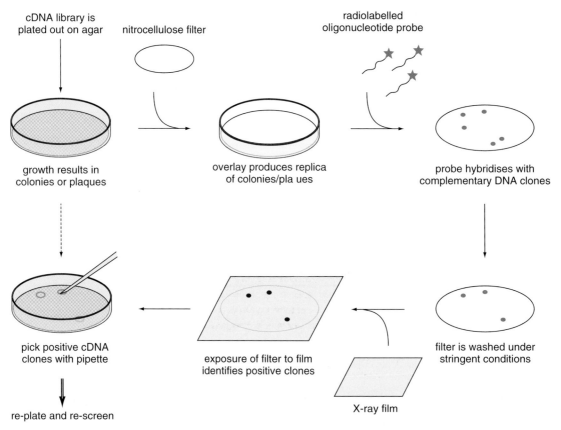

Figure 2.4 The diagram illustrates the first round of screening a cDNA library. Pure recombinant cDNA clones are obtained through several rounds of screening, whereby the isolated clones are re-plated at lower densities.

Certainly, the success of this approach depends largely on the quality – or specificity – of the oligonucleotide used in the screening process. Another important factor is the wash conditions, which remove the excess or unspecifically-bound probe. Highly-stringent wash conditions favour strong probe/cDNA hybrids and may facilitate the isolation of the clone of interest. Lower stringencies, on the other hand, may also save those hybrids, which have formed with less sequence complementarity; it is a possibility to detect homologous sequences.

Cloning using a specific antibody

This screening process identifies a cDNA clone, which may encode the protein of interest, through immunological detection rather than hybridisation with a DNA-based probe. It requires a cDNA expression library and the presence of a target-specific antibody, which has been generated previously against an isolated yet uncharacterised protein antigen. Such a library allows the inducible expression of cDNA clones, to generate heterologous proteins in the host cells, which can be screened with the antibody. For this, the expression library is constructed in a vector (e.g. bacteriophage λgt11) that fuses individual cDNAs with a protein-encoding sequence (e.g. β-galactosidase; see Figure 2.5), which can be expressed from the vector.

Screening of an expression library with an antibody is very similar to screening a cDNA library with an oligonucleotide. The main difference is that, prior to generating the replica, the nitrocellulose filter is soaked in an inducer of the promoter that drives the expression of the fusion protein, for example, isopropyl β-D-thiogalactopyranoside (IPTG) in the case of the well-characterised *lac* promoter (Figure 2.5).

The subsequent overlay of the impregnated filter onto the Petri dish induces expression from the bacteriophage vector, and binds the fusion proteins, with the replica being a mirror image of the plaque pattern. The controlled induction is a precautious step, which ensures the synthesis of sufficient amounts of proteins, while the viability of the host cells is maintained. An uncontrolled rise of high levels of the heterologous proteins may otherwise exert toxic effects on the bacteria.

The proteins on the filter can be detected by incubation with the specific, primary antibody, followed by an appropriate secondary antibody, which is conjugated to an enzyme (e.g. horseradish peroxidase) or a fluorochrome (e.g. fluorescein) to enable the localisation of the antigen-antibody complex. Positive cDNA clones are identified by comparing the signal(s) on the nitrocellulose filter with the original culture in the Petri dish. These are picked, re-plated at a lower density, and re-screened until a single, pure recombinant is obtained. An example of this approach is the discovery of the synapse-associated protein SAP90 from rat brain (Kistner et al., 1993). Here, the authors used a polyclonal antiserum against purified synaptic proteins to screen an expression library. The fusion protein from the isolated clones later enabled the affinity purification of primary antibodies, which were utilised in Western blots on brain extracts and in immunostaining.

It should be noted that the cloning of DNA fragments into vectors is an essentially random process. Only one in six inserts will have the correct orientation and reading frame (of which there are six; three on each strand of the cDNA) to produce an in-frame fusion of the drug target and β-galactosidase.

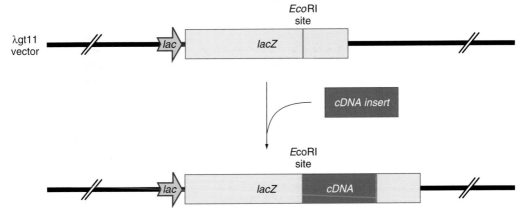

Figure 2.5 Cloning of cDNAs into the *Eco*RI restriction site of the bacteriophage vector λgt11 to produce fusion proteins with β-galactosidase, which is encoded by the *lacZ* gene.

Cloning using a functional assay

Cloning using a functional assay requires either a cDNA library in a vector, from which RNA can be synthesised *in vitro*, or one that can be transfected into mammalian cells. In the former case, pools of the cDNA library are individually subjected to *in vitro* transcription, with an appropriate RNA polymerase, and the produced RNA molecules are microinjected into oocytes from the frog *Xenopus laevis*, where the translation occurs. Besides their large size, which facilitates the microinjection and the successive assay, another advantage of this eukaryotic expression system is its ability to post-translationally modify and insert the protein into the membrane, if it is membrane-bound.

The drug target can be detected 24 to 48 hours later using an appropriate electrophysiological assay, such as ion-channel activity from either an implanted LGIC or voltage-gated ion channel, or the coupling of certain implanted GPCRs to an endogenous oocyte channel. The latter is thought to be mediated by the activation of phospholipase C, which liberates inositol trisphosphate causing the release of intracellular calcium and the consequent activation of an endogenous calcium-activated chloride current (see Chapter 3, for details). If a pool of RNAs yields a positive signal, then it is subdivided into smaller pools, which can be re-tested in exactly the same way until a single clone is obtained.

Alternatively, expression cloning can be performed by transfecting a cDNA library into mammalian cells, followed by testing membranes for binding activity using a suitable radioligand. This process is known as 'panning'. Again, individual pools of the library are transfected into mammalian cells, which are later tested. If a positive pool is identified through binding, it is subdivided and retested. This process is repeated until a single cDNA is obtained that, when transfected, produces a protein with the ability to bind the radiolabelled compound (for examples, see Masu et al., 1987; Kieffer et al., 1992).

Cloning using Polymerase Chain Reaction

The recently sequenced genomes of human and other organisms have significantly facilitated and accelerated the isolation of cDNA clones. The time-consuming isolation and sequencing of protein fragments, as well as the screening of libraries are no longer necessary to obtain (partial) sequence information. Specific oligonucleotide primers can be designed to recognise the flanking regions of an mRNA that specifies a drug target, if the 5'- and 3'-ends can be found in the nucleotide sequence database.

These primers can be used in the PCR (Mullis and Faloona, 1987; Saiki et al., 1988), a process that amplifies DNA molecules with the help of a heat-stable DNA polymerase, commonly the *Taq* DNA polymerase from the bacterium *Thermus acquaticus*. All that is required, in addition, is single-stranded cDNA that has been synthesised from RNA isolated from a source expressing the drug target. An amplicon of the desired molecular size can be identified after the PCR, through gel electrophoresis, and cloned into a vector.

The only problem with this approach is that, unless the entire coding sequence of the target is known, it is often difficult to recognise the extreme 5'- and 3'-untranslated sequences of the corresponding mRNA in databases.

2.5 What information can DNA cloning provide?

The ultimate aim of studies involving molecular cloning may be the functional and pharmacological characterisation of a drug target. However, as mentioned earlier, already the sequence of the isolated cDNA can reveal interesting information or entirely unexpected findings. This was particularly true for the discoveries in the early years of molecular cloning.

Information on the secondary structure

The cloning of a cDNA provides the primary sequence of a protein, which is obtained by simply translating the cDNA sequence. Often, by analysing the primary sequence with computer algorithms, it is possible to gain information on the secondary structure, including hydrophobic regions, which may represent membrane-spanning domains and indicate the topology, as well as potential sites for glycosylation, phosphorylation, and so on. For instance, the number and location of the membrane-spanning domains within each GABA$_A$ receptor subunit were predicted from the amino-acid sequence (Schofield et al., 1987).

Membrane-spanning domains are hydrophobic regions that comprise 20 to 22 amino acids, for example valine, leucine, isoleucine, methionine, phenylalanine, tryptophan and tyrosine. These domains typically have an α-helical conformation, and they can be predicted using so-called hydropathy plots (Figure 2.6). The computer programme that generates these plots attributes a score to each amino acid according to its hydrophilic or hydrophobic nature, and analyses the entire sequence in a stepwise manner with a set window length (e.g. 17 amino acids, as shown below). The distance between

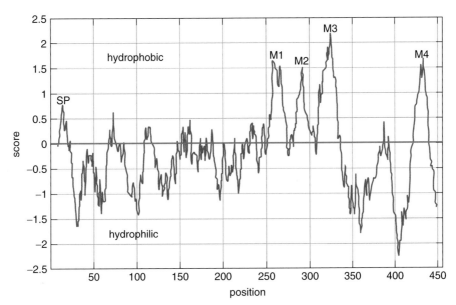

Figure 2.6 Hydropathy plot for the 456 amino acids of the bovine GABA$_A$ receptor α1-subunit showing the presence of four membrane-spanning domains (M1 to M4) and a signal peptide (SP). The plot was generated using the parameters described by Kyte and Doolittle (1982). See text for details.

the predicted membrane-spanning domains can also be estimated from hydropathy plots.

In the case of the GABA$_A$ receptor, a multi-subunit protein, it is evident that each subunit possesses four membrane-spanning domains and a signal peptide. The latter is a hydrophobic sequence of 20 to 30 amino acids found at the extreme amino-termini of some proteins. It ensures the correct insertion of the new protein into the membrane, as it is synthesised on the rough endoplasmic reticulum. The signal peptide is cleaved off after membrane insertion and is not part of the mature protein.

Furthermore, the orientation of the protein in the membrane, that is, the topology, can often be deduced from the hydropathy plot. For the bovine GABA$_A$ receptor α1 subunit (Figure 2.7), with a length of 456 amino acids, the presence of a signal peptide indicates that the amino-terminus is located extracellularly and some 220 residues long. This is followed by three membrane-spanning domains, a sequence of ~100 amino acids that is intracellular and, finally, a fourth membrane-spanning domain very close to the carboxy-terminus.

The hydropathy plot of a GPCR, for example the 477 amino acids of the human β$_1$-adrenergic receptor; (Figure 2.8), shows the characteristics that are typical for this group of receptors (Chapter 3): seven membrane-spanning domains, with an extracellular

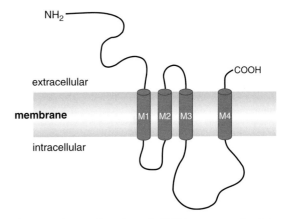

Figure 2.7 Proposed topology of a GABA$_A$ receptor subunit in the membrane. Both, the amino (NH$_2$) terminus and the carboxy (COOH) terminus are located on the extracellular side.

amino-terminus, an intracellular carboxy-terminus and a large intracellular loop between the fifth and sixth transmembrane domains (Figure 2.9).

If the topology of the protein can be deduced, then the amino-acid sequence can be scanned to predict the location of glycosylation and phosphorylation sites. Potential amino-linked glycosylation sites, which are found extracellularly in all membrane proteins, have

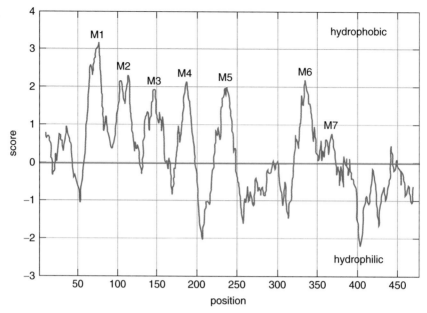

Figure 2.8 Hydropathy plot for the 477 amino acids of the human β_1-adrenergic receptor, a GPCR, according to the method by described by Kyte and Doolittle (1982). It shows the presence of seven membrane-spanning domains (M1-M7).

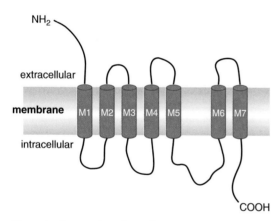

Figure 2.9 Proposed topology of a GPCR in the membrane.

the following consensus sequence: Asn (asparagine)-Xaa (any amino acid)-Ser/Thr (serine or threonine). In contrast, phosphorylation sites, which are recognised by a plethora of kinases (e.g. protein kinase A, protein kinase C), are found intracellularly. The position of these sites is of interest, since membrane proteins, such as the voltage-dependent calcium channels at the presynaptic terminals of neurons, are regulated by phosphorylation/ dephosphorylation.

However, cDNA cloning does not provide insight into the tertiary (three dimensional) and quaternary (the association of polypeptides in a multi-subunit protein) structures of a drug target. This information would be invaluable to the pharmaceutical industry because a tertiary structure permits the discovery of new drugs by molecular modelling. Unfortunately, the majority of drug targets are receptors and ion channels, which can not easily be purified in large quantities, and so their crystal structures are not always available. Currently, a large effort is on-going to determine the three-dimensional structures of proteins, such as GPCRs (Chapter 3).

Predicting the topology of a given drug target from a hydropathy plot is not infallible. Therefore, the proposed structure has to be established by experimentation. One approach is to utilise antibodies against the protein of interest. They are generated in mice (monoclonal antibodies) and/or rabbits (polyclonal), which have been immunised with chemically-synthesised peptides corresponding to different parts of the target protein. Such peptide sequences can be chosen to correspond to extracellular or intracellular regions.

The specific antibodies are usually applied on transfected mammalian cells, which express the cDNA encoding the receptor. Antibodies that recognise extracellular antigens bind to the receptor when it is expressed on the mammalian cell surface, while those directed at intracellular sites do not. Permeabilisation of the host cells with detergent, however, allows antibodies that are raised against intracellular domains to access and to bind the respective sites on the cytoplasmic side.

Information on protein subtypes and gene families

Molecular cloning also provides information on the existence of protein subtypes and gene families. Based on 'traditional' pharmacological techniques, using agonists and antagonists, pharmacologists have been able to deduce (in some cases) that more than one type of a given receptor, so-called subtypes, exists. For example, it has long been known that at least two pharmacologically-distinct types of dopamine receptor and two types of muscarinic receptor were present on cells. However, molecular cloning has subsequently revealed that five subtypes of each receptor are present within the human genome.

It is now evident that there are numerous subtypes of receptors, ion channels, neurotransmitter transporters, enzymes, and so on. The different subtypes may be coupled to different cellular signalling pathways, may be expressed at different developmental stages, or may be found in different tissues or cell types. This is exemplified by the four forms of the adenosine receptor (A_1, A_{2A}, A_{2B} and A_3), all of which are GPCRs. Here, the A_{2A} and A_{2B} receptor subtypes couple to G_s proteins and result in stimulation of adenylyl cyclase upon activation, whereas the A_1 and A_3 receptors couple to G_i proteins and mediate inhibition of this enzyme. The five subtypes of the somatostatin receptor (SST_{1-5}), on the other hand, all bind the same agonist and couple to G_i proteins, but they differ in their expression pattern and their rates of internalisation.

Likewise, diversity is a characteristic of the multigene family of $GABA_A$ receptors. Early studies including receptor autoradiography implied that, at most, two types of this ionotropic receptor exist (Sieghart and Karobath, 1980). However, the receptors are heteropentamers and can be assembled from 16 different subunits ($\alpha 1$-$\alpha 6$, $\beta 1$-$\beta 3$, $\gamma 1$-$\gamma 3$, δ, ϵ, π and θ; see Chapter 4) in mammals! Even given the restriction that the majority of receptors comprise two α, two β and one γ polypeptide, the various subunits can associate to form over 100,000 receptor subtypes. While this large number is not believed to exist *in vivo*, it seems likely that at least 20 to 30 different subtypes are present, and these bind different therapeutic compounds with distinct affinities (Whiting, 2003).

Finally, comparative analysis of sequences from molecular cloning has identified amino-acid regions or motifs, which are remarkable conserved among various groups of receptors. It led to the discovery of gene superfamilies, such as the GPCR family and the LGIC family, followed by the introduction of receptor classifications, which are largely based on amino-acid similarity. All GPCRs share common structural features, including seven membrane-spanning domains, an extracellular amino-terminus of variable length, and an intracellular carboxy-terminus. The LGIC superfamily includes the nicotinic acetylcholine receptors found in muscle and brain, and the serotonin/5-hydroxytryptamine type 3 (5-HT$_3$) receptor, which are all cation selective, as well as the $GABA_A$ and glycine receptors, which are selective for anions (mainly chloride). Each of these channels has a pentameric structure with a central ion channel, and each of the five receptor subunits is characterised by having four membrane-spanning domains (the second of which forms the lining of ion-selective pore), a long extracellular amino-terminus and a short extracellular carboxy-terminus. It is now evident that the GPCR and ligand-gated ion-channel families each evolved by a process of gene duplication and subsequent sequence divergence (e.g. Darlison et al., 2005).

The specific physiological roles of a subtype *in vivo* can be investigated through genetic engineering, such as the knockout of the respective gene in mice (see Chapter 10). Alternatively, subtype-selective compounds can be used to determine the *in vivo* functions of particular subtypes, but the development of such agents is hampered by the high degree of sequence similarity between them (typically around 70% amino-acid identity).

2.6 Comparing the pharmacologic profile of the 'cloned' and the 'native' drug target

To pharmacologically characterise the 'cloned' drug target, the corresponding cDNA can be expressed in a suitable cell system, which results in the production of the protein of interest: Mammalian cells are used for radioligand binding experiments to determine drug affinities, to investigate intracellular signalling, and for other experiments such as the measurement of enzymatic properties, while *Xenopus* oocytes are the preferred system for electrophysiological studies. The pharmacologic profile of the 'cloned' drug target can, thus, be compared with that of the 'native' protein, which has been studied *in vivo* with 'traditional' pharmacological methods. It is vitally important to establish whether the physiological properties – and hence pharmacological profiles – of the 'cloned' and the 'native' drug targets are identical. If the outcome is negative, it may be because not all of the components of a given target have yet been cloned. In this case, it would not be recommended to pursue with a screen for novel therapeutic compounds using the 'cloned' target.

A good example that demonstrates the need to identify all of the components of a given target is the $GABA_A$ receptor, which is the major inhibitory neurotransmitter receptor in brain. Upon exposure to the agonist GABA, an integral ion channel in the receptor opens and chloride ions pass the membrane; the channel closes when GABA is removed. The direction of flux is dependent on the concentration gradient of chloride ions across the cell membrane but, usually, the ions flow into neurons and cause hyperpolarisation. This influx can be increased through the therapeutically-important group of benzodiazepines (BZs), such as diazepam. This modulator of $GABA_A$ receptors potentiates the response to GABA by increasing the frequency of channel opening.

Initially, two $GABA_A$ receptor cDNAs were isolated (Schofield et al., 1987), which encoded an α and a β subunit. Neither of these cDNAs alone directed the formation of GABA-activated ion channels, when their *in vitro*-transcribed RNA was injected into *Xenopus* oocytes. Channels were only formed when the α- and β-subunit RNAs were co-injected. However, unexpectedly, diazepam had no effect on the expressed receptor. This lead to a search for a 'missing component', a cDNA for a third type of subunit (i.e. γ subunit), which was isolated a few years later (Pritchett et al., 1989). Finally, when RNAs for the α, β and γ subunits were co-injected into *Xenopus* oocytes, the resultant recombinant receptor did respond to diazepam, and the expected increased current through the channel was observed. This showed that a γ subunit is required for BZ modulation of the $GABA_A$ receptor. The reason for this was later recognised, through mutagenesis on the cDNA clones, when the BZ binding site was located at the interface between α and γ subunits (Wieland et al., 1992).

Another example is the $GABA_B$ receptor, a GPCR that couples to G_i and G_o proteins. Its activation inhibits the enzyme adenylyl cyclase leading to a reduction in intracellular cyclic AMP (cAMP) levels, activates a particular class of potassium channels (called inwardly-rectifying potassium channels), and inhibits calcium channels (for details, see Chapter 3). This receptor proved difficult to 'clone' as it could not be easily purified, and no anti-$GABA_B$ receptor antibody existed. However, a cDNA was eventually isolated using the functional expression approach known as 'panning' (Kaupmann et al., 1997). In fact, the encoded receptor ($GABA_B R1$) was found to exist in two forms (called $GABA_B R1a$ and $GABA_B R1b$) that arise from alterative splicing of the primary gene transcript.

Since, at that time, GPCRs were considered to be single subunit receptors, it was believed that the $GABA_B$ receptor had finally been 'cloned'. However, when a cDNA for either $GABA_B R1a$ or $GABA_B R1b$ was transfected into mammalian cells, agonists had a 100- to 150-fold lower potency at the recombinant receptors than was observed for the 'native' receptor. Furthermore, while activation of the receptor led to the inhibition of adenylyl cyclase, and the activation of calcium channels, neither $GABA_B R1$ receptor coupled to potassium channels.

Eventually, as a result of searching nucleotide sequence databases, a second cDNA was isolated that encoded a protein with a similar sequence to $GABA_B R1$ (Kaupmann et al., 1998). When the cDNA of this $GABA_B R2$ named receptor was expressed alone in mammalian cells, the resultant receptor did not bind either agonists or antagonists, and it did not couple to potassium channels. Co-expression of the cDNAs for $GABA_B R2$ and either of the $GABA_B R1$ splice variants, however, recreated the properties of the 'native' receptor. In fact, $GABA_B R2$ has also been shown to help translocate the $GABA_B R1$ protein to the cell surface. These data indicated that the $GABA_B$ receptor existed as a dimer – a discovery, which has led to a revolution in our thinking about GPCRs. Most GPCRs are now thought to be present *in vivo* as dimers (Chapter 3). This clearly has important implications for drug development.

2.7 Reverse pharmacology illustrated on orphan GPCRs

Historically, therapeutically-active drugs were identified through forward pharmacology, where the given compound was tested on animal models or isolated tissues, with the attempt to positively modulate the physiological phenotype. Frequently, with this approach, the molecular target and the mode of action continued to be obscure until the introduction of molecular biology techniques.

A different challenge arose with the availability of huge amounts of sequence data, from the human genome project or, in earlier years, from expressed sequence tag (EST) databases. ESTs are nucleotide sequences which are obtained by randomly sequencing the 5′- and 3′-ends of clones from cDNA libraries. These data could now be screened for 'druggable' gene products, that is, proteins with structural motifs, which potentially could be modulated by small molecules (Hopkins and Groom, 2002). However, a novel drug target qualifies as such only if its role in (patho)physiological processes is of significance. Indeed, the sequence explosion led to the discovery of a number of possible drug targets with yet unknown functions. For example, there are 'orphan' GPCRs, that is, receptors that have sequence similarity to GPCRs but for which the endogenous ligand (agonist) is unknown; similarly, there are 'orphan' transporters and 'orphan' transcription factors.

Alternatively, new gene products have been discovered through PCR using degenerate oligonucleotide primers. These primers have been designed on the basis of conserved protein sequences found in known proteins. In the case of receptors, the conserved protein sequences that have typically been used are membrane-spanning domains, which are usually highly conserved in sequence between different members of a receptor family.

Among the 'druggable' targets, the 'orphan' GPCRs provide a rich resource for the pharmaceutical industry, because approximately 30% of all approved drugs modulate GPCR function (see Chapter 1; Overington et al., 2006). They will be looked at in more detail in the next section.

'Deorphanisation' through reverse pharmacology

To be of use as a pharmaceutical target, any 'orphan' GPCR must be 'deorphanised', that is, its natural, endogenous, activating ligand must be identified (Figure 2.10; Wise et al., 2002). Then the physiological function(s) of the novel receptor must be determined in order to identify in which disease condition(s) it might be an appropriate target. The methodology for doing this is referred to

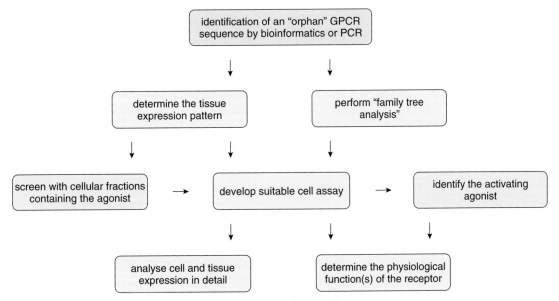

Figure 2.10 The steps involved in reverse pharmacology (see text for details).

Table 2.1 A list of some of the first 'orphan' GPCRs for which the activating agonist was identified, and the research group or company that carried out the work.

Year	Receptor / agonist	Company or research group
1995	LC132/ORL1 binds orphanin FQ/nociceptin	Hoffman-La Roche (Reinscheid et al.) and the group of Meunier et al.
1998	hGR3 binds prolactin-releasing peptide	Takeda Chemical Industries (Hinuma et al.)
1998	HFGAN72 and one other 'orphan' GPCR bind orexins (orexin-A and -B)	Sakurai et al.
1999	SLC-1 binds melanin-concentrating hormone	Bächner et al., Saito et al., AstraZeneca, SmithKline Beecham and Takeda Chemical Industries
1999	GPR14 binds urotensin-II	SmithKline Beecham (Ames et al.), Takeda Chemical Industries (Mori et al.) and Merck Research Laboratories (Liu et al.)

as 'reverse pharmacology', and a brief history of the 'deorphanisation' of 'orphan' GPCRs is presented in Table 2.1. As can be seen, the first 'orphan' GPCR to be characterised was known as LC132 or ORL1 (opioid receptor like 1 receptor; Bunzow et al., 1994; Mollereau et al., 1994), and the natural agonist has been called orphanin FQ and nociceptin (Meunier et al., 1995; Reinscheid et al., 1995).

After identifying the sequence of the 'orphan' GPCR, it is usual to search for other closely related and well-characterised GPCRs, for which the endogenous agonist is known. This can be done by further database searching and 'family tree analysis', and the outcome may already indicate whether the agonist is an amine, a nucleotide, a peptide, a fatty acid, a glycoprotein hormone, and so on.

Next, it is essential to know in which tissue or organ the 'orphan' GPCR is found, because it is reasonable to assume that the activating ligand is also present there. When this has been achieved, for example through Northern blotting, a full-length receptor cDNA can be cloned (if necessary), expressed in an appropriate cell system and a suitable assay can be devised to detect the presence of the endogenous agonist (for details, see Chapter 3). The latter is often the most challenging aspect, since the G-protein to which the 'orphan' GPCR couples is usually unknown at that stage.

Once the endogenous agonist is identified, a detailed analysis of the tissue- and cell-specific expression of the receptor can be performed, using techniques such as *in situ* hybridisation and immunocytochemistry. And, finally, the physiological function(s) of the 'orphan' GPCR can be studied using a variety of methods, including the disruption ('knockout') of the gene in mice (see Chapter 10).

Example: 'deorphanisation' of the opioid receptor like 1 receptor

Prior to 1995, three opioid receptor cDNAs, that encoded different subtypes of this receptor, called μ, δ and κ, had been cloned (Kieffer et al., 1992). The importance of these GPCRs lies in their ability to bind morphine and synthetic opioids, and to mediate analgesia; all three receptors couple to G_i proteins. In 1994, two groups cloned a cDNA for an 'orphan' GPCR, named either LC132 or ORL1 (Bunzow et al., 1994; Mollereau et al., 1994). It had strong sequence similarity to opioid receptors but did not bind any of the available opioid peptides or opioid receptor ligands. To 'deorphanise' this receptor, two assumptions were made (Reinscheid et al., 1995): firstly, that the natural agonist was a peptide (as is the case for the μ-, δ- and κ-opioid receptors) and, secondly, that LC132/ORL1 coupled to the same type of G-protein as the μ-, δ- and κ-opioid receptors, that is, a G_i protein.

The activity of G_i-coupled GPCRs can be monitored in mammalian cells, after transfecting the appropriate cDNA, by incubating with forskolin. This compound can penetrate cells and increase the intracellular levels of cAMP by stimulating adenylyl cyclase. The elevated cAMP level, however, is reduced – and can be measured – when an agonist activates the expressed G_i-coupled receptor. This screen was used to 'deorphanise' the LC132/ORL1 receptor, and the hypothalamus served as source of the agonist, as the gene encoding the 'orphan' GPCR is highly expressed here.

A peptide extract was obtained from the hypothalamus and fractionated using cation-exchange high-performance liquid chromatography (HPLC). Eighty fractions were collected from the column, and these were

Orphanin FQ	F	G	G	F	T	G	A	R	K	S	A	R	K	L	A	N	Q
Dynorphin A	Y	G	G	F	L	R	R	I	R	P	K	L	K	W	D	N	Q
Alpha-endorphin	Y	G	G	F	M	T	S	E	K	S	Q	T	P	L	V	T	
Dynorphin B	Y	G	G	F	L	R	R	Q	F	K	V	V	T				
Leu-enkephalin	Y	G	G	F	L												

Figure 2.11 Comparison of the amino-acid sequence of orphanin FQ with those of some opioid peptides. Residues that are found, in the same position, in orphanin FQ and the opioid peptides are highlighted in red.

applied to Chinese Hamster Ovary cells expressing the LC132/ORL1 receptor. Intracellular cAMP levels were subsequently measured. The two fractions that gave the largest decrease were pooled, further fractionated using reversed-phase HPLC and finally tested in the cell system. A final purification step yielded a homogenous substance that was analysed by mass spectrometry and sequenced by Edman degradation. The active peptide was named orphanin FQ (Figure 2.11).

To confirm that the identified peptide was, indeed, the natural agonist of the LC132/ORL1 receptor, it was chemically synthesised and tested. It was found to inhibit forskolin-stimulated cAMP accumulation with high potency. Radioligand binding studies were also performed on the expressed receptor using a Tyr^{14}-substituted orphanin FQ analogue (i.e. the leucine at position 14 was replaced by a tyrosine residue) that was labelled with $[^{125}I]$. This compound displayed saturable and displaceable binding, to membranes from transfected cells.

These first series of experiments verified orphanin FQ as the native, endogenous agonist of the LC132/ORL1 receptor. In addition, it confirmed that this GPCR coupled to a G_i protein, but with a pharmacologic profile quite distinct from those of the three other opioid receptors. LC132/ORL1 was, therefore, renamed orphanin FQ receptor. However, its physiological function remained to be elucidated. For this, the peptide was injected into the brains of mice, followed by a variety of behavioural tests. The peptide was found to decrease horizontal and vertical locomotor activity in a dose-dependent manner.

Surprisingly, when the pain sensitivity of the mice was assessed in the hot-plate test, orphanin FQ only showed an effect at the highest concentration. However, in a second assay, orphanin FQ decreased the time that the mice took to respond to a heat source. These data strongly suggested that rather than causing analgesia (as is the case for activation of opioid receptors), stimulation of the orphanin FQ receptor results in hyperalgesia (a greater sensitivity to pain). The lack of effect of orphanin FQ

in the hot-plate test, except at the highest concentration, is thought to have been due to the decreased locomotor activity induced by this peptide.

In conclusion, although the orphanin FQ receptor is similar in structure and sequence to opioid receptors, and couples to the same type of G-protein (i.e. G_i), it has a unique agonist. Furthermore, its activation does not induce the same physiological responses that are characteristic for the stimulation of opioid receptors, that is, analgesia, respiratory depression and euphoria. Indeed, activation of the orphanin FQ receptor seems to cause effects opposite to those induced by opioid peptides (e.g. hyperalgesia).

2.8 Summary

The introduction of molecular cloning in the 1970s has revolutionised the field of pharmacology. The new scientific approaches, in particular the ability to express cloned cDNA fragments in cell systems and characterise the encoded protein *in vitro*, have greatly enhanced our knowledge of the number of drug targets and their response to natural or synthetic ligands. However, it also made us aware of the diversity of signalling molecules, the complexities of signalling pathways – and the lack of specific compounds. It enabled the establishment of high-throughput screens and facilitated the discovery of novel therapeutic compounds. However, molecular cloning has also limitations in that it does not reveal the tertiary or quaternary structure of a drug target.

References

Ames RS, Sarau HM, Chambers JK, Willette RN, Aiyar NV, Romanic AM, Louden CS, Foley JJ, Sauermelch CF, Coatney RW, Ao Z, Disa J, Holmes SD, Stadel JM, Martin JD, Liu WS, Glover GI, Wilson S, McNulty DE, Ellis CE, Elshourbagy NA, Shabon U, Trill JJ, Hay DW, Ohlstein EH, Bergsma DJ and Douglas SA (1999). Human urotensin-II is a potent vasoconstrictor and agonist for the orphan receptor GPR14. Nature 401: 282–286.

Bächner D, Kreienkamp H, Weise C, Buck F and Richter D (1999). Identification of melanin concentrating hormone (MCH) as the natural ligand for the orphan somatostatin-like receptor 1 (SLC-1). FEBS Letters 457: 522–524.

Baltimore D (1970). RNA-dependent DNA polymerase in virions of RNA tumour viruses. Nature 226: 1209–1211.

Bunzow JR, Saez C, Mortrud M, Bouvier C, Williams JT, Low M and Grandy DK (1994). Molecular cloning and tissue distribution of a putative member of the rat opioid receptor gene family that is not a mu, delta or kappa opioid receptor type. FEBS Letters 347: 284–288.

Cohen SN, Chang ACY and Hsu L (1972). Nonchromosomal antibiotic resistance in bacteria: genetic transformation of E. coli by R-factor DNA. Proceedings of the National Academy of Sciences USA 69: 2110–2114.

Cohen SN, Chang ACY, Boyer HW and Helling RB (1973). Construction of biologically functional bacterial plasmids in vitro. Proceedings of the National Academy of Sciences USA 70: 3240–3244.

Danna K and Nathans D (1971). Specific cleavage of simian virus 40 DNA by restriction endonuclease of *Hemophilus influenza*. Proceedings of the National Academy of Sciences USA 68: 2913–2917.

Darlison MG, Pahal I and Thode C (2005). Consequences of the evolution of the GABA(A) receptor gene family. Cellular Molecular Neurobiology 25: 607–624.

Hinuma S, Habata Y, Fujii R, Kawamata Y, Hosoya M, Fukusumi S, Kitada C, Masuo Y, Asano T, Matsumoto H, Sekiguchi M, Kurokawa T, Nishimura O, Onda H and Fujino M (1998). A prolactin-releasing peptide in the brain. Nature 393: 272–276.

Hopkins AL and Groom CR (2002). The druggable genome. Nature Reviews Drug Discovery 1: 727–730.

Jackson DA, Symons RH and Berg P (1972). Biochemical method for inserting new genetic information into DNA of simian virus 40. Proceedings of the National Academy of Sciences USA 69: 2904–2909.

Kaupmann K, Huggel K, Heid J, Flor PJ, Bischoff S, Mickel SJ, McMaster G, Angst C, Bittiger H, Froestl W and Bettler B (1997). Expression cloning of GABA(B) receptors uncovers similarity to metabotropic glutamate receptors. Nature 386: 239–246.

Kaupmann K, Malitschek B, Schuler V, Heid J, Froestl W, Beck P, Mosbacher J, Bischoff S, Kulik A, Shigemoto R, Karschin A and Bettler B (1998). GABA(B)-receptor subtypes assemble into functional heteromeric complexes. Nature 396: 683–687.

Kieffer BL, Befort K, Gaveriaux-Ruff C and Hirth CG (1992). The delta-opioid receptor: Isolation of a cDNA by expression cloning and pharmacological characterization. Proceedings of the National Academy of Sciences USA 89: 12048–12052.

Kistner U, Wenzel BM, Veh RW, Cases-Langhoff C, Garner AM, Appeltauer U, Voss B, Gundelfinger ED and Garner CC (1993). SAP90, a rat presynaptic protein related to the product of the Drosophila tumor suppressor gene dlg-A. Journal of Biological Chemistry 268: 4580–4583.

Kyte J and Doolittle RF (1982). A simple method for displaying the hydropathic character of a protein. Journal of Molecular Biology 157: 105–132.

Linn S and Arber W (1968). Host specificity of DNA produced by Escherichia coli, X. In vitro restriction of phage fd replicative form. Proceedings of the National Academy of Sciences USA 59: 1300–1306.

Liu Q, Pong SS, Zeng Z, Zhang Q, Howard AD, Williams DL Jr,, Davidoff M, Wang R, Austin CP, McDonald TP, Bai C, George SR, Evans J Fand Caskey CT (1999). Identification

of urotensin II as the endogenous ligand for the orphan G-protein-coupled receptor GPR14. Biochemical Biophysical Research Communications 266: 174–178.

Masu Y, Nakayama K, Tamaki H, Harada Y, Kuno M and Nakanishi S (1987). cDNA cloning of bovine substance-K receptor through oocyte expression system. Nature 329: 836–838.

Meunier JC, Mollereau C, Toll L, Suaudeau C, Moisand C, Alvinerie P, Butour JL, Guillemot JC, Ferrara P, Monsarrat B, Mazarguil H, Vassart G, Parmentier M and Costentiná J (1995). Isolation and structure of the endogenous agonist of opioid receptor-like ORL1 receptor. Nature 377: 532–535.

Mollereau C, Parmentier M, Mailleux P, Butour JL, Moisand C, Chalon P, Caput D, Vassart G and Meunier JC (1994). ORL1, a novel member of the opioid receptor family. Cloning, functional expression and localization. FEBS Letters 341: 33–38.

Mori M, Sugo T, Abe M, Shimomura Y, Kurihara M, Kitada C, Kikuchi K, Shintani Y, Kurokawa T, Onda H, Nishimura O and Fujino M (1999). Urotensin II is the endogenous ligand of a G-protein-coupled orphan receptor, SENR (GPR14). Biochemical Biophysical Research Communications 265: 123–129.

Mullis K.B and Faloona FA (1987). Specific synthesis of DNA in vitro via a polymerase-catalyzed chain reaction. Methods in Enzymology 155: 335–350.

Noda M, Takahashi H, Tanabe T, Toyosato M, Furutani Y, Hirose T, Asai M, Inayama S, Miyata T and Numa S (1982). Primary structure of alpha-subunit precursor of Torpedo californica acetylcholine receptor deduced from cDNA sequence. Nature 299: 793–797.

Olsen RW, Meunier JC and Changeux JP (1972). Progress in the purification of the cholinergic receptor protein from Electrophorus electricus by affinity chromatography. FEBS Letters 28: 96–100.

Overington JP, Al-Lazikani B and Hopkins AL (2006). How many drug targets are there? Nature Reviews 5: 993–996.

Pritchett DB, Sontheimer H, Shivers BD, Ymer S, Kettenmann H, Schofield PR and Seeburg PH (1989). Importance of a novel GABA$_A$ receptor subunit for benzodiazepine pharmacology. Nature 338: 582–585.

Reinscheid RK, Nothacker HP, Bourson A, Ardati A, Henningsen RA, Bunzow JR, Grandy DK, Langen H, Monsma FJ Jr, and Civelli O (1995). Orphanin FQ: a neuropeptide that activates an opioidlike G protein-coupled receptor. Science 270: 792–794.

Saiki RK, Gelfand DH, Stoffel S, Scharf SJ, Higuchi R, Horn GT, Mullis KB and Erlich HA (1988). Primer-directed enzymatic amplification of DNA with a thermostable DNA polymerase. Science 239: 487–491.

Saito Y, Nothacker HP, Wang Z, Lin SH, Leslie F and Civelli O (1999). Molecular characterization of the melanin-concentrating-hormone receptor. Nature 400: 265–269.

Sakurai T, Amemiya A, Ishii M, Matsuzaki I, Chemelli RM, Tanaka H, Williams SC, Richardson JA, Kozlowski GP, Wilson S, Arch JR, Buckingham RE, Haynes AC, Carr SA, Annan RS, McNulty DE, Liu WS, Terrett JA, Elshourbagy NA, Bergsma

DJ and Yanagisawa M (1998). Orexins and orexin receptors: a family of hypothalamic neuropeptides and G protein-coupled receptors that regulate feeding behavior. Cell 92:573–585.

Sambrook J and Russel DW (2001). Molecular Cloning: A Laboratory Manual, (3rd ed) CSH Press, USA.

Sanger F, Nicklen S and Coulson AR (1977). DNA sequencing with chain-terminating inhibitors. Proceedings of the National Academy of Sciences USA 74: 5463–5467.

Schofield PR, Darlison MG, Fujita N, Burt DR, Stephenson A, Rodriguez H, Rhee LM, Ramachandran J, Reale V, Glencorse TA, Seeburg PH and Barnard EA (1987). Sequence and functional expression of the GABA$_A$ receptor shows a ligand-gated receptor super-family. Nature 328: 221–227.

Sieghart W and Karobath M (1980). Molecular heterogeneity of benzodiazepine receptors. Nature 286: 285–287.

Smith HO and Wilcox KW (1970). A restriction enzyme from Hemophilus influenza. I. Purification and general properties. Journal of Molecular Biology 51: 379–391.

Temin HM and Mizutani S (1970). RNA dependent DNA polymerase in virions of Rous sarcoma virus. Nature 226: 1211–1213.

Ullrich A, Coussens L, Hayflick JS, Dull TJ, Gray A, Tam AW, Lee J, Yarden Y, Libermann TA, Schlessinger J, Downward J, Mayes EVV, Whittle N, Waterfield MD and Seeburg PH (1984). Human epidermal growth factor receptor cDNA sequence and aberrant expression of the amplified gene in A431 epidermoid carcinoma cells. Nature 309: 418–425.

Whiting PJ (2003). GABA-A receptor subtypes in the brain: A paradigm for CNS drug discovery? Drug Discovery Today 8: 445–450.

Wieland HA, Lüddens H and Seeburg PH (1992). A single histidine in GABA$_A$ receptors is essential for benzodiazepine agonist binding. Journal of Biological Chemistry 267: 1426–1429.

Wise A, Gearing K and Rees S (2002). Target validation of G-protein coupled receptors. Drug Discovery Today 7: 235–246.

Zimmerman SB, Little JW, Oshinsky CK and Gellert M (1967). Enzymatic joining of DNA strands: a novel reaction of diphosphopyridine nucleotide. Proceedings of the National Academy of Sciences USA 57: 1841–1848.

3 G Protein-coupled Receptors

3.1 Introduction to G protein-coupled receptors

G protein-coupled receptors (GPCRs) represent the largest group of membrane-bound receptor proteins in mammals, with the human genome containing $\sim$800 genes for this family. They are so called due to their interaction with heterotrimeric G-proteins. The basic function of GPCRs is to detect extracellular signals and through G-protein activation trigger intracellular signal transduction cascades that lead to cellular responses. As such GPCRs regulate a wide variety of physiological processes.

Approximately 400 GPCRs are classified as olfactory receptors since they are involved in the detection of smell and taste, with the remainder defined as non-olfactory. The potential number of receptor proteins is increased further if you take into account post-transcriptional modifications such as alternative splicing of pre-mRNA (some GPCR genes contain introns; covered later in this chapter)

and RNA editing. It has been estimated that an individual cell may express as many as 100 different GPCRs. In this chapter we will cover GPCR structure and signal transduction pathways together with more recent developments in the field of GPCR research including GPCR dimerisation, splice variants and allosteric modulators.

The physiological importance of GPCRs is underlined by the fact that >30% of all small-molecule pharmaceutical drugs bind to GPCRs (Overington et al., 2006). At present these are grouped into two broad categories: agonists – drugs which bind to and promote receptor activation leading to a pharmacological response, or antagonists – drugs which block the effect of an agonist by interacting with the same orthosteric binding site of the receptor. The orthosteric binding site is the region that selectively binds the endogenous ligand(s) for the receptor. A third class of drug is allosteric modulators which bind to GPCRs at sites that are distinct from the orthosteric binding site (see section 3.8).

Molecular Pharmacology: From DNA to Drug Discovery, First Edition. John Dickenson, Fiona Freeman, Chris Lloyd Mills, Shiva Sivasubramaniam and Christian Thode.
© 2013 John Wiley & Sons, Ltd. Published 2013 by John Wiley & Sons, Ltd.

Table 3.1 Examples of GPCRs as pharmaceutical drug targets.

Brand name	Generic name	Position in Top 200 pharmaceuticals[a]	Therapeutic application	GPCR target
Toprol	Metoprolol	3	High blood pressure	β_1-AR antagonist
Proventil	Aibuterol	10	Asthma	β_2-AR agonist
Singulair	Montelukast	11	Asthma plus other allergies	$CysLT_1$ receptor antagonist
Zyrtec	Cetirizine	15	Hayfever plus other allergies	H_1R antagonist
Diovan	Valsartan	31	High blood pressure, heart failure	AT_1 receptor antagonist

[a]Source: Pharmacy Times, Top 200 Prescription Drugs of 2006 (http://www.pharmacytimes.com).

At present only ∼30 of known GPCRs are targeted pharmaceutically and hence there is considerable potential for the future development of drugs that target other members of this receptor super-family. A few well known examples of GPCRs as therapeutic targets are given in Table 3.1. It is noteworthy that GPCRs are also the targets of many recreational drugs of abuse including heroin, LSD (D-lysergic acid diethylamide) and cannabis.

GPCRs can be activated by photons (via rhodopsin, the light-trapping receptor located in the retina), and a diverse range of ligands including ions (Ca^{2+}), catecholamines (e.g. adrenaline, noradrenaline, dopamine), biogenic amines (e.g. histamine, 5-hydroxytryptamine), nucleotides (e.g. ATP, UTP), peptides (e.g. endothelin, bradykinin, neuropeptide Y), glycoprotein hormones (e.g. thyrotropin, luteinising hormone, follicle-stimulating hormone) and lipids (e.g. prostaglandins, leukotrienes, anandamide).

Many endogenous GPCR agonists activate multiple subtypes within a given receptor family. For example, at least nine different GPCRs are activated by adrenaline, five by acetylcholine and at least 12 by 5-hydroxytryptamine (5-HT). GPCR families well-known to pharmacologists are listed in Table 3.2. For a comprehensive and up-dated guide to the nomenclature of GPCRs see Alexander et al. (2009) or visit the website of the International Union of Pharmacology (IUPHAR) at www.iuphar.org.

For many so-called 'orphan' GPCRs (>100) the endogenous ligand(s) are unknown. The identification of orphan receptor ligands (termed de-orphanisation) is an intense area of molecular pharmacology research, which may lead to the identification of novel therapeutic targets (see review by Chung et al. (2008) and Chapter 2 for more details).

Molecular structure of GPCRs

GPCRs are single polypeptide chains which vary considerably in amino acid number, from 318 for the human A_3 adenosine receptor up to 1,212 for the human $mGlu_5$ receptor. The predominant structural characteristic of GPCRs are the seven transmembrane (TM1-7) hydrophobic α-helices, each containing 25–35 amino acids. Due to the presence of these α-helices GPCRs are also known as 7TM, serpentine or heptahelical receptors. Three extracellular loops (designated e1, e2 and e3) and three intracellular loops (i1, i2 and i3) connect the transmembrane α-helices, with the NH_2-terminus being extracellular and the COOH-terminus being intracellular. Recent X-ray crystallography studies have revealed the presence of an additional α helix (helix 8; Huynh et al., 2009) which is located at the start of the C-terminus and appears to lie parallel with the cell membrane. For some GPCRs, the helix 8 domain is attached to the cell membrane through a lipid anchor (Figure 3.1). Most GPCRs also contain at least one concensus N-glycosylation site (an asparagine residue) located in N-terminus or extracellular loop 2. Depending on the specific GPCR the function(s) of this post-translational modification include regulation of cell surface expression and protein folding, ligand recognition and receptor-G-protein coupling. Another notable feature of GPCRs is the phosphorylation sites located predominantly in the third intracellular loop and C-terminus. These are the targets for second messenger-dependent protein kinase (PKA and PKC)

Table 3.2 Well-known members of the GPCR family.

Receptor family	Endogenous agonist(s)	Subtypes	G-protein coupling
5-HT	5-hydroxytryptamine	5-HT_{1A}, 5-HT_{1B}, 5-HT_{1D} 5-HT_{1F}	G_i/G_o G_i/G_o
		5-HT_{2A}, 5-HT_{2B}, 5-HT_{2C}	G_q
		5-HT_4, 5-HT_5, 5-HT_7	G_s
Adenosine	Adenosine	A_1, A_3	G_i/G_o
		A_{2A}, A_{2B}	G_s
Adrenoceptors	Adrenaline	α_{1A}, α_{1B}, α_{1C}	G_q
	Noradrenaline	α_{2A}, α_{2B}, α_{2C}	G_i/G_q
		β_1, β_2, β_3	G_s
Angiotensin	Angiotensin II	AT_1	G_q
		AT_2	Unknown[a]
Cannabinoid	Anandamide[b]	CB_1, CB_2	G_i/G_o
Dopamine	Dopamine	D1, D5	G_s
		D2, D3, D4	G_i/G_o
$GABA_B$	γ-aminobutyric acid	$GABA_{B1}$, $GABA_{B2}$	G_i/G_o
Glutamate	L-glutamate	$mGlu_1$, $mGlu_5$	G_q
(metabotropic)	L-aspartate	$mGlu_2$, $mGlu_3$, $mGlu_4$	G_i/G_o
		$mGlu_6$, $mGlu_7$, $mGlu_8$	G_i/G_o
Histamine	Histamine	H_1	G_q
		H_2	G_s
		H_3, H_4	G_i/G_o
Muscarinic	Acetylcholine	m1, m3, m5	G_q
		m2, m4	G_i/G_o
Opioid	Enkephalins	Delta (δ; DOR)	
	β-endorphin	Kappa (κ; KOP)	All G_i/G_o
	Dynorphins	Mu (μ; MOR)	
Somatostatin	Somatostatin-14	sst_1, sst_2, sst_3,	All G_i/G_o
	Somatostatin-28	sst_4, sst_5	

[a] Activates several G-protein independent signalling pathways.
[b] Several other endogenous agonists have also been identified.

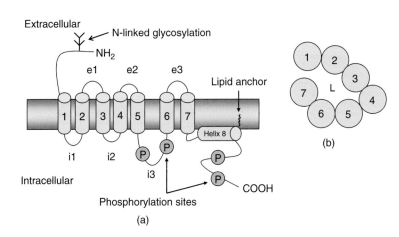

(a)

(b)

Figure 3.1 G protein-coupled receptor structure. (a) Schematic model of a typical GPCR showing the seven transmembrane domains (1–7) and helix 8. Three extracellular loops (e1, e2 and e3) and three intracellular loops (i1, i2 and i3) connect the transmembrane α-helices. (b) The seven transmembrane domains are arranged in a circular fashion which for Class A GPCRs creates a ligand (L) binding pocket.

and G protein-coupled receptor kinase (GRK) mediated phosphorylation and are important in regulating receptor desensitisation and in some cases G-protein coupling (see section 3.6). For reviews on GPCR structure and signal transduction see Marinissen and Gutkind (2001) and Lefkowitz (2004).

Protein sequence alignment analysis has revealed two important amino acid sequences which are highly conserved amongst the Class A rhodopsin-like GPCR family (the classification of GPCRs is discussed later in this chapter). First is the sequence E/DRY (single letter amino acid code) which is found at the cytoplasmic end of TM3 (Rovati et al., 2007). The second is NPxxY (where × is any amino acid), which is located at the end of TM7. Both these sequences are involved in the conformational changes associated with receptor activation and G-protein coupling. Mutation of the glutamic acid and/or aspartic acid residue within the E/DRY motif results in constitutively active receptors, a topic to be covered later in this chapter.

For members of the Class A GPCR family the circular arrangement of the seven TM domains creates a central core or ligand binding pocket (Figure 3.1). The orientation of the α-helices domains was initially determined from low-resolution electron diffraction studies using frog rhodopsin. These experiments revealed that TM domains 4, 6 and 7 are probably perpendicular to the plasma membrane, whereas TM domains 1, 2, 3, and 5 are tilted. In 2000 the high-resolution X-ray diffraction structure of bovine rhodopsin (resolution 2.8 Å; 1 Å = 0.1 nm) was obtained revealing for the first time the architecture of the seven TM domains (Palczewski et al., 2000). To put some perspective on these measurements bond lengths between two atoms in a molecule are usually in the order of 0.1–0.2 nm and a typical GPCR has dimensions of 75 × 45 × 30 Å.

GPCR structural studies: X-ray crystallography and NMR spectroscopy

Modern drug discovery programmes require detailed structural information of the intended drug target. For many soluble proteins such as enzymes this is readily achieved via the combined use of X-ray crystallography and NMR spectroscopy. However, for large transmembrane proteins such as GPCRs X-ray analysis this has proved extremely challenging since they are difficult to grow as crystals due to their structural instability. Despite these hurdles the last decade has seen the reporting in the literature of seven different GPCR crystal structures: bovine rhodopsin, avian β_1-adrenergic

receptor, human β_2-adrenergic receptor (Cherezov et al., 2007; Rasmussen et al., 2007; Rosenbaum et al., 2007), human A_{2A} adenosine receptor (Jaakola et al., 2008), human dopamine D3 receptor (Chien et al., 2010), human CXCR4 receptor (Wu et al., 2010), and human histamine H_1 receptor (Shimamura et al., 2011). In order to overcome the inherent instability problem associated with GPCR structure researchers have adopted several different approaches. These include replacing the third intracellular loop sequence with that of bacteriophage T4 lysozyme or more recently the use of point mutations to increase thermostability (Lebon et al., 2011). GPCR-T4 lysozyme fusion proteins are more structurally stable since they lack part of the receptor that is associated with G-protein coupling. Furthermore, until very recently the vast majority of GPCR crystal structures have been obtained with the receptor bound either to an inverse agonist (Figure 3.2) or antagonist in order to aid stabilisation during crystal formation. However, in 2011 the crystal structure

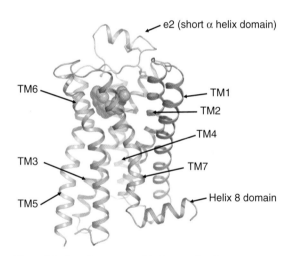

Figure 3.2 Crystal structure of the human β_2-adrenoceptor. The image below reveals the crystal structure of the human β_2-adrenoceptor bound to partial inverse agonist carazolol (green). The positions of the seven transmembrane domains (TM1-7) and the helix 8 domain are indicated. The extracellular loop 2 (e2) contains a short α-helix domain that is stabilised by intra- and inter-loop disulphide bonds (yellow). Ligand binding involves polar and hydrophobic interactions with specific amino acids in TM domains 3, 5, 6 and 7. In order to obtain crystals of the β_2AR several modifications were made including stabilisation of TM5/TM6 achieved by replacing the third intracellular loop with bacteriophage T4 lysozyme, truncating the flexible C-terminus, and removal of N-linked glycosylation sites. Image kindly donated by Professor Brian K. Kobilka, Stanford University, USA.

of the agonist-bound human A_{2A} adenosine receptor was reported by two groups revealing for the first time structural changes associated with active receptors (Xu et al., 2011, Lebon et al., 2011). Another major breakthrough in the field of GPCR structural biology has been the crystallisation of the agonist-occupied β_2-adrenergic receptor in complex with the heterotrimeric G_s-protein (Rasmussen et al., 2011). This significant achievement, from the research team lead by Professor Brian Kobilka, will hopefully provide a greater understanding of how GPCRs function at the molecular level thus aiding future drug discovery programmes involving *in silico* screening. In the future as methodology and techniques for purifying and stabilising GPCR complexes continues to develop we can expect further crystal structures of GPCRs bound to the other members of the heterotrimeric G-protein family (e.g. G_i and G_q) and ultimately other GPCR interacting proteins. For more detailed information on the crystal structures of GPCRs, see Kobilka and Schertler (2008), Mustafi and Palczewski (2009), Rosenbaum et al. (2009) and Katritch et al. (2012).

Whilst X-ray crystallography yields a wealth of structural information it only provides a static rather in-active view of protein structure. Recently GPCR structure has been analysed using NMR spectroscopy which enables the dynamics of GPCR activation and ligand binding to be studied. For example, Bokoch et al. (2010) used NMR spectroscopy to explore the conformational changes that occur around a salt bridge (a noncovalent interaction between amino acids involving either electrostatic interactions or hydrogen bonding) between extracellular loops 2 and 3 of the β_2-adrenergic receptor. This region was chosen because it is extremely variable amongst GPCRs and therefore may represent a suitable target for developing novel receptor subtype-specific allosteric modulators. These studies required the isotopic-labelling of purified β_2-adrenergic receptors on lysine[305], which is located near the salt bridge, with a ^{13}C-methyl group in order to carry out NMR analysis. The results obtained revealed conformational coupling between the extracellular surface of the receptor and the transmembrane domains associated with orthosteric ligand binding. In the future drugs that target the extracellular surface(s) of GPCRs may be able to act as allosteric modulators of orthosteric ligand binding and therefore provide novel therapeutic opportunities. Structural studies of GPCRs using X-ray crystallography and NMR spectroscopy seem certain to expand in the future and become routine tools for studying the complex conformational changes that occur following ligand binding.

Classification of GPCRs

Since the completion of the human genome project several GPCR classification systems have been proposed and one of the most frequently used is the A, B, C, D, E and F grouping. This system covers both vertebrate and invertebrate GPCRs and hence includes some families that do not occur in humans (namely groups D and E). The vast majority of mammalian GPCRs belong to Class A and ligand binding occurs predominantly within the seven TM domains. Class B receptors are a small family with little sequence homology to Class A or Class C receptors. Ligand binding to Class B receptors involves the long extracellular N-terminus region. Class C is the smallest family and contains metabotropic glutamate receptors (mGlu), Ca^{2+}-sensing receptors, $GABA_B$ receptors and the sweet and umami taste receptors (T1R1-3). This class is also characterised by a large N-terminus which contains a Venus flytrap (VFT) module important in ligand binding. Agonist binding causes the VFT domain to close (hence its name), promoting receptor activation. A notable feature of Class C receptors is that they exist as constitutive dimers (this will be covered later in this chapter). The structural differences between Class A, B and C GPCRs are illustrated in Figure 3.3.

More recently an alternative classification system has been proposed which is based on GPCRs in the human genome. This divides GPCRs into five main families named Glutamate (G), Rhodopsin (R), Adhesion (A), Frizzled/Taste2 (F), and Secretin (S) and is known as the GRAFS system (Table 3.3). For more detailed information on GPCR classification see Lagerström and Schiöth (2008).

Activation of GPCRs

The predominant mechanism associated with GPCR activation is agonist binding which induces a conformational change within the receptor that allows coupling to heterotrimeric G-proteins. However there are two exceptions to this rule; the light sensing receptor rhodopsin and proteinase-activated receptors (PARs). Rhodopsin is activated when a photon of light causes the isomerisation and hydrolysis of covalently bound 11-*cis*-retinal to 11-*trans* retinal. This results in the disruption of a salt bridge (weak ionic bond) between TM3 (retinal is bound to a lysine residue within this domain) and TM7 resulting in a conformational change that enables G-protein coupling.

Proteinase-activated receptors represent a novel class of GPCRs which are activated by a distinct mechanism that involves proteolytic cleavage of the N-terminal tail

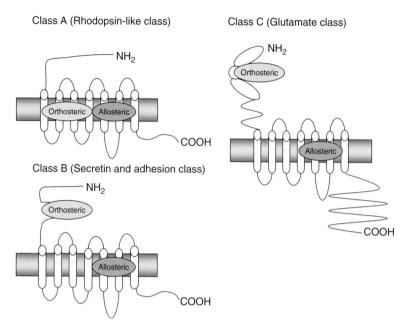

Class A (Rhodopsin-like class)

Class C (Glutamate class)

Class B (Secretin and adhesion class)

Figure 3.3 Structural differences between Class A, B and C GPCRs. For most class A receptors the endogenous orthosteric ligand binding site resides within seven TM domains, whereas for class B and C receptors endogenous ligands bind to the large N-terminal domains which are a characteristic feature of these receptors. Putative allosteric modulator binding sites are shown for each receptor class.

by protease agonists. The coagulation protease thrombin promotes platelet aggregation via the activation of PARs. Agonist protease hydrolysis results in the unmasking of a short N-terminal amino acid sequence which then functions as a 'tethered agonist'. The tethered agonist interacts with the second extracellular loop promoting a conformational change which leads to receptor activation. The problem with this mode of activation is that the receptor cannot be de-activated and stimulated again as is the case with the majority of GPCRs. Following activation PARs are rapidly desensitised (covered later in this chapter), removed from the cell surface via endocytosis and replaced with newly synthesised receptors.

The binding or coupling of GPCRs to G-proteins involves specific regions of the receptor, predominantly the second and third intracellular loops together with the C-terminal. It is interesting to note that interactions with heterotrimeric G-proteins have not been experimentally proven for the vast majority of receptors classified as GPCRs! Indeed, there is evidence that certain GPCRs can signal independently of G-proteins. Molecular pharmacologists are able to explore the conformational changes involved in GPCR activation using a variety of biophysical

and biochemical techniques (Wess et al., 2008). Such studies have revealed that conformational changes occur within TM domains 3, 5, 6, 7 and helix 8, which subsequently alter the conformation of intracellular loops i2 and i3 and enable G-protein coupling (Unal and Karnik, 2012). Deletion or mutation of the i3 generates receptors that can still bind ligands (agonists and antagonists) but are not capable to producing cell signalling responses.

3.2 Heterotrimeric G-proteins

Heterotrimeric G-proteins (guanine nucleotide binding proteins) can be considered as the middle management in the organisation of GPCR-mediated cell signalling. They link GPCR activation to the stimulation or inhibition of enzymes and ion channels that are involved in the regulation of intracellular levels of second messengers (for example cyclic AMP and IP_3) and ions (Ca^{2+}, Na^+ and K^+).

The G-protein superfamily includes monomeric G-proteins, for example Ras, and heterotrimeric

Table 3.3 GPCR classification: the GRAFS and A-F systems.

	Glutamate	Rhodopsin	Adhesion	Frizzled/Taste2	Secretin
	C	A	B[a]	F	B[a]
Number of full-length proteins	22	672[b]	33[c]	36	15
Number of orphan receptors	7	63[d]	30	21[e] (Taste 2)	0
Examples of endogenous ligands	Glutamate GABA Ca^{2+}	Light Peptides Amines Purines Lipids Proteases	TGase GAGs	Wnt[f] Bitter tasting compounds	Calcitonin CRF Glucagon PTH, VIP
Extended N-terminus	Yes	No	Yes	Yes	No

[a]The GRAFS system split family B into the adhesion and secretin families.
[b]includes an estimated 388 olfactory receptors.
[c]Only three Adhesion GPCRs have been de-orphanised.
[d]not including olfactory receptors.
[e]The human genome contains 25 taste 2 receptor (TR2) genes many of which are still orphan receptors. They are involved in the detection of bitter compounds.
[f]Wnt glycoproteins signal through a group of 10 frizzled receptors and are involved in the regulation of developmental processes (see Wang et al., 2006 for more information about this class of GPCR). Abbreviations: CRF, Corticotropin-releasing factor; GABA, γ-aminobutyric acid; GAGs, Glycosaminoglycans; PTH, parathyroid hormone; TGase, Tissue transglutaminase; VIP, vasoactive intestinal peptide.

G-proteins, which are associated with GPCRs. As their name suggests heterotrimeric G-proteins consist of three different protein subunits, alpha (Gα), beta (Gβ) and gamma (Gγ), with the guanine nucleotides (GTP or GDP) binding to the α-subunit. The G-protein subunits are anchored to the cell membrane via lipid side chains (see below). Humans possess 21 Gα subunits (encoded by 16 genes), 6 Gβ (encoded by 5 genes) and 12 Gγ subunits.

Lipid modifications of heterotrimeric G-proteins

Many membrane associated proteins are post-translationally modified through the covalent attachment of lipid groups to specific amino acid residues. These lipid modifications include 14-carbon (myristate) and 16-carbon (palmitate) saturated fatty acids or 15-carbon (farnesyl) and 20-carbon (geranylgeranyl) isoprenoids. Such modifications aid in membrane association, subcellular trafficking and interactions with other proteins.

Heterotrimeric G-proteins exhibit three types of lipid modification. All Gα subunits are modified either by myristoylation (addition of myristate to a glycine residue located at the N-terminus) or by palmitoylation (addition of palmitate to a cysteine residue located near the N-terminus), and in some cases both. In contrast Gγ subunits are modified by prenylation, which involves the attachment of geranylgeranyl to a cysteine residue located near the C-terminus. For more detailed information on the role and function of lipid modifications of heterotrimeric G-proteins, see Chen and Manning (2001).

Activation of heterotrimeric G-proteins

Conformational changes within the agonist-occupied GPCR promote heterotrimeric G-protein coupling. However, this paradigm may change since recent evidence using fluorescence resonance energy transfer (FRET) measurements has revealed that certain GPCRs may already be pre-coupled to G-proteins prior to receptor activation. In the resting or basal state the G-protein has GDP bound to the Gα subunit. Following coupling to the receptor the Gα subunit undergoes a conformational

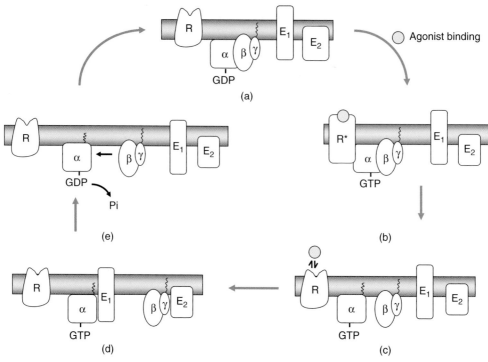

Figure 3.4 GPCR-mediated activation of heterotrimeric G-proteins. (a) As detailed in the text heterotrimeric G-proteins comprise of three subunits (α,β,γ) with GDP bound in the basal or inactive state. (b) The activated agonist-occupied receptor (R*) undergoes a conformational change which enables G-protein coupling, promoting GDP bound to the α subunit to be replaced with GTP. (c) The G-protein α-GTP and $\beta\gamma$ subunits dissociate from each other and from the activated receptor. (d) The α-GTP and $\beta\gamma$ subunits interact with target effector proteins (E_1, E_2) such as phospholipase C, adenylyl cyclase or ion channels. (e) The intrinsic GTPase activity of the α subunit increases when bound to effector molecules resulting in the hydrolysis of GTP to GDP with the release of inorganic phosphate (Pi). This causes the α-GDP and $\beta\gamma$ subunits to recombine and terminates the cycle.

change which results in the release of GDP and the binding of GTP (Figure 3.4). The G-protein complex dissociates releasing $G\alpha$-GTP and $G\beta\gamma$ subunits which then independently activate and/or inhibit various enzymes and ion channels; collectively known as effector proteins. The active $G\alpha$-GTP is eventually inactivated by the hydrolysis of GTP back to GDP via the intrinsic GTPase activity of the $G\alpha$-subunit. The $G\alpha$-GDP dissociates from the target effector protein and recombines with the $G\beta\gamma$ subunit. This completes the G-protein cycle (Figure 3.4). For a comprehensive review on heterotrimeric G-protein activation see Oldham and Hamm (2008).

The intrinsic GTPase activity of the $G\alpha$ subunit can be enhanced by GTPase activating proteins (GAPs). The effectors phospholipase C-β and adenylyl cyclase V (both covered later in this chapter) acts as GAPs for $Gq\alpha$ and $Gs\alpha$, respectively. More recently a family of proteins named regulators of G-protein signalling (RGS) have

been discovered to act as GAPs for $Gi\alpha1$, $Gi\alpha2$, $Gi\alpha3$, $Gi\alpha1$, $Go\alpha$, and $Gq\alpha$ but not $Gs\alpha$. More than 20 different RGS proteins have been identified and in addition to their GAP role they also directly interact with GPCRs, adenylyl cyclase, phospholipase C-β, Ca^{2+} channels and G-protein gated inwardly rectifying potassium channels (GIRKs). Due to their wide roles in regulating GPCR signalling they may represent an important future drug target (for a review on RGS protein see Hurst and Hooks, 2009).

Heterotrimeric G-protein families

To date there are more than 20 known subtypes of $G\alpha$ subunit, six of $G\beta$ and 12 of $G\gamma$. Despite the large number of $G\alpha$ subunits they are grouped or classified into four main families (G_s, $G_{i/o}$, G_q and $G_{12/13}$), which show selectivity for specific GPCR subtypes and effector proteins.

The G_s family containing α_S is primarily associated with the stimulation (G_s for stimulatory) of the enzyme

Table 3.4 G-protein families and their effector protein targets.

Family	Subtypes	Distribution	Effectors
G_s	α_s	Ubiquitous	↑ Adenylyl cyclase
	α_{olf}	Olfactory cells, brain	↑ Adenylyl cyclase
$G_{i/o}$	α_{i1}	Widely expressed	↓ Adenylyl cyclase
	α_{i2}	Ubiquitous	↓ Adenylyl cyclase
	α_{i3}	Widely expressed	↓ Adenylyl cyclase
	α_{o1}	Neuronal	↑ VGCC, ↑ GIRK
	[a]α_{o2}	Neuronal	↑ VGCC, ↑ GIRK
	α_z	Neuronal, platelets	↓ Adenylyl cyclase
	α_{gust}	Taste and brush cells	Unknown (↑ PDE?)
	α_{t-r}	Retinal rods, taste cells	↑ PDE type 5
	α_{t-c}	Retinal cones	↑ PDE5 type 5
G_q	α_q,	Ubiquitous	↑ Phospholipase C-β
	α_{11},	Ubiquitous	↑ Phospholipase C-β
	α_{14},	Kidney, lung, spleen	↑ Phospholipase C-β
	[b]$\alpha_{15/16}$	Haematopoietic cells	↑ Phospholipase C-β
$G_{12/13}$	α_{12},	Ubiquitous	↑ PDZ-RhoGEF
	α_{13}	Ubiquitous	↑ PDZ-RhoGEF
			↑ p115-RhoGEF

[a]Splice variant of α_{o1},
[b]Mouse (α_{15}) and human (α_{16}) orthologues
Abbreviations: VGCC, voltage-gated calcium channel; GIRK, G-protein regulated inward-rectifier potassium channel; PDE, phosphodiesterase; PDZ-RhoGEF, PSD95-Disc-Large-ZO-1; RhoGEF, Rho guanine nucleotide exchange factor. ↑ = activates; ↓ = inhibits; ? = possible effector.

adenylyl cyclase, whereas the $G_{i/o}$ family containing several different α subunits (α_{i1}, α_{i2}, α_{i3}, α_{o1}, α_{o2} and α_z) mediates the inhibition (G_i for inhibitory) of adenylyl cyclase. Some GPCRs couple to G_s and activate adenylyl cyclase (G_s-PCR) whereas others couple to $G_{i/o}$ and inhibit adenylyl cyclase (G_i-PCR).

The third main heterotrimeric G-protein family is G_q. It contains several different α subunits (α_q, α_{11}, α_{14}, $\alpha_{15/16}$) all of which activate the enzyme phospholipase C-β. The fourth family is G_{12}, which contains the α_{12} and α_{13} subunits, and effector protein targets include guanine nucleotide exchange factors (GEFs) for monomeric G-proteins such as RhoA. Downstream targets of active RhoA include Rho kinase which is involved in the regulation of many cellular functions including muscle contraction, cell migration, cell adhesion and angiogenesis. The main G-protein families and their associated effectors are summarised in Table 3.4.

Until recently it was generally accepted that G-protein signalling only involved the Gα subunit and that the Gβγ subunit was in effect an innocent bystander. This initial view has now changed and Gβγ subunits, especially those released from activated $G_{i/o}$ proteins, play a vital role in the regulation of effector proteins. Effector proteins modulated by Gβγ include activation of adenylyl cyclase isoform 1 (AC1), inhibition of adenylyl cyclase isoforms 2 and 4 (AC2 and AC4), phospholipase C-β, phospholipase A_2 and phosphoinositide 3-kinase-γ (PI-3K). In addition to modulating enzyme activity GPCRs can also control ion channel function via Gα and βγ subunits. For example voltage-gated Ca^{2+} channels and G-protein regulated inward-rectifier potassium channels are regulated via Gβγ subunits.

Modification of heterotrimeric G-proteins by bacterial toxins

Several bacterial toxins, including cholera toxin produced by the bacterium *Vibrio cholerae*, are known to modify heterotrimeric G-protein signalling. Cholera toxin catalyses the ADP-ribosylation of Gα$_s$ subunits which inhibits the intrinsic GTPase activity resulting in sustained G_s-protein activation and cyclic AMP production independent of receptor activation. This causes excessive fluid loss from cells lining the small intestine resulting in life-threatening diarrhoea. Another bacterial toxin is pertussis toxin which is produced by the bacterium *Bordetella pertussis* responsible for whooping cough. It specifically catalyses the ADP-ribosylation of $G\alpha_{i/o}$ subunits blocking GPCR coupling to this class of G-proteins. Cholera toxin and pertussis toxin are used experimentally to investigate the roles of G_s and $G_{i/o}$-proteins, respectively.

3.3 Signal transduction pathways

As already detailed previously GPCRs modulate a wide range of signal transduction pathways involving numerous phospholipases, ion channels and protein kinases. In this section we shall cover two prominent pathways namely phospholipase C and adenylyl cyclase and learn how to measure the second messengers produced by these important effector proteins.

Phospholipase C

Phospholipase C (PLC) catalyses the hydrolysis of the membrane-bound phospholipid, phosphatidylinositol biphosphate (PIP_2), generating the second messengers' inositol 1,4,5-trisphosphate (IP_3) and diacylglycerol (DAG). The water-soluble IP_3 triggers the release of Ca^{2+} from intracellular stores, whereas DAG, which remains membrane bound, activates protein kinase C (PKC) leading to changes in protein phosphorylation (Figure 3.5).

There are 13 isoforms of PLC grouped into seven distinct classes based on structure and activation mechanisms. These are PLCβ1 to β4; PLCγ1 and γ2; PLCδ1, δ3 and δ4; PLCε, PLCζ; PLCη1and η2. $G_{q/11}$ proteins activate the PLC-β isoforms.

The second messengers IP_3 and DAG are rapidly deactivated and used to regenerate PIP_2 via the phosphoinositide cycle. IP_3 is sequentially dephosphorylated to inositol by the activity of inositol phosphatases, whereas DAG undergoes phosphorylation to produce phosphatidic acid (PA). PA and inositol recombine to produce phosphatidylinositol, which is phosphorylated by lipid kinases to regenerate PIP_2. Lithium blocks this recycling pathway by inhibiting inositol 1-phosphatase activity. The effect of lithium on phosphoinositide synthesis is thought to account for the therapeutic benefits of lithium when used to control manic depression.

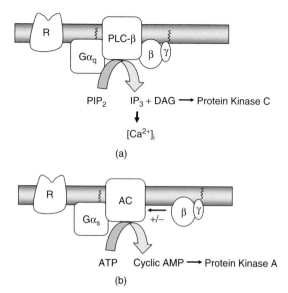

Figure 3.5 GPCR-mediated activation of phospholipase C and adenylyl cyclase. (a) GPCRs coupled to $G_{q/11}$ proteins stimulate phospholipase C (PLC-β) activation via $G\alpha_q$-GTP. Gβγ subunits released from $G_{i/o}$-PCRs can also stimulate PLC-β. For details see text. (b) GPCRs coupled to G_s-proteins stimulate adenylyl cyclase (AC) via $G\alpha_s$-GTP. βγ subunits can also stimulate or inhibit certain isoforms of AC. GPCRs coupled $G_{i/o}$-proteins inhibit AC via $G\alpha_{i/o}$-GTP (not shown). For details see text.

Measurement of phospholipase C activation

A range of experimental methods have been developed to measure PLC activation. Indirect approaches include monitoring IP_3-induced increases in intracellular Ca^{2+}. This is easily achieved using calcium-sensitive fluorescent dyes such as fura-2. Alternatively the accumulation of inositol phosphates in response to GPCR activation can be measured using radiolabelled ^3H-*myo*-inositol.

The ^3H-*myo*-inositol is readily taken up by cells and becomes incorporated into inositol-containing phospholipids, namely phosphatidylinositol, phosphatidylinositol 4-phosphate and PIP_2. Activation of PLC-β following G_q-PCR stimulation releases [^3H]-inositol 1,4,5-trisphosphate (^3H-IP_3) into the cytosol. [^3H]-IP_3 is metabolised by various intracellular phosphatases to produce a range of different [^3H]-inositol phosphate compounds. The addition of lithium inhibits a number of these steps, but most importantly, it can prevent the conversion of ^3H-inositol monophosphates to free ^3H-inositol. This produces an accumulation of ^3H-inositol monophosphates which can be separated from ^3H-inositol using anion-exchange chromatography.

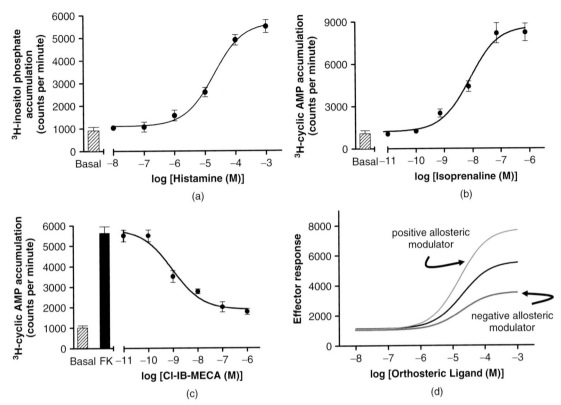

Figure 3.6 Experimental measurement of phospholipase C and adenylyl cyclase activity. Theoretical concentration response curves for (a) histamine stimulated [^{3}H]- inositol phosphate accumulation via the histamine H_1 receptor , (b) isoprenaline stimulated [^{3}H]-cyclic AMP accumulation via the β_2-adrenoceptor and (c) Cl-IB-MECA mediated inhibition of forskolin-stimulated [^{3}H]-cyclic AMP accumulation via the A_3 adenosine receptor. The hatched column in (c) is the accumulation of cyclic AMP induced by forskolin alone (i.e. in the absence of Cl-IB-MECA). The filled column in each panel represents the accumulation of inositol phosphates or cyclic AMP measured in the absence of agonist or forskolin and represents the so-called basal value. (d) Effect of positive (red curve) and negative (green curve) allosteric modulators on orthosteric agonist efficacy (black curve; in absence of allosteric modulator). The maximal functional responses (E_{max}) are altered without a significant change in agonist potency (EC_{50}). For more details see text.

The level of radioactivity in each sample can be determined using scintillation counting and is proportional to the amount of ^{3}H-inositol phosphates (Figure 3.6).

A scintillation proximity assay for high throughput measurement of inositol phosphates in cell extracts has also been developed which eliminates the chromatography step. This method uses positively charged yttrium silicate microscopic beads that bind inositol phosphates. The beads are coated with a scintillant that emits light when stimulated with the β-particles released from the radio-labelled material. The emitted light is then detected using a conventional scintillation counter.

When measuring agonist-mediated GPCR responses it is normal practice to produce $\log_{10}$ concentration-response curves which are then plotted using computer assisted curve fitting programmes (Figure 3.6). A widely used software package is GraphPad Prism. When plotted on a logarithmic scale this produces a sigmoidal curve with the majority of the response occurring over two orders of magnitude of concentration.

Adenylyl cyclase

G_s and $G_{i/o}$-proteins are primarily associated with the stimulation and inhibition of adenylyl cyclase, respectively. Adenylyl cyclase, of which there are nine isoforms (AC1 to AC9), stimulates the synthesis of the second messenger cyclic AMP from ATP. Increases in cyclic AMP trigger the activation of protein kinase A (PKA), which phosphorylates specific target proteins on serine or threonine residues leading to a biological response (Figure 3.5).

Cyclic AMP is rapidly broken down by a family of enzymes called phosphodiesterases (PDEs), which catalyse its hydrolysis into AMP. As such PDEs play a major role in regulating the intracellular levels of cyclic AMP and cyclic GMP. There are 11 PDE isoenzymes (PDE1-11) which exhibit differing substrate specificity (some are cyclic AMP or cyclic GMP specific) and tissue distribution. There is considerable interest in the development PDE3 inhibitors for congestive heart failure and PDE4 inhibitors for inflammatory airway disease. PDE5 inhibitors (sildenafil or Viagra) have proved to be effective in the treatment of erectile dysfunction. For a comprehensive review on PDE inhibitors see Boswell-Smith et al. (2006).

Measurement of adenylyl cyclase activation and inhibition

Several methods for the detection of cyclic AMP in cells and tissue samples are currently in use. One widely used technique involves the use of ^{3}H-adenine to radiolabel endogenous ATP. Water-soluble ^{3}H-cyclic AMP can easily be isolated from cell and tissue samples using anion-exchange chromatography and the amount of radioactivity determined using scintillation counting. Such experiments are usually carried out in the presence of a PDE inhibitor, which increases the size of the response by preventing the normal breakdown of cyclic AMP to AMP. Figure 3.6b depicts ^{3}H-cyclic AMP accumulation in response to the non-selective β-adrenoreceptor agonist isoprenaline. Nonradioactive-based approaches are becoming increasingly popular, including an ELISA-based assay, which uses an antibody against cyclic AMP, and several fluorescent, luminescent and reporter gene-based assays.

How do we measure $G_{i/o}$-protein coupled receptor responses? To achieve this it is necessary to pre-activate adenylyl cyclase and then determine whether an appropriate $G_{i/o}$-PCR agonist is able to inhibit such a response. Activation of adenylyl cyclase can be achieved either by stimulating with a G_s-PCR agonist or more usually with forskolin (a plant derived compound), which is a direct activator of adenylyl cyclase and produces increases in cyclic AMP independent of receptor activation. An illustration of $G_{i/o}$-PCR induced inhibition of forskolin-stimulated cyclic AMP accumulation is shown in Figure 3.6c.

Novel GPCR screening assays

Historically GPCR drug screening programmes have involved radioligand binding studies or second messenger-based assays that measure changes in intracellular cyclic AMP, inositol phosphate or Ca^{2+} levels (see above). However, the discovery of alternative strategies to target GPCRs (allosteric modulators, biased ligands, bivalent ligands to name but a few and covered later in this chapter) will require the development of novel assays to screen for these exciting new categories of drug. Many existing GPCR assays are dependent upon G-protein coupling and involve the measurement of second messenger production using various indicators and labels. In this section two novel approaches for assaying GPCRs in living cells will be discussed; one measures GPCR activation kinetics whilst the other enables label-free detection of GPCR pharmacology. Both have the potential to be extremely useful for large-scale drug screening programmes in the future.

Measurement of GPCR activation kinetics using fluorescence-based assays in living cells

Fluorescence-based techniques have recently been developed that allow pharmacologists to measure conformational changes in GPCRs in living cells. These assays are based on the measurement of FRET (see section 3.10) between protein donor (CFP; cyan fluorescent protein) and protein acceptor (YFP; yellow fluorescent protein) fluorophores that have been inserted into the third intracellular loop and C-terminus of the receptor under investigation (Figure 3.7). In the absence of agonist binding to the receptor FRET will occur between the two fluorophores located at these two different positions. However, the binding of an agonist to the receptor causes a conformational change which increases the distance between the fluorescent donor protein and fluorescent acceptor protein thus reducing the FRET signal. Using this change in FRET response it is possible to calculate the kinetics of receptor activation for different agonists at the same receptor. This FRET-based GPCR activation approach has been refined by replacing the large fluorescent protein YFP (which may interfere with G-protein coupling) with the six amino acid sequence Cys-Cys-Pro-Gly-Cys-Cys which binds the small fluorescent reagent FlaSH-EDT$_2$ (Figure 3.7). This fluorescein-based reagent only becomes fluorescent when it binds to recombinant proteins containing the six amino acid tetracysteine motif. This approach was used to investigate α_{2A}-adrenergic receptor and muscarinic receptor

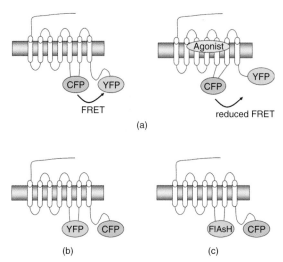

Figure 3.7 FRET-based approaches to measure GPCR activation in living cells. (a) FRET signals between donor (CFP; cyan fluorescent protein) and acceptor (YFP; yellow fluorescent protein) fluorophores inserted into the third intracellular loop and C-terminus of the receptor. Agonist-induced conformational changes in the receptor increase the distance between the fluorescent donor and acceptor causing a decrease in FRET signal. (b) Similar measurements can be obtained if the positions of the fluorophores are switched around. (c) FRET measurements using FlAsH technology and CFP.

(M_1, M_3 and M_5 subtypes) activation and revealed marked kinetic differences between different agonists for the same receptor (Ambrosio et al., 2011; Ziegler et al., 2010). These observations support the idea that different agonists induce varying states of GPCR activation which may correspond to the stimulation of different signalling pathways. In summary, these exciting cell-based assays enable the measurement of ligand binding on receptor conformation that is independent of downstream coupling to G-proteins and signal transduction. Hopefully this technology can be used during drug screening programmes to identify novel ligands that induce conformational changes distinct from known agonists.

Label-free detection of GPCR pharmacology in living cells

At present the majority of cell-based GPCR assays involve the use of a range of different reagents and detection systems to monitor predominantly ligand-induced changes in signal transduction pathways. In marked contrast label-free assay systems, as their name suggests, do not require the addition of detection reagents but instead measure ligand-induced changes in cell behaviour such as adhesion and morphology. From a drug discovery perspective label-free assays are extremely sensitive thus enabling GPCR screenings to be carried out using cells isolated from native tissue instead of traditional recombinant cell-line models. Some label-free instruments developed to date are more amenable to the study of GPCR pharmacology since they are able to distinguish between G_s, G_i and G_q-protein mediated responses. What are the principles behind label-free detection systems? At present there are two main techniques for label-free detection of cell behaviour; impedance-based biosensors and optical-based biosensors (Figure 3.8). Impedance-based biosensors are designed to measure the impedance to current flow between two electrodes located at the bottom of a microtiter well plate containing a confluent cell monolayer. The flow of alternating current between the two electrodes is dependent upon the level of cell adherence; increased cell adherence impedes the flow of alternating current and vice versa. An agonist-stimulated GPCR will activate cell signalling pathways that will promote changes in cell morphology, volume, adherence and cell-cell interactions. These changes in cell behaviour influence the flow of current through the cell and therefore produce measureable changes in impedance. In contrast, optical-based biosensors are designed to measure the wavelength of light that is reflected by a grating surface that is located at the bottom of a microtiter plate (Figure 3.8). The wavelength of light reflected is extremely sensitive to changes in the concentration and distribution of biomolecules within the adjacent cell monolayer. The activation of GPCRs triggers subtle changes in cell morphology, volume, adherence and reorganisation of the cytoskeleton that result in the movement and redistribution of biomolecules. However, the biochemical and signal transduction pathways responsible for these changes are not fully understood, but evidence suggests that the modulation of actin cytoskeleton plays a key role both in impedance and optical-based label-free readouts of GPCR activation. When compared to traditional technologies label-free assays offer several advantages for future high-throughput screening programmes. These include the ability to detect receptors that activate G_s, G_i and G_q-protein signalling and perhaps more importantly, due to their high sensitivity, the ability to screen GPCR responses using nonrecombinant cell models such as primary cell lines or even human cells acquired from patients. For a comprehensive review on the potential use label-free assays see Scott and Peters (2010).

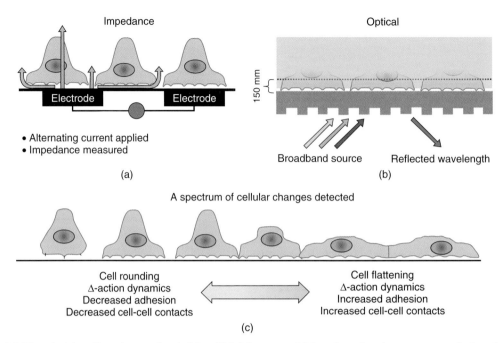

Impedance

- Alternating current applied
- Impedance measured

(a)

Optical

150 mm

Broadband source   Reflected wavelength

(b)

A spectrum of cellular changes detected

Cell rounding
Δ-action dynamics
Decreased adhesion
Decreased cell-cell contacts

Cell flattening
Δ-action dynamics
Increased adhesion
Increased cell-cell contacts

(c)

Figure 3.8 The principles of impedance and optical-based label-free assays. (a) Impedance-based assays measure the impedance to current flow between two electrodes located at the bottom of a specialised microtiter well plate. (b) Optical-based biosensors measure the wavelength of light reflected by a grating surface located at the bottom of a specialised microtiter well plate. (c) The cellular changes detected by label-free assays. Reprinted from Drug Discovery Today (2010), Scott CW and Peters MF, Label-free whole cell assays: expanding the scope of GPCR screening, 15: 704–716 with permission from Elsevier.

3.4 Desensitisation and down-regulation of GPCR signalling

The ability to regulate and control signal transduction is a key requirement for maintaining normal tissue and cell physiology. GPCR-mediated cell signalling is 'switched-off' at many different levels within the overall cascade. Since GPCRs are important pharmaceutical targets there is considerable interest in understanding the regulatory mechanisms that control GPCR responses. Indeed chronic drug (agonist) treatment often leads to a greatly reduced therapeutic response. For example prolonged use of β_2-adrenoceptor agonists significantly decreases their effectiveness in the treatment of asthma. Similarly, analgesic tolerance and dependence to morphine and related opioids involves reduced responsiveness of the μ-opioid receptor.

Removal of agonist and second messenger breakdown

The actions of some agonists are rapidly terminated by enzymatic degradation. For example acetylcholine is degraded by acetylcholinesterase into choline and acetate and peptide agonists are hydrolysed by membrane-bound peptidases. Many agonists, especially neurotransmitters such as dopamine, noradrenaline, 5-HT and glutamate, are transported back into the neuron from the synapse via specific membrane bound transporters. These transporters represent important therapeutic targets for the treatment of several disorders including depression (see Chapter 5). A second line of defence for 'switching off' GPCR signalling involves the rapid degradation of the second messengers. Inositol phosphatases and phosphodiesterases terminate the actions of IP_3 and cyclic AMP, respectively. A third line of defence is the intrinsic GTPase activity of the $G\alpha$ protein subunit which hydrolyses GTP and terminates heterotrimeric G-protein function.

Role of GPCR phosphorylation in desensitisation

In addition to the above mechanisms the GPCR itself is also the target for regulation. It is a well known phenomenon that the continuous or repeated stimulation of a GPCR reduces subsequent responsiveness

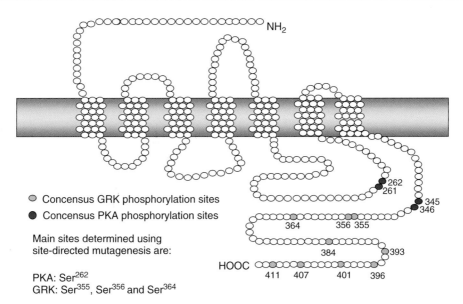

○ Concensus GRK phosphorylation sites

● Concensus PKA phosphorylation sites

Main sites determined using
site-directed mutagenesis are:

PKA: Ser^{262}
GRK: Ser^{355}, Ser^{356} and Ser^{364}

Figure 3.9 PKA and GRK phosphorylation sites within the human β_2-adrenoceptor. The schematic representation of the human β_2-adrenoceptor showing concensus phosphorylation sites for protein kinase A (PKA; blue) and G-protein coupled receptor kinase (GRK; red) within the third intracellular loop and C-terminal. The numbers refer to the specific amino acid number within the receptor protein. Complex site-directed mutagenesis experiments have identified the specific amino acid sites phosphorylated by PKA and GRK.

to an agonist (termed desensitisation or tachyphylaxis). Two types of GPCR desensitisation have been characterised; agonist-specific (termed homologous desensitisation) and agonist non-specific (heterologous desensitisation). Both types of desensitisation involve GPCR phosphorylation (see Figures 3.9 and 3.10). Homologous desensitisation is mediated by phosphorylation of specific serine and threonine residues located primarily within the carboxyl-terminal tail of the agonist-activated receptor by G-protein coupled receptor kinases (GRKs). In contrast, heterologous desensitisation mainly involves phosphorylation of specific serine and threonine residues within the third intracellular loop of the receptor by second-messenger dependent kinases such as protein kinase A (PKA) or protein kinase C (PKC). Given the prominent role of GRKs in regulating GPCR signalling there is growing interest in the therapeutic potential of GRK inhibitors. For example, inhibition of GRK2 may help restore β_1-adrenoceptor signalling in patients with chronic heart failure, who exhibit increased levels of GRK2 protein expression.

The next step in homologous desensitisation is the binding of proteins called β-arrestins to the phosphorylated GPCR. Arrestins uncouple the receptor from the

G protein and initiate GPCR endocytosis via a clathrin-coated pit-dependent pathway. This is also referred to as internalisation or sequestration. β-arrestins facilitate internalisation by interacting with proteins associated with the endocytic pathway including clathrin and clathrin adaptor protein (AP-2).

The fate of internalised GPCRs

Internalised GPCRs are either de-phosphorylated and returned to the plasma membrane (termed re-sensitisation) or targeted for degradation leading to the loss of receptor from the cell and down-regulation. GPCR degradation can occur either by lysosomes or via the 26S proteasome and in some cases involving ubiquitination (Figure 3.11). For more detailed information on the regulatory mechanisms associated with GPCR desensitisation and down-regulation, see the following review articles Böhm et al., 1997; Ferguson, 2001 and Marchese et al., 2008.

3.5 Constitutive GPCR activity

Initial attempts to explain G-protein activation resulted in the development of the two-state or ternary complex

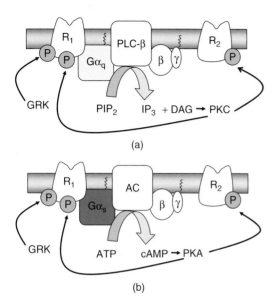

(a)

(b)

Figure 3.10 Heterologous GPCR desensitisation. (a)
G_q-coupled and (b) G_s-coupled GPCRs are rapidly desensitised
through GRK-mediated phosphorylation of the
agonist-occupied receptor (R_1). In certain cases PKC (for
G_q-linked) and PKA (for G_s-linked) also play a role in the
desensitisation of R_1 but in addition may also phosphorylate
agonist-unoccupied GPCR subtypes (R_2) resulting in the
phenomenon of heterologous desensitisation. PKC and PKA
phosphorylation is thought to sterically inhibit the receptor
coupling to G-protein rather than promote arrestin binding
and internalisation. P = phosphate group.

hypothesis. This simple model proposes that GPCRs exist
in equilibrium between two states; an active conformation
(denoted R^*) and an inactive conformation (R). The R
form does not couple to G-proteins, whereas R^* can
couple and activate G-proteins. Switching between R
and R^* states involves conformational changes within
TM domains 3,6,7 and helix 8. Agonists (A) bind preferentially to R^* and stabilise the active conformation.
The A/R^* complex is now able to bind and activate
G-proteins (G) forming the ternary complex ($A/R^*/G$).
This is summarised in Figure 3.12.

GPCRs can also switch between R and R^* conformations independent of agonist binding. This property is
known as constitutive activity and results in the activation
of G-protein signalling independent of receptor activation
(referred to as basal activity). The constitutive activity of a
particular GPCR can increase as a consequence of genetic
mutations, single nucleotide polymorphisms (SNPs) and

splice variants (for reviews see de Ligt et al., 2000; Bond
and Ijzerman, 2006).

Inverse agonists

Inverse agonists preferentially bind and stabilise the
inactive R conformation which results in a decrease in
constitutive activity. In contrast, the term neutral antagonist is now used to describe an antagonist which has
no inverse agonist activity and hence does not alter the
R/R^* equilibrium. It is likely that the vast majority of
antagonists (85%) may actually be inverse agonists. Several clinically used drugs have been demonstrated to be
inverse agonists (Table 3.5).

A number of human diseases/conditions are associated with naturally occurring GPCR mutants which
display increased constitutive activity (Table 3.6). Interestingly the genomes of several herpes-viruses including
the human cytomegalovirus (HCMV) encode constitutively active GPCRs which appear crucial for infection
and may prove to be effective future therapeutic targets
(Vischer et al., 2006).

Clinical use of inverse agonists

Since the discovery of inverse agonism there has been
considerable interest in applying the concept to future
drug discovery and current therapeutic strategies. For
example pathological conditions that involve constitutive
active GPCR mutants (Table 3.6) would clearly benefit
from inverse agonists since neutral antagonists would
have no effect on the enhanced basal activity. Inverse
agonists may also prove useful for treatment of
autoimmune diseases that involve GPCR auto-antibodies
that behave as agonists. Agonist auto-antibodies against
the type 1 angiotensin receptor (AT_1) are involved
in allograft rejection in renal transplantation patients.
Treatment with an AT_1 receptor inverse agonist such as
losartan may prove useful.

It is known that the prolonged treatment with an
inverse agonist leads to the increased expression (up-
regulation) of the GPCR involved, a characteristic not
observed with neutral antagonists. In certain situations
increased receptor expression could be problematic and
may be linked to drug tolerance. However, there are
examples where inverse agonist induced up-regulation of
GPCR expression appears to be clinically beneficial.

β_1-adrenoceptor antagonists ('β-blockers') are used to
treat chronic heart failure. Their clinical success is thought
to be due in part to the re-sensitisation of the β_1 cardiac

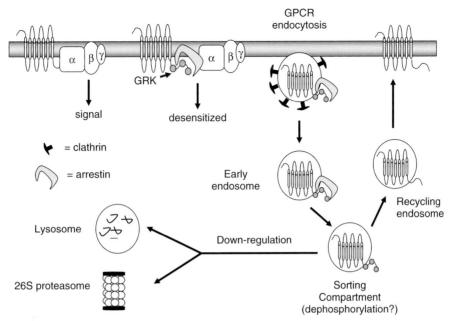

Figure 3.11 GPCR internalisation and down-regulation. Agonist-occupied GPCRs are rapidly phosphorylated (red circles) by GRKs promoting arrestin binding and G-protein uncoupling. The desensitised receptor is subsequently internalised via clathrin-coated pit mediated endocytosis. Internalised receptors are either de-phosphorylated and returned to the plasma membrane or targeted for degradation by lysosomes or the 26S proteasome.

contractile system, which is compromised due to the elevated levels of noradrenaline associated with chronic heart failure. The high levels of noradrenaline would cause a significant decrease in β_1-adrenoceptor expression due to receptor down-regulation. Clinical evidence suggests that the β_1-adrenoceptor inverse agonists, metoprolol and carvedilol are more effective at reducing mortality than the neutral antagonist bucindolol. This may be due to increased levels of β_1-adrenoceptor expression. When screening for novel GPCR antagonists it may be important to incorporate assays that can distinguish between inverse agonists and neutral antagonists.

Endogenous inverse agonists

Melanocortin type 4 receptors (MC_4), which are activated by the peptide hormone melanocyte-stimulating hormone, play a major role in regulating body weight. Interestingly, the MC_4 receptor displays constitutive activity and mutations in the gene encoding this receptor have recently been discovered that reduce constitutive activity in obese patients. It is also notable that the constitutive activity of the MC_4 receptor is regulated by an

endogenous inverse agonist called agouti-related peptide (Adan, 2006). This suggests that regulation of MC_4 receptor constitutive activity is essential for regulation of body weight and hence of physiological relevance. The identification of agouti-related peptide as an endogenous inverse agonist raised the question; are other constitutively active GPCRs regulated in a similar way? There is evidence that constitutively active opioid receptors and $mGlu_1$ receptors are regulated by calmodulin and homer 3 proteins, respectively. Thus the regulation of constitutive receptor activity by endogenous inverse agonists adds further fine control and modulation of GPCR signalling.

3.6 Promiscuous G-protein coupling

It was traditionally assumed that GPCRs couple exclusively to only one of the four main families of heterotrimeric G-proteins. However it is now apparent that many GPCRs exhibit promiscuous coupling and activate more than one class of G-protein. For example, the β_2 adrenoceptor, which is classically associated with G_s coupling and mediates signalling via the PKA/cyclic AMP

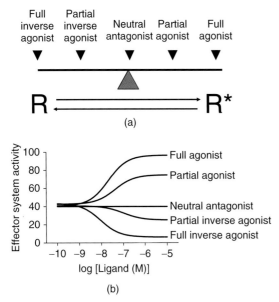

Figure 3.12 Constitutive GPCR activity and inverse agonism. (a) The ternary complex model proposes that GPCRs exist in equilibrium between two states; an inactive conformation (R) and an active conformation (R*). Agonists preferentially bind to R* and stabilise the active conformation, whereas inverse agonists preferentially bind to R and stabilise the inactive conformation. GPCRs can also switch between R and R* independent of agonist binding, a phenomenon known as constitutive activity. Neutral antagonists bind but do not alter the R/R* equilibrium. Partial agonists and partial inverse agonists display lower efficacies and hence only partially influence the position of the R/R* equilibrium. (b) Theoretical concentration-response curves for drugs with different efficacies in a receptor system displaying constitutive activity. The constitutive activity of the receptor results in a high level of basal effector activity due to R* coupling to heterotrimeric G-proteins independent of agonist binding. Agonists promote R* formation and hence G-protein coupling and effector activation, whereas inverse agonists promote R formation and reduce basal G-protein coupling and effector activation. Neutral antagonists do not influence R/R* and therefore have no effect on basal effector activity. Figure modified from Seifert and Wenzel-Seifert (2002) Naunyn Schmiedebergs Arch Pharmacol 366: 381–416.

pathway, can also couple to G_i and G_q. Coupling to different G-proteins increases the complexity of cell signalling pathways modulated by individual GPCR family members. In the case of the β_2 adrenoceptor, phosphorylation of the receptor by PKA causes a switch from G_s coupling to G_i coupling (Figure 3.13). For a review on G-protein switching see Lefkowitz et al. (2002).

Table 3.5 Clinically used drugs proven to be inverse agonists.

Brand name	Generic name	Therapeutic use	GPCR target
Toprol	Metoprolol	High blood pressure	β_1-adrenoceptor
Pepcidine	Famotidine	Peptic ulcers	Histamine H_2 receptor
Cozaar	Losartan	High blood pressure and heart failure	Angiotensin AT_1 receptor

Table 3.6 Constitutive active GPCRs associated with human disease.

GPCR	Medical condition	G-protein	Effect of constitutive
Rhodopsin	Congenital night blindness	G_t	Enhanced PDE activity
LHR	Male precocious-puberty	G_s	Enhanced basal activity of AC
CaSR	Autosomal dominant hypo-calcemia	G_q	Enhanced basal activity of PLC

Abbreviations: AC; adenylyl cyclase, CaSR; Calcium-sensing receptor, LHR; luteinising hormone receptor, PDE; phosphodiesterase, PLC; phospholipase C.

3.7 Agonist-directed signalling

Whilst it is known that different agonists for a given receptor can display marked differences in efficacy there is growing evidence for the idea of agonist-directed signalling (also referred to as agonist-directed trafficking; Perez and Karnik, 2005). Agonist efficacy refers to the variation in the size of response produced by different agonists even when occupying the same number of receptors. For example high-efficacy agonists trigger maximal responses whilst occupying a lower proportion of receptor sites compared to low efficacy agonists which cannot elicit the same maximal response even if occupying all available receptor sites. Compounds displaying low efficacy are referred to as partial agonists (Figure 3.12).

Agonist-directed signalling involves different agonists for the same receptor stimulating diverse signalling

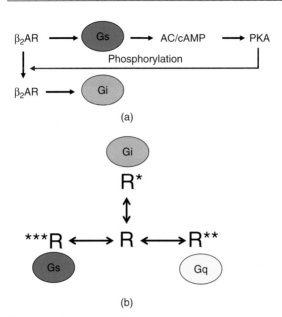

(a)

(b)

Figure 3.13 Promiscuous G-protein coupling and agonist-directed signalling. (a) The β_2-adrenoceptor (β_2AR) is associated with G_s-protein coupling and the subsequent activation of protein kinase A (PKA) via adenylyl cyclase (AC) mediated cyclic AMP production. When the receptor is phosphorylated by PKA, G_s-protein coupling is reduced, whereas G_i-protein coupling increases. This PKA-mediated switching of G-protein coupling has also been reported for other G_s-coupled receptors. (b) GPCRs may adopt different active conformations (R^*, R^{**}, R^{***}) each of which couples to a different G-protein. Agonist-directed signalling involves different agonists for the same receptor stimulating diverse signalling pathways possibly via the activation of different G-proteins. Coupling to different G-proteins may involve the receptor adopting agonist-specific conformations.

pathways possibly via the activation of different G-proteins (Figure 3.13). Coupling to different G-proteins may involve the receptor adopting agonist-specific conformations. Specific examples of agonist-directed signalling are illustrated in Table 3.7. Agonist-directed signalling may also be a consequence of 'arrestin-dependent signalling' a topic that is covered in Chapter 11 (section 11.5).

Agonist-directed signalling has many implications for drug development and discovery. Firstly, it may be possible to develop drugs that selectively activate signalling pathways that produce the desired therapeutic effect whilst preventing adverse side effects, which may be through a different signalling pathway activated by the same receptor. Secondly, high-throughput screening

Table 3.7 Agonist-directed signalling.

Receptor	Agonist	Signalling pathway preferentially activated
5-HT$_{2C}$	TFMPP	Phospholipase C
	LSD	Phospholipase A$_2$
D2 dopamine	p-tyramine	GTPγS binding to G$_o$-protein
	Dopamine	GTPγS binding to G$_{12}$ and G$_o$-protein
CB$_1$ receptor	CP-55940	G$_i$-protein coupling
	WIN-552-12-2	G$_i$ and G$_s$-protein coupling

assays need to be carefully designed in order not to miss any potentially novel drugs if screening is done using a particular assay that is not relevant to the clinically desired effect. Similarly, using the wrong assay may also lead to false positives and therefore it may be useful to screen each compound against a range of different signalling pathways.

3.8 Allosteric modulators of GPCR function

The majority of synthetic ligands that target GPCRs are classified as agonists or antagonists which bind to the orthosteric site on the receptor for endogenous ligands. More recently there has been considerable interest in the development and therapeutic use of allosteric modulators which bind to GPCRs at sites that are topographically distinct from the orthosteric binding site (Conn et al., 2009; Langmead and Christopoulos, 2006). This concept is illustrated in Figure 3.3. Examples of allosteric modulators for all three major classes of GPCRs are shown in Table 3.8. There are three categories of allosteric modulator:
1. Allosteric modulators that affect the binding affinity of orthosteric ligands (both agonists and antagonists).
2. Allosteric ligands that modulate the efficacy of orthosteric agonists.
3. Allosteric ligands which are capable of modulating GPCR activity independently of orthosteric ligand binding. Such compounds can be classed as allosteric agonists and allosteric inverse agonists.

Allosteric modulators of GPCR function have traditionally been explored using complex orthosteric-radioligand binding assays. Such assays can detect

Table 3.8 Allosteric modulators of class A, B and C GPCRs.

Receptor	Allosteric modulator	Effect on receptor Pharmacology
Class A GPCRs		
A_1 adenosine receptor	PD81723	Increased agonist binding affinity
CB_1 receptor	Org27569	Reduced efficacy of orthosteric agonist WIN552122
m1 muscarinic receptor	AC42	Agonist activity independent of orthosteric site
Class B GPCRs		
CRF_1 receptor	NB127914	Decreased peptide agonist binding (non-competitive antagonist)
Class C GPCRs		
$mGlu_5$ receptor	CDPPB	Increased agonist potency and efficacy
Calcium-sensing receptor	AMG073 (Cinacalcet)	Increased Ca^{2+} binding

allosteric compounds that either increase or decrease the affinity of the orthosteric ligand but do not allow for the identification of modulators that influence receptor function independent of orthosteric ligand binding. Functional assays that measure GPCR signal transduction allow for the detection of allosteric modulation of orthosteric agonist efficacy. Some allosteric modulators behave as negative regulators of orthosteric agonist efficacy, whereas some enhance agonist efficacy and are classed as positive regulators. Allosteric modulators that inhibit orthosteric agonist binding, reduce agonist efficacy, or in some cases both are also referred to as noncompetitive antagonists. The overall effect of an allosteric modulator will depend on whether the conformational changes that occur within the receptor following allosteric ligand binding influence the orthosteric binding site or alter conformational changes associated with receptor activation. Allosteric modulation of orthosteric agonist efficacy is shown in Figure 6d.

Clinical use of allosteric modulators

At present two allosteric modulators are currently on the market; cinacalcet and maraviroc. Cinacalcet is classed as a positive allosteric modulator of Ca^{2+} ion binding to the calcium-sensing receptor (CaSR). It is used clinically to treat hyperparathyroidism since activation of the CaSR inhibits the release of parathyroid hormone and protects against osteoporosis. Maraviroc is an allosteric inhibitor of the chemokine receptor subtype CCR5 and is used to treat HIV infections. The CCR5 receptor functions as a co-receptor for the entry of HIV into cells and maraviroc causes conformational changes in the CCR5 receptor that block interaction with HIV. The use of allosteric modulators to fine-tine GPCR function represents an exciting avenue for future drug development with many other allosteric modulators already in different phases of clinical trial.

Allosteric modulation of GPCR interactions with heterotrimeric G-proteins

Small molecule ligands that disrupt or allosterically modulate protein-protein interactions involved in Bcl-2 and p53 function are under clinical trial (see Chapter 11). Attempts are also being made to develop novel therapeutics that modulate protein-proteins interactions associated with GPCR signalling. For example a family of molecules known as pepducins have been developed which target the interaction between GPCR and heterotrimeric G-protein. Pepducins are synthetic peptides based on the intracellular loop sequences of GPCRs that are associated with G-protein coupling. Depending on their structure they can possess agonist or antagonist activity and to facilitate cell entry and membrane attachment they are synthesised with an N-terminal lipid tail. Such peptide-based drugs have been developed to modulate members of the proteinase-activated receptor (PAR) family including PAR1 and PAR4. The PAR family, which are activated by proteolytic cleavage and generation of a tethered ligand, are involved in mediating the biological effects of thrombin and represent important clinical targets. For example, PAR1 pepducin antagonists have been shown in preclinical trials to be effective in killing breast cancer cells. Indeed, high PAR1 expression is a feature observed in a number of cancers of epithelial cell origin such as breast and lung cancer. The development of these novel PAR ligands holds considerable promise since developing small-molecule antagonists against these important therapeutic targets has proven very difficult to date.

3.9 Pharmacological chaperones for GPCRs

The endoplasmic reticulum (ER) is an intracellular organelle involved in the synthesis and post-translational

Table 3.9 GPCR mutations associated with congenital disease.

GPCR	Disease
Thyroid stimulating hormone receptor	Congenital hypothyroidism
Luteinizing hormone receptor	Male pseudohermaphroditism
Adrenocorticotropic hormone receptor	Familial adrenocorticotropic hormone resistance
Calcium sensing receptor	Familial hypocalciuric hypercalcemia
Rhodopsin	Retinitis pigmentosa
Gonadotropin-releasing hormone receptor	Hypogonadotropic hypogonadism
Endothelin B receptors (ET_B)	Hirschsprung's disease
Melanocortin 4 (MC_4) receptor	Obesity
V_2 vasopressin receptor	Nephrogenic diabetes insipidus

modification of secretory and membrane proteins. Following their synthesis in the ER correctly folded membrane proteins are trafficked to the cell surface via the Golgi. The ER also functions as a quality control centre to ensure that incorrectly folded proteins are not processed and trafficked but instead are targeted for degradation. It is now recognised that naturally occurring mutations in GPCRs that cause their misfolding and retention in the ER are linked to several congenital diseases (a disease that exists at birth). This is similar to Class II mutations in the CFTR that result in ER trafficking defects (see Chapter 6.3). Some key examples of GPCR mutations and their associated disease states are shown in Table 3.9. The retention of GPCRs in the ER will not only result in loss of function due to a decrease in cell surface expression but also ER stress due to the accumulation of mutant proteins. Recent structural studies suggest that the helix 8 domain located at the start of the C-terminus together with several conserved amino acids in TM2, TM6 and TM7 are critical for the correct folding of many Class A (rhodopsin-like) GPCRs. Experimental deletion of helix 8 or mutation of these conserved amino acids results in the ER retention of GPCRs (recently reviewed by Nakamura et al., 2010).

Within the last few years several small molecule orthosteric ligands have been discovered to possess the capacity to rescue ER-trapped GPCRs allowing their trafficking to the cell membrane. These so called 'pharmacological chaperones' bind to the misfolded mutant protein promoting their correct folding and subsequent transport out of the ER (Figure 3.14). For example antagonists for the V_2 vasopressin receptor, agonists and antagonists for the δ-opioid receptor, agonists for rhodopsin and finally antagonists for the gonadotropin-releasing hormone receptor are all able to rescue their respective ER-trapped mutant receptors (see review by Bernier et al., 2004). The development of such ligands may provide therapeutic opportunities for the treatment of congenital conditions such as retinitis pigmentosa and nephrogenic diabetes insipidus. The use of small molecule orthosteric ligands to rescue ER-trapped mutant misfolded GPCRs, whilst of therapeutic potential, does have some drawbacks. For example, the use of agonist-based chaperones may result in the inappropriate activation of successfully trafficked GPCRs, whilst antagonist-based chaperones may block the activation of rescued receptors by endogenous agonists. A promising development in this area has been the report of a small-molecule allosteric agonist that promotes the cell surface expression of misfolded ER-trapped luteinising hormone (LH) receptors (Newton et al., 2011). The successful use of an allosteric ligand to rescue mutant misfolded LH receptors offers the prospect of developing this approach for other ER-trapped GPCR mutants.

3.10 GPCR dimerisation

Many proteins involved signal transduction function as dimers. Examples include tyrosine kinase receptors, such as the epidermal growth factor (EGF) receptor, which dimerise in response to ligand activation. Such receptors are single transmembrane spanning proteins and dimerisation is essential for activation of down-stream cell signalling pathways.

It has also emerged that GPCRs exist as dimers involving either the same receptor subtype (termed homodimerisation) or different GPCR subtypes (heterodimerisation). It is apparent that dimerisation influences many aspects of GPCR life including pharmacology, cell signalling, desensitisation/down-regulation and cell surface expression (trafficking of GPCRs from the endoplasmic reticulum). Because of this dimerisation is a 'hot topic' in the field of GPCR biology. There are several excellent reviews on GPCR dimerisation (Devi, 2001; Milligan, 2004; Prinster et al., 2005; Pin et al., 2007;

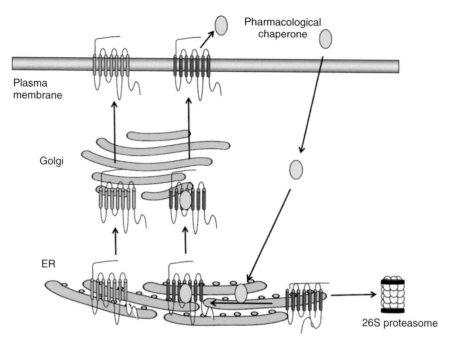

Figure 3.14 ER transport of mutant GPCRs by pharmacological chaperones. Following synthesis in the endoplasmic reticulum (ER) GPCRs that are correctly folded (highlighted in green) move through the Golgi en-route to the plasma membrane. Misfolded mutant GPCRs (highlighted red) are retained in the ER and targeted for proteasomal degradation. Pharmacological chaperones bind to misfolded GPCRs promoting conformational changes that enable the receptor to escape from the ER and be transported to the plasma membrane.

Dalrymple et al., 2008; Milligan, 2009; Visher et al., 2011; Maurice et al., 2011).

Methods to study GPCR dimerisation

A variety of biochemical and biophysical methods are used to study GPCR dimerisation (Table 3.10). However it is important to realise that the vast majority of the research exploring GPCR dimerisation is performed using heterologous expression systems involving cloned GPCRs often tagged with immunological epitopes or fluorescent proteins. However the use of transfected cell lines is problematic and raises many issues regarding the validity of the results obtained. One concern is that the phenomenon of GPCR dimerisation could simply be an artefact due to the over-expression of receptor protein(s) when compared to endogenous levels of GPCR expression. Evidence for endogenous GPCR dimerisation comes from atomic-force microscopy studies which have revealed orderly rows of rhodopsin dimers arranged within retinal disc membranes (Fotiadis et al., 2003). An important characteristic of these membranes is that they exhibit extremely high levels of rhodopsin protein expression.

Biochemical techniques
Differential epitope tagging

Immunoprecipitation of epitope-tagged receptors has been extensively used to demonstrate GPCR dimerisation. Immunoprecipitation involves the interaction between a protein and its specific antibody and the separation of these immune complexes using Protein A/G-sepharose beads. This technique is a rapid and simple method to separate a specific protein or protein complex from all the other proteins in a cell. Immunoprecipitated proteins are then visualised using SDS-PAGE followed by Western blotting.

Epitope-tagged constructs (or fusion proteins) for the receptor of interest are generated using recombinant DNA technology and transfected into an appropriate cell line (Figure 3.15). The epitope is a short peptide sequence of typically 6–12 amino acids that can easily be recognised using a commercially available anti-epitope antibody. Commonly used epitopes are listed in Table 3.11. Epitope tags are usually located at the N-terminus of the GPCR. Can you think of a reason why this might be important? It is possible using recombinant DNA technology to locate

Table 3.10 Techniques used to study GPCR dimerisation.

Approach	Example of GPCR dimerisation
Biochemical techniques	
Differential epitope tagging	δ-opioid receptor/μ-opioid receptor
	β_2-adrenoceptor/δ-opioid receptor
Biophysical techniques	
BRET	β_2-adrenoceptor/δ-opioid receptor
FRET	sst_4/sst_5
BiFC	A_{2A} adenosine receptor/ dopamine D2
BRET/FRET BiFC	A_{2A} adenosine receptor (trimer)
BiFC/BiLC	β_2-adrenoceptor/dopamine D2 (tetramers)
Functional complementation	
Chimeric mutants	α_2-adrenoceptor/muscarinic m3
Deletion mutants	sst_1-sst_5 and sst_5/dopamine D2

Abbreviations: BRET; bioluminescence resonance energy transfer, FRET; fluorescence resonance energy transfer, BiFC; bimolecular fluorescence complementation, BiLC; bimolecular luminescence complementation, sst; somatostatin.

Table 3.11 Frequently used epitope tag sequences.

Name of epitope tag	Amino-acid sequence of the epitope
c-myc	Glu-Gln-Leu-Ile-Ser-Glu-Glu-Asp-Leu
Heamagglutinin (HA)	Tyr-Pro-Tyr-Asp-Val-Pro-Asp-Tyr-Ala
FLAG	Asp-Tyr-Lys-Asp-Asp-Asp-Asp-Lys
Hexahistidine	His-His-His-His-His-His

Abbreviations: Asp; aspartic acid, Gln; glutamine, Glu; glutamate; His ; histidine, Ile; isoleucine, Leu; leucine, Lys; lysine, Pro; praline, Ser; serine, Tyr; tyrosine, Val; valine

the epitope tag at virtually any position within the GPCR sequence. However, researchers generally locate the epitope within the N-terminus of the receptor, since location within the C-terminus may influence G-protein coupling.

If the GPCR under investigation forms homodimers when expressed in a model cell line then the following epitope-tagged combinations are theoretically possible: *c-myc*-GPCR/*c-myc*-GPCR, HA-GPCR/HA-GPCR

and *c-myc*-GPCR/HA-GPCR together with *c-myc*-GPCR and HA-GPCR monomers (Figure 3.15). Differential epitope tagging involves the isolation of protein complexes using an antibody to one of the epitopes (via immunoprecipitation) and the subsequent visualisation of associating tagged receptors using an antibody to the second epitope (via SDS-PAGE/Western blotting). Using this approach β_2-adrenoceptor homodimers were detected which provided the first biochemical evidence that GPCRs can exist as dimers. However, there are concerns that the solubilisation of hydrophobic membrane proteins prior to immunoprecipitation of receptor complexes causes artificial aggregations.

Biophysical techniques

A number of biophysical techniques have been developed that allow for the visualisation of protein-protein interactions in living cells. These include fluorescence resonance energy transfer (FRET) and bioluminescence resonance energy transfer (BRET). Although these techniques avoid some of the complications associated with biochemical approaches they still require genetic manipulation and heterologous expression systems. Both techniques involve the transfer of energy from an acceptor to a donor. For FRET and BRET to occur effectively the distance between the donor and acceptor is typically 50 to 100 angstroms (Å; 1 Å = 0.1 nm).

Bioluminescence resonance energy transfer

BRET is a naturally occurring phenomenon involving the transfer of energy between a luminescent donor protein and a fluorescent acceptor protein. The sea pansy *Renilla reniformis* is a bioluminescent soft coral which displays blue-green bioluminescence. This is achieved using the enzyme luciferase (the luminescent donor; Rluc), which in the presence of oxygen catalyses the degradation of the substrate luciferin to produce blue light. The generated blue light is then transferred to green fluorescent protein (GFP; the fluorescent acceptor) which emits green light giving the coral their blue-green appearance.

When using BRET to study GPCR dimerisation it is again necessary to transfect appropriate cell lines with cDNA plasmids that encode luciferase and fluorescent protein fusion constructs. Changes in BRET signal can be monitored in response to agonist stimulation using a fluorescent plate reader (Figure 3.16). However, a major concern when measuring BRET is how to distinguish between agonist-induced dimerisation of GPCR monomers (discussed later) and agonist-induced changes in receptor conformation of pre-existing dimers, which

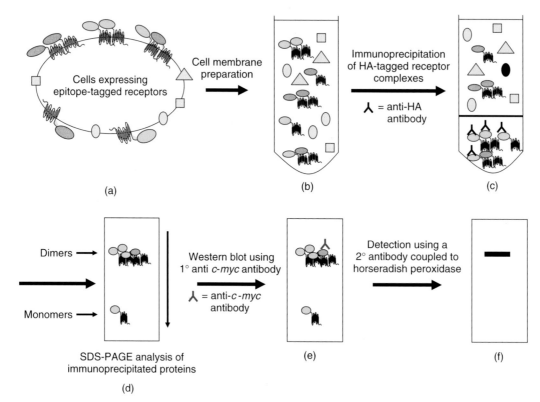

Figure 3.15 Visualisation of GPCR dimers using differential epitope tagging. (a) A suitable cell line is transfected with cDNA constructs that encode for the epitope tagged receptors. These constructs could encode for the same receptor or different GPCR subtypes to monitor homodimerisation or heterodimerisation, respectively. When expressed at the cell surface several combinations of epitope-tagged receptor protein complexes are theoretically possible: *c-myc*-GPCR/*c-myc*-GPCR, HA-GPCR/HA-GPCR and *c-myc*-GPCR/HA-GPCR together with *c-myc*-GPCR and HA-GPCR monomers (orange oval; *c-myc*, yellow oval; HA). (b) Using a cocktail of biochemical detergents hydrophobic membrane proteins are isolated and solubilised to produce a cell membrane preparation. (c) Receptor protein complexes containing the HA-epitope are immunoprecipitated using a commercially available anti-HA antibody. (d) Immunoprecipitated GPCR complexes consisting of monomers and dimers (HA/HA and HA/*c-myc*) are separated using SDS-PAGE and (e) analysed by Western blotting using an anti-*c-myc* antibody. (f) Detection of immune complexes using a secondary antibody coupled to horseradish peroxidase. Secondary antibody binding can be visualised using chemiluminescent-based approaches which emit light that can then be detected using photographic film.

may be sufficient to promote a change in BRET signal. Furthermore, the addition of extra protein sequence, (for example *Renilla* luciferase and YFP are 314 and 238 amino acids in length, respectively) to the C-terminus may influence G-protein coupling or receptor pharmacology. For these reasons, it is essential to characterise the pharmacological and cell signalling properties of any GPCR fusion protein generated.

Fluorescence resonance energy transfer

FRET involves a fluorophore in an excited state (donor) transferring its excitation energy to an adjacent fluorophore (acceptor) via a dipole-dipole interaction. It is an essential requirement that the emission spectra of the donor fluorophore and the excitation spectra of the acceptor overlap. Exploring GPCR dimerisation by means of FRET can be achieved using several different experimental designs. One approach uses variants of GFP fused to the GPCR(s) of interest. In recent years a number of GFP variants have been generated, using site-directed mutagenesis, which emit light at wavelengths distinct from the native GFP. These variants include cyan (CFP) and yellow (YFP) fluorescent proteins. The Nobel Prize in Chemistry 2008 was awarded to Dr Osamu Shimomura, Dr Martin

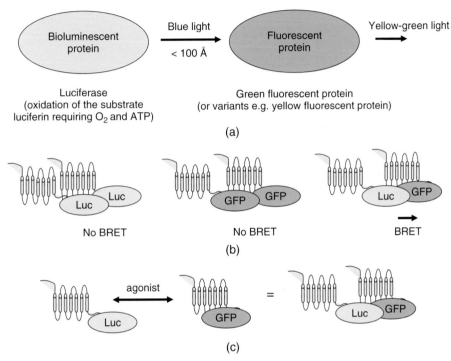

Figure 3.16 Visualisation of GPCR dimers using BRET. (a) Bioluminescence resonance energy transfer (BRET) between a luminescent donor protein (luciferase; Luc) and a fluorescent acceptor protein (green fluorescent protein; GFP). (b) BRET signals from constitutive GPCR dimers or (c) GPCR dimerisation following agonist stimulation. Both cases result in the donor and acceptor proteins being in close enough proximity for BRET to occur.

Chalfie and Dr Roger Y. Tsien for their work relating to the discovery and development of GFP as a tagging tool for bioscience research. A popular combination when studying GPCR dimerisation is YFP and CFP (Figure 3.17).

An alternative fluorescent-based approach, which does not involve fusion proteins, is to use small molecule fluorophores conjugated to antibodies, typically fluorescein (donor) and rhodamine (acceptor). For this antibodies against epitope-tagged GPCRs (HA and *c*-Myc; see above) are used, since receptor-specific antibodies often lack specificity. Finally GPCR oligomerisation can be explored using fluorescently labelled ligands. This approach has the distinct advantage of allowing endogenous GPCR interactions to be studied. For more detailed information on the application of BRET and FRET-based techniques to study GPCR dimerisation see Pfleger and Eidne (2005).

Fluorescent and bioluminescent protein-fragment complementation

Conventional FRET and BRET analysis of protein-protein interactions in living cells is restricted to the detection of binary complexes. Emerging developments combine BRET/FRET with protein-fragment complementation assays, enabling the detection of ternary and quaternary protein complexes. Protein-fragment complementation assays involve fragments of fluorescent or luminescent proteins, recombining to form a functional protein when in close proximity. They are commonly known as bimolecular fluorescence complementation (BiFC) and bimolecular luminescence complementation (BiLC) assays. GPCR dimerisation has been observed using fusion proteins containing amino (N) and carboxyl (C) terminal fragments of YFP attached to the carboxyl-terminus of the GPCR (Figure 3.18 and Figure 3.19).

By combining BRET or FRET with BiFC it is possible to detect and monitor in living cells GPCR complexes containing more than two partners. For example, BRET/FRET-BiFC approaches have both shown that the A_{2A} adenosine receptor exists as a homo-oligomer containing at least three receptors (Figure 3.19b). Extending this technique has enabled the detection of β_2 adrenoceptor and dopamine D2 receptor homotetramers

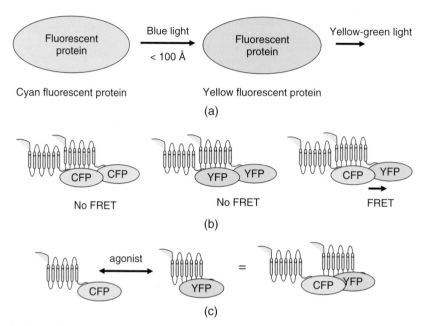

Figure 3.17 Visualisation of GPCR dimers using FRET. (a) Fluorescence resonance energy transfer (FRET) between a fluorescent donor protein (in this case CFP) and a fluorescent acceptor protein (YFP). Transfer of fluorescence energy only occurs if the emission spectrum of the donor and the excitation spectrum of the acceptor overlap and the distance between the two is < 100 Å. (b) GPCR dimerisation will result in the donor and acceptor proteins being in close enough proximity for FRET to occur.

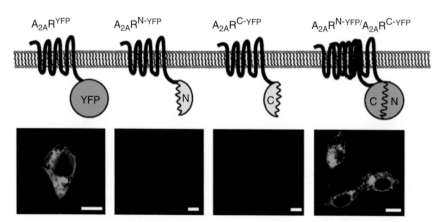

Figure 3.18 Visualisation of A_{2A} adenosine receptor homodimers using the bimolecular fluorescence complementation (BiFC) technique. Mammalian HEK293 cells were transfected with cDNA encoding the A_{2A} adenosine receptor fused either to YFP ($A_{2A}R^{YFP}$), the amino (N) terminus of YFP ($A_{2A}R^{N\text{-}YFP}$), the carboxyl (C) terminus of YFP ($A_{2A}R^{C\text{-}YFP}$), or $A_{2A}R^{N\text{-}YFP}$ plus $A_{2A}R^{C\text{-}YFP}$. These $A_{2A}R$ fusion proteins are illustrated schematically in the upper panel. When the cells were visualised using confocal microscopy green fluorescence was observed on the plasma membrane of cells expressing $A_{2A}R^{YFP}$ and $A_{2A}R^{N\text{-}YFP}$ plus $A_{2A}R^{C\text{-}YFP}$. These results show that $A_{2A}R$ homodimerisation enabled the YFP fragments to recombine and generate fluorescence. In contrast cells transfected with the $A_{2A}R$ fused to the YFP fragments did not show any fluorescent signal. Scale bar: 10 μm. Reprinted from FEBS Letters 582: Gandia et al., Detection of higher-order G protein-coupled receptor oligomers by a combined BRET-BiFC technique, 2979–2984 (2008) with permission from Elsevier.

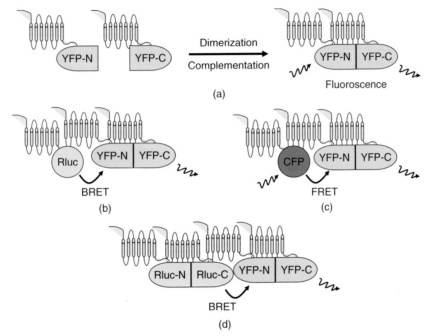

Figure 3.19 Visualisation of GPCR oligomers using Fluorescent and Bioluminescent protein-fragment complementation. (a) GPCR dimerisation can be visualised using protein-fragment complementation assays involving nonfunctional fragments of fluorescent proteins (in this example the N-terminus and C-terminus of YFP) that recombine to form a functional protein when in close proximity. Resonance energy transfer techniques can be combined with protein-fragment complementation to monitor trimeric protein complexes using either (b) BRET/BiFC or (c) FRET/BiFC. (d) GPCR tetramers can be observed using a BiFC-BiLC approach. This involves monitoring BRET between complemented luminescent (Rluc) and fluorescent proteins. See text for more detail.

using a combined BiFC-BiLC approach (Figure 3.19d). For a detailed account on fluorescent and bioluminescent protein-fragment complementation assays see Vidi and Watts (2009).

Functional complementation techniques

Functional complementation techniques involve the heterologous expression of mutant nonactive GPCRs, generated by recombinant DNA technology, which combine to form functional units.

Chimeric GPCR mutants

One of the first reports to indicate the possibility that GPCRs exist as dimers involved the use of muscarinic M_3 receptor and α_{2C}-adrenoceptor chimeras; namely $\alpha_{2C}(TM1-5)/M_3(TM6-7)$ and $M_3(TM1-5)/\alpha_{2C}(TM6-V7)$. To create these mutants TM domains 6 and 7 from the α_{2C}-AR were exchanged for domains 6 and 7 from the M_3 receptor and vice versa (Figure 3.20). As would be expected the chimeric receptors when individually expressed in separate cell lines did not bind their selective

agonists or antagonists. However, co-expression of the chimeric receptors restored ligand binding suggesting that α_{2C} and M_3 muscarinic receptors physically interact to form a functional heterodimer.

Deletion mutants

Deletion mutants can also be used as a tool for exploring GPCR dimerisation. A C-terminal deletion mutant of the somatostatin 5 receptor (sst_5; $\Delta318$) was used to identify heterodimerisation with the dopamine D2 receptor. Somatostatin and dopamine are two important neurotransmitters whose receptors are often co-localised in specific brain regions. The sst_5 mutant ($\Delta318$; truncated at amino acid 318) is missing the last 46 amino acids from its C-terminal. When heterologously expressed the sst_5 ($\Delta318$) mutant does not couple to the inhibition of adenylyl cyclase (this would be expected since the C-terminal is important for G-protein coupling), but it still displayed agonist binding. However, co-expression of the sst_5 ($\Delta318$) mutant with the dopamine D2 receptor, restored the ability of somatostatin to inhibit adenylyl

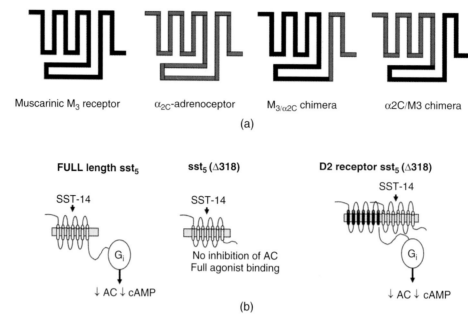

Figure 3.20 Functional complementation techniques to study GPCR dimers. (a) Schematic representation of muscarinic M₃ receptor and α_{2C}-adrenoceptor chimeric mutants; α_{2C}(TM1-5)/M₃(TM6-7) and M₃(TM1-5)/α_{2C}(TM6-V7). (b) The use of deletion mutants to study GPCR dimerisation. The SSTR5 receptor couples to G_i-protein and when activated inhibits adenylyl cyclase (AC) reducing intracellular cyclic AMP levels. The SSTR5 Δ318 mutant is missing the last 46 amino acids from its C-terminal and does not couple to G_i-protein but still retains agonist binding (SST-14). Co-expression of the dopamine D2 receptor restores the ability of SST-14 to inhibit adenylyl cyclase.

cyclase (Figure 3.20). The pharmacological of the sst₅-D2 heterodimer is discussed later in this chapter.

GPCR homodimerisation

Although there has been an explosion of research into GPCR dimerisation in recent years, earlier studies also provided indirect evidence that GPCRs may exist as dimers or even oligomers. These observations included data from ligand-binding studies and estimates of receptor complexes obtained from gel filtration chromatography.

Despite many Class A GPCRs reportedly forming homodimers (see Table 3.12), very little is known about the region(s) of the receptor involved in such interactions. However, several different experimental approaches have shown that the hydrophobic TM domains are involved in Class A GPCR receptor homodimerisation.

GPCR dimers are classified as either: (a) contact dimers involving interactions which maintain the ligand (L) binding pocket or (b) domain swapped dimers in which the two ligand binding pockets are formed by the exchange of TM domains from each receptor (Figure 3.21). The

specific TM domains responsible vary according to which GPCR is involved but studies have indicated roles for TM4-5 (D2 receptor; contact dimers), TM5-6 (histamine H₁ receptor; domain swapping dimers) and TM6 for the β_2-adrenoceptor. Complex BiFC studies have revealed that the α_{1B}-adrenoceptor exists as an oligomer involving TM domains 1 and 4 (Figure 3.21c). In some cases GPCRs dimerise in the response to agonist stimulation, whilst others exist as constitutive dimers. There are also reports of agonist-induced monomerisation. Examples of GPCR homodimers and the consequences of agonist activation on the levels of homodimer are given in Table 3.12.

Despite the numerous reports that have described homodimerisation of Class A GPCRs, their existence and function is still an area of intense debate and contention amongst researchers working in this field. Many of the reported agonist-mediated changes (both increases and decreases) in the levels of homodimers have been observed using FRET or BRET based techniques. However, the results from these experiments should be treated with caution since increases or decreases in energy transfer may occur due to changes in receptor conformation

Table 3.12 GPCR homodimerisation: consequences of agonist activation.

GPCR	Effect of agonist on the levels of homodimerisation	Functional implications of homodimerisation/monomerisation
β_2-adrenoreceptor	Increase	Required for G_s coupling
Bradykinin B_2	Increase	Not necessary for cell signalling but required for internalisation
Ca^{2+}-sensing receptor	Increase	Ca^{2+} activation and cell signalling
DOR	Decrease	Agonist-induced monomerisation. Needed for internalisation.
NPY Y_4 receptor	Decrease	Activation and down-regulation?
CCK_1	Decrease	?
KOR	No effect	?
Muscarinic m3	No effect	?

Abbreviations: CCK_1; cholecystokinin type 1 receptor, DOR; delta opioid receptor, KOR; kappa opioid receptor, NPY; neuropeptide Y.

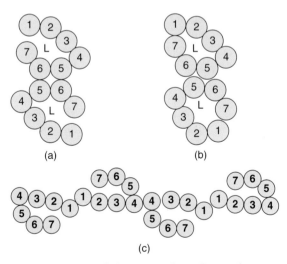

Figure 3.21 Models of Class A GPCR homodimer and oligomer formation. (a) contact dimers; (b) domain-swapped dimers; and (c) oligomer formation of the α_{1B}-adrenoceptor.

of existing dimers rather than actual changes in the levels of dimer. For an excellent review discussing this area in depth see Gurevich and Gurevich, 2008.

There is no doubt that Class C GPCRs exist as constitutive homo- and heterodimers (discussed in the next section). Class C GPCRs include metabotropic glutamate receptors (mGlu$_1$ to mGlu$_8$), Ca^{2+}-sensing receptors (CaSR), GABA$_B$ receptors and the sweet and umami taste receptors (T1R1-3). They are characterised by a large N-terminus which contains a Venus flytrap (VFT) module and in the case of mGlu and CaSR receptors, a cysteine-rich domain (CRD) located between the VFT and the seven TM domains. Class C receptors form stable dimers via adjacent VFT/VFT interactions and disulphide (S-S) bonds between cysteine residues located in the CRD (Figure 3.22).

Members of Class B GPCRs including vasoactive intestinal peptide receptors (VPAC$_1$, VPAC$_2$), and CRF$_1$ receptor also form homodimers. In addition the calcitonin and calcitonin receptor-like receptors dimerise with receptor activity modifying proteins (RAMPs; discussed in Chapter 11).

GPCR heterodimerisation

Although GPCR homodimerisation generated considerable interest, it is the concept of heterodimerisation that has captured the imagination of academics and pharmaceutical companies. To date there are numerous examples of heterodimers between GPCRs from the same family, for example κ- and δ-opioid receptor dimers. There are also many reports of functional heterodimers between GPCRs from different families, for example both the κ- and δ-opioid receptor dimerise with the β_2-adrenoreceptor. Since these heterodimers often exhibit distinct pharmacological properties, there is substantial clinical interest in GPCR heterodimerisation as an area for the development of novel therapeutic drugs. Some key examples of GPCR heterodimers are given in Table 3.13. The vast majority of heterodimers have been detected using co-immunoprecipitation, FRET and BRET based techniques.

Functional consequences of GPCR heterodimerisation

It is apparent that GPCR heterodimerisation influences pharmacology, cell signalling, desensitisation/down-regulation and cell surface expression (trafficking of GPCRs from the endoplasmic reticulum). Specific examples from each of these areas are discussed below.

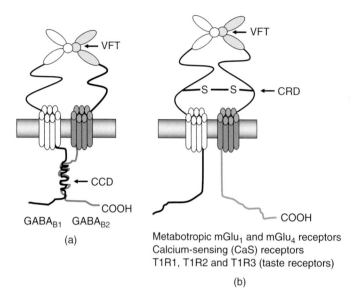

GABA$_{B1}$ GABA$_{B2}$

(a)

Metabotropic mGlu$_1$ and mGlu$_4$ receptors
Calcium-sensing (CaS) receptors
T1R1, T1R2 and T1R3 (taste receptors)

(b)

Figure 3.22 Class C GPCR homo- and heterodimers. (a) The GABA$_{B1}$ and GABA$_{B2}$ receptor heterodimer involves interactions between adjacent Venus flytrap (VFT) domains located in the N-terminus and coiled-coil domain (CCD) in the C-terminus. (b) homodimers for mGlu receptors and CaS receptors and heterodimers for taste receptors involve disulphide bonds between adjacent cysteine rich domains (CRD) as wells as VFT interactions.

Effect on GPCR cell surface expression

Many GPCRs do not reach the cell membrane following heterologous expression in model cell lines. This is illustrated by the G$_{i/o}$-coupled GABA$_B$ receptor which is a Class C GPCR and when stimulated inhibits adenylyl cyclase and activates G-protein activated inward rectifying K$^+$ channels (GIRKs). The GABA$_B$ receptor was cloned in 1997 by Kaupmann et al. but when heterologously expressed it failed to signal properly due to low levels of expression at the cell surface. The cloning of a second GABA$_B$ receptor (the GABA$_{B2}$) was subsequently reported, which must be co-expressed with the GABA$_{B1}$ in order to help it reach the cell surface. This represented the first example of a GPCR heterodimer. How does the GABA$_{B2}$ aid GABA$_{B1}$ expression? The GABA$_{B1}$ receptor contains an endoplasmic reticulum (ER) retention signal within its C-terminus preventing cell surface expression. However, the coiled-coil domain of the GABA$_{B2}$ 'masks' the ER retention signal allowing the release of the GABA$_{B1}$/GABA$_{B2}$ heterodimer from the ER. The trafficking of the GABA$_{B1}$/ GABA$_{B2}$ heterodimer to the cell surface is summarised in Figure 3.23.

Agonist binding occurs at the GABA$_{B1}$ receptor, whereas G-protein coupling is through the GABA$_{B2}$ receptor (Figure 3.23). These observations partly answer two important questions about GPCR dimerisation; i) is agonist binding to both receptor partners (protomer) in the dimer required for G-protein activation? and ii) once activated do both receptors in the dimer couple to a G-protein?

Many Class A receptors also fail to reach the cell surface when expressed in model cell lines including the α_{1D}-adrenoceptor, which requires heterodimerisation with the α_{1B}-adrenoceptor for transport to the cell surface. The vast majority of olfactory receptors, which constitute almost half of all GPCRs in the human genome, also remain in the ER when heterologously expressed. This has proved a major obstacle for the study of this large group of Class A GPCRs.

Effect on GPCR pharmacology

The effect on receptor pharmacology represents one of the most interesting consequences of GPCR heterodimerisation. Changes in receptor pharmacology may result from allosteric interactions between the receptor partners. This is certainly the case with the GABA$_{B1}$/GABA$_{B2}$ heterodimer in which the GABA$_{B2}$ subunit increases the agonist affinity of the GABA$_{B1}$. Alternatively, changes in receptor pharmacology may be a consequence of TM domain swapping between the monomers of the dimer to create a novel binding site. Several prominent examples from the current literature are discussed below.

There are three cloned opioid receptors, delta (δ; DOR), kappa (κ; KOR) and mu (μ; MOR). The opioid receptor system modulates several important physiological processes including analgesia and the MOR is the main target for the analgesic effect of morphine. It is noteworthy that there are more endogenous opioid receptor peptides (for example β-endorphin, met-enkephalin, Leu-enkephalin and dynorphin) than there are cloned

Table 3.13 Some key examples of GPCR heterodimers.

Receptor Pair	Effect of heterodimerisation
Class A GPCRs from the same family	
DOR-KOR	Pharmacology and cell signalling
DOR-MOR	Pharmacology and cell signalling
β_1-β_2 adrenoceptors	Pharmacology, signalling, internalisation
α_{1B}-α_{1D} adrenoceptors	Pharmacology, cell surface expression
CCR2-CXCR4 or CCR5	Signalling, reduction in HIV infection
Class A GPCRs from different families	
sst_5-dopamine D2	Pharmacology
δ-opioid-β_2 adrenoceptor	Internalisation
Adenosine A_{2A}-dopamine D2	Signalling, internalisation
Angiotensin AT_1-β_2 adrenoceptor	Signalling
Angiotensin AT_1-Bradykinin B_2	Pharmacology, internalisation
Class C GPCRs	
$GABA_{B1}$/$GABA_{B2}$	Required for cell surface expression
T1R2-T1R3	Detection of sweet taste compounds
T1R1-T1R3	Detection of umami taste compounds
Class A and Class C GPCRs	
Adenosine A_1R-mglu$_1$	Cell signalling

Abbreviations: DOR; delta opioid receptor, KOR; kappa opioid receptor, MOR, mu opioid receptor, CCR2/CXCR4/CCR5, chemokine receptors.

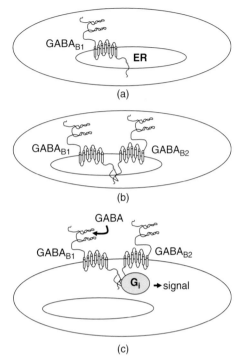

(a)

(b)

(c)

Figure 3.23 GPCR heterodimerisation is required for cell surface expression. (a) The $GABA_{B1}$ receptor is retained in the endoplasmic reticulum (ER) due the presence of an ER retention sequence within its C-terminus (red section). (b) The coiled-coil domain of the $GABA_{B2}$ 'masks' the ER retention signal enabling the $GABA_{B1}$/$GABA_{B2}$ heterodimer to be released from the ER and expressed at the cell surface (c).

opioid receptor genes. However, pharmacological-based evidence indicates that there are several subtypes for each known receptor (μ_1, μ_2, δ_1, δ_2, κ_1, κ_2, and κ_3).

The DOR-KOR heterodimer displays distinct pharmacological properties when compared to DOR and KOR homodimers (Levac et al., 2002). Selective DOR and KOR agonists and antagonists have reduced binding affinities, whereas nonselective opioid receptor antagonists' show increased affinity. The pharmacology of the DOR-KOR heterodimer is similar to the κ_2 subtype. The DOR-MOR heterodimer also creates a novel binding site with reduced affinity for selective synthetic agonists (including morphine), but increased affinity for endogenous opioid peptides (endomorphin-1 and Leu-enkephalin).

A major problem associated with morphine treatment for pain relief is the development of opioid tolerance following chronic use. A large body of evidence indicates that the DOR is involved in the development of morphine tolerance and that blocking the DOR enhances MOR analgesia. Bivalent ligands that target the DOR-MOR heterodimer have been developed and consist of a MOR agonist linked by a chemical spacer to a DOR antagonist (Daniels et al., 2005) Such bivalent ligands may represent a novel strategy for future development of analgesics without the common side-effects. It is interesting to note that an endogenous bivalent agonist has been reported, bovine adrenal medulla peptide 22 (BAM22), which binds to DOR/sensory neuron-specific receptor-4 (SNSR4) heterodimers. Bivalent ligands are also of use experimentally to confirm the existence of specific GPCR heterodimers in native tissue.

The opioid receptor family has provided clear evidence that GPCR heterodimerisation produces pharmacologically distinct binding sites. There are many other examples of Class A GPCRs from the same family forming heterodimers which have pharmacology properties different from the individual monomers (Table 3.13). Dimerisation has also been observed between GPCRs that are activated by completely different endogenous ligands, for example, sst_5-D2 heterodimers. The binding affinity of the sst_5 receptor agonist somatostatin-14 (SST-14) is enhanced by the D2 receptor agonist quinpirole, but decreased in the presence of the D2 receptor antagonist sulpiride. Overall, these observations suggest that conformational changes induced by dopamine D2 receptor ligands modulate SST-14 binding.

Effect on GPCR signalling

GPCR heterodimerisation has also been shown to influence cell signalling pathways including alterations in G-protein coupling. For example, the DOR-MOR heterodimer triggers pertussis toxin-insensitive inhibition of adenylyl cyclase which suggests coupling to G_z protein. When expressed alone both the MOR and DOR mediate pertussis toxin-sensitive inhibition of adenylyl cyclase. With the notable exception of G_z-protein, pertussis toxin catalyses the ADP-ribosylation of $G_{i/o}$-protein

family members. The G_s-protein coupled dopamine D1 receptor and the G_i-protein coupled dopamine D2 receptor form heterodimers which couple to $G_{q/11}$-protein.

Effect on GPCR desensitisation

The majority of GPCRs undergo agonist-induced internalisation into the cell via endocytosis as part of the process of desensitisation (see section 3.4). In the case of GPCR homodimers it is not clear if agonist-occupancy of both receptor partners is necessary for internalisation. With heterodimerisation there are many examples of co-desensitisation which involve the internalisation of both receptors in the dimer following stimulation with one partner agonist. Stimulation of the DOR-β_2-adrenoceptor heterodimer with the β_2 agonist isoprenaline induces DOR internalisation. Similarly, the β_2-adrenoceptor undergoes internalisation when DOR-β_2 dimers are stimulated with the opioid agonist etorphine. This may represent a common mechanism for heterologous desensitisation of GPCR signalling independent of receptor phosphorylation. In contrast, β_2-adrenoceptors do not internalise when associated with the KOR (see Figure 3.24).

Although internalisation plays a major role in switching off GPCR signalling it is also required in

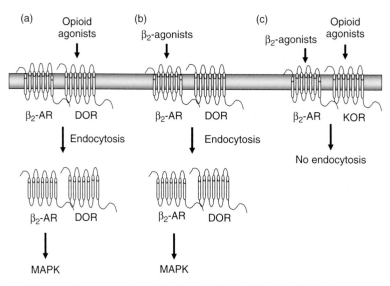

Figure 3.24 GPCR heterodimers regulate receptor internalisation and cell signalling. (a) The β_2-adrenoceptor undergoes internalisation when DOR-β_2 dimers are stimulated with the opioid agonists. (b) The DOR internalises when DOR-β_2 dimers are stimulated with β_2 agonists. In both cases β_2-adrenoceptor internalisation is required for the activation of the mitogen-activated protein kinase (MAPK) pathway by β_2 agonists. (c) KOR-β_2 dimers do not internalise when challenged with β_2 or opioid agonists and indeed KOR expression reduces β_2-adrenoceptor stimulation of MAPK.

certain cases for the activation of GPCR signalling. For example β_2-adrenoceptor internalisation is necessary for the activation of the mitogen-activated protein kinase (MAPK) pathway by β_2 agonists, which is reduced in cells co-expressing the KOR. Hence GPCR heterodimerisation represents a novel mechanism of regulating receptor signalling.

The above examples clearly illustrate how GPCR heterodimerisation can influence GPCR pharmacology and cell signalling. As such targeting GPCR heterodimers with bivalent ligands represents an intriguing and exciting target for future drug design (Kent et al., 2007; Bergue-Bestel et al., 2008).

Clinical and pathophysiological relevance of GPCR heterodimerisation

Since GPCRs are the target of >30% of all pharmaceutical drugs is there any evidence that GPCR heterodimerisation has clinical significance? As already discussed targeting the MOR-DOR heterodimer with bivalent ligands may prove useful for the treatment of pain (Dietis et al., 2009).

The clinical relevance of GPCR heterodimerisation is also illustrated by elegant studies on chemokine receptors. Chemokines belong to the cytokine peptide family of ligands and are involved in the recruitment and activation of white blood cells including $CD4^+$ T-lymphocytes. Two chemokine receptors, CXCR4 and CCR5, function as co-receptors for the entry of HIV into cells and both form heterodimers with the CCR2 chemokine receptor. Interestingly a single nucleotide polymorphism in CCR2, which is linked with a decrease in AIDS progression, increases CCR2/CCR5 and CCR2/CXCR4 heterodimerisation. Hence the ability of CCR2 to form heterodimers with CCR5 and/or CXCR4 appears to be of clinical significance with regards to HIV infection. Promoting the formation of such heterodimers by using chemokine receptor agonists or antibodies may be of use in the treatment of HIV infection.

The first report linking GPCR heterodimerisation with the pathogenesis of a human disorder appeared in 2001. It was noted that the levels of heterodimers between the angiotensin AT_1 receptor and the bradykinin B_2 receptor increased in pre-eclamptic pregnancies compared to normotensive pregnancies. The increased levels of the AT_1-B_2 heterodimer resulted in an increased response to the vasopressor angiotensin II causing an increase in blood pressure and hence hypertension. These examples highlight the importance of GPCR heterodimers in potentially modulating disease progression and also as distinct therapeutic targets.

3.11 GPCR splice variants

The protein coding regions of many eukaryotic genes (generally referred to as exons) are often interrupted by sequences of noncoding DNA called introns. Genomic DNA is transcribed into precursor RNA (containing both introns and exons) which then undergoes RNA splicing to remove the introns. RNA splicing can also result in different combinations of exons being spliced together through a process known as alternative splicing. In some cases RNA splicing results in specific introns being retained in the mature mRNA (intron retention) and thus coding for additional protein sequence (Figure 3.25). These post-transcriptional modifications involve a specialised complex of proteins and RNA termed the spliceosome which recognises specific sequences at the exon-intron border. It is highly regulated process and is often cell and/or tissue specific.

The occurrence of spice variants in GPCRs was first reported for the dopamine D2 receptor in 1989. Excluding olfactory receptors bioinformatic analysis of the human genome has revealed that 52% of GPCRs contain at least two exons in their open reading frame, indicative of an intron and hence the possibility of splice variants. However, the presence of introns within a GPCR gene does not always produce a splice variant(s). For reviews GPCR splice variants see Kilpatrick et al. (1999), Minneman (2001) and Markovic and Challiss (2009).

The majority of GPCR splice variants occur within the C-terminal tail and third intracellular loops and as such are likely to influence G-protein coupling and downstream effector activation. Some splice variants are species-specific which has important implications when comparing pharmacological data across different species. Furthermore, some GPCR splice variants are differentially distributed which suggests distinct physiological roles for certain isoforms.

Influence of splice variants on GPCR function

It is apparent that GPCR splice variants influence pharmacology, cell signalling, constitutive activity and desensitisation/down-regulation. Specific examples from each of these areas are discussed.

Effect on ligand binding

Ligand binding to the vast majority of Class A GPCRs involves the seven TM spanning domains. At present splice variants within the seven TM regions are unusual.

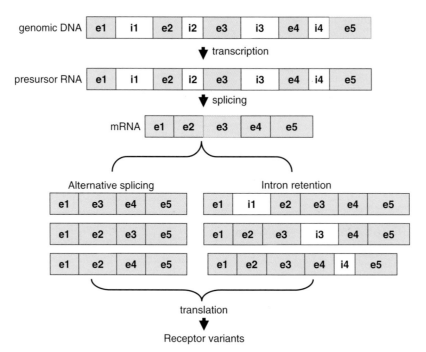

Figure 3.25 Generation of splice variants from a hypothetical gene containing five exons (e1-e5) and four introns (i1-i4).

However, there are examples of N-terminus and C-terminus GPCR splice variants that do exhibit differences in agonist and antagonist binding.

Effect on cell signalling: activation of different pathways

Splice variants can have dramatic effects on the cell signalling pathways activated by the receptor. One of the first reports showing the influence of splice variants on GPCR-mediated cell signalling involved the rat PAC_1 receptor, which is stimulated by the neuropeptide pituitary adenylate cyclase-activating polypeptide (PACAP) and couples to both G_q and G_s-proteins. Spengler et al. (1993) reported the existence of five splice variants within the third intracellular loop of the rat PAC_1 receptor which regulate adenylyl cyclase and phospholipase C differently. Four of the splice variants activated both adenylyl cyclase (G_s) and phospholipase C (G_q), whereas one variant only activated adenylyl cyclase. An additional rat PAC_1 receptor splice variant which differs from the wild-type receptor in TM4 does not activate adenylyl cyclase or phospholipase C. However it does stimulate increases in intracellular $[Ca^{2+}]_i$ by activating voltage-gated Ca^{2+} channels.

Alternative splicing of the calcitonin receptor generates a splice variant with a 14 amino acid deletion in TM7. The shorter form of the receptor couples to cyclic AMP production but not inositol phosphate accumulation. In contrast the longer form of the receptor stimulates both cyclic AMP production and inositol phosphate accumulation. These intriguing examples suggest that alternative splicing of GPCRs represents a mechanism for modulating G-protein coupling.

Effect on G-protein coupling efficiency

Changes in GPCR coupling efficiency are usually associated with variations in the intracellular domains of GPCRs. The majority of reported cases involving changes in coupling efficiency can be explained by changes in the affinity of ligands for the receptor. However, there are examples of splice variants which do not alter agonist/antagonist binding but do influence the coupling of receptors to G-proteins and hence effector proteins (adenylyl cyclase, phospholipase C, ion channels etc.). These can be classified into three groups.

Coupling to cell signalling pathways is abolished

There are some GPCR splice variants which no longer couple to heterotrimeric G-proteins. A splice variant of

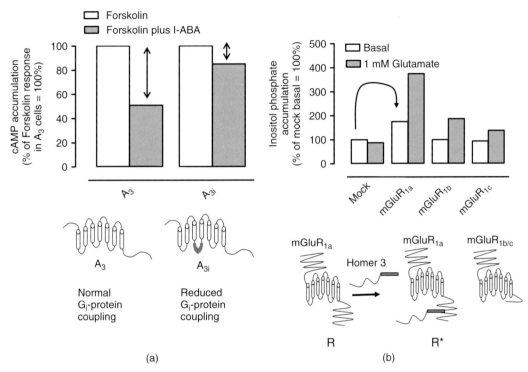

Figure 3.26 GPCR splice variants influence G-protein coupling and constitutive activity. (a) A splice variant of the adenosine A_3 receptor (A_{3i}) displays reduced ability to inhibition forskolin-stimulated cyclic AMP accumulation. See text for more detail. Data adapted from Sajjadi FG et al. (1996) FEBS Letts 382: 125–129. (b) The mGluR$_{1a}$ receptor splice variant, which has a long C-terminus, is constitutively active when compared to mGlu$_{1b/c}$ variants which have a short C-terminus. The constitutive activity of the mGluR$_{1a}$ is regulated by Homer 3 which promotes R* formation. The graph shows basal inositol phosphate accumulation in the absence (basal) and presence of the agonist glutamate. Data adapted from Prézeau L et al. (1996) Molecular Pharmacology 49: 422–429.

the neuropeptide Y (NPY) Y_1 receptor (termed Y_1-beta), which lacks part of TM7 and has no C-terminal tail, does not couple to any of the second messenger systems tested (inhibition of adenylyl cyclase, release of intracellular Ca^{2+} release or stimulation of mitogen-activated protein kinase) when compared to the NPY$_1$-alpha form of the receptor. The question then arises of what is the function of the Y_1-beta isoform which still binds NPY? It is possible that the apparent inactive version of the NPY$_1$ receptor is used to remove NPY from the extracellular environment and in doing so modulate the levels of this important neurotransmitter.

Coupling is maintained but efficiency is reduced

There are examples of splice variants which modify the efficiency of coupling to second messenger pathways. A splice variant of the rat A_3 adenosine receptor (A_{3i}), which

has a 17 amino acid insertion in the second intracellular loop, couples poorly to $G_{i/o}$-proteins when compared to the receptor without the insert (Figure 3.26a; highlighted in red). As illustrated in Figure 3.26a, the selective A_3 adenosine receptor agonist I-ABA produced less inhibition of forskolin-induced cyclic AMP accumulation in cells expressing the A_{3i} splice variant indicating less efficient coupling to $G_{i/o}$-proteins.

Similarly, four splice variants of the human PAC$_1$ receptor have been identified which differ in their maximal response for inositol phosphate accumulation. Thus although the EC$_{50}$ value for the agonist PACAP-38 is similar for each variant the maximal response (efficacy) varies significantly. The EC$_{50}$ represents the molar concentration of an agonist which produces 50% of the maximum possible response for that agonist. These examples indicate that splice variants of GPCRs represent a mechanism for fine-tuning the level of GPCR coupling to G-proteins.

Influence on GPCR constitutive activity

There are a number of reports describing differences in constitutive activity arising from splice variants located within the C-terminal. An alternatively spliced variant of the $mGluR_1$ (termed $mGluR_{1a}$), which has a long C-terminus, displays higher levels of constitutive activity compared to the short $mGluR_{1b}$ and $mGluR_{1c}$ variants. When heterologously expressed the $mGluR_{1a}$ generates a high basal level of inositol phosphate accumulation which is independent of agonist binding (Figure 3.26b). In contrast, expression of $mGluR_{1b}$ and $mGluR_{1c}$ produces basal inositol phosphate levels that are similar to untransfected (mock) cells. The constitutive activity of the $mGluR_{1a}$ is regulated by Homer 3 (a GPCR interacting protein; see later) which interacts with the homer binding sequence found within long C-terminus and promotes the active R^* conformation independent of agonist binding (Figure 3.26b).

Similar observations have been reported for splice variants of the $G_{i/o}$-protein linked prostanoid EP_3 receptor. The $EP_{3\alpha}$ variant is constitutively active and shows high levels of adenylyl cyclase inhibition in the absence of agonist, whereas the $EP_{3\beta}$ isoform shows no agonist-independent activity. Two splice variants of the $5\text{-}HT_4$ receptor, with short C-terminal sequences ($5\text{-}HT_{4(e)}$ and $5\text{-}HT_{4(f)}$), display higher levels of constitutive activity when compared to a variant with a long C-terminal ($5\text{-}HT_{4(a)}$). These examples illustrate that splice variants can modify the constitutive activity of G_q- ($mGluR_1$ variants), G_i- (EP_3 receptor variants) and G_s-protein ($5\text{-}HT_4$ receptor variants) coupled receptors.

Influence of splice variants on GPCR desensitisation

GPCRs interact with a host of other proteins called GPCR interacting proteins (GIP). They are involved in the modulation of GPCR signalling, the targeting of GPCRs to the correct subcellular compartment, the regulation of GPCR trafficking to the plasma membrane, receptor desensitisation/resensitisation and the formation of GPCR signalling complexes. The topic of GIPs will be expanded in Chapter 11. Some of these proteins are transmembrane proteins and include other GPCRs (dimerisation), ion channels, and single transmembrane proteins (e.g. RAMPs). However, the vast majority of GIPs are soluble cytoplasmic proteins that predominantly interact with the C-terminal tail. PDZ domain containing proteins are the most common GIP and they usually interact with the extreme end of the C-terminus (typically the last 3–4 amino acids). PDZ domains obtained their name from the repeat sequences first identified in three separate proteins: <u>P</u>ost synaptic density (PSD) protein PSD-95, <u>D</u>iscs large protein and tight junction protein <u>Z</u>O-1. PDZ proteins are involved in protein trafficking and scaffolding multi-protein complexes. There are three classes of consensus PDZ binding motifs; class I (S/TxØ; Ø represents a hydrophobic amino acid and × any amino acid), class II (ØxØ) and class III (E/DxØ). For comprehensive reviews on GIPs see Bockaert et al. (2004) and Bockaert (2010).

Some PDZ proteins modulate receptor endocytosis (internalisation) whilst others influence recycling back to the plasma membrane. Hence the kinetics of GPCR desensitisation and re-sensitisation may be 'fine-tuned' depending on the type of PDZ protein interacting with the C-terminal.

Several C-terminal splice variants of GPCRs display differences in desensitisation. For example C-terminal spliced variants of the μ-opioid receptor (MOR1 and MOR1B) and $mGluR_1$ ($mGluR_{1a}$ and $mGluR_{1b}$) exhibit different rates of internalisation. In both cases the shorter receptor variants (MOR1B and $mGluR_{1b}$) show a greater loss from the cell surface following prolonged agonist exposure. These differences may reflect the selective binding of GIPs involved in receptor desensitisation/resensitisation to specific splice variants.

Proteomic experiments using a combination of peptide-affinity chromatography, two-dimensional electrophoresis and mass spectrometry identified 13 GIPS (predominantly PDZ proteins) that interact with mouse $5\text{-}HT_{4(a)}$ and $5\text{-}HT_{4(e)}$ splice variants (Figure 3.27). Ten of these proteins interact solely with the $5\text{-}HT_{4(a)}$ variant including sorting nexin (SNX27) which is involved in escorting the $5\text{-}HT_{4(a)}$ to early endosomes for desensitisation. The $5\text{-}HT_{4(a)}$ receptor also interacts with NHERF (Na^+/H^+ exchanger regulator factor) and this is responsible for trafficking the receptor to microvilli, which is consistent with its role in cytoskeleton remodelling. The $5\text{-}HT_{4(b)}$ does not contain a PDZ protein binding domain and is not located at microvilli. These observations highlight how GPCR splice variants regulate receptor subcellular localisation and possibly rates of receptor desensitisation.

Clinical and pathophysiological relevance of GPCR splice variants

A number of reports link specific GPCR splice variants with the development or progression of a pathophysiological condition. For example an alternative spliced isoform of the CCK_B receptor has been implicated in the

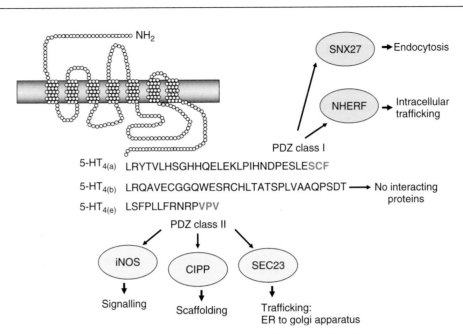

Figure 3.27 Proteins interacting with the C-terminus of 5-HT$_4$ receptor splice variants. The schematic representation shows the C-terminal amino acid sequences (single letter codes) for the mouse 5-HT$_{4(a)}$, 5-HT$_{4(b)}$ and 5-HT$_{4(e)}$ receptor splice variants. The 5-HT$_{4(a)}$ and 5-HT$_{4(e)}$ variants both contain a PDZ binding domain sequence (highlighted) in their C-terminus, whereas 5-HT$_{4(b)}$ does not. Synthetic peptides based upon the C-terminal sequences were used as baits for peptide affinity chromatography isolation of interacting proteins. Proteomic analysis has identified a number of PDZ proteins which differentially interact with these PDZ-containing variants. This may provide a basis for splice variants of the same receptor exhibiting different rates of desensitisation, cell signalling properties and sub-cellular location. iNOS; inducible nitric oxide synthetase. Figure adapted with permission from Joubert L et al. (2004) Journal of Cell Science 117: 5367–5379.

development and progression of colon cancer. Certain splice variants of the dopamine D3 receptor have been linked to schizophrenia. In the future these differences may be exploited pharmaceutically with the development splice variant specific ligands especially for isoforms which display distinct pharmacological properties and differential tissue distribution.

3.12 Summary

Drugs that target GPCRs represent a significant proportion of the current pharmaceutical market and generate annual revenues estimated to be in excess of £25 billion. Although the human GPCR genome contains more than 800 members only approximately 30 GPCRs are currently exploited as drug targets. The challenge for future drug development will be not only to exploit newly discovered GPCR family members but also to make use of the exciting developments and discoveries in

the field of GPCR biology that have been described in this chapter.

References

Adan RAH (2006). Endogenous inverse agonists and constitutive receptor activity in the melanocortin system. Trends in Pharmacological Sciences 27: 183–186.

Alexander SPH, Mathie A and Peters JA (2009). Guide to Receptors and Channels (GRAC). 4th edn. British Journal of Pharmacology 158 (Suppl. 1): S1-S254.

Ambrosio M, Zürn A and Lohse MJ (2011). Sensing G protein-coupled receptor activation. Nueropharmacology 60: 45–51.

Bernier V, Bichet DG and Bouvier M (2004). Pharmacological chaperone action on G-protein-coupled receptors. Current Opinion in Pharmacology 4: 528–533.

Berque-Bestel I, Lezoualc'h F and Jockers R (2008). Bivalent ligands as specific pharmacological tools for G protein-coupled receptor dimers. Current Drug Discovery Technologies 5: 312–3118.

Bockaert J, Fagni L, Dumuis A, Marin P (2004). GPCR interacting proteins (GIP). Pharmacology and Therapeutics 103: 203–221.

Bockaert J, Perroy J, Bécamel C, Marin P and Fagni L (2010). GPCR interacting proteins (GIPs) in the nervous system: roles in physiology and pathologies. Annual Review of Pharmacology and Toxicology 50: 89–109.

Böhm SK, Grady EF and Bunnett NW (1997). Regulatory mechanisms that modulate signalling by G-protein-coupled receptors. Biochemical Journal 322: 1–18.

Bokoch M, Zou Y, Rasmussen SGF, Liu CW, Nygaard R, Rosenbaum DM, Fung JJ, Choi H-J, Thian FS, Kobilka TS, Puglisi JD, Weis WI, Pardo L, Prosser RS, Mueller L and Kobilka BK (2010). Ligand-specific regulation of the extracellular surface of a G protein coupled receptor. Nature 463: 108–112.

Bond RA and IJzerman AP (2006). Recent developments in constitutive receptor activity and inverse agonism, and their potential for GPCR drug discovery. Trends in Pharmacological Sciences 27: 92–96.

Boswell-Smith V, Spina D and Page CP (2006). Phosphodiesterase inhibitors. British Journal of Pharmacology 147: S252-S257.

Chen CA and Manning DR (2001). Regulation of G proteins by covalent modification. Oncogene 20: 1643–1652.

Cherezov V, Rosenbaum DM, Hanson MA, Rasmussen SG, Thian FS, Kobilka TS, Choi HJ, Kuhn P, Weis WI, Kobilka BK and Stevens RC (2007). High-resolution crystal structure of an engineered human β_2-adrenergic G protein-coupled receptor. Science 318: 1258–1265.

Chien EY, Liu W, Zhao Q, Katritch V, Han GW, Hanson MA, Shi L, Newman AH, Javitch JA, Cherezov V and Stevens RC (2010). Structure of the human dopamine D3 receptor in complex with a D2/D3 selective antagonist. Science 330: 1091–1095.

Chung S, Funakoshi T and Civelli O (2008). Orphan GPCR research. British Journal of Pharmacology 153: S339-S346.

Conn PJ, Christopoulus A and Lindsley CW (2009). Allosteric modulators of GPCRs: a novel approach for the treatment of CNS disorders. Nature Reviews: Drug Discovery 8: 41–54.

Daniels DJ, Lenard NR, Etienne CL, Law P-Y, Roerig SC and Portoghese PS (2005). Opioid-induced tolerance and dependence in mice is modulated by the distance between pharmacophores in a bivalent ligand series. Proceedings of the National Academy of Sciences USA 102: 19208–19213.

Dalrymple MB, Pfleger KDG and Eidne KA (2008). G protein-coupled receptor dimers: Functional consequences, disease states and drug targets. Pharmacology and Therapeutics 118: 359–371.

Devi LA (2001). Heterodimerization of G-protein-coupled receptors: pharmacology, signaling and trafficking. Trends in Pharmacological Sciences 22: 532–537.

Dietis N, Guerrini R, Calo G, Salvadori S, Rowbotham DJ and Lambert DG (2009). Simultaneous targeting of multiple opioid receptors: a strategy to improve side-effect profile. British Journal of Anaesthesia 103: 38–49.

Ferguson SSG (2001). Evolving concepts in G protein-coupled receptor endocytosis: the role in receptor desensitization and signaling. Pharmacological Reviews 53: 1–24.

Gurevich VV and Gurevich EV (2008). How and why do GPCRs dimerize? Trends in Pharmacological Sciences 29: 234–240.

Hurst JH and Hooks SB (2009). Regulator of G-protein signalling (RGS) proteins in cancer biology. Biochemical Pharmacology 78: 1289–1297.

Huynh J, Thomas WG, Aguilar M-I and Pattenden LK (2009). Role of helix 8 in G protein-coupled receptors based on structure-function studies of the type 1 angiotensin receptor. Molecular and Cellular Endocrinology. 302: 118–127.

Jaakola VP, Griffith MT, Hanson MA, Cherezov V, Chien EY, Lane JR, Iizerman AP and Stevens RC (2008). The 2.6 angstrom crystal structure of a human A_{2A} adenosine receptor bound to an antagonist. Science 322: 1211–1217.

Katritch V, Cherezov V and Stevens RC (2012). Diversity and modularity of G protein-coupled receptor structures. Trends in Pharmacological Sciences 33: 17–27.

Kaupmann K, Huggel K, Heid J, Flor PJ, Bischoff S, Mickel SJ, McMaster G, Angst C, Bittiger H, Froestl W and Bettler B (1997). Expression cloning of $GABA_B$ receptors uncovers similarity to metabotropic glutamate receptors. Nature 386: 239–246.

Kent T, McAlpine C, Sabetnia S and Presland J (2007). G-protein-coupled receptor heterodimerization: assay technologies to clinical significance. Current Opinion in Drug Discovery Development 10: 580–589.

Kilpatrick GJ, Dautzenberg FM, Martin GR and Eglen RM (1999). 7TM receptors: the splicing on the cake. Trends in Pharmacological Sciences 20: 294–301.

Kobilka B and Schertler GFX (2008). New G-protein-coupled receptor crystal structures: insights and limitations. Trends in Pharmacological Sciences 29: 79–83.

Langmead CJ and Christopoulos A (2006). Allosteric agonists of 7TM receptors: expanding the pharmacological toolbox. Trends in Pharmacological Sciences 27: 475–481.

Lagerström MC and Schiöth HB (2008). Structural diversity of G protein coupled receptors and significance for drug discovery. Nature Reviews Drug Discovery 7: 339–357.

Lebon G, Warne T, Edwards PC, Bennett K, Langmead CJ, Leslie AGW and Tate CG (2011). Agonist-bound adenosine A_{2A} receptor structures reveal common features of GPCR activation. Nature 474: 521–525.

Lefkowitz RJ, Pierce KL and Luttrell LM (2002). Dancing with different partners: protein kinase A phosphorylation of seven membrane-spanning receptors regulates their G protein-coupling specificity. Molecular Pharmacology 62: 971–974.

Lefkowitz RJ (2004). Historical review: a brief history and personal retrospective of seven-transmembrane receptors. Trends in Pharmacological Sciences 25: 413–422.

Levac BAR, O'Dowd BF and George SR (2002). Oligomerization of opioid receptors: generation of novel signaling units. Current Opinion in Pharmacology 2: 76–81.

de Ligt RAF, Kourounakis AP and IJzerman AP (2000). Inverse agonism at G protein-coupled receptors: (patho)physiological relevance and implications for drug discovery. British Journal of Pharmacology 130: 1–12.

Marchese A, Piang MM, Temple BRS and Trejo J (2008). G protein-coupled receptor sorting to endosomes and lysosomes. Annual Review of Pharmacology and Toxicology 48: 601–629.

Marinissen MJ and Gutkind JS (2001). G-protein-coupled receptors and signalling networks: emerging paradigms. Trends in Pharmacological Sciences 22: 368–375.

Markovic D and Challiss RAJ (2009). Alternative splicing of G protein coupled receptors: physiology and pathophysiology. Cellular and Molecular Life Sciences 66: 3337–3352.

Maurice P, Kamal M and Jockers R (2011). Asymmetry of GPCR oligomers supports their functional relevance. Trends in Pharmacological Sciences 32: 514–520.

Milligan G (2004). G protein-coupled receptor dimerization: Function and ligand pharmacology. Molecular Pharmacology 66: 1–7.

Milligan G (2009). G protein-coupled receptor heterodimerization: contribution to pharmacology and function. British Journal of Pharmacology 158: 5–14.

Minneman KP (2001). Splice variants of G protein-coupled receptors. Molecular Interventions 1: 108–116.

Mustafi D and Palczewski K (2009). Topology of Class A G protein-coupled receptors: Insights gained from crystal structures of rhodopsins, adrenergic and adenosine receptors. Molecular Pharmacology 75: 1–12.

Nakamura M, Yasuda D, Hirota N and Shimizu T (2010). Specific ligands as pharmacological chaperones: the transport of misfolded G-protein coupled receptors to the cell surface. IUBMB Life 62: 453–459.

Newton CL, Whay AM, McArdle CA, Zhang M, van Koppen CJ, van de Lagemaat R, Segaloff DL and Millar RP (2011). Rescue of expression and signaling of human luteinizing hormone G protein-coupled receptor mutants with an allosterically binding small-molecule agonist. Proceedings of the National Academy of Science 108: 7172–7176.

Oldham WM and Hamm HE (2008). Heterotrimeric G protein activation by G-protein-coupled receptors. Nature Reviews: Molecular Cell Biology 9: 60–71.

Overington JP, Al-Lazikani B and Hopkins AL (2006). How many drug targets are there? Nature Reviews: Drug Discovery 5: 993–997.

Perez DM and Karnik SS (2005). Multiple signaling states of G-protein-coupled receptors. Pharmacological Reviews 57: 147–161.

Pfleger KDG and Eidne KA (2005). Monitoring the formation of dynamic G-protein-coupled receptor-protein complexes in living cells. Biochemical Journal 385: 625–637.

Pin J-P, Neubig R, Bouvier M, Devi L, Filizola M, Javitch JA, Lohse MJ, Milligan G, Palczewski K, Parmentier M and Spedding M (2007). International Union of Basic and Clinical Pharmacology. LXVII. Recommendations for the recognition and nomenclature of G protein-coupled receptor heterodimers. Pharmacological Reviews 59: 5–13.

Prinster SC, Hague C and Hall RA (2005). Heterodimerization of G protein-coupled receptors: specificity and functional significance. Pharmacological Reviews 57: 289–298.

Rasmussen SG, Choi HJ, Rosenbaum DM, Kobilka TS, Thian FS, Edwards PC, Burghammer M, Ratnala VR, Sanishvili R, Fishetti RF, Schertler GF, Weis WI and Kobilka BK (2007). Crystal structure of the human β_2-adrenergic G-protein coupled receptor Nature 450: 383–387.

Rasmussen SG, Devree BT, Zou Y, Kruse AC, Chung KY, Kobilka TS, Thian FS, Chae PS, Pardon E, Calinski D, Mathiesen JM, Shah ST, Lyons JA, Caffrey M, Gellman SH, Steyaert J, Skiniotis G, Weis WI, Sunahara RK and Kobilka BK (2011). Crystal structure of the β_2-adrenergic receptor-Gs protein complex. Nature 477: 549–555.

Rosenbaum DM, Cherezov V, Hanson MA, Rasmussen SG, Thian FS, Kobilka TS, Choi HJ, Yao XJ, Weis WI, Stevens RC and Kobilka BK (2007). GPCR engineering yields high-resolution structural insights into β_2-adrenergic receptor function. Science 318: 1266–1273.

Rosenbaum DM, Rasmussen SGF and Kobilka BK (2009). The structure and function of G-protein-coupled receptors. Nature 459: 356–363.

Rovati GE, Capra V and Neubig RR (2007). The highly conserved DRY motif of Class A G protein-coupled receptors: beyond the ground state. Molecular Pharmacology 71: 959–964.

Scott CW and Peters MF (2010). Label-free whole-cell assays; expanding the scope of GPCR screening. Drug Discovery Today 15: 704–716.

Shimamura T, Shiroishi M, Weyand S, Tsujimoto H, Winter G, Katritch V, Abagyan R, Cherezov V, Liu W, Han GW, Kobayashi T, Stevens RC and Iwata S (2011). Structure of the human histamine H_1 receptor complex with doxepin. Nature 475: 65–70.

Spengler D, Waeber C, Pantaloni C, Holsboer F, Bockaert J, Seeburg PH and Journot L (1993). Differential signal transduction by five splice variants of the PACAP receptor. Nature 365: 170–175.

Unal H and Karnik SS (2012). Domain coupling in GPCRs: the engine for induced conformational changes. Trends in Pharmacological Sciences 33: 79–88.

Vidi P-A and Watts VJ (2009). Fluorescent and bioluminescent protein-fragment complementation assays in the study of G protein-coupled receptor oligomerization and signaling. Molecular Pharmacology 75: 733–739.

Vischer HF, Leurs R and Smit MJ (2006). HCMV-encoded G-protein-coupled receptors as constitutively active modulators of cellular signaling networks. Trends in Pharmacological Sciences 27: 56–63.

Vischer HF, Watts AO, Nijmeijer S and Leurs R (2011). G protein-coupled receptors: walking hand-in-hand, talking hand-in-hand? British Journal of Pharmacology 163: 246–260.

Wang H, Liu T and Malbon CC (2006). Structure-function analysis of Frizzleds. Cellular Signalling 18: 934–941.

Wess J, Han S-J, Kim S-K, Jacobson KA and Li JH (2008). Conformational changes involved in G-protein-coupled receptor activation. Trends in Pharmacological Sciences. 29: 616–625.

Wu B, Chien EY, Mol CD, Fenalti G, Liu W, Katritch V, Abagyan R, Brooun A, Wells P, Bi FC, Hamel DJ, Kuhn P, Handel TM, Cherezov V and Stevens RC (2010). Structures of the CXCR4 chemokine GPCR with small-molecule and cyclic peptide antagonists. Science 330: 1066–1071.

Xu F, Wu H, Katritch V, Han GW, Jacobson KA, Gao ZG, Cherezov V and Stevens RC (2011). Structure of an agonist-bound human A_{2A} adenosine receptor. Science 332: 322–327.

Ziegler N, Bätz J, Zabel U, Lohse MJ and Hoffmann C (2011). FRET-based sensors for the human M_1-, M_3-, and M_5-acetylcholine receptors. Bioorganic and Medicinal Chemistry 19: 1048–1054.

Useful Web sites

International Union of Pharmacology (IUPHAR): 2012 http://www.iuphar.org
A very informative website which includes an up-to-date database on GPCR nomenclature.2012

4 Ion Channels

4.1 Introduction

Ion channels allow the passage of ions and other small substances through membranes. Their opening and closing can be regulated by changes in the charge (voltage) across the membrane or the binding of a ligand.

A comparison between the structure of the different ion channel subunits has revealed a remarkably similar basic topology (see Figure 4.1). If we start with the voltage-gated K^+ channel (K_v). It comprises of six transmembrane segments (TMS) of which two line the pore (TMS_{5-6}) and one is a voltage sensor (TMS_4). These six TMS form a transmembrane domain (TMD). Variations of this TMD are found in many other types of ion channel receptors (e.g. BK_{Ca}, SK_{Ca}, HCN, CNG, TRP, catSper). During evolution this TMD has undergone two duplication events. This first has given rise to the two pore channels (TPC) and the second to voltage-gated Na^+ and Ca^{2+} channels (Na_v and Ca_v). Interestingly all of these receptors function with a total of 24 TMS, that is those with a single TMD form tetramers, those with two TMD form dimers and those with four TMD are monomers.

Another duplication event also occurred in one of these single TMD (six TMS) channels. Except this time the terminal TMS_{5-6} were duplicated giving rise to the outwardly rectifying K^+ ion channel subunits (e.g. YORK, TOK1). Rather than requiring 24 TMS for activity these ion channels contain only 16 TMS. This is because like the aforementioned voltage-gated ion channels, its pore is composed of eight TMS and hence the subunits need only to dimerise for functionality. There is some debate in the literature as to whether TMS_4 of some members of this family still has voltage sensitivity (Lesage et al., 1996) raising the possibility that this function has been lost during evolution.

The inwardly rectifying K^+ channels (K_{ir}) subunits only have two TMS that appear to be similar to TMS_{5-6} of the voltage-gated ion channels mentioned above. Whether they evolved from each other is difficult to determine. They are similar to the outwardly rectifying K^+ ion channel subunits in that eight TMS are required and hence a tetrametric structure is needed for activity. Two-pore K^+ channels (K_{2p}) are closely related to K_{ir} channels in that they have their two TMS that appear to be duplicated to give a subunit with four TMS. Two subunits combine to yield a channel with eight TMS.

Subunits for the acid sensing ion channels (ASIC) and endothelial Na^+ channel (ENaC) appear to be very similar to the K_{ir} channels except the re-entrant loop between each TMS has expanded into a large extracellular loop. In addition, three subunits rather than four as in K_{ir}, are required for functionality. This is also true for the ligand-gated P2X family suggesting that it is closely related in evolutionary terms to ASIC and ENaC.

Molecular Pharmacology: From DNA to Drug Discovery, First Edition. John Dickenson, Fiona Freeman, Chris Lloyd Mills, Shiva Sivasubramaniam and Christian Thode.
© 2013 John Wiley & Sons, Ltd. Published 2013 by John Wiley & Sons, Ltd.

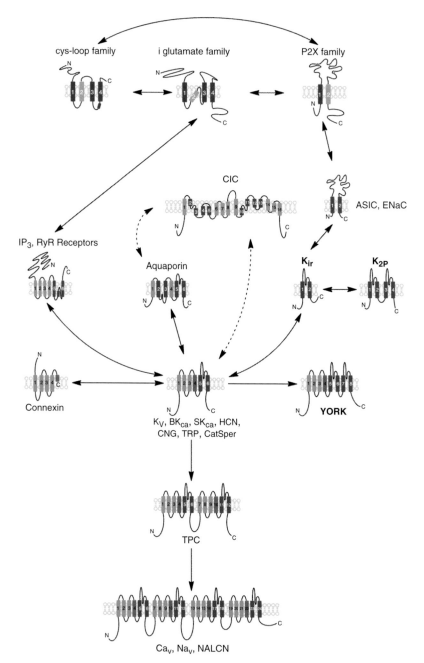

Figure 4.1 Topology of different members of the ion channel family. The ligand-gated ion channels (cys-loop, i glutamate and P2X) consist of TMS that forms the pore (orange) and other TMS (green). The voltage gate ion channels are depicted with the TMS pore forming domains (blue), voltage sensing TMS (red) and other TMS (turquoise). Full arrows indicate a possible evolution link between different classes of ion channels whereas dashed arrows are suggestive of a more tenuous evolutionary link. BK_{Ca}, Ca^{2+}-activated K^+ channels with big conductances; SK_{Ca}, Ca^{2+}-activated K^+ channels with small conductances; HCN, hyperpolarisation-activated cyclic nucleotide-gated channels; CNG, cyclic nucleotide-gated channel; CIC, chloride selective ion channel; TRP, transient receptor potential channels; catSper, cation channels in sperm; TPC, two pore channels; Na_v, voltage-gated Na^+ channels; Ca_v, voltage-gated Ca^{2+} channels; K_{ir}, inwardly rectifying K^+ channels; ASIC, acid sensing ion channels, ENaC, endothelial Na^+ channel; IP_3, Inositol triphosphate; RyR, ryanodine receptors; K_{2P}, two-pore potassium channels; K_v, voltage-gated K^+ channels; NALCN, sodium leak channel non-selective protein; YORK, yeast outward rectifying K^+ channel.

All of the ligand-gate ion channels assemble as either trimers (P2X), tetramers (i glutamate) or pentamers (cys-loop) with TMS_2 forming the pore which is suggestive of a common ancestor. However, TMS_2's structure in members of the i glutamate family is a re-entrant loop and similar to that found in IP_3 and RyR receptors as well as K_v channels, which implies that this ligand-gated ion channel evolved from voltage gated ion channels. Whether IP_3 and RyR receptors and i glutamate receptors evolved independently is unclear.

The aquaporin subunit is interesting as it contains three TMS (two of which are similar to the classic TMS pore forming domain) that appears to have been duplicated and inverted during evolution. Even though each subunit contains four TMS that form their own water channel, four subunits oligermerising are needed for function. This four-pore structure may reflect the channel's need for the bulk movement of water. The connexins have also broken away from 'tradition' because six subunits oligermise to form a hemi-channel, which might serve to expand the pore size for the relatively large cargo transported by gap junctions. They also appear to have lost the classic TMS_{5-6} pore lining domain. Since this domain has a re-entrant loop between each TMS that confers ion selectivity upon the channel its omission may reflect the large and diverse cargo that passes through. There is an α-helix structure at the subunits amino terminal that can serve as a gate and in some isoforms has voltage sensitivity.

Like the aquaporins, chloride selective ion channels (CICs) have an inverted repeat structural topology (see Figure 4.23). Both types of ion channels require more than one subunit for functionality with each subunit forming its own pore. That is, aquaporins have four separate ion channels and CICs have two. Like all voltage-sensitive ion channels, CICs have a classic re-entrant loop that helps form the pore and plays a role in ion selectivity. The inverted repeat structural topology of CICs is reminiscent of transporters (see Chapter 5). Until recently all members of the CIC family were considered to be classic ion channels, in that they permit the flow of ions through a membrane spanning pore. However, several members have now been shown to act as H^+/Cl^- transporters. In fact, point mutation studies have shown that the substrate biding pocket of some of these H^+/Cl^- transporters can essentially be converted into a Cl^- selective ion channel that completely traverses the membrane. This is indicative of an evolutionary link between transporters and ion channels (Accardia and Alessandra, 2010) and is perhaps unsurprising given that they both serve to facilitate the movement of ions and small molecules across biological membranes.

4.2 Voltage-gated ion channels

Ion channels are proteins that contain a pore for the passage of ions across membranes. Opening and closing of the pore, otherwise known as gating, can be controlled by a number of different factors. This includes binding of ligands such as neurotransmitters (ligand-gated ion channels; LGIC) which are discussed later in this chapter. Some ion channels can be 'stretched' open, a type of K^+ ion channel in cochlear hair cells being an example of this. These receptors detect changes in sound wave pressures which results in their channel being physically 'stretched' open. The opening and closing of various ion channels can be elicited by certain chemical modifications such as phosphorylation whilst a number of ion channel types are sensitive to changes in the membrane potential. In this section we shall concentrate on these latter types of ion channels which are also known as voltage-gated receptors; basically they detect changes in the local electrochemical gradient across membranes which is measured in volts hence their name.

Generation of membrane potential

In Chapter 11 we will see how membranes can partition cellular compartments. Membranes in most living cells are polarised, that is, they have an uneven distribution of ions and hence charge across them. Normally there is a higher concentration of Na^+, Ca^{2+} and Cl^- ions outside and K^+ ions inside the cell because these ions cannot usually diffuse freely across membranes. This electrochemical concentration gradient develops because a number of transporters (see Chapter 5) actually pump these ions in or out of the cell against their concentration gradient. This distribution of charge is known as the membrane potential (V_m) and its value can change depending upon membrane permeability. Ion channels embedded in the membrane can open, allowing these ions to diffuse across the membrane, down their concentration gradient. However, ions have charge (valency) which creates an electrostatic (electrogenic) pull or repulsion that can either facilitate or hinder diffusion. This means that there will be no net movement of ions across a membrane when the diffusion charge equals the electrostatic pull. When this occurs the difference in charge (potential difference) across the membrane is known as the equilibrium potential (E) for that particular ion (E_{ion};

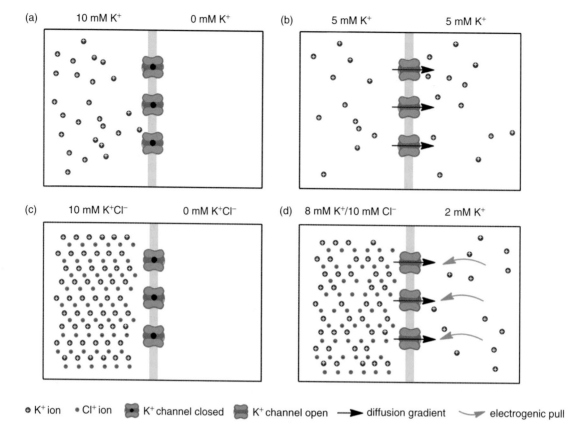

Figure 4.2 Diagram illustrating the effect of electrogenic pull on the diffusion gradient. (a) K$^+$ ions are unable to cross the membrane because K$^+$ channels are closed. (b) Opening of K$^+$ channels allows K$^+$ ions to diffuse down their concentration gradient into the other chamber until the concentration on both sides of the membrane are the same. (c) When KCl is introduced into the first chamber it dissociates into its components; K$^+$ and Cl$^-$ ions. (d) K$^+$ channels open so K$^+$ ions diffuse into the other chamber. However, Cl$^-$ ions remain in the first chamber resulting in a higher concentration of negative charge. This charge attracts the positive charge K$^+$ ions (electrogenic pull) preventing some K$^+$ ions diffusing down its gradient into the second chamber so that the concentration of K$^+$ ions in each chamber will never be equal. The resultant difference in charge distribution across the membrane gives rise to the equilibrium potential (e) for K$^+$ (E_K) which is measured in volts. In reality, biological membranes have a number of different ions so the membrane potential (V_m) will depend upon the E_{ion} of all the ion species present.

see Figure 4.2). The E_{ion} for each ion species can be used to calculate the V_m.

Ions, like all charged particles, create an electric field. Since membranes are relatively thin ($\sim$100 Å $= 0.1 \times 10^{-9}$ cm) the electric field due to 0.1V would create an electric field of 1,000,000,000 V cm^{-1}. This property is important in the activity of voltage-gated ion channels where changes in the V_m value are detected and used to open or close the channels.

Structure of voltage-gated ion channels

Voltage-gated ion channels consist of four TMD, with each subunit containing six trans-membrane segments (TMS). As illustrated in Figure 4.3, the first four TMS are thought to act as the voltage sensor and the last two form the central ion pore. The loop between TMS$_5$ and TMS$_6$ acts as a selectivity filter and determines which ion or ions can enter the pore (e.g. Na$^+$, K$^+$ or Ca^{2+}). TMS$_4$ has a three amino acid residue motif that is repeated between four and seven times. This motif contains a positively charged amino acid (usually arginine) followed by two hydrophobic amino acid residues. Mutagenesis studies have identified that four of the arginine residues are crucial for channel opening. Basically they interact with negative charges on the other TMS. The application of a strong electric field which is produced by the resting V_m

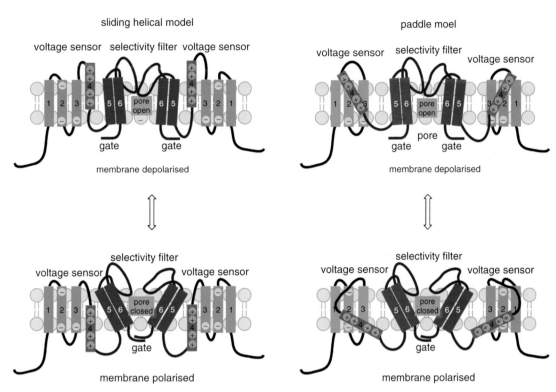

Figure 4.3 Proposed mechanisms of voltage-gated ion channel opening and closing. In both models positive charged arginine residues in TMS_4 interact with negative charges in TMS_2 and TMS_3. The electric field affects this interaction. Low electric fields are seen during membrane depolarisation and result in TMS_4 moving through the membrane so that it pulls on the pore forming domains, $TMS_{5/6}$, which move away from adjacent $TMS_{5/6}$ of the other subunits thereby facilitating pore opening. The loop between TMS_5 and TMS_6 serves as a selectivity filter for determining which ions can enter and transverse the pore. At resting membrane potentials, the electric field is higher and this causes TMS_4 to move downwards resulting in pore closure due to $TMS_{5/6}$ of each subunit being closer and their carboxyl terminuses forming a gate. How TMS_4 moves in the membrane is under debate with two mechanisms proposed. In the sliding helical model, TMS_4 rotates like a cork screw up and down in the plane of the membrane, but in the paddle model TMS_4 moves adjacent to the plane of the membrane. Voltage-gated ion channels are composed of four TMD but for clarity only two TMD are shown.

can enhance these interactions and prevent the pore from opening. But during depolarisation, when the electric field decreases, this electrostatic force is released allowing the pore to open. There is considerable debate in the literature as to how the TMS interact to form a functional ion channel. These include: the 'paddle model' which has the TMS_4 moving away from the pore subunits thereby allowing the channels to open, or the 'sliding helical model' where TMS_4 rotates according to the electric field enabling the channels to open or close. (Catterall, 2010; Francisco, 2005; Payandeh et al., 2011). Never the less, mutations in the critical arginine residues in TMS_4 or the negatively charged residues that they interact with can have profound effects on receptor function.

Voltage-gated ion channels in health and disease

The major types of voltage-gated ion channels can be classified according to the ion(s) that they conduct (Table 4.1). The voltage-gated Na^+, K^+ and Ca^{2+} ion channels are primarily regulated by membrane depolarisation. Some members of this family are included due to the presence of the voltage-sensing TMS_{1-4}. This means that although their primary activator is ligand binding, certain members have the potential to be modulated by changes in membrane potential. For example, hyperpolarisation-activated cyclic nucleotide-gated channels (HCN) are sensitive to cyclic AMP or cyclic GMP binding but can also open in response to hyperpolarising

Table 4.1 Voltage-gated ion channel members.

Name	Ion(s)	Examples
voltage-gated calcium channels	Ca^{2+}	$Ca_v1.1$- $Ca_v3.3$
voltage-gated sodium channels	Na^+	$Na_v1.1$ - $Na_v1.9$
voltage-gated potassium channels	K^+	$K_v1.1$ - $K_v12.3$
calcium-activated potassium channels	Ca^{2+}	$K_{Ca}1.1$ - $K_{Ca}5.1$
catSper and two-pore channels	Ca^{2+}	CatSper1 - CatSper4 TPC1 - TPC4
inwardly rectifying potassium channels	K^+	$K_{ir}1.1$ - $K_{ir}7.1$
two-pore potassium channels	K^+	$K_{2p}1.1$ - $K_{2p}18.1$
cyclic nucleotide-regulated channels	Ca^{2+}, Na^+, K^+	CNGA1 - CNGB3 HCN1 - HCN4
transient receptor potential channels	Ca^{2+}, Na^+, K^+	TRPA1 TRPC1 - TRPC7 TRPM1 - TRPM8 TRPML1 - TRPML3 TRPP1 - TRPP3 TRPV1 - TRPV6

Table 4.2 Families of conotoxins that target voltage-gated ion channels.

Superfamily	Family	Channel modulation
A	κA-Conotoxins	K^+ channel inhibitor
I	L-Conotoxins	Na^+ channel agonist
	κI-Conotoxins	K^+ channel inhibitor
J	κJ-Conotoxins	K^+ channel inhibitor
M	μ-Conotoxins	Na^+ channel inhibitor
	κM-Conotoxins	K^+ channel inhibitor
	μO-Conotoxins	Na^+ channel inhibitor
O	ω-Conotoxins	Ca^{2+} channel inhibitor
	κ-Conotoxins	K^+ channel inhibitor
	δ-Conotoxins	Na^+ channel inactivation inhibitor
T	T1-Conotoxins	Na^+ channel inhibitor

membrane potentials. Many of these channels are associated with human disease particularly neuronal and muscular pathologies.

The venoms of cone sea snails, conotoxins, have proved invaluable tools for dissecting the roles of various voltage-gated ion channels in health and disease. Table 4.2 shows the six super-families of conotoxins that specifically target voltage-gated ion channels. Conotoxins have the ability to discriminate between closely related isoforms of receptors and their activational states. This specificity means that certain conotoxins have proved useful in the treatment of conditions, such as chronic pain, with minimum nonspecific effects. However, some conotoxins are too toxic for use or they are rapidly inactivated by peptidases *in vivo*. This has led to the development of conotoxin-derived drugs that are less toxic and more stable (Raffa, 2010).

Voltage-gated ion channels and neurotransmission

The three main ions transported by voltage-gated ion channels are Na^+, K^+ and Ca^{2+}, and their role in neurotransmission has been studied extensively. Voltage-gated Na^+ (Na_v) and K^+ (K_v) channels playing important roles in action potential propagation along the axon/dendrite and pre-synaptically located voltage-gated Ca^{2+} channels (Ca_v) can indirectly control neurotransmitter release. Figure 4.5 illustrates how an action potential travels down the axon, activating Na_v and K_v channels until it reaches the Ca_v channels located in the presynaptic bouton. All three types of ion channels are activated by membrane depolarisation around their locality; Na_v and K_v channel opening cause membrane depolarisation which activates Ca_v channels. The influx of Ca^{2+} ions into the presynaptic neurone initiates a chain of events that leads to neurotransmitter release. The neurotransmitter can then diffuse across the synaptic left and activate its cognate receptor in the post-synaptic cell. If the receptor is involved in excitatory neurotransmission it will cause the post-synaptic membrane to depolarise which is detected by Na_v and K_v channels in the dendrite. The whole cycle starts again with an action potential passing down the dendrite to the axon and subsequent neurotransmitter release at the next synapse. The resting V_m is restored by the action of the Na^+/K^+ (Figure 4.4) and Ca^{2+}/Na^+ pumps. The opening, duration of opening and closing of voltage-gated ion channels in neurones can be manipulated to a degree. The best studied example is ω-conotoxins which inhibits N-type Ca^{2+} channels ($Ca_v2.2$).

Voltage-gated ion channels and muscle contraction

Striated muscle such as skeletal and cardiac contains myofibrils that are enveloped by a plasma membrane known as the sarcolemma. This plasma membrane invaginates into the muscle via T-(transverse) tubules. Sandwiched between these T-tubules, in a triad arrangement, is the sarcoplasmic reticulum (SR) where Ca^{2+} ions are stored. Usually skeletal muscle contraction is initiated by stimulating a motor nerve that drives activity in the muscle. An action potential is generated in the nerve and neurotransmitter released as described in the previous section (Figure 4.6). However, the interface between this neurone and the skeletal muscle is called the neuromuscular junction rather than a synapse. Acetylcholine is the major neurotransmitter involved in neuromuscular transmission and activation of nicotinic receptors on the plasma membrane results in Na^+ ion influx and K^+ ion efflux (see section 4.2) causing the plasma membrane to depolarise. The 'wave' of depolarisation is propagated to the T-tubules and is detected by voltage sensitive L-type Ca^{2+} channels (also known as voltage-operated calcium channels; VOCC) within their membrane. These slow opening L-type Ca^{2+} channels are also called DHP channels due to their sensitivity to dihydropyridines such as verapamil and nifedipine. They are arranged in groups of four (tetrads) in the plasma membrane. Depolarisation of the T-tubule membrane causes these channels to open as well as enabling the tetrads to interact with, and activate, a Ca^{2+} channel located on the SR membrane. These Ca^{2+} channels are also known as ryanodine receptors (RyR) because of their sensitivity to the plant alkaloid, ryanodine. Ca^{2+} ions are rapidly released from the SR via RyRs, and interact with the excitation-contraction coupling machinery to illicit muscle contraction. The RyR can

also be activated by increases in the local concentration of Ca^{2+} ions due to the opening of the L-type Ca^{2+} channels; a mechanism known as Ca^{2+}-induced Ca^{2+} release (CICR) (Snyders, 1999).

In skeletal muscle, CICR is not important for muscle contraction. However, in cardiac muscle, CICR plays an important role in controlling cardiac output. This is because Ca^{2+} ions entry from the lumen of the T-tubules plays a role in activation of cardiac RyR through CICR; whereas in skeletal muscle, depolarisation of the T-luminal membrane alone is sufficient for activation of the L-type channels and its interaction with, and activation of, the RyR. Since RyRs stays open longer than the L-type Ca^{2+} channels they are active for far longer and hence can make more of a contribution to the increase in intracellular Ca^{2+} ions necessary for excitation-contraction coupling.

Smooth muscle has caveoli rather than T-tubules (see Figure 4.7). There is evidence suggesting that L-type Ca^{2+} channels located in the caveoli membrane can either directly interact with RyRs on the SR to cause release of Ca^{2+} ions from the SR or mediate their activation by increasing the local intracellular Ca^{2+} ion levels and thereby facilitate CICR. However, the structure of smooth muscle is not as regimented as striated muscle so that L-type Ca^{2+} channels and RyR interaction is greatly reduced and likely only to play a minor role in excitation-contraction coupling. The L-type Ca^{2+} channels do not have the ability to increase intracellular concentration by themselves because the extracellular concentration of Ca^{2+} ions is insufficient. It appears that the IP_3 receptor (which is another SR located Ca^{2+} channel) plays a greater role in smooth muscle contraction.

Voltage-gated Ca^{2+} channels

Typical of voltage-gated ion channels, the voltage-gated Ca^{2+} channels (Ca_v) are composed of four domains, each of which contain a voltage sensor (TMS_{1-4}) and pore forming region (TMS_{5-6}). A glutamate motif (EEEE) in the selectivity filter confers Ca^{2+} ion selectivity upon these channels. Ca_v are composed of α1, α2, β, δ, and γ subunits (see Figure 4.9). The α2, β, δ and γ subunits are accessory proteins that modulate activity of the α1 subunit. The α1 subunit is responsible for channel gating and many pharmacological properties of these channels. These ion channels can be classified according to their Ca^{2+} ion conductance because pharmacological and electrophysiological studies have identified six different voltage-gate Ca^{2+} currents: L (long-lasting), N (neuronal), P (Purkinje), Q (granule cell), T (transient)

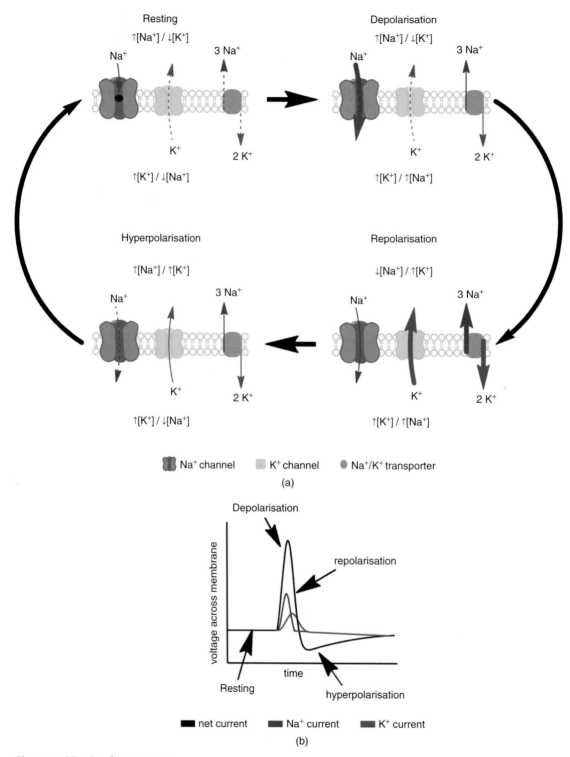

Figure 4.4 (*Continued on next page*)

Table 4.3 Physiology and pathologies associated with voltage-gated Ca^{2+} ion channels.

Ca^{2+} current	α1 subunit	Location	Function	Pathologies
L	$Ca_v1.1$	Skeletal muscle	EC-coupling CREB activity	Hypokalaemia associated muscle weakness
	$Ca_v1.2$	Cardiac and smooth muscle Neuronal soma and dendrites	EC-coupling Endocrine secretion Activation of 2nd messenger pathways Regulation of enzyme activity CREB activity	Hypotension Cardiac arrhythmia Developmental abnormalities Autism
	$Ca_v1.3$	Cardiac tissue (e.g. sino arterial node) Neuronal soma and dendrites	Regulate heart rate Endocrine secretion neurotransmission	Cardiac arrhythmias Parkinson's disease
	$Ca_v1.4$	Retina	Visual transduction	Night blindness
P/Q	$Ca_v2.1$	Presynaptic bouton Dendrites	Neurotransmitter release	Migraine Ataxia Epilepsy
N	$Ca_v2.2$	Presynaptic bouton Dendrites	Neurotransmitter release	Pain
R	$Ca_v2.3$	Presynaptic bouton Dendrites	Neurotransmitter release	Pain Epilepsy
T	$Ca_v3.1$	Cardiac myocytes Brain	Pace-making and Repetitive firing	Epilepsy Hypertension Sleep disorder
	$Ca_v3.2$	Cardiac myocytes Brain	Pace-making Repetitive firing	Sleep disorder Epilepsy Pain
	$Ca_v3.3$	Brain Peripheral nervous system	Pace-making Repetitive firing	Sleep disorder Epilepsy Pain

EC = excitation-contraction.

and R (toxin-resistant). They can also be further classified according to which α1 subunit is present. So far 10 genes that encode the α1 subunits have been identified in mammals (Ca_v1-3), each with distinct physiological roles (see Table 4.3). The Ca_v1 subfamily is involved in initiating muscle contraction, endocrine secretion, regulation of gene expression and integration of synaptic inputs. Members of the Ca_v2 subfamily are responsible for initiation of fast synaptic transmission. Finally, the Ca_v3 family plays an important role in the rhythmic firing of action potentials in cardiac cells and thalamic neurones.

Five characteristic Ca^{2+} currents that are based on their relative opening times are associated with these channels, of which four can be studied in isolation due to specific antagonists: dihydropyridines (DHP) such as verapamil and nifedipine inhibit L-type; the conotoxin,

Figure 4.4 (*Continued*) The role of Na_v and K_v channels in action potential generation. (a) During resting, Na_v channels are closed and the membrane remains polarised. A small amount of current 'leakage' is due to the activity of K^+ channels. However, the Na^+/K^+ transporter maintains the membrane potential by exporting Na^+ ions and importing K^+ ions. During membrane depolarisation the Na_v channels rapidly open allowing the influx of Na^+ ions. The K_v channels initially remain closed but slowly respond to the membrane depolarisation by opening just as the Na_v channels close. This enables the membrane to repolarise. The Na^+/K^+ transporter also helps to restore the membrane potential. Because the K_v channels are open for such a relatively long period of time the membrane becomes hyperpolarised before returning to the resting potential. (b) Illustration of the ionic currents involved in the generation of an action potential.

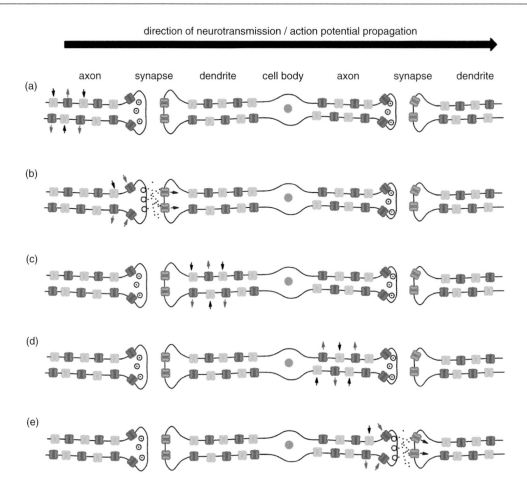

Figure 4.5 The role of voltage-gated Na$^+$, K$^+$ and Ca^{2+} channels in action potential propagation and neurotransmission. (a) Na$^+$ ions influx into the axon vial Na$^+$ channels, resulting in membrane depolarisation (reduced V$_m$). The reduction in V$_m$ is also detected by K$_v$ channels but their response is much slower and lasts longer compared to the Na$_v$ channels. This allows the membrane to be repolarised ready for another action potential to arrive as well as enabling the wave of membrane depolarisation to travel down the axon to the synapse. (b) Pre-synaptically located Ca$_v$ channels detect the reduction in V$_m$ and open allowing Ca^{2+} ion influx which initiates the cascade of events involved in release of neurotransmitter into the synaptic cleft. The neurotransmitter can activate its cognate receptor. If the receptor is involved in excitatory neurotransmission the post-synaptic membrane will depolarise. Membrane depolarisation is detected by Na$_v$ and K$_v$ channels in the dendrite (c) followed by the axon (d) of the post-synaptic cell. When the signal reaches that neurones pre-synaptic compartment, Ca$_v$ channels are activated (e) as in (b) and the cycle of neurotransmission and action potential propagation starts again.

ω-CTx-GVIA, targets N-type; the funnel web spider venom, ω-Agatoxin IVA, blocks P/Q-type; and the tarantula venom, SNX-482, acts at R-type channels.

The Ca$_v$1 family play a significant role in excitation-contraction coupling in muscle. Interestingly, although both cardiac and skeletal muscle is striated, only calcium-induced calcium release (CICR) plays a significant role in cardiac tissue. The utilisation of different ion channel subtypes (Ca$_v$1.1 in skeletal and Ca$_v$1.2 in cardiac) is a significant contributing factor. Another contributing factor is different members of the ryanodine receptor (RyR) embedded in the SR

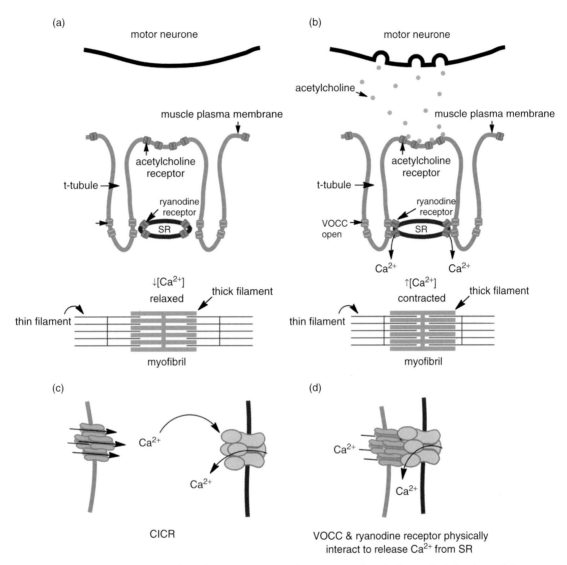

Figure 4.6 Muscle contraction in striated muscle. (a) No activity at the neuromuscular junction results in low intracellular concentrations of Ca^{2+} ions. The degree of cross over between thick and thin filament in the myofibril is low and the muscle is relaxed. (b) Acetylcholine released from the motor neurone activates nicotinic acetylcholine receptors causing depolarisation of the muscle plasma membrane which is propagated down the T-tubules. L-type Ca^{2+} channels (VOCC) open allowing Ca^{2+} ions to flow into the cytoplasm. This increase in Ca^{2+} ion concentration can activate ryanodine receptors (RyR) on the SR (sarcoplasmic reticulum) causing them to open and release more Ca^{2+} ions into the cytosol; a mechanism known as Ca^{2+}-induced Ca^{2+} release (CICR). This initiates a cascade of events where the thick and thin filament of the myofibril move over each other so that its length decreases and hence the muscle contracts. Increased cytosolic Ca^{2+} can occur due to two mechanisms (c) CICR and (d) physical interaction of a tetramer of VOCC with each foot of a ryanodine receptor to stimulate Ca^{2+} ion release from the SR.

membrane that interact with the Ca^{2+} ion channel tetramer (see Figure 4.6d); $Ca_v1.1$ with RyR1 and $Ca_v1.2$ with RyR2. Since smooth muscle has fewer SR compared to cardiac tissue the role of $Ca_v1.2$ here

may be to modulate secondary pathways involved in IP_3 receptor activation (see Figure 4.7) and endocrine secretions. Activation of these secondary pathways can also initiate binding of transcription factors such as

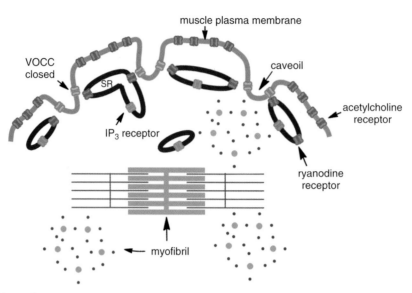

Figure 4.7 Smooth muscle contractions. The plasma membrane of smooth muscle has caveoli rather than T-tubules. In addition, the contribution made by VOCC and ryanodine receptors to cytosolic Ca^{2+} ion levels is insignificant; the ligand gated IP_3 receptor is mainly responsible for Ca^{2+} ion release from the SR. Although the tissue is not striated, which means the myofibril occur in many different planes, it is the intracellular Ca^{2+} ion concentration that controls myofibril length as in striated muscle.

CREB to their responsive elements (see section 8.3). The dihydropyridine antagonist nifedipine, targets these receptors and is used to treat hypertension. It works by stabilising the inactivated state of the channel. Since the duration of depolarisation is longer in arterial vascular smooth muscle compared to cardiac muscle, nifedipine has longer to interact with the inactive conformation of the receptor. Hence nifedipine is more likely to bind to the receptor located in the smooth muscle to cause vasodilation. In addition the $Ca_v 1.2$ ion channel is alternatively spliced and the variant expressed in smooth muscle is more receptive to nifedipine block than the cardiac located variant. This means that at low concentrations nifedipine has a vasodilatory effect whereas at higher concentrations it can cause arrhythmias and depressed cardiac output. On the other hand, phenylalkylamines, such as verapamil, interact with the channel in its open conformation causing it to enter the inactivated conformation. It also increases the time for recovery for the inactive conformation thereby increasing the receptor's refractory time. So, during increased stimulation frequencies, when the depolarisation time is reduced, fewer $Ca_v 1$ channels are open. Thus verapamil can be used to treat arrhythmias associated with high heart rates, which is in addition to its vasodilation and reduced cardiac output effect (Striessnig

et al., 1998). Rhythmic activity of neurones and some non-neuronal tissue is an important factor with $Ca_v 1.3$ (and $Ca_v 3$ channels) capable of controlling heart rate by modulating the rate of contraction via the various cardiac pace-makers (e.g. sino arterial node, atrioventricular node) or thalamic activity which can control motor outputs such as the coordination of limbs during walking.

The $Ca_v 2$ channels are the most extensively characterised because of their ability to modulate neurotransmitter release. Mutations in the gene for $Ca_v 2.1$ have been associated with migraines where this channel is considered to cause increased neocortical excitability and abnormal cerebral blood flow. Zolmitriptan, a P/Q-type channel inhibitor, has proved to be effective in the treatment of migraines. $Ca_v 2.2$ channels are involved in neurotransmitter release. They have been associated with pain because of their abundance in the dorsal horn of the spinal cord where they regulate the release of glutamate and substance P, both of which are involved in processing of nociceptive stimuli. A synthetic version of the ω-conotoxin MVIIA, ziconotide, targets the $Ca_v 2.2$ channel and is an effective treatment for chronic pain. However, due to its ability to target $Ca_v 2.2$. channels in other parts of the nervous system, it has severe side-effects and for this reason it can only be administered directly into the spine using a micro-infusion pump. A splice variant of the $Ca_v2.2$ channel which has an exon inserted in the cytosolic loop between domains II and III shows some brain region specific locations. Whether this variant has a specific role within these locations remains to be determined. However, it does indicate a further level of receptor specificity that could be exploited to treat particular diseases as well as reduce drug side-effects. Targets of $Ca_v2.3$ channels are being developed as anti-convulsives. The tarantula venom, SNX-482, acts at these receptors but the peptide lacks sufficient stability to be considered as a serious therapy. Currently synthetic derivatives are being developed to address this problem (Catterall, 2011; Gao, 2010). Several splice variants of Ca_v2 are expressed. Interestingly $Ca_v2.2$ transcripts with exon deletions in the loop between domains II and III have been identified which appear to have a role in determining intracellular targeting/trafficking and hence cellular function.

The Ca_v3 channels have been associated with epilepsy. These channels have a lower membrane potential threshold for opening, are rapidly inactivated and take longer

to deactivate. This means that there is an overlap in the formation of the activated and inactive receptor states so that at any given time a small fraction of Ca_v3 channels are open and do not inactivate at the resting membrane potential. This property enables cells to maintain a sustained increase in cytosolic Ca^{2+} ion levels in excitable tissues like muscle and neurones. Anti-epileptics such as valproic acid and ethosuximide are thought to target thalamic-cortical Ca_v3 channels to reduce the impact of this low but sustained Ca^{2+} current (T-type) that is characteristic of absent epilepsies.

Voltage-gated Na+ channels

Voltage-gated Na^+ channels (Na_v) are required for generation of action potentials in nerves which leads to the release of neurotransmitters at the synapse and neuromuscular junction (see Figures 4.5–4.7) leading to neuronal pathway activation and muscle contraction respectively. They also initiate contraction of cardiac tissue (see Figure 4.8). Therefore their role in pain perception, neuronal pathway activity and cardiac output

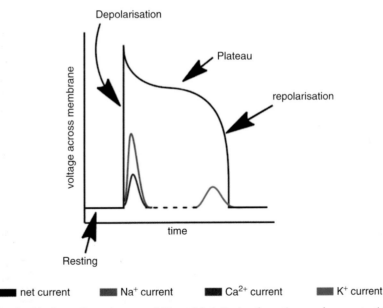

Figure 4.8 Currents involved in the cardiac action potential (ventricles). During the resting membrane potential the heart is in diastole (ventricular relaxation). Rapid depolarisation is due to Na^+ and Ca^{2+} channels opening. This is followed by a transient period of rapid repolarisation as both the Na^+ and Ca^{2+} channels close as well as the transient K^+ channels opening. The membrane voltage then plateaus for a short period of time because some Ca^{2+} channels remain open. Repolarisation occurs mainly due to activation of slow voltage-gated K^+ channels as well as ligand-gated K^+ channels (e.g. inwardly rectify K^+ channels (GIRK), ATP (K_{ATP}) and transient K^+ channels). The characteristic action potential for the ventricles is shown but other heart regions utilise these currents with different V_m / time characteristics.

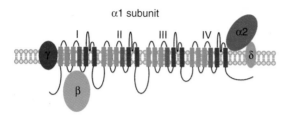

α1 subunit

Figure 4.9 Structure of voltage-gated Ca^{2+} channels. The α1 subunit is responsible for opening and closure of the channel. It has four domains (I-IV) where Ca^{2+} channel modulating drugs bind and hence dictate their pharmacological properties. The α2, β, δ and γ subunits are accessory proteins that modulate activity of the α1 subunit.

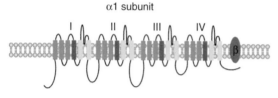

α1 subunit

Figure 4.10 Voltage-gated Na^{+} channel structure. The channel has the characteristic four transmembrane domains (I-IV) each consisting of six transmembrane segments (TMS); the first four TMS are the voltage sensors and the last two TMS form the pore. The accessory protein, β, functions to modify the channel activity. CNS located channels have two β-subunits whereas skeletal muscle has only one β-subunit.

makes them important targets for local anaesthetics, anti-convulsants and antiarrhythmics.

Like all voltage-gated ion channels, these channels are composed of four domains, each of which contain a voltage sensor (TMS_{1-4}) and pore forming region (TMS_{5-6}). These are called the Na_vα1 subunits. An aspartate/glutamate/lysine/alanine (DEKA) motif in the selectivity filter confers Na^{+} ion selectivity upon these channels (see Figure 4.10). To date nine members of this family (Na_v1.1-1.9) have been identified in humans (see Table 4.4). In most family members the voltage-sensing TMS_{1-4} in domains I-III play an important role in pore opening whereas the one in domain IV is involved in inactivating the channel milliseconds after its activation. Na_v channels also have a single β-subunit in skeletal muscle and two β-subunits in the CNS. There are four β-subunit isoforms and their function is to modify the kinetics and voltage dependence of the channel. In fact mutations in β1 have been associated with epilepsy.

Unlike other voltage-gated ion channel families, the Na_v α-subunits share over 50% identity making their pharmacology very similar. So diseases/conditions associated abnormalities in Na_v activity are primarily related to their expression profile rather than differences in their pharmacology. Since they all contribute to action potential initiation, drugs that act at Na_v channels can affect other physiological systems that are not the primary target with severe consequences. In an attempt to identify target specific drugs, venoms have been used extensively to study these channels. It has been shown that a significant number of these toxins that act at Na_v channels appear to interfere with the movement of TMS_4 through the membrane in response to different membrane potentials. Consequently these TMS_4 targeting toxins can also influence the transmembrane movement of TMS_4 in other types of voltage-gated ion channels and hence their ion conductance (see Figure 4.3). Hence drugs that do not target the TMS_4 of Na_v channels would be desirable.

Puffer fish are considered a delicacy in Japan but unfortunately, if not prepared correctly, they can be lethal. This is due to bacteria in the liver and ovaries of this fish (and other marine species) that produce a potent toxin; tetrodotoxin (TTX), which targets Na_v channels. No other voltage-gated ion channel is affected by TTX because it binds to the selectivity filter rather than the voltage sensor. Also, apart from inhibiting Na^{+} ion movement, it does not alter the channels conductance characteristic because it does not bind to the pore domains. In addition, since TTX has a high affinity for fast inactivation Na_v channels compared to slow inactivation ones (e.g. Na_v1.5, Na_v1.8, Na_v1.9) this is a potential avenue for the development of drugs with greater specificity.

Na_v1.5 is the major Na_v found in the heart and it is associated with the depolarisation characteristic of the cardiac action potential (Figure 4.8). It is expressed abundantly in portions of the conducting apparatus of the heart such as the bundle of His, its branches and the Purkinje fibres, and not in the sinoartial and atrioventricular nodes which are associated with cardiac pacing. Thus dysfunction of Na_v1.5 is a cause of ventricular arrhythmias. Patients with mutations in the gene for Na_v1.5 have been associated with a condition called long QT syndrome. Basically the time for ventricle depolarisation and its subsequent repolarisation is elongated. This leads to reduced heart rates (bradycardia) and hence cardiac output which can cause palpitations, fainting and sudden death. Most mutations of Na_v1.5 disrupt the channel's fast inactivation so that the channel re-opens resulting in a persistent inward current during the plateau phase of the cardiac action potential which delays the repolarisation phase (see Figure 4.8). The Na_v blocker, mexiletine, has been used to treat long

QT syndrome but there is evidence that the drug only targets the mutated form of $Na_v1.5$. Hence it is ineffective in patients whose symptoms are not due to an alteration in this gene (Remme and Bezzina, 2010).

Lidocaine, which blocks Na_v channels, is commonly used as an effective local anaesthetic. However, it cannot be used as a general anaesthetic due to inhibition of cardiac Na_v channels. So a number of strategies have been developed to increase target specificity. For example, the design of drugs that cannot cross the blood brain barrier and hence target only peripheral Na_v channels. An alternative approach is to use another receptor, like TRPV1 (see section 4.3), for drug access so that a drug which only targets intracellular Na_v domains can gain entry into the neurone. In this example capsaicin can be used to open the receptor's channel thereby allowing a lidocaine derivative (e.g. QX-314) to enter and only inactivate neuronal Na_v channels thus preventing cardio-related side-effects.

Because of their role in neurotransmission, Na_v channels are targets for pain management. Pain can be perceived due to noxious, thermal and mechanical or chemical stimuli. These stimuli are conveyed to the dorsal root ganglia within the spinal cord by four major types of neurons: Aα, Aβ Aδ and C (Figure 4.11). There are two distinct phases involved in pain perception. The first is an initial sharp sensation which involves the fast conducting fibres responsible for mechano-reception: Aβ and Aδ. This is followed by a more prolonged dull ache due to activation of the slow conduction, nociceptive, C-fibres. Each type of fibre has slightly different characteristic Na^+ ion currents which are thought to be due to the expression of different Na_v channel members. The Na^+ ion currents of C fibres typically have a slightly longer-lasting action potential that has an inflection during the falling phase. There is a preponderance of $Na_v1.8$ and $Na_v1.9$ subtypes in C fibres and this is thought to contribute to this distinctive action potential 'shape'. Evidence suggests that in chronic pain there is an up-regulation of these channels within the dorsal root ganglion. In addition, mediators of inflammation such as prostaglandin E_2 (PGE_2) have been shown to increase the activity of $Na_v1.9$ channels (Rush,

Table 4.4 Na_v channels and their related pathologies.

α1-subunit	Location	Function	Pathologies
$Na_v1.1$	CNS Heart	Initiate AP Repetitive firing EC coupling in cardiac tissue	Epilepsy
$Na_v1.2$	CNS	Initiate and conductance of AP Repetitive firing	Epilepsy
$Na_v1.3$	Embryonic nervous system CNS Heart	Initiate and conductance of AP Repetitive firing	Epilepsy
$Na_v1.4$	Skeletal muscle	Initiate and conductance of AP in skeletal muscle	Periodic paralysismyotonias
$Na_v1.5^*$	Heart	Initiate and conductance of AP	Long QT syndrome Arrhythmias
$Na_v1.6$	Spinal cord Brain	Initiate and conductance of AP	Neurological dysfunction Neuromuscular dysfunction
$Na_v1.7$	Spinal cord	Initiate and conductance of AP	Abnormal pain perception
$Na_v1.8^*$	Spinal cord	Generation of action potential	Hypoalgesia Sensory hypersensitivity
$Na_v1.9^*$	Spinal cord	Sensory perception	Pain

* slow inactivation rates and relatively insensitive to tetratoxin. AP = action potential; EC = Excitation-contraction.

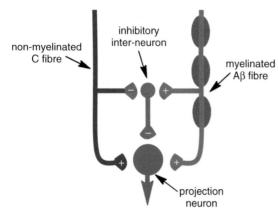

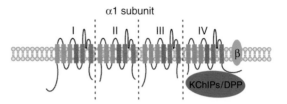

Figure 4.12 Structure of voltage-gated K$^+$ channels. K$_v$ channels are tetramers with the characteristic voltage sensor (TMS$_{1-4}$) and pore forming (TMS$_{5-6}$) domains. Other proteins can alter their activity such as K$^+$ channel interacting proteins (KChIPs) and dipeptidyl aminopeptidase protein (DPP).

Figure 4.11 Pain perception and the role of different neurones in the spinal cord (dorsal root ganglion). Normally, nociceptive C fibres are activated first. It synapses onto the projection neurone which sends an impulse to the pain perception areas in the brain and we perceive pain. The C-fibre also sends out a branch to an inhibitory interneuron. This synapse is inhibitory (as indicated by red) so that the inhibitory interneuron is not activated. When the mechano-receptive Aβ fibres are activated they too stimulate the projection fibre. However, the output of the projection neuron is reduced because a branch of the Aβ fibre also activates the inhibitory interneuron which reduces the projection neuron's activity. So the amount of pain perceived is a balance between C fibre and Aβ activity.

Cummins and Waxman, 2007; Theile and Cummins, 2011). As Figure 4.11 shows, an increase in the activity of the C fibres results in greater pain perception because of its ability to increase the projection neurone output by preventing inhibitory neurons from damping down projection neurone activity. This increased signal results in greater pain perception by enhancing activity in areas of the brain responsible for processing this type of signal.

The μO-conotoxin, MrVIB, has been shown to have very high selectivity for Na$_v$1.8 channels. Derivatives of this venom are currently being developed for treatment of neuropathic pain. No specific toxins that target Na$_v$1.9 have been identified. However, whilst there is a high degree of identity between Na$_v$ members, Na$_v$1.9 shows the least similarity and is thus an exciting avenue for development of drugs involved in pain management (Theile and Cummins, 2011).

Voltage-Gated K$^+$ channels

The fruit fly, drosophila melanogaster, has provided an invaluable insight into the function of many genes. Mutated genotypes have produced some interesting phenotypes which have immortalised these genes with names

such as dishevelled and sexy. One gene that produced flies with an abnormal response to anaesthetics, whereby their legs shook, was called 'shaker'. This gene turned out to be a voltage-gated K$^+$ channel (K$_v$) and was the first K$_v$ channel to be cloned. Since then 40 K$_v$ genes have been identified and grouped into 12 classes: K$_v$1-K$_v$12 (Table 4.5). Like all voltage-gated ion channels, K$_v$'s are composed of four subunit domains (I-IV; α1 subunit) with each domain consisting of voltage-sensing TMS$_{1-4}$ and TMS$_{5-6}$ pore forming regions (see Figure 4.12). As with other K$^+$ channels, K$_v$ channels have a tripeptide sequence motif, glycine(tyrosine/phenylalanine)glycine (GY/FG) in the selectivity filter loop between TMS$_{5-6}$ that confers K$^+$ ion selectivity. There is considerable functional diversity between members of the K$_v$1, K$_v$7 and K$_v$10 families because not only can they form homotetramers, but they can also form heterotetramers between different subunits within the same family. Furthermore, members of K$_v$4, K$_v$5, K$_v$8 and K$_v$9 can form heterotetramers with members of the K$_v$2 family to modify their activity. In addition, the α1-subunit (K$_v$) can interact with a number of accessory proteins which can alter the channel's activity. Another source of K$_v$ diversity is due to some genes having the potential to produce alternative splice variants (e.g. K$_v$3, K$_v$4, K$_v$6, K$_v$7, K$_v$9, K$_v$10 and K$_v$11).

Channels, like many membrane proteins, have a number of conformational states. The three basic states include: activated, non-activated and inactivated. This is important because some drugs will only bind to a particular conformation. For example, K$^+$ ion channels inactivate after their initial activation which means that depolarisation is maintained but no ions are conducted through the pore. At least two distinct inactivation states have been identified for K$_v$ channels. The first is where the N-terminus of the protein subunits quickly interacts with the cytosolic side of the pore in a 'ball and chain' fashion (C-type). The second type involves a slow but

Table 4.5 K_v channels function and related pathologies.

α1-subunit	Location	Function	Pathologies
K_v1 (8)*	CNS, Node of Ranvier, lymphocytes ($K_v1.3$), cardiac, skeletal and smooth muscle	Neurotransmission Ca^{2+} signalling in lymphocytes Cardiac and vascular activity movement	Seizures/epilepsy Pain Diabetes Arrhythmias
K_v2 (2)*	CNS, pancreas, cardiac, skeletal and smooth muscle	Neurotransmission Metabolism	Diabetes Hypertension
K_v3 (4)*	CNS, pancreas, skeletal muscle	Neurotransmission Metabolism	Ataxia Epilepsy
K_v4 (3)*	Heart, CNS, smooth muscle	Neurotransmission Cardiac and vascular activity	Inflammatory pain Arrhythmias Epilepsy
K_v5 (1)*	Interact with K_v2 subunits to modify or silencers their activity.		
K_v6 (4)*	Interact with K_v2 subunits to modify or silencers their activity.		
K_v7 (5)*	Heart, ear, skeletal muscle, CNS, auditory hair cells	Ventricular contraction neurotransmission	Diabetes Deafness Pain Arrhythmias
K_v8 (2)*	Interact with K_v2 subunits to modify or silencers their activity.		
K_v9 (3)*	Interact with K_v2 subunits to modify or silencers their activity.		
K_v10 (2)*	CNS, muscle, heart	Neurotransmission	Cancers Seizures
K_v11 (3)*	Heart, endocrine	Neurotransmission Heart rate	Arrhythmias Cancer
K_v12 (3)*	CNS	Neurotransmission	Epilepsy

*indicates the number of family members.

incomplete constriction of the pore (N-type) (Snyders, 1999). Drugs that act at the N-type inactivated channel will allow a slow K^+ ion current leak whereas those that target C-type inactivation will stop any current. Both types of inactivation are of physiological relevance. That is, if you need to maintain a membrane potential without depolarisation, the partial activation of a few K^+ ion channels is necessary; whereas, on the other hand, if you want fast recovery from inactivation in neurones that have high firing rates this C type inactivation would be inappropriate. In the cardiac action potential both types of inactivation play a critical role in the plateau and repolarisation phases, while slow inactivation receptors are involved in endocrine secretions.

K_v1 channels play vital roles in neurotransmission by maintaining the membrane potential. They also help to control neuronal excitability by affecting the duration, intensity and frequency of action potentials. Indirectly they can influence neurotransmitter release by hyperpolarising the membrane and thus preventing Ca_v channels from opening. Since members of this family tend to form heterotetramers rather than homotetramers there is a huge range of functional K_v1 channels each with slightly different kinetics. In neurons, $K_v1.2$ type channels are the most abundantly expressed type followed by $K_v1.1$. Both of these subtypes are axonally located, low-voltage activated channels that function to increase the threshold for depolarisation.

RNA editing plays a role in $K_v1.1$ function. In mammals, a highly conserved isoleucine within the pore of the channel can be changed to a valine. This substitution results in a channel with a recovery time from inactivation approximately 20 times faster and hence an ability to sustain much higher firing rates. In fact,

$K_v1.1$ channels containing this valine are found in brain regions with extremely fast firing rates like the medulla, thalamus and spinal cord (Gonzalez et al., 2011). Other congenital mutations in $K_v1.1$ result in problems with coordination, balance and speech which are probably related to a decrease in the ability of certain neurones to fire sufficiently fast.

The $K_v1.3$ channel has been implicated in the regulation of a host of physiological functions, such as neuronal excitability, neurotransmitter release, regulation of cell volume, cell proliferation and apoptosis. $K_v1.3$ channels also play a role in T-lymphocyte cell activation and hence immune surveillance. Basically a rise in intracellular Ca^{2+} ions is essential for activation of the T-cell. This increase in Ca^{2+} ions is due to release from internal stores as well as an influx through Ca^{2+} channels. The $K_v1.3$ channels can open because they have a sigmoidal voltage dependence response, allowing K^+ ions to efflux whilst maintaining the membrane potential. In other words, $K_v1.3$ channels function to sustain a Ca^{2+} ions influx without depolarising the membrane. This makes the $K_v1.3$ channel an attractive target for development of therapies for chronic inflammation and autoimmune disorders (Cahalan and Chandy, 2009). Some venoms from scorpions and sea anemone target the $K_v1.3$ channel. However, these peptides appear to behave slightly differently in rodents compared to humans and may partially explain why they lack specificity or potency to be effective immunosuppressive treatments.

The $K_v1.3$, $K_v1.4$, $K_v1.6$, $K_v2.1$, and $K_v3.2$ subunits are expressed in pancreatic β-cells. These K_v channels function to counter the depolarising action of increased intracellular Ca^{2+} ion levels whilst maintaining the membrane potential. They therefore play a role in controlling the secretion of insulin. $K_v1.3$ is of particular interest as a novel target for boosting insulin production in the treatment of type 2 diabetes. Since mutations in the gene for $K_v1.3$ also decrease body weight in normal and obese animal models, this gene is considered a target for anti-obesity drugs (Choi and Hahn, 2010).

Atrial fibrillation can cause cardiac arrhythmias that if untreated can increase the risk of stroke as well as congestive heart failure. However, ventricular fibrillation is far more prevalent and can lead to sudden death. K_v4 activity results in a transient outward current and is involved in the early phase of repolarisation whereas strong inwardly rectifying currents are responsible for the latter phase of cardiac repolarisation. Manipulation of the ultra-rapidly activating $K_v1.5$ channel, which is an inwardly rectifying current, can alter the duration of repolarisation. Therefore it is a possible candidate for the treatment of atrial fibrillation. And since it is expressed in atria and not the ventricles it will have no effect on ventricular output (Islam, 2010).

A number of congenital diseases are associated with the K_v7 family. These channels have a reduced threshold, are slowly activating and deactivating, and do not inactivate. Therefore they limit the amount of repetitive firing in neurones. A reduction in firing rates explains their contribution to epilepsy ($K_v7.2$), deafness ($K_v7.3$) and age-related hearing loss ($K_v7.4$). Linopiridine and its derivatives have K_v7 selectivity and have been shown to improve cognition in rodents. However the nonspecific characteristics of this blocker are an impetus for development of drugs that target specific K_v7 members. (Miceli et al., 2008).

The channel $K_v10.1$ (and $K_v1.3$) is involved in cell proliferation. Normally it is expressed exclusively in neuronal tissue but it is present in over 70% of all tumours, including ones of non-neuronal origin, suggesting a role in tumour progression. K_v10 inhibitors have also been shown to reduce tumour progression. Whether it helps in maintaining depolarisation of the cell membrane during the G1 phase of the cell cycle and somehow 'helps' uncontrolled cell growth remains to be determined. Nevertheless, it may prove useful as a potential biomarker for cancerous tissue (Stühmer and Walter, 2006).

$K_v11.1$ plays a similar role to $K_v1.5$ in atrial repolarisation and has been implicated in long and short QT syndrome. It has also been shown to be involved in endocrine secretions, cell proliferation, neuronal outgrowth and cardiac function.

An array of accessory proteins that can modulate K_v activity have been identified and have been shown to play just as an important role in K_v activity as the α1 (K_v) subunit. For example $K_vβ$ family members cause the rapid inactivation of some K_v channels that are usually resistant to inactivation as well as conferring pathological phenotypes (e.g. in combination with shaker; $K_v1.1$). In mammals, three genes encode for the $K_vβ$ family (β1-β3) to produce a number of splice variants that can interact with members of the K_v1 and K_v2 families. In general the $K_vβ$ subunits not only influence activation and inactivation times, they can also facilitate $K_vα$ trafficking and responses to drugs.

K^+ channel interacting proteins (KChIPs) and dipeptidyl aminopeptidase protein (DPP) are other accessory proteins that can alter the activity of K_v4 channels. Whilst all members of the KChIPs family (1–4) and DDP (6 and 10) can inactivate the K_v channel, subtle changes in duration of channel opening, rates of activation and inactivation can give rise to a multitude of K_v4 channels with slightly different gating properties. Interestingly, since K_v4 plays a major role in both the timing and frequency of neuronal excitability as well as the cardiac action potential, alteration in their activity could reduce the threshold potential for opening and hence action potential firing. Other accessory proteins include calmodulin and mink which can modulate the activity of the K_v10 and K_v11 families respectively.

4.3 Other types of voltage-gated ion channels

Determining the crystalline structure of membrane embedded proteins is difficult because the conditions for crystallisation either favour the hydrophilic or hydrophobic moieties. Since bacterial homologues usually have a simpler structure, with fewer post-translational modifications they are easier to crystallise. The bacterial K^+ channel, KcsA, has provided invaluable insight into how the pore of this channel functions. Like the K_v channels, KcsA channels are tetramers. Basically the pore region of a KcsA subunit consists of two TMS with an re-entrant loop (P-loop) that helps form the channel between both TMS. There are up to five K^+ ion binding sites within the pore/selectivity filter that facilitate K^+ ions conductance.

Subsequent studies have shown that this pore structure is common to all K^+ channels as well as being similar for Na^+ and Ca^{2+} channels. Interestingly many of these other ion channels are not voltage dependent but require the binding of a ligand/modulator for activation. It appears that these channels have evolved from a common ancestor which has the pore domain consisting of 2 TMS and a P-loop and that sequences have been added to confer different mechanisms of activation: for example, a voltage sensor (TMS_{1-4}), a Ca^{2+} ion binding domain or a ligand binding domain. Alterations in the ion-specific sequence motif in the selectivity filter of these channels can all determine which ions are conducted through the channel. These other types of K^+ channels are discussed in the next sections.

Ca²⁺-activated K⁺ channels

Ca^{2+}-activated K^+ (K_{Ca}) channels contain the voltage sensitive TMS_{1-4} regions but most family members are not activated by changes in the membrane voltage. Instead they respond to changes in the intracellular Ca^{2+} ion concentration. When activated they allow K^+ ions to efflux to either repolarise or hyperpolarise the cell membrane. This causes Ca_v channels to become deactivated (and stimulates the Na^+/Ca^{2+} exchanger to pump Ca^{2+} ions out of the cytosol) thereby limiting the intracellular

concentration of Ca^{2+} ions. Therefore K_{Ca} channels play a role in determining the amplitude and duration of Ca^{2+} transients and the downstream signalling pathways that perturbations in Ca^{2+} ion concentration influence.

Eight members of the K_{Ca} family have been identified, but three of them ($K_{Ca}4.1$, $K_{Ca}4.2$ and $K_{Ca}5.1$) are not regulated by Ca^{2+} ions and are only included by virtue of the fact they share considerable structural homology with the other K_{Ca} channel. Despite this, K_{Ca} channels can be grouped into two classes based on their conductance and voltage sensitivity. Members of the BK_{Ca} family, like $K_{Ca}1.1$, have big K^+ ion conductance which is membrane potential dependent. Whereas SK_{Ca} members, such as $K_{Ca}2$ and $K_{Ca}3$, are regulated by changes in Ca^{2+} ion concentration, have small K^+ ion conductance and their activation/inactivation is voltage-independent.

Scorpion toxins, charybdotoxin and iberiotoxin, block BK_{Ca} channels and have proved useful in determining their properties. In smooth muscle, BK_{Ca} channels operate to reduce the activity of Ca_v1 channels and hence promote muscle relaxation. BK_{Ca} channels also contain a β accessory subunit of which there are four types ($BK\beta1$-4) that serve to modulate channel activity as well as trafficking. BK_{Ca} channels in many tissues such as the brain or adrenal glands are either associated with or without a $BK\beta$ subunit. Cells containing $BK_{Ca}/BK\beta$ channels are involved in repetitive or tonic firing patterns because their activity produces a pronounced after-hyperpolarisation which causes Na_v channels to exit their inactive state and depolarise the membrane. In contrast, other cells with BK_{Ca} channels that possess no $BK\beta$ accessory subunit are rapidly inactivated and therefore create only a small after-hyperpolarisation and hence a more phasic pattern of firing. Evidence is emerging where the BK_{Ca} channels actually participate in a complex with the Ca_v channels at presynaptic membranes to enhance signal transduction between each receptor type (Berkefeld, Fakler and Schulte, 2010).

Whilst BK_{Ca} channels have a Ca^{2+} ion sensing/binding domain in the cytosolic loop after TMS_6, SK_{Ca} channels utilise the Ca^{2+} dependent protein, calmodulin, as its Ca^{2+} sensor at this site (see Figure 4.13). Since there are a number of intermediate steps leading to channel activation and the fact that calmodulin is not rapidly inactivated once Ca^{2+} ions dissociate, the SK_{Ca} channel opens more slowly, and for longer. So physiologically, the SK_{Ca} channel can function as a pacemaker to reduce firing rates in central neurons. Since it can also respond to low rises in Ca^{2+} ion concentration it can limit Ca^{2+} ion post-synaptic influx to fine tune the excitatory post-synaptic potential. This is seen in neurones undergoing NMDA

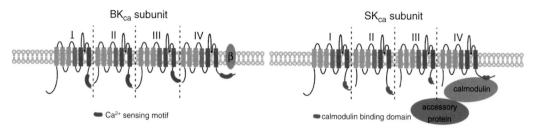

Figure 4.13 Structure of Ca^{2+}-activated K^+ channels. BK_{Ca} have a Ca^{2+} ion sensor whereas SK_{Ca} respond to the Ca^{2+} dependent protein, calmodulin.

receptor-mediated synaptic plasticity (see section 4.4). Here membrane depolarisation removes a Mg^{2+} ion block for the NMDA receptor allowing Ca^{2+} ions to influx through the receptor's channel. But the hyper-polarising effect of SK_{Ca} channel activity can stop this Ca^{2+} current because the Mg^{2+} ion can interact with the NMDA receptor again to block the NMDA receptors' Ca^{2+} channel. SK_{Ca} channels can also interact with accessory proteins that can alter the channel's activity. Like its activator, calmodulin, many of these accessory proteins are also targets of kinases. This can explain why activation of GPCRs like β-adrenergic receptors can reduce SK_{Ca} channel activity; the G-protein interacts with an accessory protein which in turn reduces calmodulin's affinity for Ca^{2+} ions. The ability of other receptor types to alter SK_{Ca} activity is an exciting avenue for drug development (Berkefeld, Fakler and Schulte, 2010).

CatSper channels

CatSper receptors derived their name from the fact that they were first isolated as putative cation channels in sperm. Four members have so far been identified: catSper1-4. Each subunit has the classical six TMS which comprises of voltage sensitive and channel-forming domains. The voltage sensor appears to be functional as it has a charged residue every third position in TMS_4. In addition, the amino end of TMS_1 in catSper1 contains a histidine rich region that can act as an indicator of pH. The pore-forming TMS_{5-6} domain has a selectivity filter that is classic for Ca^{2+} ion permeability. CatSper channel subunits are expressed as monomers (Ren and Dejian, 2010) and like all other voltage sensitive channels form a tetrameric subunit structure (see Figure 4.14). A number of accessory proteins have been associated with catSper channels including catSperβ, catSperδ and catSperγ. In addition, catSper channels have been shown to cluster around other types of receptors: for example GCPR and CNG (cyclic nucleotide-gated ion channels) (Brenker,

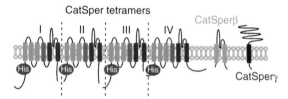

Figure 4.14 Structure of a catSper channel (catSper1) with accessory proteins catSperβ and catSperγ. Four subunits are required for functionality.

2012). This may allow activation of secondary messenger Ca^{2+} ion signalling pathways that are independent of receptor ligand binding.

CatSper1 and 2 are found in the tail of sperm cells and there is growing evidence that they play a vital role in male fertility. For reproduction to be successful sperm must swim to, and fertilise, the ovum. The tail region of sperm contains Ca^{2+}-dependent motor proteins that facilitate this process. In many cells the endoplasmic reticulum functions as a Ca^{2+} ion store so that there is a readily available source of Ca^{2+} ions. However, sperm do not possess an endoplasmic reticulum and instead the mitochondria can act as a small intracellular Ca^{2+} ion store. Since 'swimming' requires a significant amount of energy the mitochondria's primary function is to produce ATP rather than as a Ca^{2+} ion store; high mitochondrial Ca^{2+} ion concentrations destabilise the electron transport chain and hence interfere with oxidative phosphorylation. Therefore an external source of Ca^{2+} ions is required and this is where catSper channels come into play. Their channel's voltage sensor detects a change in membrane potential due to the slightly alkaline environment within the Fallopian tubes, causing them to open, and thus allowing for Ca^{2+} ion influx. In man, polymorphisms in catSper channels have been linked with male infertility. Therefore an understanding of catSper channels pharmacology could lead to treatments for male infertility.

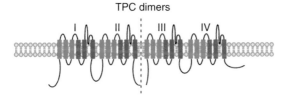

Figure 4.15 Structure of TPC. Two subunits need to dimerise for functionality.

Two-pore channels

Since K_v, catSper and transient receptor (TRP) channels have one TMD whereas Na_v and Ca_v channels have four TMD it is believed that Na_v/Ca_v channels evolved from K_v, catSper, TRP or a similar ancestral gene (see Figure 4.1). For this to have occurred, two duplication events must have occurred. The two pore calcium channels (TPC) have two TMD and are thought to have arisen due to the first duplication event. TPCs, like the aforementioned channels consist of four TMD, each of which is composed of six TMS. That is, functional TPC assemble as dimers (see Figure 4.15).

Three TPC channels (TPC1-3) have been cloned so far. However, TPC3 is not expressed in man or other primates. They have a similar structure to catSper channels but they are expressed in high levels in kidney, liver and lung tissue. Emerging evidence suggests that they play a role in Ca^{2+} ion release from acidic organelles such as endosomes, lysomes and secretory vesicles. They are thought to mediate Ca^{2+} ion release in a similar manner to the IP_3 receptor in that they increase cytosolic Ca^{2+} ion concentrates by enabling release from internal stores in response to the metabolic demands of the cell. TPC1 (and TPC3) are primarily associated with endosomal release whereas TPC2 controls Ca^{2+} ion release from lysomes. Interestingly TPC2 has two binding sites for the metabolite NAADP (a derivative of NADP, which is an important factor in metabolism); a low and a high affinity site (Patel, 2011). This means that they can mediate biphasic Ca^{2+} ion release as in the case of calcium induced calcium release (CICR) as seen in cardiac muscle (see Figure 4.6; (Zhu, 2010). TPC have also been implicated in sperm motility and hence fertility. Whether this is due to interplay between catSper channels and TPC remains to be determined.

Inwardly rectifying K⁺ channels

The inwardly rectifying K^+ (K_{ir}) channels (Figure 4.16), like other K^+ channels' family members, are responsible for K^+ ion efflux. They play an important role in

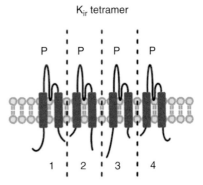

Figure 4.16 K_{ir} structure. Each subunit has two TMS and a re-entrant P loop. Four subunits are required for functionality.

maintaining neuronal activity by establishing and maintaining the membrane potential. In the cardiac cycle, K_v channels play a predominant role in the initial repolarisation of cardiac myocytes (Figure 4.8), but toward the end of this phase it is the activity of K_{ir} channels which re-establish the membrane potential and muscle relaxation. K_{ir} channels are expressed in glial cells, neurones, epithelia and endothelial cells, osteoclasts, oocytes, blood cell, as well as cardiac myocytes.

Since G-protein gated K^+ (K_G) and ATP-sensitive K^+ (K_{ATP}) channels facilitate the efflux of K^+ ions they are also members of the K_{ir} family. So far, 15 genes encoding K_{ir} subunits for seven subfamilies ($K_{ir}1.x$- $K_{ir}7.x$) have been identified and these can be assigned to one of four groups based on their function: classical K_{ir} channels ($K_{ir}2.x$), K_G channels ($K_{ir}3.x$), K_{ATP} channels ($K_{ir}6.x$) and K^+-transport channels ($K_{ir}1.x$ $K_{ir}4.x$ $K_{ir}5.x$ and $K_{ir}7.x$). Functional channels can be formed by hetero- or homo-tetramerisation within subfamilies, giving rise to a myriad of K_{ir} channel types with slightly different properties. Interestingly the $K_{ir}4.1$ and $K_{ir}5.1$ subunits are an exception to this as they can only hetero-tetramerise to form active K_{ir} channels. (Ashcroft and Gribble, 2000)

K_{ir} channels become active at hyperpolarising but not depolarising membrane potentials. Hence they have voltage-related activity. Since these channels only allow the flow of K^+ ions out of the cell, they are known as rectifying channels. This directional conductance is due to the interaction of Mg^{2+} ions and/or polyamines with motifs within the pore which prevent K^+ ions from inffluxing. Other factors also regulate the size of the K^+ ion conductance through K_{ir} channels. For example, decreasing the extracellular concentration of K^+ ions decreases the current. Protein kinases can also ameliorate K_{ir} channel function as well as the presence of the anchoring protein, phosphatidylinositol 4,5-bisphosphate (PIP_2). And some scaffolding proteins like, PSD_{95}, play a role in determining subcellular compartment distribution.

K_{ATP} channels ($K_{ir}6$) are regulated by ATP with high intracellular concentration of ATP causing the channel to close and low concentrations (or high nucleotide-diphosphate levels) facilitating its opening. K_{ATP} channels need to complex with an atypical transporter (see Chapter 5) called the sulfonylurea receptor (SUR) for functionality. Basically when the concentration of glucose is high, ATP levels are high due to oxidative phosphorylation. If this occurs in pancreatic β-cells then the elevated ATP production causes K_{ir} channel closure and the membrane starts to depolarise due to K^+ ion leakage. This is detected by Ca_v channels which open. The elevation in intracellular Ca^{2+} ion concentration results in the exocytosis of vesicles containing insulin and its secretion into the blood stream. Conversely, reduced glucose levels means less insulin secretion due to K_{ir} opening as a consequence of low ATP levels. For this reason SURs and $K_{ir}6$ channels have been implicated in hypoglycaemia and noninsulin-dependent (type 2) diabetes mellitus.

K_{ATP} ($K_{ir}6.x$/SUR) channels also function in cardiac muscle. Here the channel is usually closed but in periods of low ATP levels, such as increased work load, hypoxia or ischaemia, binding of ADP to the nucleotide binding domain (NBD) of SUR causes the channels to open. The resultant K^+ ion efflux hyperpolarises the membrane and prevents Ca_v channels from opening. This reduces cardiac output by decreasing cardiac action potential duration as well as ATP utilisation. A similar scenario is seen with smooth muscle and promotion of relaxation.

Like $K_{ir}6$, SURs are encoded by two genes (SUR1 and SUR2) and a number of splice variants are expressed with slightly different properties. They are considered atypical transporters because even though they have the classic ABC transporter structure (see section 5.4) there is no evidence that they actually transport substrates across membranes. They are thought to sense the concentration of ATP/ADP through their NBD. This, coupled with binding of ATP directly to the $K_{ir}6$ channel, is thought to enhance sensitivity to the metabolic status of the cell.

Inhibitors including sulfonylureas are used exclusively for diabetes treatment. Interestingly, the effects on other physiological systems are minimal. This specificity is probably due to the fact that $K_{ir}6.1$/SUR1 are preferentially expressed in pancreatic cells, $K_{ir}6.2$/SUR2A in the heart, $K_{ir}6.1$/SUR2B in smooth muscle and $K_{ir}6.2$/SUR1/SUR2 in the brain. Stimulators of K_{ATP}

channels are known as K^+ channel openers (KCO) and include pinacidil, nicroandil and diazoxide. These are used to treat heart and vascular disease as they can reduce cardiac muscle contraction as well as induce vasodilation for the treatment of hypertension and its related diseases. Whilst KCOs are used predominately to treat cardiovascular pathologies a few have been used to treat baldness. Minoxidil was initially developed for the management of high blood pressure but at sub-therapeutic anti-hypertensive concentrations it is thought to aid vascularisation of the hair follicle and thus promote hair growth (Hibino et al., 2010).

There are four genes ascribed to the K_G ($K_{ir}3$) family with each expressing numerous splice variants. Basically the activation of pertussis toxin sensitive G_i-protein coupled receptors (GPCR) results in the release of G-protein α and βγ subunits, with the latter activating K_G ($K_{ir}3$) channels. For this reason K_G channels are also known as GIRKs (G-protein-gated inwardly rectify K^+) channels. K_G channel activation leads to an efflux of K^+ ions and hyperpolarisation of the membrane. For example activation of muscarinic cholinergic receptors leads to βγ subunit release and subsequent K_G-mediated hyperpolarisation. If this occurs at the neuromuscular junction then there is no Ca^{2+} influx through Ca_v channels and hence no muscle contraction. So, depending upon the type of muscle, this could result in decreased cardiac output (cardiac), decreased movement (skeletal) or vasodilation (smooth). In addition, the pace-making areas of the heart can be altered due to reduced excitability/conductance. Activation of GPCR and subsequent K_G channel activation can also interfere with neurotransmission by reducing neurotransmitter release pre-synaptically or preventing action potential propagate in the post-synaptic neurone.

There is evidence that the $K_{ir}3$ channels, upon activation, cluster in lipid raft/caveoli (see section 11.10) with their GPCR (e.g. $GABA_B$, dopamine, acetylcholine receptors) as well as Ca_v channels. This compartmentalisation gives rise to more effective signal transduction that can efficiently couple GCPR action to Ca^{2+}-mediated neurotransmitter or peptide release through altered $K_{ir}3$ activity. The duration of K_G channel activity is dependent upon how long the βγ-subunit remains dissociated from the α-subunit with a number of factors that can delay or enhance re-association. These factors are discussed in Chapter 3.

$K_{ir}3.4$/$K_{ir}3.1$ heterotetramers are expressed in cardiac tissue and the hypothalamus where they are involved in controlling cardiac output and pituitary secretions whereas heterotetramers of $K_{ir}3.1$/$K_{ir}3.2$, $K_{ir}3.2$/$K_{ir}3.3$,

$K_{ir}3.1/K_{ir}3.3$ and homotetramers of $K_{ir}3.2/K_{ir}3.2$ are expressed in the brain. These neuronal located $K_{ir}3$ channels are associated with problems in neuronal firing rates leading to conditions such as epilepsy, Parkinson's disease and ataxia. Interestingly, the $K_{ir}3.2$ gene is located on chromosome 21 and sufferers of Down's syndrome have an extra copy of this gene. And since animal models with an extra $K_{ir}3.2$ have abnormal hyperpolarising currents that are mediated by $GABA_B$ receptors it is thought that this gene duplication may contribute to the abnormal brain functions/development associated with Down's syndrome. However care should be taken with the interpretation of these results as chromosome 21 contains many other genes. Clustering of dopamine or opioid receptors with $K_{ir}3$ channels in the reward pathway have raised the possibility that they could be involved in the development of drug addiction. Removal of the genes that encode for $K_{ir}3$ subunits gives rise to mice with reduced drug addictive phenotypes adding credence to this theory (Luscher and Slesinger, 2010).

The other members of the K_{ir} channel family ($K_{ir}1$, $K_{ir}4$, $K_{ir}5$ and $K_{ir}7$) make up the remaining subfamily: K^+ transport channels. $K_{ir}1.1$ and $K_{ir}4.1/K_{ir}5.1$ channels play vital roles in urine and blood homeostasis by closely regulating the movement of ions such as K^+, Na^+ and Cl^- across the renal medullary membrane. Basically $K_{ir}1$ and $K_{ir}4.1/K_{ir}5.1$ channels maintain the K^+ ion gradient which is vital for $Na^+/K^+/2Cl^-$ symporter and Na^+/K^+-ATPase activity respectively (transporters are discussed in Chapter 5). Gene mutations in the $K_{ir}1.1$ subunit lead to Bartter's syndrome which is a loss of function disease where patients have impaired kidney function owing to an inability to reabsorb Na^+ ions due to the diminished K^+ ion gradient. Like $K_{ir}1.1$, $K_{ir}7.1$ has been shown to cluster with the Na^+/K^+ ATPase transporter in epithelia cells but little is known about its physiological function.

The 'recycling of K^+ ions' by $K_{ir}4$ and $K_{ir}5.1$ channels also occurs in the ear. Here they function to maintain a higher concentration of K^+ ions in the endolymph (cytosol) compared to the perilymph (extracellular) compartments of the cochlear. This is important for maintaining the membrane potential and impairment of these channels' activity leads to deafness. These channels can also cluster with aquaporins (AQP) so that as K^+ ions efflux, water molecules also move out of the cell via their AQP channel due to osmotic pull. This movement of water helps maintain the osmotic pressure of the extracellular and intracellular fluids. $K_{ir}4$ and $K_{ir}5.1$ channels, that are clustered with AQP at sites adjacent to

blood vessels, facilitates the movement of water into the extracellular space and its entry into the blood stream.

$K_{ir}4.1/K_{ir}5.1$ channels help maintain the ionic and osmotic composition of the extracellular space. During neuronal excitation the concentration of K^+ ions is high, so these K_{ir} channels are activated enabling the K^+ ions to move down this gradient into the glial cells, otherwise the high extracellular K^+ ion concentration would destabilise the membrane potential resulting in continuous depolarisation. There is evidence that $K_{ir}4.1$ channels also cluster with the glutamate transporter (see section 5.4) in glial cells which symports two Na^+ and one H^+ and antiports an ion K^+ during glutamate uptake. Here the K_{ir} channel would maintain a K^+ ion gradient to facilitate glutamate uptake.

Transient receptor potential channels

Transient receptor potential (TRP) channels are cation channels that comprise of 28 members that can be grouped into six subfamilies: canonical, TRPC; vanilloid, TRPV; melastatin, TRPM; ankyrin, TRPA; polycystin, TRPP; and mucolipin, TRPML (see Table 4.6). Generally TRP channels are nonselective for K^+, Na^+ or Ca^{2+} ions although some can be more selective for Ca^{2+} (TRPV5 and TRPV6) or Na^+ ions (TRPM4 and TRPM5). TRPML1 and TRPV6 can also conduct Fe^{2+} and Mg^{2+} ions respectively. All TRP channels have the characteristic TMS_4 for voltage sensitivity. However, there are fewer charged arginine residues in this region than the Ca_v, K_v and Na_v channels and hence their sensitivity to membrane potential is severely diminished. Most TRP channels respond to changes in temperature and hence their roles in thermoception and inflammation. TRP channels usually assemble as homotetramers although there are a few examples of heterotetramers (Figure 4.17).

The TRP channel family play roles in a diverse number of physiological processes which include nociception, control of bladder function, skin physiology and respiration, as well as all aspects of sensation, including vision, olfaction, mechanosensation, thermosensation and nociception. Since they have relatively low protein identity between family members compared to other voltage-gated ion channels there is greater potential to develop drugs that target specific members. In fact TRP channels are a huge target for drug development by pharmaceutical companies with a number of compounds already in clinical trials as discussed below.

Probably the best known TRP channel is TRPV1 because of its role in perceiving the spicy hot flavour in chilli peppers (capsaicin). As well as developing TPRV1

Table 4.6 Classification of TRP channels and associated pathophysiology.

TRP channel Family	Members	Functions/Pathologies
Canonical TRPC	TRPC1-7	↑weight, ↓saliva secretions, altered sexual/mating behaviour, ataxia, altered vascular function, ↓anxiety
Vanilloid TRPV	TRPV1-6	Abnormal osmolarity ⇒ associated problems, ↓inflammation-mediate hyperalgesia, ↓bladder function, immunocompromised, skin problems, abnormal thermosensation, renal problem, ↓bone density, sensitivity to capsaicin (chillies)
Melastatin TRPM	TRPM1-8	Immunocompromised, visual defects, abnormal thermosensation, embryonic development
Ankyrin TRPA	TRPA1	↓skin sensations, ↑inflammation-mediate hyperalgesia
Polycystin TRPP	TRPP1-3	Polycystic kidney disease, embryonic development
Mucolipin TRPML	TRPML1-3	Mucolipidosis, motor defects, visual defects

Adapted by permission from Macmillan Publishers Ltd: Nature, Moran, copyright 2011.

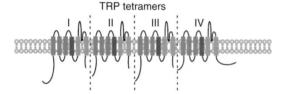

TRP tetramers

Figure 4.17 TRP channel structure. Four subunits (I-IV) need to combine to form a functional channel.

specific agonists and antagonists, pharmacologists have tried to exploit the fact that TPRV1 rapidly desensitise by designing compounds that encourage the channel to enter into, and stay in, the inactive form. Such drugs can then be used as analgesics for the management of pain. In fact, topical application of capsaicin and similar compounds in creams has been used for many years in the treatment of muscular pain. However, clinical trials with systemic antagonists have failed because TPRV1 channels also mediate thermoception; inhibiting the channel can cause potentially life threatening hyperthermia. Interestingly TRPM8 channels are co-located with TPRV1 channels in the skin and rather than responding to high temperatures they play a role in sensing cold temperatures. This means that both channels can act in concert to detect the full range of environmental temperatures.

The TRPV3 channel is also implicated in inflammatory pain. It is thought to act as a convergence point for multiple pathways involved in pain perception. For example, histamine and bradykinin (GPCR agonists) and alterations in Ca^{2+} ion concentrations can ameliorate TRPV3 activity. Drugs that target TRPA1 channels have also been developed to treat pain associated with inflammation because of the link between mutations in the gene and heightened pain perception in cold, fasting and fatiguing situations.

TRPV1 and TRPV4 are found in the bladder where they are activated by physical stretching when the bladder is full as well as the presence of hypo-osmotic urine. They function via sensory neurones to tell us when our bladder is full and hence facilitate micturition. Development of drugs that target these channels may be useful in the treatment of urinary retention and incontinence. Currently the agonist, resiniferatoxin is used to treat daily incontinence by desensitising the TRPV1 channel within the bladder and thereby effectively increasing the bladder's capacity. Resiniferatoxin therapy may also be an effective treatment for the pain and increased frequency of urination associated with interstitial cystitis.

TRP channels, particularly TRPV1 and TRPV3, play a major role in the skin where they are involved in temperature sensation, mediating and detecting inflammation, differentiation, proliferation and apoptosis of the various cell types, production of the epidermal barrier (in addition to TRPV4 and TRPV6), and mediating hair growth. TRPM7 is associated with melanogenesis whilst TRPC1 and TRPC4 may have an anti-tumour effect. So, targeting of these receptors with topical creams could have a beneficial effect on general skin health.

In the lungs, TRP channels are found in the smooth muscle of the airways (TRPC3 and TRPV4) and blood vessels (TRPC6) where they facilitate constriction or relaxation due to the movement of Ca^{2+} ions through their channel. This means that the volume of air entering the lungs and the volume of blood passing through the lungs is in accordance with the body's requirements. In addition, the alveolar membrane permeability can be altered (e.g. TRPC1, TRPC4 and TRPV4) to enhance or depress gaseous exchange. TRP channels also play a role in the removal of foreign objects and irritants. Here they are either found in sensory neurones (TRPA1 and TRPV1) and their activation results in altered vagal output and hence changed respiratory pattern, blood flow and coughing or located in alveolar macrophages (TRPV2 and TRPV4) for initiation of an immune response. Whether the TRP channels can be exploited as a potential therapy for abnormalities associated with any of the aforementioned factors remains to be determined.

Several channelopathies in man have been associated with TRP channel mutations. These include TRPM8 and prostate cancer; TRPC3, TRPC6 and TRPM4 with cardiovascular disease; and TRPM5 and TRPV1 with impaired glucose tolerance (Moran, 2011; Wu, 2010).

Two-pore potassium channels

The two-pore potassium (K_{2P}) channels (Figure 4.18) are a major contributor to background or 'leak' K^+ currents that contribute to the resting membrane potential. They are expressed ubiquitously through the body. Structurally K_{2P} channels are dimers, with each subunit being composed of the two pore domains, minus the voltage-sensing TMS_{1-4} regions typical of voltage-gated ion channels (see Figure 4.3). Fifteen genes encode the K_{2P} family and this can be subdivided into six groups based on structure and function (see Table 4.7).

Their activity can be regulated by numerous factors including voltage, temperature, physical stretching, protons, fatty acids and phospholipids. However, the actual mechanism of pore opening, inactivation and closure is not really known. In many cells they function to prevent elevation in intracellular Ca^{2+} ion concentration and so contribute to muscle relaxation, reduced neurotransmitter release and depressed endocrine secretions. However under certain conditions such as hypoxia, factors (e.g. H^+ or vasoconstricting peptide) are produced to inhibit the activity of K_{2P} channels. This causes membrane depolarisation and hence Ca_v channel opening. The resultant

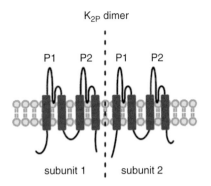

Figure 4.18 K_{2P} structure. Each subunit consists of four TMS that are thought to be derived from a duplication event of TMS_{1-2} during evolution; P1 and P2. Each P region has a classic re-entrant loop two between the TMS. Two subunits are required for activity.

elevated cytosolic Ca^{2+} ion concentration can facilitate neuronal firing, muscle contractions or hormone secretions. Conversely, the drug treprostinil stimulates PKA activity which in turn phosphorylates the $K_{2P}3.1$ channel. This leads to membrane hyperpolarisation and decreased cytosolic Ca^{2+} ion levels and ultimately vasodilation. Hence dysfunction of the K_{2P} channels leads to a myriad of pathophysiological conditions such as cardiac problems, mental retardation, depression, memory problems, migraine, pain disorders, tumorigenisis and male infertility (Es-Salah-Lamoureux, Steele and Fedida, 2010).

Cyclic nucleotide-regulated cation channels

This group of channels have the classic voltage sensitive TMS_{1-4} and pore forming TMS_{5-6} regions (see Figures 4.3 and 4.19) that can conduct Na^+ and K^+ ions, and in some cases Ca^{2+} ions. They can be divided into two groups: cyclic nucleotide-gated (CNG) and hyperpolarisation-activated cyclic nucleotide-gated (HCN) channels. CNG channels are activated by cyclic AMP or cyclic GMP binding whereas HCN channels are voltage operated. HCN channels differ from K_v channels in that they are activated by hyperpolarising, not depolarising, membrane potentials. Also the TMS_4 sensor causes pore opening by moving through the plane of the membrane in the opposite direction to voltage-gated ion channels (see Figure 4.3). Whilst CNG channels also possess the voltage sensing regions, how/if they facilitate pore opening remains to be determined (Biel, 2009; Hofmann, Biel and Kaupp, 2005).

Table 4.7 Role of K_{2p} channels in human disease.

K_{2p} subunit	Old name	Physiological/pathological roles
$K_{2p}1.1$	TWIK	Modulation of the aggressiveness and metastasis of tumours
$K_{2p}6.1$		Contribution to the deafness-associated sensitisation of the neural auditory pathway
$K_{2p}2.1$	TREK	Mechanosensitivity
$K_{2p}10.1$		
$K_{2p}4.1$	TRAAK	Thermosensitivity
		Nociception
		Neuroprotection
		Depression
		Anaesthesia
		Cytoskeletal remodelling in neonatal neurons
		Cardioprotection
		Vasodilatation
		Bladder relaxation
		Proliferation of cancer cells
$K_{2p}3.1$	TASK	Acidosis, hypercapnia and hypoxia sensors
$K_{2p}5.1$		Vasodilatation
$K_{2p}9.1$		Regulation of aldosterone secretion
		Immunomodulation
		Epilepsy
		Promotion of the survival of cancer cells
$K_{2p}17.1$	TALK	Contribution to bicarbonate reabsorption
		Control of the decrease of apoptotic volume (kidney proximal cells)
$K_{2p}18.1$	TRESK	Temperature detection in neurons
		Nociception
		Migraine and migraine-related disorders
		Immunomodulation

Many family members have not been characterised yet and hence are not included in this table. Adapted from Es-Salah-Lamoureux, Steele and Fedida, 2010.

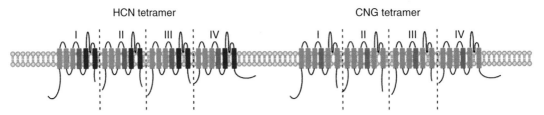

Figure 4.19 Cyclic nucleotide-regulated cation channels structure. Both have the voltage sensor but only HCN channels are voltage sensitive.

Hyperpolarisation-activated cyclic nucleotide-gated (HCN) channels

There are four subunits that comprise the HCN sub-family (HCN1-4) and they are expressed in neuron and cardiac cells. These subunits can form functional hetero-or homotetramers with different pharmacological and electrophysiological properties. There is a gradation of HCN channel opening kinetics with HCN1 being the fastest followed by HCN2, then HCN3 and finally HCN4 which is the slowest. HCN channels contribute to a current seen at hyperpolarising membrane potential: I_h. This I_h current plays a role in determining the rate of firing of pace-making tissues such as the sino arterial node of the heart or rhythmically active thalamocortical circuits of the brain. The I_h current is achieved by permitting an influx of Na^+ ions through the HCN channel after the termination of an action potential. This leads to the membrane slowly depolarising. In the heart, sympathetic activity in the vagus nerve increases cyclic AMP levels in the sino arterial node which enhances the I_h current, increases the rate of depolarisation during diastole and thereby accelerates the heart rate. Conversely, activity of muscarinic receptors reduces cyclic AMP levels, diminishes the I_h current and hence slows down the heart rate. In neurons, as well as mediating pacemaker activity, the I_h current contributes to the membrane potential, dendritic integration, and synaptic transmission (Biel et al., 2009).

Whilst HCN channels are primarily operated by hyperpolarisation, other factors like cyclic AMP or cyclic GMP can act as co-agonist to facilitate opening by binding to the intracellular loop between TMS_6 and TMS_1 of adjacent subunits and hence modifying the channel's activity. Hormones and neurotransmitters that alter cyclic AMP levels can alter HCN channel activity. That is, at high cyclic AMP levels the channels open faster and more completely, whereas at low cyclic AMP concentration the opposite is true. So membrane potential and cyclic AMP levels play a huge role in whether the HCN will open and for how long. Like cyclic AMP, cyclic GMP can also influence voltage-dependent HCN channel opening but its physiological role remains unclear. This is illustrated by the fact that the secondary messenger, nitric oxide (NO), can facilitate neurotransmitter release in the brain and reduce smooth muscle contraction by enhancing cyclic GMP levels. Whether HCN channels are not part of the protein complex involved in signal transduction at these two sites or they are ineffective because of membrane depolarisation remains to be seen. Another factor could be that HCN channels have an affinity for cyclic GMP that is an order of magnitude lower than cyclic AMP.

A number of auxiliary proteins and factors can also modulate HCN channel activity. These include: H^+ and Cl^- ions, kinases (e.g. Src kinase, p38 MAP kinase) and scaffolding proteins. HCN channels and their associated subunits are also found to cluster into lipid rafts.

Within cardiac tissue the HCN4 subunit is the most prominent subunit expressed, whereas the HCN2 subunit is the most commonly expressed subunit throughout the brain, with the other HCN channels showing some level of brain region-specific expression: HCN1, hippocampus;

HCN3, olfactory bulb and hypothalamus; HCN4, thalamus. Studies in mouse models where the genes encoding these subunits have either been deleted or mutated have revealed a correlation between brain region and altered phenotype. Specifically: HCN1 and impaired memory formation; HCN2 with the development of epilepsy and ataxia (and sinus node dysfunction); and HNC4 mice die in utero due to nonformation of SA pacemaker cells.

Cyclic nucleotide-gated (CNG) channels

CNG channels are nonspecific cation channels. Whilst they are more permeable to the influx of Na^+ compared to Ca^{2+} ions, the predominant current is Ca^{2+}. This is because during conductance both Ca^{2+} and Na^+ ions bind to a site within the channel but the Ca^{2+} ion dissociates much slower thereby blocking Na^+ influx. CNG channels were first identified in retinal photoreceptors and in chemo-sensitive cilia of olfactory sensory neurons (OSN) where they aid in the transduction of light or chemical stimuli into a cellular response. They are composed of four subunits derived from six genes: A1-4, B1 and B3. Functional CNG channels contain a combination of these subunits rather than being homotetramers. Channel opening is regulated by cyclic AMP and cyclic GMP, with four cyclic AMP/cyclic GMP molecules per receptor required for full activity.

CNG channels are found in the outer segment of the retinal photocell (CNG1 in rods and CNG3 in cones). Here they play a major role in photo-transduction (see Figure 4.20). Basically cyclic GMP binds to the CNG channels allowing Na^+ and Ca^{2+} ions to influx and K^+ ions to efflux. In dark conditions the cellular concentration of cyclic GMP is high due to its synthesis by guanylyl cyclase (GC), so that CNG channels are open. The resultant membrane depolarisation is detected by Ca_v channels resulting in constant release of the neurotransmitter glutamate from the photocells. Glutamate can then stimulate or inhibit activation of the post-synaptic neurone (bipolar cells) depending upon which type of glutamate receptor is present (see section 4.4). Stimulation of a photocell with light causes membrane hyperpolarisation. This is because CNG channels are no longer open due to the activity of the cyclic GMP hydrolysing enzyme, phosphodiesterase (PDE). Light stimulation causes photo-pigments such as retinal to transform from a cis- to a trans-structure. This conformational change is detected by the photoreceptor rhodopsin (Class A GPCR) which subsequently activates the heterotrimeric G-protein transducin promoting the release of α and $\beta\gamma$ subunits. The α-subunit activates

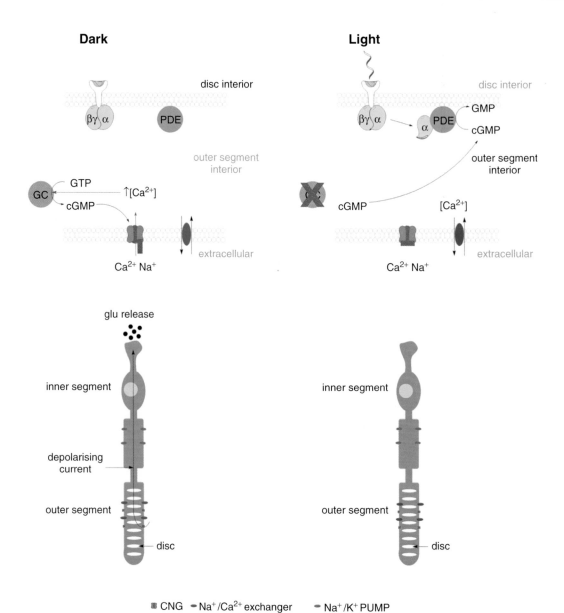

Figure 4.20 Role of CNG channels in photocells. In the dark photocells continually release glutamate (glu). This is because guanylyl cyclase (GC) is constitutively active. GC converts GTP to cyclic GMP which binds to CNG causing the channel to open. Na^+ and Ca^{2+} ions influx into the cytoplasm of the outer segment. This causes a wave of depolarisation to travel down the cell, ultimately resulting in neurotransmitter release. The cytosolic concentrations of Na^+, Ca^{2+} and K^+ ions are maintained by the Na^+/Ca^{2+} exchanger in the outer segment and the Na^+/K^+ pump in the inner segment. The Ca^{2+} ion influx inhibits GC activity and thereby regulates cyclic GMP levels. Light causes the photoreceptor (rhodopsin) embedded in the disc membrane to activate the heterotrimeric G-protein transducin promoting the release of α subunits, which stimulate phosphodiesterase (PDE) to hydrolyse cyclic GMP. With no cyclic GMP the CNG channels close. The photocell membrane is hyperpolarised due to K^+ channel activity and no neurotransmitter is released. Since the intracellular concentration of Ca^{2+} ion drops, GC is no longer inhibited and begins to synthesis more cyclic GMP in preparation for the next dark phase.

PDE and thereby reduces cyclic GMP levels. The resting membrane potential is quickly re-established due to activity of the $Na^+/Ca^{2+}/K^+$ exchanger which exudes Ca^{2+} and Na^+ ions and imports K^+ ions. Since the Na^+ ion gradient is the driving force for this transporter's activity the membrane becomes hyperpolarised (see Chapter 8). HCN1 channels also contribute to this hyperpolarisation. The net effect is the cessation of glutamate release.

Tight regulation of the activity of GC or PDE can fine tune the level of cyclic GMP and hence membrane potential. GC activity is sensitive to Ca^{2+} ion levels so that during dark conditions (high $[Ca^{2+}]$) GC activity is inhibited due to feedback inhibition but in the light (low $[Ca^{2+}]$) it is stimulated to produce more cyclic GMP. In addition, Na^+ ion influx via CNG stimulates activity of the $Na^+/Ca^{2+}/K^+$ exchanger and so can contribute to rapid photocell activation and inactivation. This cycling allows the photocell to respond rapidly to changes in light intensity and hence the 'picture' in view at any one moment. Increased photo-sensitivity is also achieved due to the fact that CNG channels do not become desensitised by ligand binding making them able to respond rapidly to fluctuations in cyclic GMP (and cyclic AMP) cellular levels, thus making them able to respond to single photos of light. In fact gene mutations in the CNG channel subunits can cause colour blindness and retinal degeneration.

The CNG subunits CNG2 and CNG4 are found in OSN cells. A similar scenario of activation is seen in OSN cells compared to photocells, except that CNG activation is mainly due to cyclic AMP. Here the inwardly flowing Ca^{2+} current leads to opening of Ca^{2+} activated Cl^- (Cl_{Ca}) channels and Cl^- ion movement. Another difference is that CNG channels in the retina can discriminate between cyclic AMP and cyclic GMP, whereas those in the OSN respond equally to both cyclic AMP and cyclic GMP (Kaupp and Seifert, 2002). Recently other members of the CNG family have been identified in bacteria and marine invertebrates but their pharmacology appears to be quite different to those of its mammalian counterparts (see Cukkemane, Seifert and Kaupp, 2011 for further information).

Acid-sensing ion channels

Acid-sensing ion channels (ASICs) are proton-activated Na^+ ions channels whose activity is voltage-independent. Hence they are chemoreceptors that detect changes in pH. They are primarily involved in pain perception due to tissue acidosis. Damaged cells release protons and thereby reduce extracellular pH. This increase in acidity is detected by transient receptor potential channels (TRPs)

and ASIC which are located on nociceptive neurons. Basically H^+ ions bind causing opening of their channels, Na^+ ions influx, and the membrane depolarises. This is detected by voltage-gated ion channels (e.g. Na_v and K_v) which elicit neuronal activity. Activation of ASIC expressed in the spinal cord can activate central pain pathways within the central nervous system and pain is perceived. ASIC expressed in presynaptic terminals are involved in enhancing neurotransmitter release because ASIC-mediated membrane depolarisation is detected by Ca_v channels. Whether some ASICs can also conduct Ca^{2+} ions remains to be determined.

ASICs belong to the epithelial sodium channel (ENaC)/degenerin superfamily of ion channels. Six subunits from four ACIS genes have been identified: ASIC1a;1b;2a;2b;3;4. Each subunit comprises of two TMS and a large intracellular loop. Three subunits are required for functionality (see Figure 4.21) with most being capable of forming hetero- and homotrimers. The extracellular domain has been likened to a clenched hand that is formed from subdomains referred to as: finger, thumb, palm, knuckle, and β-turn. Proton binding causes rotation of the extracellular domain as well as movement between the thumb and finger domains. This causes the two TMS to twist so that the channel opens (Yang et al., 2009).

ASICs are not active at physiological pH (7.4) but activity increases as the pH lowers. Different ASICs have diverse pH sensitivities and inactivation kinetics. Activity can be measured in terms of the pH that causes 50% maximal activation (pH0.5). ASIC1 has a pH0.5 ranging from pH 5.9 to pH 6.5 whereas ASIC3 is ~pH 4.4. These different sensitivities enable ASIC to respond to specific stimuli. For example ASIC3 is involved in mediating pain

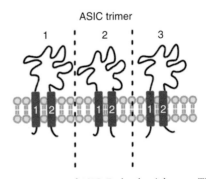

ASIC trimer

Figure 4.21 Structure of ASIC. Each subunit has two TMS and a large extracellular loop. Three subunits are required for a functional channel.

due to lactosis in skeletal and cardiac muscles or acidosis in the gastro-intestinal tract. And ASIC1 is involved in activation of central pain pathways in the spinal cord. Both ASIC1 and ASIC3 can respond to narrow changes in pH (e.g. from pH 7.4 to pH 7.2; Deval et al., 2010).

In addition to peripheral pain perception, ASICs expressed in the central nervous system are involved in synaptic plasticity which underlies many behaviours such as learning and memory, and drug addiction. Here they can modulate NMDA receptor activity in central synapses as well as those in the spinal cord, which are also involved in processing painful stimuli. They are also implicated in neurodegeneration because traumatic brain injury, inflammation or ischaemia causes acidosis due to reduced oxidative phosphorylation which can trigger excitotoxicity (see section 5.5). Nonsteroidal anti-inflammatory drugs are negative allosteric modulators of ASIC function. Heavy metals interfere with the function of ASICs. The diverse role of ACISs makes them attractive targets for drug design.

Epithelial Na⁺ channels

Epithelial Na$^+$ channels (ENaC, Figure 4.22) are constitutively active and are involved in reabsorbing Na$^+$ ions across epithelial membranes primarily in the kidney, gut and lungs. Recently studies have indicated that ENaC resembles the structure of ASIC (see previous section); a trimer with a clenched hand configuration. Emerging evidence suggests that these trimers can then further oligomerise to form a trimer-on-trimer structure within the membrane (Stewart, 2011). Four ENaC subunits (α, β, γ and δ) have been identified with the α, β and γ subunits forming the canonical channels. In vitro studies have shown that all subunits are capable of forming homotrimers although whether this occurs in vivo is

unknown. Each subunit has two TMS, a larger extracellular loop and intracellular carboxyl and amino termini. The α subunit is essential for channel function whereas the β and γ subunits enhance its activity. The δ subunit was first identified in primate neurones and subsequent studies have revealed that two spice variants are expressed in humans. This subunit shares a degree of similarity with the α subunit but its physiological role remains to be determined (Wesch, 2011).

Gain of function mutations in either the β or γ subunit resulting in severe hypertension that is mainly resistant to conventional antihypertensives (Liddle syndrome). Hypertension is due to excessive ENaC activity in the kidney leading to reduced urine output and hence water retention. Basically ENaC located in the renal collecting duct serve to reabsorb Na$^+$ ions that have passed into the tuble lumen. If this did not happen then the body would lose too many Na$^+$ ions and this would alter the composition of intracellular and extracellular fluid with grave consequences. Water is also reabsorbed along with Na$^+$ ions due to osmotic pull. If ENaCs are reabsorbing too much Na$^+$ ions then more water will be returned to the cardiovascular system and hence blood pressure will rise. The hormones, insulin and aldosterone can also enhance ENaC activity. Aldosterone works at the mineralocorticoid receptor (a nuclear receptor; see section 8.4 and Figure 8.8) to induce expression of ENaC so that more channels are inserted into the renal collecting duct and hence more Na$^+$ ions are reabsorbed. A loss of function mutation in ENaC causes pseudohypoaldosteronism where the extracellular volume is depleted leading to hypotension. Insulin, on the other hand, can interact directly with ENaC or indirectly by stimulating the PI-3K pathway so that more ENaCs are translocated to the apical membrane of the collecting duct for greater Na$^+$ ion reabsorption. Obviously perturbations in the levels/activities of these hormones can also have a profound effect on blood pressure.

ENaC is also expressed in the colon where it functions to aid the reabsorption of Na$^+$ ions and consequently water. Here the nuclear receptor ligand, glucocorticoid can enhance ENaC protein expression in a similar manner to aldosterone in the kidney. Exocrine secretions such as sweat also rely on ENaC activity. ENaCs located in the lung serve to maintain the composition of epithelia secretions involved in many aspects of lung function. Again this is achieved through the movement of Na$^+$ ions and the osmotic and electrochemical pull that this process generates. Interestingly ENaC have been investigated as a potential target for the treatment of abnormal mucous

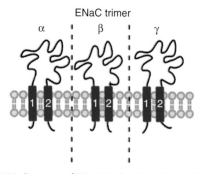

Figure 4.22 Structure of ENaC. Each subunit has two TMS and a large extracellular loop. Three subunits are required for a functional channel.

production in the lungs of cystic fibrosis sufferers (see Chapter 6) (Schild, 2010). Here ENaC activity is increased so that the lungs produce smaller volumes of mucous with increased viscosity that the mucociliary find difficult to remove. Amiloride is a relatively selective blocker of ENaC which has been used as an aerosol to improve the quality of mucous production with some success. However, its inability to improve pulmonary function in severely affected sufferers has led to its discontinuation in clinical trials. RNA interference (RNAi; see Chapter 8) has also been used to reduce ENaC expression in the lungs. Currently delivery vectors are being developed to improve RNAi distribution without evoking an inflammatory response.

Chloride channels

This group is an amalgamation of rather under-explored, integral membrane proteins, with diverse structural and functional characteristics. However, their common and essential feature is the selectivity for anions, which enables them to regulate and facilitate the movement of chloride ions (Cl^-) across membranes. The physiological significance of this has become apparent in recent years, with the study of various genetic diseases and the discovery of underlying channelopathies. These disorders have provided valuable insights into the role of channels, whose functional characterisation poses technical challenges (Planells-Cases and Jentsch, 2009).

These channels can be divided into three classes according to the mechanisms, which determine their opening and closing, that is, voltage-gated chloride channels (ClCs), calcium-activated chloride channels (CaCCs) and cAMP activated cystic fibrosis transmembrane conductance regulator (CFTR).

ClCs

This extraordinary class consists of nine family members (ClC-1 to ClC-7, ClC-Ka and ClC-Kb), which are structurally similar and yet can be subdivided into two physiologically distinct groups of proteins, that is, Cl^- channels and Cl^-/H^+ exchange transporters. The structural differences that separate both groups appear to be surprisingly small; for example, a highly conserved glutamate residue in the selectivity filter of the channels is important for the gating process (Waldegger and Jentsch, 2000).

All ClCs are dimers with a double-barrel architecture that forms two ion pores. Unusually there is also the topology of the individual subunits, as inferred from crystallographic data of the bacterial homolog EcClC (Dutzler et al., 2002). Each subunit has 16 α-helical segments of variable lengths (see Figure 4.23), which either fully or partially span the membrane, often tilted at an angle of 45°. Within a dimer, the segments of each subunit arrange into two antiparallel domains that shape the ion pore, while the loops between the α-helices form the ion selectivity filter.

Among the chloride channels are ClC-1, ClC-2, ClC-Ka and ClC-Kb; they are located in the cell membrane. ClC-1 is voltage-dependent and found in skeletal muscle, where it mediates a large Cl^- conductance that contributes to

CIC dimer

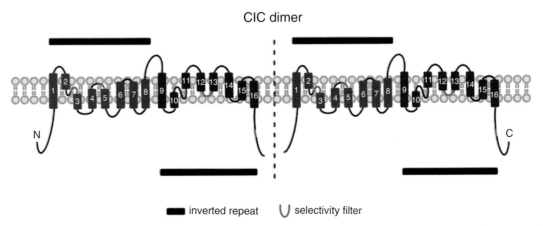

■■■ inverted repeat   ∪ selectivity filter

Figure 4.23 Structure of the chloride selective ion channel (CIC). Each subunit consists of 16 TMS that are essentially an inverted repeat of two smaller TMDs; TMS_{1-8} and TMS_{9-16}. The re-entrant loops formed by TMS_{4-5} and TMS_{12-13}, along with TMS_{2-3} forms the pore and is involved in Cl^- ion selectivity. Two subunits are required for functionality with each subunit forming its own channel (i.e. each CIC has two separate ion channels).

the repolarisation after action potentials. Dysfunction of ClC-1 is associated with recessive and dominant forms of myotonia, an impairment of muscle relaxation. In contrast, the widely distributed ClC-2 is activated by hyperpolarisation, mild extracellular acidification and cell swelling. It is believed to be involved in transepithelial transport of Cl^-, to regulate cell volume and to stabilise membrane potential. Mutations in human ClC-2 have been linked to idiopathic generalised epilepsy, although these mutations do not impair channel function in vitro. The channels ClC-Ka and ClC-Kb reabsorb Cl^- in the nephrons of the kidney and in the inner ear. However, they require barttin, another integral membrane protein, as accessory subunit for the trafficking to the plasma membrane. Mutations in barttin cause severe renal salt loss (Bartter's syndrome type 4) and deafness.

ClC-3, ClC-4 and ClC-5 have been identified in the endosomal membranes of numerous tissues. They potentially act as electrogenic antiporters and acidify endosomes, by exchanging two Cl^- for each H^+. Some *in vitro* studies suggest that they operate in a voltage-dependent manner, but supporting *in vivo* data are currently lacking. Dent's disease, which is accompanied by proteinuria and kidney stones, is linked to dysfunction of ClC-5.

Little is known about ClC-6 and ClC-7, which are also found in the endosomes in many tissues and possibly act as electrogenic transporters. Mutations in ClC-7 affect its function in osteoclasts and lead to increased but fragile bone mass.

CaCCs

These channels exist throughout the animal kingdom in excitable and nonexcitable cells, where they produce outward rectifying currents, in response to cytosolic calcium. They participate in diverse physiological processes, such as epithelial Cl^- secretion, neuronal and cardiac excitation, smooth muscle contraction, oocyte fertilisation and sensory signal transduction (Kunzelmann et al., 2009). Remarkably, the existence of CaCCs has been known from electrophysiological recordings for decades, but their molecular identities are still not fully clear. To date, only two protein families have been identified, which include members that convince as authentic calcium-activated chloride channels, that is, bestrophins and transmembrane protein with unknown function 16A (TMEM16A).

Bestrophin 1 is the best-studied member within a family of four integral membrane proteins (BEST1-4). It is highly expressed in the retinal pigment epithelial cells and, if mutated, believed to cause loss of vision in Best

vitelliform macular dystrophy (Best disease). However, its physiological role is not fully understood. Likewise, although all bestrophins can generate calcium-activated Cl^- currents, it is currently debated whether they act as Cl^- channels or also regulate other ion channels.

TMEM16A (anocatmin 1) is a widely expressed protein that was identified as CaCC in 2008. Hydropathy plots suggest that this and nine related proteins (TMEM16A-K; anoctamin 1–10) possess eight transmembrane-spanning segments with the N and C termini on the intracellular side. The putative pore-forming region is located between TMS5 and TMS6, and characterised by relatively high sequence conservation. It contains a large extracellular portion with four smaller loops, one of which partially penetrates the membrane as a re-entrant loop. Basic amino acids within this region are likely to confer the anion selectivity.

CFTR

Since its discovery in 1989, this channel protein has raised much attention, as it has been linked to cystic fibrosis, a common and lethal genetic disease. CFTR is a cAMP-activated channel in the airways epithelial cells, where it produces outwardly rectifying Cl^- currents and inhibits the activity of the epithelial sodium channel (ENaC). This induces fluid secretion on the surface of the airways and, thus, contributes to the vital processes of trapping and removing foreign particles from the airways. A large number of mutations in CFTR can result in disturbances to the electrolyte transport and mucus secretion, which are associated with pathological features in several organs. (CFTR and cystic fibrosis have been covered in great detail in Chapter 6).

IP₃ receptors

Inositol triphosphate (IP₃) receptors mediate Ca^{2+} ion release from internal stores such as the endoplasmic- and sarcoplasmic-reticulum and they play a major role in Ca^{2+} signalling (see Chapter 6). There are three members of the IP₃ receptor family (IP₃R1-3) and numerous splice variants. Four subunits that are either hetero- or homo-oligermerise are required for receptor activity. Each subunit has six TMS with the two terminal TMS (TMS$_{5-6}$) forming the pore and selectivity filter that is also found in voltage-gated ion channels (see Figure 4.24). Interestingly, these pore-forming domains and the large cytosolic domain are reminiscent of the ligand-gated iGluR and KcsA receptors (see Figure 4.32). Basically the pore of all three has a re-entrant loop that is flanked by two TMS: TMS$_2$ (M-loop) in iGluRs, and

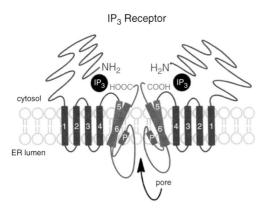

IP$_3$ Receptor

Figure 4.24 Structure of the IP$_3$ receptor. Four subunits are required for activity but only two are shown for clarity. IP$_3$ interacts with moieties at the carboxyl terminal. TMS$_{5-6}$ and a re-entrant loop (P) lines the pore. Cations move from the endoplasmic reticulum (ER) lumen into the cytosol. The amino and carboxyl termini are targets for modulation of receptor activity.

P-loops in KcsA and IP$_3$ receptors. The centre of the pore is narrow due to TMS tapering and the presence of M- or P-loops. This determines the channels selectivity for the conductance of specific ions. In fact the selectivity filter sequence in IP$_3$ receptors includes a GGVGD motif which is similar to that found in KcsA's P-loop. Despite this KcsA channels are selective for K$^+$ ions whereas IP$_3$ receptors are nonselective cation channels. However, IP$_3$ receptors are mainly associated with Ca^{2+} ion conductance due to this cation having the only appreciable gradient across membranes where IP$_3$ receptors are expressed.

The TMS$_1$ domain of the IP$_3$ receptor is similar to that seen in iGluR receptors (see Figure 4.32) in that it is very large and appears to allow a pocket to form for its substrate (IP$_3$) to bind. The two domains that contribute to this clam-like structure are known as the α and β domains. There are no known IP$_3$ receptor specific antagonists making it difficult to evaluate these receptors pharmacologically, although some semi-specific compounds have yielded interesting results. These include the competitive IP$_3$ receptor antagonist heparin that unfortunately also acts as ryanodine receptors (RyR; see next section) as well as uncoupling GPCRs. Caffeine blocks IP$_3$ receptors and RyR, as well as inhibiting cyclic nucleotide phosphodiesterases. This has hampered the design of specific ligands to treat IP$_3$ receptor-related pathologies. In addition, since several different types of GCPR are coupled to IP$_3$ production if any were to dysfunction they could indirectly affect IP$_3$ receptor function.

Studies have shown that binding of IP$_3$ is required for the activation of IP$_3$ receptors that leads to a further increase in cytosolic Ca^{2+} ion levels. These IP$_3$ receptors can then form small clusters within the membrane. The receptors are now sensitive to the elevated cytosolic Ca^{2+} ion levels and can mediate further Ca^{2+} ion release that is known as Ca^{2+} induced Ca^{2+} release (CICR). This property is shared by RyR and plays an important function in cardiac and skeletal muscle contraction (see Figure 4.6). Whether membrane depolarisation is primarily responsible for further Ca^{2+} ion release or whether Ca^{2+} ions bind directly to the IP$_3$ receptor ligand binding site, an intermediate (e.g. calmodulin; CaM) or via the receptor's channel is as yet not known. But it should be noted that high and low affinity Ca^{2+} ion binding sites have been located within the receptor and that very high Ca^{2+} ion concentrations can inhibit the channel's activity. Some researchers have argued that under normal conditions Ca^{2+} ions block IP$_3$ receptor activity and activation of the receptor by IP$_3$ binding relieves this block and thereby allows the receptor to become fully activated by Ca^{2+} ion binding (Taylor and Tovey, 2010).

The three IP$_3$ receptors have different affinities for IP$_3$ (IP$_3$R2 > IP$_3$R1 >> IP$_3$R3) due to the presence and activity of an IP$_3$ suppressor domain in the amino terminal that interacts directly with the core-IP$_3$ binding domain. A number of proteins have been found to interact with both cytosolic domains. These include cytochrome c and huntingtin-associated protein 1A (HAP1A) at the carboxyl terminal and Homer at the amino terminal; obviously factors that bind to the amino terminal have the potential to have a profound effect on the receptor's affinity for IP$_3$ and hence activity. No diseases in man have been directly associated with mutations in any of the IP$_3$ receptor genes. Studies did show that deletions in the IP$_3$R1 gene appear to correlate with spinocerebellar ataxia. However, it was subsequently found that this deletion was not responsible for the condition since the adjacent gene (SUMO) also had deletions. Nevertheless, knockout animals and site-specific mutational studies have revealed physiological roles for the three IP$_3$ receptors. Both IP$_3$R2 and IP$_3$R3 receptors play important roles in pancreatic and glandular secretions as mutant mice have abnormal metabolism as well as reduced salivary gland activity. Removal of the IP$_3$R1 receptor produces neuronal cells with abnormal dendritic architecture that can be 'recovered' by the addition of brain derived neurotrophic factor (BDNF). BDNF plays an important role in many cognitive functions and this finding suggests a role for IP$_3$R1 in the mechanisms that underlie synaptic plasticity. In fact there appears to be a relationship between the ligand-gated NMDA receptor (an iGluR receptor) and metabotropic glutamate receptors (mGluR) where they work in concert to ensure homeostatic cytosolic Ca^{2+} ion levels. (Mikoshiba, 2007).

Ryanodine receptors

Ryanodine receptors (RyR, see Figure 4.25) are Ca^{2+} ion channels and they are very similar to IP_3 receptors in that they are tetramers, the subunits have a similar topology, mediate Ca^{2+} ion release from the sarcoplasmic and endoplasmic reticulums and participate in CICR. However, they are almost twice as large as IP_3 receptors and they are sensitive to the plant alkaloid, ryanodine (hence their name) rather than IP_3. A number of splice variants are expressed by all three of the genes that encode for RyR (RyR1-3). Whereas RyR1 and RyR2 are primarily found in muscle, all three types of RyR are expressed in neurones where they are thought to play a role in neurotransmitter release.

Figure 4.6 in section 4.2 illustrates the role played by RyR in striated (skeletal and cardiac) muscle contraction; RyR located in smooth muscle play an insignificant role in contractions. Basically release of neurotransmitter (e.g. acetylcholine) at the neuromuscular junction results in depolarisation of the muscle plasma membrane that is propagated down the T-tubules. Depolarisation is detected by L-type Ca^{2+} channels (Ca_v1) and their activation allows Ca^{2+} ions to flow into the cytoplasm. This increase in Ca^{2+} ion concentration can activate RyRs on the sarcoplasmic reticulum causing them to open and release more Ca^{2+} ions into the cytosol via CICR. Thus a cascade of events is initiated resulting in muscle contraction. RyR located in striated muscle can actually physically interact with the L-type Ca^{2+} channels in the wall of the T-tubules of the muscle cell to stimulate Ca^{2+} ion release from the sarcoplasmic reticulum. So elevated Ca^{2+} ion levels sufficient to illicit a muscle contraction can be due to an initial increase in Ca^{2+} ion influx through L-type Ca^{2+} channels leading to RyR activation (CICR) and/or the physical interactions between L-type Ca^{2+} channels and RyR. In reality CICR only plays a significant role in cardiac muscle contraction. This is partly due to the utilisation of different ion channel subtypes; $Ca_v1.1$ in skeletal and $Ca_v1.2$ in cardiac that physically interact with RyR1 and RyR2 respectively.

Mutations in RyR1 are associated with complications related to inhalation anaesthetics as well as skeletal muscle myopathies. Here anaesthetics such as halothane can cause malignant hyperthermia due to uncontrolled Ca^{2+} ion release from the sarcoplasmic reticulum of skeletal muscle that leads to muscle rigidity, muscle hypoglycaemia, acidosis and heat generation. Dantrolene is a RyR channel blocker and used with some success to counter the effects of anaesthetic-induced malignant hyperthermia. Conversely mutations in RyR1 that reduce Ca^{2+} ion release from the sarcoplasmic reticulum lead to muscle weakness.

Dysfunction of RyR2 has been associated with cardiomyopathies. These include a potential life-threatening arrhythmia due to catecholamine release induced by stressful situations (catecholaminergic polymorphic ventricular tachycardia; CPVT). Excessive catecholamine release is often seen in response to conditions such as a cardiac infarction or viral myocarditis and this has a similar impact on the heart as CPVT can lead to heart failure. In both cases mutations in the RyR2 means that some of the factors that can normally modulate RyR function (e.g. CaM, ATP, PKA, Ca^{2+}, Mg^{2+}) are unable to interact with it and hence there is a malfunction in the RyR-mediated response (Zalk et al., 2007).

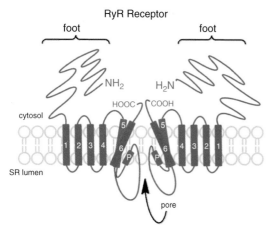

Figure 4.25 Structure of RyR receptor. Four subunits are required for activity but only two are shown for clarity. Artificial agonists such as ryanodine interact with moieties at the carboxyl terminal. TMS_{5-6} and a re-entrant loop (P) lines the pore. Cations move from the sarcoplasmic reticulum (SR) lumen into the cytosol. The foot of each subunit can interact with the cytosolic domains of other Ca^{2+} channels such as the Ca_v1 channels to enhance Ca^{2+} ion release. The amino and carboxyl termini are targets for modulation of receptor activity.

Connexins and pannexins

Gap junctions play a vital role in regulating metabolic and electrical coupling between adjacent cells. Such cell-to-cell communication is important for a number of physiology functions including cardiac and smooth muscle contraction, visual adaptation and hearing (Sáez et al., 2003). Gap junctions allow the passive diffusion from one cell to another of a variety of small molecules (up to 1 kDa in size) such as ions, small metabolites, neurotransmitters, nucleotides (ATP) and second messengers (cyclic AMP, IP_3 and Ca^{2+}). Structurally they consist of proteins called connexins (Cx) of which there are 21 known subtypes (Cx23, Cx25, Cx26, Cx30, Cx30.2, Cx30.3, Cx31, Cx31.1, Cx31.9, Cx32, Cx36, Cx37, Cx40, Cx40.1, Cx43, Cx45, Cx46, Cx47, Cx50, Cx59 and Cx62; the numbers refer to their molecular weight in kDa). The functions of specific connexins are highlighted in Table 4.8.

Connexin proteins contain four transmembrane spanning domains, two extracellular loops, one intracellular loop and the COOH-termini located in the cytoplasm. At the NH_2-terminal there is a helical structure (NTH) located in the membrane region which forms the pore funnel (Figure 4.26). Closure of the channel is due to the NTH moving within the pore to physically block it. Some

Connexin hexamers

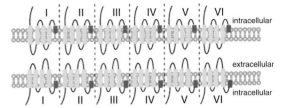

Figure 4.26 Connexion/pannexin structure. Each subunit is composed of four TMS (yellow) with a N-terminal helix (NTH; red). Six subunits hexamerise to form a functional hemi-channel that can interact with another hemi-channel in the opposing membrane. The six NTH in each hemi-channel form the pore funnel. The NTH can be voltage sensitive. Channel closure is due to the NTH moving into the channel and physically blocking it.

NTH have voltage sensitivity and thus share similarities with the classic voltage-sensitive TMS_4 domain characteristic of K_v, Ca_v and Na_v channels. Whether the NTH is an evolutionary precursor or procursor of the TMS_4 domain remains to be seen. Interestingly, six rather than four subunits are required to form a functional channel and this may be due to the fact that gap junctions can conduct much larger molecules than other members of the voltage-gated ion channel family. Variations in the amino acid length of the C-terminal tail account for the varying molecular mass of connexion family members. Connexins assemble into hexameric complexes called connexons or hemichannels and the interaction between connexons on adjacent cells leads to the formation of a gap junction channel (Figure 4.27). Until recently hemichannels were considered to function solely as components of gap junction formation. However, it is now apparent that the hemichannels independently regulate a wide range of cellular functions via their role in Ca^{2+} homoeostasis and signalling (Figure 4.28; Burra and Jiang, 2011; Evans et al., 2006). Several triggers for hemichannel opening have been identified including changes in cytoplasmic Ca^{2+} concentration and pH (Figure 4.27). Furthermore, using synthetic peptides (named Gap 26 and Gap 27) it is now possible to separate out the physiological functions of gap junctions and hemichannels (Evans et al., 2006). These mimetic peptides are based on the second extracellular loop of the relevant connexin protein and studies have revealed that short term exposure times (minutes)

Table 4.8 Physiological function of selected connexins.

Connexin	Location and physiological function
Cx43	Predominant gap junction protein in the heart and involved in electrical conductance
Cx40	Atrial cardiomyocytes and responsible for coordinating spread of electrical activity
Cx36	Pancreatic β-cells and involved in insulin secretion
Cx32	Expressed in myelinating Schwann cells and involved in nerve conduction
Cx30.2	Expressed in the inner ear and involved in signal transduction associated with hearing
Cx26	Expressed in the cochlea and involved in auditory hair cell excitation

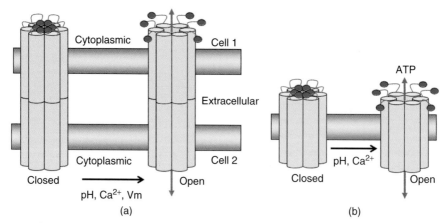

Figure 4.27 Schematic representation of hemichannel and gap junction structure. (a) Six connexin molecules assemble to form a connexon or hemichannel and two connexons on adjacent cells interact to form a gap junction. (b) Connexin hemichannels also regulate cell function independently of their role in gap junction formation. The opening (gating) of gap junctions and hemichannels is regulated by changes in pH, Ca^{2+} and membrane potential (V_m).

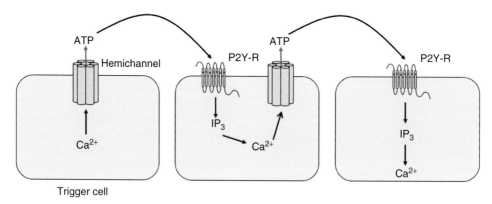

Figure 4.28 Connexin hemichannels and propagation of Ca^{2+} signalling. In response to increases in cytoplasmic Ca^{2+} concentration hemichannels open in 'trigger cells' enabling ATP to diffuse out into the extracellular space. Released ATP activates G-protein coupled P2Y receptors on adjacent cells which stimulate phospholipase C activation resulting in IP_3-mediated release of Ca^{2+} from intracellular stores. The released Ca^{2+} opens hemichannels promoting the release of ATP which activates P2Y receptors on an adjacent cell. This chain of events enables the propagation of Ca^{2+} signals. A similar mechanism may operate using pannexin hemichannels.

selectively blocks hemichannel function whereas longer exposure times (hours) are required for gap junction inhibition. This temporal difference in mimetic peptide sensitivity is most likely due to the connexin protein being more accessible in hemichannels than in gap junctions.

Connexons can be formed from either one type of connexin (termed homomeric) or a combination of two types of connexin (termed heteromeric). Gap junctions may involve two homomeric connexons each containing different connexins (heterotypic channels) or two different heteromeric connexons (heteromeric-heterotypic

channels). The level of gap junction channel communication between adjacent cells is influenced by a number of factors that include the number of gap junctions, the probability that each connexon channel is open and the conductance properties of each connexon. Indeed, the opening or gating of gap junctions is regulated by changes in pH, intracellular Ca^{2+} and membrane potential (V_m). The conformational change between the closed and open state of a channel is called gating. The heterogeneity in connexion composition generates gap junctions with differing functional and structural properties such as pore size, pH dependence, open probability, voltage dependence and molecule preference (both size and charge).

Mutations in connexins and human disease

Given their ubiquitous distribution and prominent role in cell physiology it is no surprise that mutations in connexin genes are associated with several pathologies which are classified into seven groups: neuropathic or myelin disorders, nonsyndromic deafness (hearing loss with no other signs or symptoms), syndromic deafness (hearing loss with abnormalities in other parts of the body), skin diseases, cataracts, oculodentodigital dysplasia (a condition that affects the eyes, teeth and fingers) and atrial fibrillation. For a comprehensive review on mutations in connexin genes and disease see Pfenniger et al., 2011. Some examples of connexin-associated diseases are shown in Table 4.9.

Therapeutic potential of gap junctions and hemichannels

There is considerable interest in targeting gap junction channels as a novel therapeutic approach for cardiovascular diseases (De Vuyst et al., 2011). Gap junctions play a critical role in the co-ordinated contraction of cardiac muscle by facilitating the spread of electrical activity from one cell to another. It is no surprise therefore that disruption of gap junction channel communication leads to ventricular arrhythmias which block the coordinated contraction of cardiac muscle leading to cardiac arrest

Table 4.9 Connexin associated diseases.

Disease	Associated Connexin
Oculodentodigital dysplasia	Cx43
Atrial fibrillation	Cx40
Cataract	Cx46, Cx50
Hearing loss	Cx26, Cx30, Cx31
Myelin-related diseases	
X-linked Charcot-Marie-Tooth disease (CMTX)	Cx32
Pelizaeus-Merzbache-like disease	Cx46, Cx47
Skin disorders	
Keratitis ichthyosis deafness (KID) syndrome	Cx26, Cx30
Vohwinkel syndrome	Cx26
Clouston syndrome	Cx30

and sudden death. A family of anti-arrhythmic peptides (AAP) have been identified which increase gap junction communication and therefore reduce the risk of arrhythmias (De Vuyst et al., 2011). These peptides (e.g. AAP10 and ZP123) indirectly enhance gap junction communication through a mechanism that involves activation of protein kinase C (PKCα isoform) and subsequent phosphorylation of connexin 43. This signalling pathway is triggered via their interaction with a putative GPCR (De Vuyst et al., 2011). ZP123 did enter Phase II clinical trials but these were abandoned due to the development of GAP-134. This peptide, which is an orally active analogue of ZP123 has successfully completed Phase I clinical trials in healthy volunteers. In animal models GAP-134 attenuates ischaemia/reperfusion-induced arrhythmias and infarct size.

During cardiac ischaemia there is increased release of ATP from the cells through hemichannels which open under ischaemic conditions. Physiologically this is designed to enhance coronary blood flow via adenosine-induced vasodilation (ATP is rapidly degraded into adenosine following release). However, the prolonged release of ATP during ischaemia leads to cell death of cardiac muscle cells. Studies using the connexin mimetic peptide Gap 26 have revealed that it blocks Ca^{2+}-triggered release of ATP from hemichannels composed of Cx43. Furthermore, Gap 26 prevents ischaemia-induced cardiac myocyte cell death in a number of model systems suggesting a potential therapeutic use of this peptide in preventing ischaemia/reperfusion-induced injury following myocardial infarction. An added benefit of the anti-arrhythmic peptide GAP-134 is its ability to block hemichannel opening whilst promoting gap junction communication.

As indicated in Table 4.9 mutations in Cx26 and Cx30 are associated with several skin disorders indicating a prominent role of gap junction function in skin homeostasis. Connexins (e.g. Cx26 and Cx43) also play a major role in wound healing; a complex process requiring coordinated communication between numerous cell types including keratinocytes. Keratinocytes are the predominant cell type in the outer layer of the skin and during the wound healing process there are pronounced alterations in the expression levels of connexins in these cells; Cx43 protein expression decreases whereas Cx26 and Cx30 protein expression increases. The reduced expression of Cx43 is important for the migration of keratinocytes to the site of wound healing. Given the prominent role of connexins in wound healing they represent potential novel therapeutic targets for wound treatment. However, this would require the design and development of connexin subtype-specific drugs. One line of attack for targeting specific connexin subtypes is the use of anti-sense oligonucleotides in order to down-regulate protein expression levels. Using this approach in mice has revealed that application of an anti-sense oligonucleotide against Cx43 (to reduce Cx43 expression) enhanced the rate of wound healing (Qiu et al., 2003). Interestingly, the wound healing process in diabetic patients is slow possibly due to abnormally high levels of Cx43 protein expression at the edge of wound. The use of Cx43-specific anti-sense oligonucleotides has been suggested as a novel approach for the treatment of chronic wounds in diabetic patients which is often delayed resulting in further complications such as infection (Wang et al., 2007). In summary, gap junction and hemichannels represent possible therapeutic targets for treating ischaemia/reperfusion-induced injury and skin wounds.

Pannexins

Invertebrates express a family of genes called innexins which are evolutionary distinct from connexins but form intercellular channels similar to gap junctions. Recently, mammalian homologs of innexins have been discovered and named pannexins (Panx). To date, three pannexin genes have been identified (Panx1, Panx2 and Panx3) which are approximately 20% similar in sequence to innexins. Their topology is similar to connexins and they contain two cysteine residues in each of the extracellular loops which are required for the formation of hexameric hemichannels. A notable feature of pannexins is their glycosylation which appears to prevent them from forming gap junctions (Bedner et al., 2012; Barbe et al., 2006). The Panx1 hemichannel is both permeable to ATP and regulated by intracellular Ca^{2+} suggesting a possible role in the propagation of Ca^{2+} signals (Barbe et al., 2006; Figure 4.35). Panx1 also interacts with P2X7 receptor as discussed in the section on P2X receptors. However, the precise functional role(s) of pannexin hemichannels in cell-to-cell communication and signalling and their therapeutic potential remains to be established.

Aquaporins

Aquaporins (AQP, Figure 4.29) are channels that are important for the bulk movement of water molecules across membranes. (Tait et al., 2008). There are 13 genes that encode AQPs in mammals. Each AQP subunit comprises of six TMS which form a helical structure with a water pore in the centre. Like transporters (see Chapter 5) AQPs have a structural fold that indicates

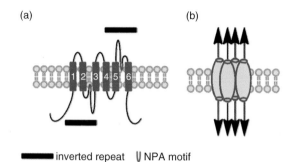

(a)   (b)

━━━━ inverted repeat   ▯ NPA motif

Figure 4.29 Structure of aquaporins (AQPs). (a) TMS_{1-3} are inverted repeats of TMS_{4-6}. The NPA (Asn-Pro-Ala) motif confers water selectivity upon the pore. (b) functional AQPs are composed of four subunits.

that it has evolved by the inverted repeating of TMS_{1-3} by TMS_{4-6}. Within the pore there are two conserved NPA (asparagine-proline-alanine) motifs between TMS_2-TMS_3 and TMS_5-TMS_6 that confers water selectivity. The re-entrant loops that consist of the NPA motif are reminiscent of the pore forming TMS_1-P-loop-TMS_2 that are characteristic of K^+ channels suggestive of a common ancestor. Functional AQP consist of four subunits, each with their own water pore. The pharmacology of AQPs is discussed in Chapter 5.

Sodium leak channels

At resting membrane potentials there is a persistent, sub-threshold, Na^+ ion current that is not reduced when the inhibitors tetrodotoxin (blocks Na_v channels) or cesium (Cs^+; inhibits K_v channels as well as voltage-gated ion channels in general) are applied. This voltage-independent Na^+ ion influx is referred to as the Na^+-leak current (I_{L-Na}). One of the channels responsible for the I_{L-Na} current have recently been identified. They are known as sodium leak channel nonselective protein (NALCN, or previously as VGCNL1) (Yu and Catterall, 2004). These channels have the classic voltage-gated channels structure of a four TMS voltage sensor and two TMS for pore formation (Figure 4.30). Although voltage-insensitivity may be due to fewer positive charges in TMS_4 (see Figure 4.3). Interestingly their selectivity filter motif is EEKEE (glutamate/glutamate/lysine/glutamate/glutamate) which appears to be a mixture of the Ca_v (EEEE) and Na_v (DEKA). This may explain why although the main ionic current is I_{L-Na}, NALCN channels are nonselective cation channels, conducting both K^+ and Ca^{2+} ions as well.

NALCN

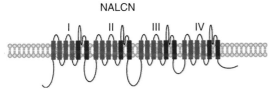

Figure 4.30 Structure of sodium leak channels (NALCN). Functional channels consist of four subunits and have a similar topology to voltage-gated ion channels.

These noninactivating NALCN channels play a role in neuronal excitability. Transgenic studies show that deletion of the gene encoding NALCN results in mice with abnormal respiratory rhythms that are only viable for 24 h (Yu and Catterall, 2004). NALCN is also expressed in the pancreas where it is thought to form a complex with muscarinic acetylcholine receptors and facilitate Ca_v mediated insulin exocytosis. As described in the section on K_{ATP} channels, higher cellular metabolism results in closure of K_{ATP} channels. The resultant membrane depolarisation is detected by Ca_v channels and triggers insulin secretion. Stimulation of the M_3 muscarinic receptor elevates intracellular Ca^{2+} ion levels via IP_3 production and subsequent Ca^{2+} ion release from internal stores (e.g. endoplasmic reticulum). So activity of NALCN channels within the M_3 receptor complex further depolarises the membrane leading to enhanced insulin release (Swayne et al., 2010). Drugs that target NALCN are under development because of their potential superiority over sulphonylureas which are the current treatment for non-insulin dependent (type 2) diabetes. Sulphonylureas act at the sulfonylurea transporter which is coupled to K_{ATP} channels and works by reducing the K_{ATP} channel conductance which leads to membrane depolarisation and hormone secretion. This means that K_{ATP} channels are closed, and insulin secreted, regardless of the glucose concentration (i.e. ATP abundance). This can result in hypoglycaemic episodes. So drugs with NALCN channel activity would only facilitate insulin secretion when glucose levels are normal or high because at low glucose levels the K_{ATP} channels are active and the I_{L-Na} current produced by the NALCN channel is too small to overcome the repolarising action of K_{ATP} channels (Gilon and Rorsman, 2009).

4.4 Ligand-gated ion channels

Members of these families can be assigned to one of three groups depending upon their topology and the number of subunits required to make functional receptors (see

Table 4.10 Different members of the ligand-gated ion channel family expressed in man.

Receptor family	Family subunits
Cys-loop superfamily	**(pentameric)**
5-HT₃	5-HT3A, 5-HT3B, 5-HT3C, 5-HT3D, 5-HT3E
Nicotinic acetylcholine	α1, α2, α3, α4, α5, α6, α7, α9, α8*, α10
	β1, β2, β3, β4
	γ, δ, ε
GABA_A	α1, α2, α3, α4, α5, α6,
	β1, β2, β3
	γ1, γ2, γ3
	δ, ε, θ, π
	ρ1, ρ2, ρ3
Glycine	α1, α2, α3, α4*
	β
Zinc-activated	ZAC
Ionotropic Glutamate family	**(tetrameric)**
AMPA	GluA1, GluA2, GluA3, GluA4
Kainate	GluK1, GluK2, GluK3, GluK4, GluK5
NMDA	GluN1, GluN2A, GluN2B, GluN2C, GluN2D, GluN3A, GluN3B
δ	GluD1, GluD2
P2X family	**(trimeric)**
P2X	P2X1, P2X2, P2X3, P2X4, P2X5, P2X6, P2X7

Subunits marked with an asterix (*) are either not expressed in man or are a pseudo-gene. Brackets indicate the number of subunits required for function receptors. Adapted from Collingridge et al., 2009.

Figure 4.31 and Table 4.10). All have extracellular ligand binding domains (LBD). The carboxyl or amino terminal binding domains can be extracellular or intracellular.

Pentameric ligand-gated ion channel family

Pentameric ligand-gated ion channels (pLGICs) are expressed in both the central and peripheral nervous systems. In humans these receptors are a major site of action for anaesthetics, muscle relaxants, insecticides and drugs that treat disorders of cognition such as Alzheimer's, drug addiction, ADHD (attention deficit hyperactivity disorder) and depression. They

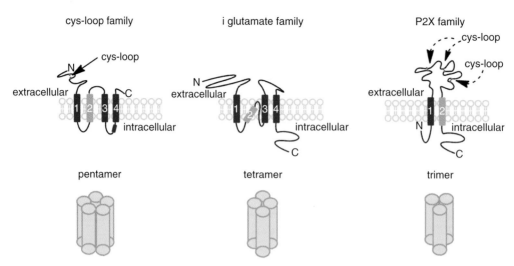

Figure 4.31 The three major structures of ligand-gated ion channels. The topology of one subunit for each group is illustrated. Their subunit assembly is shown below each example. The pore forming region is coloured orange. Cys-loops and 2PX receptors have characteristic cysteine loops (in red). Members of the cys-loops family form pentamers, i (ionotrophic) glutamate form tetramers and P2X form trimers. Adapted from Collingridge et al., 2009.

are also expressed in prokaryotes where they act as chemoreceptors. Initial information about their structure has been derived primarily from nicotinic acetylcholine receptors (nAChR) isolated from the torpedo ray fish, *Torpedo marmorata*, using cryo-electron microscopy. This receptor is expressed in their electric organ and is involved in stunning prey by electrifying them with up to 200V. Subsequent studies of other eukaryotic members of the pLGIC family have revealed that within the extracellular domain there is a highly conserved loop of 13 amino acids due to a disulphide bridge between cysteine residues (C-x-[LIVMFQ]-x-[LIVMF]-x(2)-[FY]-P-x-D-x(3)-C) and for this reason they are also known as cys-loop receptors. However, this term can be misleading as prokaryotic counter-parts do not contain these cys-loops. Members of the pLGIC family can be further divided depending upon their preferred ligand (neurotransmitter). These families include nicotinic acetylcholine (nACh), serotonin (5-HT$_3$) and zinc activated receptors (ZAC) that conduct cations, as well as GABA$_A$ and glycine (Gly) receptors which conduct anions (Baenziger and Corringer, 2011) see Table 4.10.

The crystalline structure of homologous bacterial pLGICs, *Erwinia chrysanthemi* (ELIC) and *Gloebacter violaceus* (GLIC) have been determined and used to infer the structure of mammalian pLGICs. This has revealed that five subunits are required for receptor functionality. Mostly they are heteromeric giving rise to functional

receptors that have an array of physiological and pharmacological properties. This is further complicated by differential post-translational modifications and the presence of various splice variants. All subunits are characterised by an external ligand binding domain (LBD). Here three peptide-loops from each subunit help to form the ligand binding pocket. However, not all subunits are able to contribute to this and in part this explains why some members of this family require only two whereas others need five molecules of ligand to bind for receptor activation. There are four TMS that span the whole membrane and they are the site of alcohol, anaesthetic and steroid action. TMS$_2$ forms the pore as well as helping determine which ion(s) are conducted. This selectivity filter in TMS$_2$ has the sequence alanine or proline/ alanine/arginine (A/PAR) in channels that conduct anions (e.g. gly α1, α2; GABA$_A$ α1 and β1) and glycine/glutamate/lysine or arginine (GEK/R) for cation channels (e.g. nAChR α1 and 5-HT$_{3A}$). Residues in the TMS$_1$ and the cytosolic loop between TMS$_3$ and TMS$_4$ are also involved in determining ion conductance; three arginine residues between TMS$_3$ and TMS$_4$ confer Ca^{2+} ion permeability. So these pLGICs are either excitatory or inhibitory depending upon the membrane potential and their activity is also governed by the distribution of specific ions species across the membrane. The internal loop between TMS$_3$ and TMS$_4$ is large in eukaryotes and is involved in trafficking and is also a potential site for modifying receptor activity. Lastly, the carboxyl terminus is short and extracellular (see Figure 4.31).

Protein structure is determined by covalent and noncovalent interactions between adjacent moieties. Cation–π interactions are an example of noncovalent whereby an interaction is formed between an electron-rich system (π) and an adjacent cation (e.g. Li^+, Na^+ sites on ligand). These interactions have similar strengths to hydrogen bonds and salt bridges. In pLGICs, cation–π interactions are important in ligand binding. The ligand binding pocket is electron-rich (i.e. π) and the ligand (agonist/antagonist) contributes the cation groups (i.e. Na^+ or Li^+). Since all ligands do not interact at the same sites within the pocket some ligands and pocket cation–π interactions cannot occur. Similarly the 'pocket' formed by some subunit interactions are not electron-rich and therefore also cannot contribute to a cation–π interaction. This explains why some ligands and subunit combinations have no/little ligand binding activity. In fact nAChRs expressed at the neuromuscular junction ($\alpha 1\beta 1(\gamma/\epsilon)\delta$) and the central nervous system ($\alpha 4\beta 2$) have different affinities for the artificial agonist, nicotine, and the absence of some of these cation–π interactions in the receptor may explain why cigarette smoking is pleasurable but does not cause severe muscle contractions. Another example is nicotine itself. It can be used as an insecticide because it rapidly desensitises nAChRs making them less responsive to acetylcholine. This in turn causes muscle paralysis that can ultimately lead to death. However, nicotine is far more potent at mammalian rather than insect nAChRs because at physiological pH nicotine is protonated. This protonation enables the mammalian, but not the insect, ligand binding pocket to form cation–π interactions and hence enhance receptor activation. Derivatives of nicotine which are capable of forming cation–π interactions with insect nAChRs and not mammalian nAChRs have severely reduced problems associated with over-exposure and toxicity in man. So a knowledge of how ligands interact with binding pockets can aid the design of potential therapeutics that target specific receptor subtypes (Sine et al., 2010).

Nicotinic acetylcholine receptors

Nicotinic acetylcholine receptors (nAChR) conduct Na^+ and K^+ ions and some subtypes can conduct Ca^{2+} ions with varying permeabilities. Their sensitivity to the artificial ligand, nicotine, enables them to be distinguished from metabotropic (muscarinic) acetylcholine receptors. They are found within the peripheral nervous system, primarily at the neuromuscular junction and autonomic ganglion.

The majority of neuronal nAChRs are composed of either the $\alpha 4$ subunits in combination with other types or homomeric $\alpha 7$ subunits. Heteromeric receptors containing the $\alpha 4$ subunit have a high probability of opening but they deactivate to high-affinity states that are resistant to reactivation; whereas homomeric $\alpha 7$ receptors have a low probability of activation that are easily desensitised but can rapidly reactivate. Since these receptors rapidly desensitise some agonists actually behave as antagonists because they facilitate down-regulation of the receptor. Many allosteric modulators of pLGICs bind to sites between subunit interfaces. Both alcohols and anaesthetics potentiate nAChR at low concentrations but inhibit them at high concentrations. Receptors consisting of the $\alpha 4\beta 2$ subunits are sensitive and those containing $\alpha 7$ subunits are insensitive to the anaesthetics, isoflurane and propofol. Galantamine is a positive allosteric modulator of $\alpha 4\beta 2$ and $\alpha 7$ nAChRs that is used to treat Alzheimer's disease.

The nAChRs expressed in human muscle are composed of $\alpha 1_2\beta 1\epsilon\delta$ subunits with the ϵ subunit being replaced by a γ subunit in some animal models. Activation of these receptors causes an influx of Na^+ ions which depolarises the membrane. This is detected by Ca_v channels within the T-tubules of the muscle which respond by opening and allowing a Ca^{2+} ion influx resulting in muscle contraction (see Figure 4.6). Abnormal function of the nAChRs, as seen in congenital myasthenia gravis, means that there is insufficient activation of the Ca_v channels leading to reduced muscle contraction.

The nAChRs located in neuronal tissue are mainly composed of $\alpha 4\beta 2$ as either $\alpha 4_2\beta 2_3$ or $\alpha 4_3\beta 2_2$. The $\alpha 4_2\beta 2_3$ compared to the $\alpha 4_3\beta 2_2$ combination has increased acetylcholine sensitivity and a reduced Ca^{2+} ion conductance. This suggests a different cellular/physiological role. The $\alpha 4\beta 2$ receptors, particularly $\alpha 4_2\beta 2_3$, are involved in reward and addiction as well as cognition and are a major target for drug design to ameliorate conditions associated with its dysfunction. The presence of an $\alpha 6$ subunit within nAChR accounts for a quarter of the presynaptically expressed nAChRs found within the pathway associated with drug addiction: the reward pathway. The $\alpha 6\alpha 4\beta 2\beta 3$ subtype has the greatest sensitivity to nicotine and facilitates dopamine release in the reward pathway which is the major neurotransmitter associated with drug addiction (Xiu et al., 2009). Furthermore, cocaine is a well-known drug of addiction that facilities dopamine release within the reward pathway. Cocaine is also a positive allosteric modulator of $\alpha 4\beta 2$ (and $\alpha 7$) receptors.

Defects in TMS_2 of the $\alpha 4$ or $\alpha 1$ subunits is associated with congenital childhood-onset nocturnal frontal lobe epilepsy whereby motor seizures occur at night during onset of sleep or during waking. Several mutations in the genes encoding for $\alpha 4$ and $\alpha 1$ have been associated with this condition. These mutations prolong channel opening by either decreasing desensitisation of the receptor or increasing its sensitivity to acetylcholine. So the difference in subunit composition between neuronal and muscular nAChRs means that drugs with minimal cross reactivity can be designed to greatly reduce toxic effects.

5-HT$_3$ receptor channels

There are seven main types of 5-HT (serotonin) receptors but only the 5-HT$_3$, is ligand gated. Like other cation pLGICs its pore is permeable to K^+ and Na^+ ions with some subtypes also showing selective Ca^{2+} ion conductance. They are expressed in the central and peripheral nervous systems as well as the gastric-intestinal tract. They have been shown to play a role in psychosis, anxiety and depression as well as irritable bowel syndrome. In addition some are susceptible to the allosteric modulators, alcohols and anaesthetics.

Five genes that encode for 5-HT$_3$ receptors have been identified in man and apart from 5-HT3C they all express a number of splice variants (Beate, 2011). Most studies have been conducted in rodents who only express the 5-HT3A and 5-HT3B subunits. 5-HT3B has an alternative promoter site that allows the expression of a long and short form of this gene in brain tissue. The physiological significance of this is still under investigation. Only 5-HT3A subunits can form functional homo-pentamers while 5-HT3B-E require the presence of a subunit from another grouping for functionality. Heteromeric 5-HT3A receptors have a greater Ca^{2+} ion permeability but have slower kinetics of activation, deactivation and desensitization than homomeric 5-HT3A receptors (Machu, 2011).

Radiotherapy and chemotherapeutics, such as cisplatin and doxorubicin, can cause nausea and vomiting because they induce 5-HT (serotonin) to be released in the digestive tract. Consequently 5-HT$_3$ receptors located on vagal nerve terminals are stimulated leading to activation of the vomiting centre within the brain. Setrons are antiemetics that inhibit 5-HT$_3$ receptor activity and are used to counter the nausea and vomiting associated with these treatments for cancer. 5-HT$_3$ receptors have also been associated with gastric reflux disease where the acid content of the stomach slowly erodes the lining of the oesophagus. In the central nervous system pre-synaptic 5-HT$_3$ receptors are involved in control of neurotransmitter release, with agonists enhancing dopamine and GABA release. They are also expressed in post-synaptic cells where they are excitatory. 5-HT$_3$ receptors are implicated in drug addiction. However their role in drug addiction is complicated and dependent upon the specific drug of addiction. With ethanol, boosting synaptic 5-HT levels with selective serotonin reuptake inhibitors like fluoxetine reduces ingestion, whereas 5-HT$_3$ receptor antagonist or agonism facilitates or suppresses addictive behaviour, respectively. Lesioning of serotonergic neurones within the reward pathway prevents opiate, but not cocaine, addictive behaviour. The main effect of 5-HT appears to involve alterations in motivation. So the role of 5-HT$_3$ receptors in drug addiction is not easily explained.

5-HT$_3$ receptors also mediate inflammation and chronic pain. They are expressed in sensory nerve endings and control the release of pain mediators such as substance P. The use of antagonists that prevent release of substance P from these sensory terminals are a potential target for the treatment of fibromyalgia and peripheral neuropathies. In addition to the emetic effect, stimulation of 5-HT$_3$ receptors increases anxiety levels. Therefore agonist and positive allosteric modulators of 5-HT$_3$ receptor function are of little pharmaceutical benefit (Tina, 2011).

Zinc activated receptors

Not much is known about the pharmacology or physiological function of these receptors. The zinc-activated channel (ZAC) was first identified by scanning genomic databases for other members of the pIGLC family. The gene was cloned in 2003 (Davies et al., 2003) and later two splice variants were identified (Houtani et al., 2005). They are cation channels that are activated by Zn^{2+} ions and inhibited by (+)-tubocurarine. To date, no other ZAC genes encoding for these channels have been identified so it is assumed that they function as homopentamers. Studies are hampered by the fact that no homologue has yet been identified in rodents even though they are expressed in human and other animal tissues (Houtani et al., 2005).

GABA$_A$ receptors

Molecular heterogeneity is one of the noticeable characteristics of the large group GABA-gated, anion-selective pLGICs that have been classified as γ-aminobutyric acid type A (GABA$_A$) receptors (see Table 4.10). In addition (or because of this), they are a physiologically and pharmacologically interesting family of ion channels, as they are the primary mediator of fast synaptic inhibition in the mammalian CNS and the target for a number of clinically-important drugs, including widely-prescribed benzodiazepine compounds (reviewed by Olsen and Sieghart, 2009).

Receptor subunits and their classifications

The molecular diversity of the receptor is due to 19 homologous subunits (i.e. $\alpha 1$-$\alpha 6$, $\beta 1$-$\beta 3$, $\gamma 1$-$\gamma 3$, δ, ϵ, θ, π, and $\rho 1$-$\rho 3$), which can assemble in a hitherto undetermined multitude of heteropentameric combinations (see below), referred to as receptor subtypes. The subunits have been classified based on sequence identity, accounting for 60% to 80% within a particular subunit class (e.g. $\beta 1$ and $\beta 3$), but only 30% to 40% between two classes (e.g. α and β). Sequence conservation is generally high for the four hydrophobic transmembrane segments that are typical for subunits of the pLGIC superfamily, while other regions, especially the large intracellular loop between TMS3 and TMS4, are of variable length and less conserved.

Interestingly, each $GABA_A$ receptor subunit is the product of a separate gene, but further polypeptide forms arise as a consequence of alternative splicing of primary mRNAs. A well-studied example is the 'long' version of the $\gamma 2$ subunit ($\gamma 2L$), which differs from the 'short' variant ($\gamma 2S$) by an additional eight amino acids within the aforementioned long intracellular loop. It derives from an alternatively-spliced 24-basepair exon, within the $\gamma 2$-subunit gene, and adds a consensus sequence for protein kinase C (PKC) and calmodulin-dependent Ser/Thr protein kinase II (CMPK II). Whether this affects the function of the native receptor is still not satisfactory proven. Similarly, two forms have been reported for the $\beta 2$ subunit, where the insertion of 38 amino acids into the large intracellular loop ($\beta 2L$) introduces potential phosphorylation sites for a few kinases, including PKC and CMPK II. In humans, alternative splicing also appears to generate several subunit transcripts with different 5′UTRs, but the encoded proteins are possibly nonfunctional or not incorporated into a receptor.

The inclusion of the three ρ subunits, as a class of $GABA_A$ receptors, follows structural and functional criteria and according to the Nomenclature Committee of IUPHAR (NC-IUPHAR; Barnard et al., 1998), however this circumstance was neither applauded by all researchers in the field, at the time, nor is it now (Bormann, 2000). Prior to 1998, the ρ subunits were classified as $GABA_C$ receptors, as they exhibit pharmacological and expression profiles, which are clearly distinct

from other $GABA_A$ receptor subtypes and polypeptides, respectively (see below). Even today, the term '$GABA_C$ receptors' appears frequently in the scientific literature, despite NC-IUPHARx's recommendation to disregard it. (NB $GABA_B$ receptors are GPCRs that are dealt with, in detail, in Chapter 3).

Likewise, the classification (and naming) of the ϵ and θ subunits can be queried. They have been placed in separate $GABA_A$ receptor classes, because they share $\sim$50% sequence identity with the γ and β subunit classes, respectively. However, the corresponding genes (*GABRE* and *GABRQ*) are also part of a gene cluster, as they have been identified for the great majority of $GABA_A$ receptor genes (e.g. the cluster *GABRG3–GABRA5–GABRB3* on chromosome 15q). They are located on the X chromosome, together with *GABRA3*, where they hold the positions of γ-like and β-like subunits genes (i.e. *GABRE–GABRA3–GABRQ*), respectively. This suggests that the ϵ and θ subunits are the result of high sequence divergence during evolution, but otherwise they could be placed in the γ and β subunit classes, according to their genomic locations. Noteworthy, two additional $GABA_A$ receptor polypeptides, named $\beta 4$ and $\gamma 4$, have been identified in the chicken (*Gallus gallus domesticus*; Lasham et al., 1991; Harvey et al., 1993) and they are believed to be less-divergent orthologues of the mammalian θ and ϵ subunits, respectively (see Darlison et al., 2005).

Stoichiometry of receptors and receptor subtypes

With the discovery of an increasing number of $GABA_A$ receptor subunits, until the late 1990s, emerged several questions, which have been central in the research on this ion channel family ever since (e.g. Whiting, 2003): Which stoichiometry and receptor subtypes exist *in vivo*? Do these subtypes possess specific physiological roles?

The different subunits can potentially assemble in a vast number of combinations, found at synaptic as well as extrasynaptic locations. However, each subunit gene has a unique spatio-temporal expression pattern *in vivo* – the co-assembly into a pentamer necessitates the co-localisation of the encoded polypeptides within the same cells, and appears to follow structural preferences of the combining subunits. *In situ* hybridisation and immuno-histochemical studies revealed that the $\alpha 1$, $\beta 1$-$\beta 3$ and $\gamma 2$ subunit genes are widely and abundantly expressed in the mammalian brain (Fritschy et al., 1992; Wisden et al., 1992). In contrast, the activity of other genes can be low and/or limited to a few areas or cell groups, such as the genes of the $\alpha 6$ subunit (exclusively expressed in cerebellar granule cells) and the π subunit (reproductive tissue). These initial studies were followed by the purification of GABA$_A$ receptor complexes through immunoprecipitation and immunoaffinity chromatography. Despite the technical challenges to dissect the molecular composition, today it is believed that the majority of native receptors are composed of two α subunits, two β subunits, and a single γ subunit or δ subunit.

Following this stoichiometry, the $\alpha 1\beta 2\gamma 2$ combination has been identified as the most common receptor subtype. Noteworthy, it is formed by three highly abundant subunits, which are all expressed from the same gene cluster. Together with $\alpha 1\beta 2\gamma 2$, the $\gamma 2$ subunit appears to be present in a total of $\sim 75\%$ of heteropentamers, including the less common subtypes $\alpha 2\beta \gamma 2$, $\alpha 3\beta \gamma 2$, $\alpha 4\beta \gamma 2$, $\alpha 5\beta \gamma 2$ and $\alpha 6\beta \gamma 2$ (with 'β' possibly representing any type of this subunit class). Other identified combinations (i.e. $\alpha 4\beta 2\delta$, $\alpha 4\beta 3\delta$, $\alpha 6\beta 2\delta$, $\alpha 6\beta 3\delta$), contain the δ subunit instead (Whiting, 2003; Olsen and Sieghart, 2009); these are exclusively found at extrasynaptic locations. The ρ polypeptide genes are predominantly expressed in the retina, and several studies suggest the existence of heteromers composed of $\rho 1$- and $\rho 2$-subunit there, and $\rho 2$-homomers in other CNS regions (Bormann, 2000). In addition, some evidence exists for receptor molecules containing more than one type of α subunit (i.e. $\alpha 1\alpha 6\beta \gamma 2$ and $\alpha 1\alpha 6\beta \delta$). Minor, less-studied subunits, such as the ϵ, θ and π subunits, can possibly substitute the γ and δ subunits (e.g. $\alpha \beta \theta$, $\alpha \beta \epsilon$ and $\alpha \beta \pi$).

A prediction of the absolute number of native GABA$_A$ receptor subtypes is difficult, although the identification of receptor complexes has much progressed since the molecular cloning of the subunits. This line of research is of great significance, for the combination of subunits determines the electrophysiological and pharmacological profiles of individual receptors (see next paragraph).

Physiology

Activation of the GABA$_A$ receptor requires the binding of two molecules of the neurotransmitter GABA at the interface between a α and β subunit (i.e. the GABA site). This interaction opens an intrinsic ion channel that is selective for chloride ions (Cl$^-$) and to a lesser degree to bicarbonate. In the adult brain, the opening is associated with a hyperpolarising Cl$^-$ influx and results in a reduced capability of the neuron to initiate action potentials (i.e. inhibition). However, in the developing brain, GABA has excitatory actions, since the immature neurons possess a high $[Cl^-]_i$, which carries a depolarising current out

of the cell upon GABA$_A$ receptor activation (Ben-Ari et al., 2007). The intracellular Cl$^-$ is accumulated by the Na$^+$-K$^+$-2Cl$^-$ co-transporter NKCC1, but this gradient gradually shifts to a high $[Cl^-]_o$ during brain maturation, with the appearance of the K$^+$-Cl$^-$ co-transporter KCC2, a chloride extruder. As GABA's fast excitatory actions precede those usually mediated by AMPA-type glutamate receptors, they are of physiological importance for the signalling in the developing nervous system. This depolarisation is even observed in restricted regions of the adult brain (e.g. some cortical neurons), where the local Cl$^-$ gradient is reversed.

In view of the GABA$_A$ receptor heterogeneity and their (sub)cellular locations, it is likely (but difficult to prove) that certain subtypes fulfil specific physiological roles, perhaps in functionally distinct circuits. On the other hand, there is clear evidence that the potency of GABA depends on the type of α subunit in the assembled pentamer (Mortensen et al., 2012). The $\alpha 6$-subunit containing subtype, for example, exhibits the highest sensitivity to GABA among heterologously-expressed $\alpha x\beta 3\gamma 2$ GABA$_A$ receptors. Small numbers of these receptors are typically found at extrasynaptic locations, where they respond with a tonic current to the low concentrations of GABA, which overspill from inhibitory synapses. In contrast, the synaptic-type $\alpha 2\beta 3\gamma 2$ and $\alpha 3\beta 3\gamma 2$ receptor isoforms are characterised by the lowest GABA potencies.

Pharmacology

The impact of the subunit combination on the pharmacological profiles, including undesired side effects, is of great interest, because GABA$_A$ receptors are sensitive to a wide range of clinically-relevant compounds: benzodiazepines (BZ), barbiturates and general anaesthetics, as well as endogenous neurosteroids and alcohol. These drugs target the GABA sites, where they act as agonists (e.g. muscimol) and antagonists (e.g. bicuculline), and on allosteric sites, where they competitively block (e.g. picrotoxinin), or positively or negatively modulate the receptor action. An enhanced activity of GABA is frequently associated with anxiolytic, sedative, hypnotic and/or anticonvulsive effects in the organism.

Drugs, especially the numerous BZ derivatives, have been invaluable tools in the molecular and electrophysiological characterisation of GABA$_A$ receptors subtypes. Indeed, prior to the molecular cloning of the receptor subunits, the BZs diazepam and CL218,872 contributed in receptor autoradiography studies to the identification of the BZ1 and BZ2 receptors, that is, the only two GABA$_A$ receptor isoforms believed to exist back then (Sieghart and Karobath, 1980). The BZ1 receptor showed a high affinity for CL218,827, but for type 2 it was low. Today, it is known that the BZ1 receptor represents the $\alpha 1\beta\gamma 2$ subtype, while the BZ2 receptor is composed of $\alpha 2$, $\alpha 3$ or $\alpha 5$, one β and the $\gamma 2$ subunit.

Diazepam (Valium®) is a widely-prescribed drug and, like many other BZ drugs (e.g. flunitrazepam, chlordiazepoxide), a CNS depressant. It has anxiolytic, sedative and myorelaxant properties, and can cause amnesia, in particular if potentiated by the simultaneous use of alcohol. The BZ flumazenil, on the other hand, is a negative allosteric modulator that can serve as an antidote for intoxication with flunitrazepam or BZs with similar effects. The interaction of all of these drugs with $GABA_A$ receptors requires the presence of the so-called BZ binding site. This is generally formed by a γ and an α subunit, but exhibits distinct affinities to BZs depending on the individual γ and α subunit types. The $\gamma 2$ subunit, for instance, contributes to receptor isoforms with higher sensitivities to diazepam than those containing the $\gamma 1$ polypeptide. In contrast, $\alpha 4$- and $\alpha 6$-containing receptors are insensitive to diazepam and flunitrazepam. This is due to the presence of a particular arginine residue, instead of a histidine, which otherwise can be found in the N-termini of the BZ-sensitive $\alpha 1$, $\alpha 2$, $\alpha 3$ or $\alpha 5$ subunits (see Chapter 10, section 10.5). Interestingly, genetic engineering has confirmed that certain therapeutic aspects can be attributed to defined receptor subtypes (Rudolph et al., 1999; Löw et al., 2000). The sedative and amnesic effects of diazepam are primarily mediated by $\alpha 1$ subunit-containing isoforms, the anxiolytic and possibly the myorelaxant qualities by the $\alpha 2$ subunit. Similar work may aid the discovery of receptor subtypes, which are potentially involved in BZs' negative side effects, such as drowsiness, or the mechanisms of BZ dependence, linked to long-term use.

In contrast to diazepam, the β-carboline DMCM (dimethoxy-4-ethyl-β-carboline-3-methoxylate) is an allosteric inhibitor of GABA, at the BZ binding site. This and similar molecules have raised attention, due to their ability to enhance the cognitive functions of animals in learning paradigms (Venault et al., 1986). These findings are in line with transgenic studies on the $\alpha 5$-subunit gene, which is predominantly expressed in the hippocampus, a learning-relevant brain region (Collinson et al., 2002). Here, the decrease of the subunit was accompanied by improved learning and memory performance. These studies suggest that a reduction of GABAergic transmission in specific areas may enhance cognitive functions. However, the clinical applications of

drugs like DMCM are hindered, as they lack specificity for $\alpha 5$-subunit containing subtypes. This example highlights again the importance of determining the molecular composition of existing $GABA_A$ receptors and to develop subtype-selective drugs.

The BZ binding site is also recognised by a class of nonbenzodiazepine tranquilisers, called Z drugs (e.g. zolpidem, zopiclone). They preferentially bind to $\alpha 1$ subunit-containing $GABA_A$ receptors, where they act as BZ site agonists, but with rather hypnotic, less anxiolytic effects on the body. Also this class of agents points out the pharmacological significance of the BZ site in the receptor. However, despite intensive research, endogenous benzodiazepines have not been identified, and a physiological role for this site is doubtful.

Other positive-allosteric modulators with clinical significance are barbiturates and general anaesthetics. They appear to bind to receptor sites, which differ from those for GABA and BZs, and probably involve the β subunits. Barbiturates are nonselective general depressants, whose molecular targets include $GABA_A$ receptors. Although frequently referred to as sleeping pills, their effects vary from being anaesthetic (e.g. thiopental), to sedative-hypnotic (e.g. pentobarbital) and anticonvulsive (phenobarbital), depending on their time of onset and duration of action. Also anaesthetics, such as the intravenously-administered propofol and etomidate, prolong the duration of the open $GABA_A$ receptor. They are commonly used to induce general anaesthesia, while volatile anaesthetics (e.g. halothane, enflurane) maintain this state; the latter are likely to bind to a site distinct on $GABA_A$ receptors from that of the injectable agents.

Finally, a pharmacologically very distinct group of $GABA_A$ receptor subtypes are the ρ subunit-containing isoforms (formerly: $GABA_C$ receptors). They neither respond to BZs, nor to barbiturates, bicuculline or neurosteroids that are typically active on $GABA_A$ receptors. However, they can be distinguished pharmacologically, from the latter, by the agonist CACA (cis-4-aminocrotonic acid) and antagonist TPMPA ((1,2,5,6-tetrahydropyridine-4-yl)methylphosphinic acid), which are selective for the GABA site of these subtypes.

Genetic epilepsies and receptor dysfunction

As mediators of synaptic inhibition, $GABA_A$ receptors counterbalance the actions of excitatory neurotransmitters. The functional importance of GABAergic signalling becomes apparent, if it is disturbed by mutations in the involved proteins. Dysinhibition and overexcitation may be the consequence, and they manifest themselves in the form of disorders like anxiety, depression and epilepsy.

Mutations in GABA$_A$ receptor subunit-genes have been linked to several types of idiopathic epilepsy (MacDonald et al., 2010), that is, childhood absence epilepsy, juvenile myoclonic epilepsy, generalised epilepsy with febrile seizures plus (GEFS+) and severe myoclonic epilepsy of infancy (Dravet syndrome). The severity of the disorder appears to depend on the type of mutation (nonsense, missense, frame shift), its location in the gene (promoter, protein-coding region), the affected region of the encoded protein (intra-/extracellular, transmembrane) and the affected subunit gene. Generally, the pathophysiological consequences of the mutations are impairments in the gating characteristics of the channel or receptor trafficking.

The majority of mutations have been detected in the γ2-subunit gene (*GABRG2*), one of the most ubiquitously-expressed GABA$_A$ receptor genes. Here, nonsense mutations can result in truncated versions of the encoded protein, lacking either a part of the N-terminal end (Q40X) or the fourth transmembrane-spanning segment (Q390X and Q429X). All of these have been linked to either GEFS+ or Dravet syndrome, but the underlying pathological mechanism has only been identified for Q390X (i.e. retention in the endoplasmic reticulum). Other mutations have been found in the genes encoding the α1 (*GABRA1*), the β3 (*GABRB3*) and the δ (*GABRD*) subunits. They are predominantly located in the extracellular regions of the polypeptide and have variable effects on its function and trafficking.

Considering the neurotransmitter imbalances, the use of antiepileptic drugs aims to potentiate GABA$_A$ receptor activity. These compounds enhance the concentration of GABA at the synapse by either inhibiting the degrading enzyme (GABA transaminase), inhibiting the uptake transporter or providing precursor molecules for the synthesis of this neurotransmitter.

Glycine receptors

Within the cys-loop superfamily, glycine-gated receptors represent another type of chloride-selective ion channels, besides the GABA$_A$ receptors. Although they share more structural and physiological similarities with the latter, compared to other pLGICs, they lack the molecular diversity and widespread distribution that characterises GABA$_A$ receptors. Only five glycine receptor subunits have been identified in mammals (i.e. α1-α4 and β) and, in humans, the α4 subunit gene even appears to be a pseudogene. *In vitro*, the subunits can assemble into homomeric (α polypeptides) or heteromeric (possibly

2α:3β) pentamers, and they are likely to do so *in vivo*, too (Lynch et al., 2009). The β subunits alone do not form channels that are activated by the natural ligand glycine. Neuroanatomically, glycine receptors are primarily found in the spinal cord, the brainstem and the retina, where they mediate inhibition in sensory and motor pathways. At the subcellular level, the homopentamers have been detected at extrasynaptic sites and heteropentamers at the synapse.

In the adult brain, the majority of receptor subtypes is believed to consist of the α1 or α3 and the β subunits (Malosio et al., 1991). Remarkably, the dominant receptor isoform in the embryonic and neonatal brain is the highly-conductive α2-subunit homomer. This subtype is then replaced by the heteromeric α1β and α3β combinations during the first few weeks after birth. The α3-subunit containing glycine receptors may also be of functional significance due to their location in nociceptive neurons. A study on mice suggests that these subtypes are involved in prostaglandin type E2-mediated inflammatory pain sensitisation (Harvey et al., 2004). Animals that lacked a functional α3-subunit showed a reduced perception of pain.

Apart from the agonist glycine, these ion channels can be activated by other amino acids, including β-alanine, taurine, β-aminobutyric acid and GABA, albeit with significantly-lower potencies (Lewis et al., 2003). In homomeric subtypes, they can interact with five identical sites, which are formed at the interface of two adjacent α subunits; heteromers (i.e. 2α:3β) possess three binding sites at the α/β interface. Other pharmacologically-interesting ligands are ivermectin (agonist), a drug against parasitic worms, and the highly potent and selective competitive antagonist strychnine. Like GABA$_A$ receptors, glycine-gated channels can be allosterically blocked by picrotoxin, which preferentially binds to homomeric receptors. Yet another allosteric site enables the modulation by zinc ions, that is, they increase the activity of glycine receptors at low concentrations, but have the opposite effect at high concentrations.

A number of mutations in the α1-subunit gene have been associated with startle disease (hyperekplexia), which presents itself by an exaggerated startle response. The mutation K271L/Q, for example, affects the pore-lining segment TMS2 (Shiang et al., 1993). This and all other mutations in the α1-subunit gene reduce the magnitude of glycine-induced currents.

From a clinical perspective, the glycine receptors, particularly α3-containing subtypes, are interesting drug targets. However, neither subunit-selective agonists, nor therapeutically-important drugs for glycine receptors are currently available.

Ionotrophic glutamate receptors

Glutamate receptors are the major excitatory receptors found within the brain. They consist of metabotropic and ionotropic receptors. There are four main groups within the ionotropic glutamate receptor (iGluR) family. Three of which are classified based upon their selective response to three artificial agonists: α-amino-3-hydroxy-5-methylisoxazole 4-propionic acid (AMPA), kainate and N-methyl-D-aspartate (NMDA). The other class, δ-glutamate receptors, was first identified by analysis of genomic libraries. They remain to be fully pharmacologically classified and are considered to be orphan receptors. In 2009 the crystalline structure of AMPA receptors was first described (Sobolevsky, Rosconi and Gouaux, 2009) and shown to be common to all iGluR subunits (see Table 4.10 for a list of subunits). AMPA receptors are composed of four subunits surrounding a central water-lined pore. The structure of its channel bears a striking resemblance to the bacterial K^+ channel, KcsA. Basically the pore of both has a re-entrant loop that is flanked by two TMS: TMS_2 (M-loop) in iGluRs and P-loop in KcsA. The centre of the pore is narrow due to TMS tapering and the presence of M- or P-loops. This determines the channels selectivity for conductance of specific ions. As Figure 4.32 shows, the TMS and loops of iGluR channels are inverted in KcsA channels. However the iGluRs conduct Na^+, K^+ and Ca^{2+} ions with varying permeabilities whereas KcsA is selective for K^+ ions. Identification of a bacterial iGluR channel (GluPo) which also has an 'inverted' pore that is selective for K^+ ions suggests that the glutamate binding domain and pore inversion in the iGluR family occurred earlier in evolution than loss of K^+ ion selectivity. As to why the pore became inverted one can only speculate. But simply without this inversion, the glutamate binding domain would not be extracellular. And since these receptors function to transduce an external stimulus into an intracellular signal/response an internal ligand binding domain (LBD) would prevent glutamatergic neurotransmission.

Figure 4.33 shows the major iGluR domains in each subunit. The N-terminus domain (NTD) is sometimes referred to as the LIVBP (leucine, isoleucine, valine-binding protein) domain because it is homologous to the bacterial amino acid binding domain of that name. Ligand (e.g. glutamate) binds to the LBD which is sub-divided into S1 and S2 depending upon whether they originate from TMS_1 or TMS_3 respectively. During receptor activation, the ligand is transiently 'locked' into the crevice formed in the middle of S1 and S2 like a clamshell. Although in most cases glutamate is the preferred ligand other amino acids like glycine, serine or aspartate can fit into the S1/S2 crevice to activate the receptor. The size of the S1/S2 cavity varies between subunits with, for example, GluK1 and GluK2 being much larger than GluA2. This means that the kainate subunit will be able to accommodate larger ligands. In terms of drug design, this is an important consideration because ligands that fit into the kainate but not AMPA S1/S2 cavity can be developed, thereby enhancing drug specificity. The C-terminal domain (CTD) is involved in receptor trafficking and anchoring. The CTD also has various sites for phosphorylation and protein-protein interaction. Near the tip of the M-loop there is a glutamate/arginine/asparagine (Q/R/N)

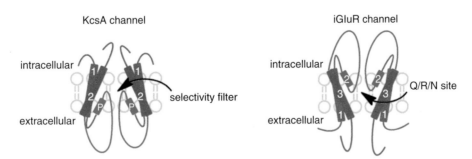

Figure 4.32 A comparison of the bacterial K^+ channel KcsA with the mammalian iGluR channel. Two subunits are shown for clarity but both types of channels are tetramers. Terminal carboxyl and amino sequences are not shown as these are not conserved between KcsA and iGluR channels. The P loop in KcsA consist of an α-helical domain (P) which forms part of the selectivity filter. Within the carboxyl loop after P is a conserved T (tyrosine) amino acid that corresponds to the Q/R/N site in iGluR receptors. This helps conserve K^+ ion selectivity on the channel. The P domain of KcsA corresponds to TMS_2 in iGluR channels.

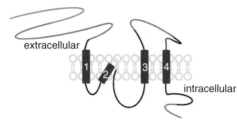

— N-terminal domain   — flip/flop domain   — Q/R/N domain
— ligand binding domain   — c-terminal domain

Figure 4.33 General structure of iGluR receptors. Each subunit has a NBD, LBD, CTD and a conserved Q/R/N sequence in TMS_2. Changing of a glutamate to arginine in the Q/R editing domain confers reduced Ca^{2+} ion permability on specific AMPA and kainate subunits/receptors. The flip/flop domain is another site for RNA editing.

site: Q/R site in AMPA/kainate receptors, N site in NMDA receptors and T (tyrosine) site in KcsA K^+ channels. This site coincides with a narrow constriction within the pore and functions as part of the ion selectivity filter. Mutation of glutamate to an arginine within this site renders the pore of kainate and AMPA receptors impermeable to Ca^{2+} ions (Wollmuth and Sobolevsky, 2004).

Four subunits are required to make a functional iGluR with the NTD and LBD having a twofold symmetry and the TMD a fourfold symmetry. If each subunit is arbitrarily referred to as A, B, C or D, then the contact between NTDs appears to be a dimer of the A/B subunits that has dimerises with that of a C/D dimer through the B and D subunits. However, within the same complex the two-fold symmetry seen at the LBD is due to A/D dimers dimerizing with B/C dimers through the A and C subunits. The linker between NTD and S1 can vary in size depending upon the exact subunit present and this can affect receptor channel opening probabilities. This domain swapping or subunit cross-over gives rise to different NTD and LBD combinations as well as iGluRs with differing gating/conductance properties that is dependent upon which subunit is present and its relative position within the receptor.

So far 18 mammalian genes that encode iGluR subunits have been identified with each gene expressing numerous splice variants (see Table 4.11). They have recently been renamed (Collingridge et al., 2009). Functional iGluRs receptors are composed of subunits from their own group. NMDA receptors mainly consist of two GluN1 and two GluN2 subunits, although the GluN3 subunit can oligomerise with GluN1 or GluN1/GluN2 to form GluN1/GluN3 or GluN1/GluN2/GluN3 receptors respectively. The AMPA receptor GluA1-4 subunits can form homo- and heteromers. Similarly, kainate receptor subunits GluK1-3 can also form homo- and heteromers, whereas GluK4 and GluK5 subunits only form heteromers when expressed with GluK1-3. The δ-type receptors can only form homotetramers and may not function solely as ion channels (see later) (Mayer, 2011).

NMDA receptor

NMDA receptors play a pivotal role in synaptic plasticity and hence remodelling of neuronal pathways. Whilst they have a voltage-dependent activity their subunits do not have the classic four TMS voltage sensor that is common to other ion channels (e.g. K_v, Na_v and Ca_v; see Figure 4.3). Instead sensitivity is derived from a moiety within the channel that binds a Mg^{2+} ion when the membrane is polarised resulting in physical blockage of the channel. Membrane depolarisation causes the Mg^{2+} ion to dissociate and move away, thereby allowing the passage of Na^+, K^+ and Ca^{2+} ions. Since the Ca^{2+} ion current is the most important feature of NMDA receptors they are also known as high conducting voltage-gated Ca^{2+} channels.

There are seven genes encoding the NMDA subunits: GluN1; GluN2A-D; GluN3A-B. For the majority, the presence of both GluN1 and GluN2 subunits are required for receptor function. Sequence comparison reveals a high degree of similarity between the GluN1 and GluN3 subunits. Pharmacological analysis has also shown that glycine or serine are the preferred ligands for GluN1 and GluN3, and glutamate for GluN2 subunits. This has led to the theory that GluN3 subunits have evolved from the GluN1 subunit. As for the GluN2 subunits, it is thought that through gene duplication these subunits have evolved with divergent pharmacological properties to provide a further level of control for receptor activity/function. Other than binding glutamate, the GluN2 subunits confer different Ca^{2+} ion conductances upon the receptor. In adult brains the majority of NMDA receptors contain the GluN2A or GluN2C subunits. However when NMDA receptors are activated they are rapidly internalised and replaced with those containing the GluN2B and GluN2D subunits respectively; cessation of synapse remodelling causes these NMDA receptors to be replaced with those containing the GluN2A and GluN2C subunits. This initial activity-dependent exchange enables greater Ca^{2+} ions influx and hence activation of secondary pathways involved in synapse remodelling. Since cytosolic Ca^{2+} ion concentrations are tightly controlled to prevent activation

Table 4.11 iGluR sub groups.

Group name	Members	Old names
NMDA	GluN1; GluN2A-D; GluN3A-B	NR1; NR2A-D; NR3A-B
Kianate	GluK1-5	GluR5-7, KA1-2
AMPA	GluA1-4	GluR1-4
δ	GluD1-2	GluR delta 1-2
Prokaryotic	GluPo	

Eighteen mammalian genes and one prokaryotic gene encode for iGLuRs. The prokaryotic GluPo receptor has proved an evolutionary link between bacterial and eukaryotic iGluRs because it has features of both ionotropic glutamate receptors and KcsA channels: that is it too has an inverted pore, is glutamate activated and a K^+ ion selective channel.

of pathways involved in neuronal death, NMDA receptor activation is tightly controlled. When the synaptic membrane is at the resting potential NMDA receptors cannot conduct ions. This is because a Mg^{2+} ion physically blocks the channel. However, if the membrane is depolarised, (by for example glutamate activating non-NMDA receptors) the Mg^{2+} ion is displaced and glutamate (and glycine) can now activate it. So for receptor activation two events that occur simultaneously are required: post-synaptic membrane depolarisation and pre-synaptic glutamate release. For this reason NMDA receptors are also known as coincidence detectors.

NMDA receptors are expressed all over the brain and in the spinal cord where they are involved in nociception. Their role in memory formation makes them attractive targets for 'smart drugs' that enhance cognition. For synapse remodelling there is a need for prolonged and sustained glutamate release and NDMA receptors play a role. The accessory and scaffolding protein, PSD_{95}, not only anchors the receptor in the membrane it also enables other proteins that contain a similar PDZ cell adhesion moiety to bind in close proximity. So when Ca^{2+} ions enter the cell they come in contact with Ca^{2+}-dependent calmodulin kinase II (CaMKII) which phosphorylates nitric oxide synthetase and enhances the production of nitric oxide. This diffusible gas travels back to the presynaptic terminal to facilitate further glutamate release. When this occurs in nociceptive neurones within the spinal cord it is known as 'wind up' and is involved in the perception of prolonged pain.

NMDA receptors are major players in excitotoxic mediated cell death (see Figure 5.21). Basically over stimulation of these receptors results in cytotoxic levels of Ca^{2+} and Na^+ ions. This creates an excess of cations within the neurone which causes an electrostatic pull and results in the inward migration of anions such as Cl^- ions. Consequently, water flows into the cell by osmosis to counter the increased ionic composition of the cytosol. The resultant increased osmotic pressure causes neuronal swelling and ultimately cell lysis. This is confounded by the rise in Ca^{2+} ions that has already activated lipases which have started to reduce membrane integrity. The excess Ca^{2+} ion concentration also disrupts oxidative phosphorylation by destabilising the mitochondrial membrane potential thereby preventing activity of the electron transport chain (see Figure 5.19). As a consequence of this, processes that are dependent upon ATP, such as the Na^+/K^+ ATPase pump (see section 5.4) transporter function, start to fail. Na^+ ions accumulate in the cytosol to such an extent that the Na^+ ion gradient is reversed. Since the glutamate transporter uses this gradient to fuel the movement of glutamate across the synaptic plasma membrane, its reversal means that glutamate is pumped out of the cell into synapses. Furthermore, the elevated Ca^{2+} ion concentrations causes further neurotransmitter release by triggering the cascade of events involved in synaptic vesicle migration down to, and fusion with, the synaptic plasma membrane. The accumulated glutamate can now trigger a new round of excitotoxicity in adjacent neurones.

There is evidence that extra-synaptic NMDA receptors play a role in neuroprotection. These receptors will only become active when excessive glutamate is released at a synapse and they function to terminate glutamate-mediated neurotransmission. Studies suggest that subunits containing the GluN2A subunit are involved and that they are coupled to different signalling pathways to those located synaptically. Naturally, pharmaceutical companies are interested in developing compounds to enhance cognition, aid neuroprotection and prevent neurodegeneration. Drugs that target the different GluN2 subunits are currently under investigation. However, these studies have proved difficult because so far the only pharmacological difference observed between these four proteins appears to be at the CTD and specifically their affinity for Zn^{2+} ions. NMDA receptors containing the GluN2A subunit have approximately 50-fold greater affinity for Zn^{2+} ions than those containing GluN2B. This has led to the development of the GluN2B-selective antagonist, ifenprodil. This compound is thought to either target the Zn^{2+} ion binding site or a site very close to it. Since ifenprodil appears to interact with other GluN2 subunits derivatives of this drug, termed 'prodils', have been synthesised. A number of these potent GluN2B-selective antagonists (e.g. MK-0657, radiprodil and traxoprodil) are in stage 2 clinical trials for the treatment of pain, Parkinson's disease and depression (Mony et al., 2009).

Other allosteric modulators of NMDA receptor activity include neurosteroids. Pregnenolone sulphate is used in the laboratory to differentiate between GluN2A/2B and GluN2C/D subunits. The NMDA receptor antagonist, memantine, is used to treat the early symptoms of Alzheimer's disease. This is achieved by preventing neurodegeneration of neurones via the excitotoxic pathway. Memantine is currently the only therapeutic compound that targets iGluR receptors in clinical use. However, it has a number of side effects due to its activity at other receptor types (e.g. 5-HT) and there appears to be little improvement in cognition.

AMPA receptor

Four genes encode the AMPA receptors subunits; GluA1-4. Figure 4.33 shows AMPA receptors contain all the major subunit domains. There is also a flip/flop site, which is only nine amino acids long, that is either spliced in or out of the mature mRNA transcript to give rise to channels with differing properties. In addition, there are also two potential RNA editing sites where the enzyme, adenosine deaminase (AD), can act; AD converts an adenosine to inosine by removing the adenosine group. The first occurs at the Q/R editing site in GluA2 subunit so that the codon for glutamate (CAG) is converted to that of arginine (CIG)(Seeburg and Hartner, 2003). This substitution introduces a charge within the channel that prevents Ca^{2+} ions from moving through the pore of homo- and heteromeric receptors. Since the GluA2 subunit is predominately expressed with an arginine in this position it renders the receptor complex impermeable to Ca^{2+} ions.

This means that most AMPA receptors only conduct Na^+ and K^+ ions. The second AD site occurs just before the flip/flop site in GluA2-4 which also yields subunits with differing properties (Nakagawa, 2010). AMPA receptors are primarily involved in glutamate-mediated synaptic transmission.

AMPA receptors are also involved in synaptic plasticity. Not only do AMPA receptors relieve the Mg^{2+} ion block of NMDA receptors by causing local membrane depolarisation, their numbers are also reduced during the re-modelling phase. This alteration in the ratio of AMPA:NMDA receptors is vital for memory formation. A number of scaffolding/auxiliary proteins are associated with AMPA receptors. Some function to modulate receptor activity while others are involved in endocytosis of the receptor. These include stargazing/TARP, cornichon 2 & 3, CKAMP44 and SOL-1. Manipulation of these protein could potentially alter the AMPA:NMDA receptor ratio and thereby affect cognitive behaviour.

AMPA receptors are associated with a whole host of neurodegenerative diseases that are related to abnormal intracellular Ca^{2+} ion handling. Basically AMPA receptors with Ca^{2+} ion permeability allow too much Ca^{2+} ion influx which triggers neuronal death via apoptotic or non-apoptotic pathways such as excitotoxicity (see Figure 5.21). The Ca^{2+} ion 'overload' can also up regulate pathways involved in cell proliferation and migration leading to tumour genesis. In fact, AMPA receptors have also been associated with glioblastoma tumour proliferation. Here there is a correlation between tumour incidence and the expression of glutamate at the Q/R/N site, which renders the receptor Ca^{2+} ion permeable. In the case of fragile-X syndrome (FXS), Ca^{2+} ions induce activity of the transcription factor CREB. This causes the expression of the fragile X mental retardation gene, FMR1. Normally this gene encodes for an RNA binding protein that negatively regulates the translation of dendritically located mRNAs. This process plays an important role in synaptic plasticity which underlies many processes such as learning and memory and neuronal pathway development. Expression of a mutated form of FMR1 causes mental retardation and cognitive impairment, both characteristics of FXS. Whether the use of drugs that inhibit AMPA receptors with Ca^{2+} ion permeability will be effective against any of these aforementioned conditions remains to be seen. However, the AMPAkine CX-516, which is a positive allosteric modulator of AMPA receptor function, is currently in phase 2 of clinical trials for the treatment of FXS. Whilst it has no side effects, initial results show that it does not appear to improve the behavioural problems associated with FXS (Bowie, 2008).

AMPAkines are also used as cognitive enhancers. This is connected to the AMPA receptors' intimate relationship with NMDA receptors and subsequent activation of pathways involved in synapse remodelling. In this scenario, activation of AMPA receptors would lead to relief of the NMDA receptor Mg^{2+} ion block and its activation. However, there is little evidence that AMPAkines actually improve memory. This is probably due to the absence of glutamate release to actually activate the NMDA receptor (Wollmuth and Sobolevsky, 2004).

Kainate receptors

There are five genes expressing kainate receptors (GluK1-5) that can be divided into two distinct groups: GluK1-3 and GluK4-5. The latter group does not form functional homotetramers and only share 45% identity with GluK1-3. In addition, their sensitivity to glutamate and kainate is different, with affinity for the GluK4-5 subunits being greater than an order of magnitude when compared to the GluK1-3 subunits. Recent findings have also revealed that homomeric kainate receptors have reduced affinity for glutamate as well as ion conductance when compared to heteromeric receptors. Whether this allows the homomeric receptor to only be activated near the site of glutamate release (that is when high glutamate concentrations are at their greatest) rather than by glutamate released from adjacent neurones which is open to speculation (Perrais, Veran and Mulle, 2010).

When compared to other iGluR subtypes very little is known about the function of kainate receptors. They are very similar in structure and pharmacology to AMPA receptors and in fact have a degree of sensitivity to AMPA. The use of ligands with high affinity for kainate receptors such as domoic acid, antibodies and construction of transgenic animals has helped give an insight into some of their functions. This has shown that both types of receptors desensitise at the same rate but kainate receptors need far longer to recover. The rate of recovery is also dependent upon the glutamate concentration with low glutamate concentrations hindering recovery; this is not true of AMPA receptors. Also Na^+ and K^+ ion binding is required for kainate receptor activation but not for AMPA receptors. Furthermore, they have much faster rates of deactivation than AMPA receptors (Jaskolski, Coussen and Mulle, 2005).

Like AMPA receptors, kainate receptors have a Q/R site which affects Ca^{2+} ion conductances. They are expressed throughout the brain at pre, post- and extra-synaptic locations to regulate the activity of neuronal networks (Jaskolski, Coussen and Mulle, 2005). The major type of kainate receptors contain GluK2 and GluK5 subunits.

Kainate receptors are thought to be involved in epilepsy because administration of kainate causes seizures in man and laboratory animals. Whereas inhibitors of receptors containing GluK1 can inhibit seizure activity. Whether inhibitors of kainate receptor activity would be superior to current therapies remains to be determined. Kainate receptors have also been implicated in nociception. Here pre-synaptic receptors regulate neurotransmitter release at glutamergic neurones within the spinal cord. Mice with the gene for GluK1 knockedout are less sensitive to persistent pain stimuli. So in theory GluK1 specific drugs could be a potential therapy for chronic pain (Bowie, 2008).

δ receptors

The δ1- and δ2-type glutamate receptors were identified by scanning mammalian genomic databases for sequences with iGluR homology. Subsequent studies showed that the δ-2 subunit is expressed in granule neurons and Purkinje neurons of the cerebellum. δ-1 subunits are expressed throughout the nervous system of juvenile mice whereas it is confined to the hippocampus of adult animals. This suggests that δ-2 subunits play a role in neuronal pathway formation. Since mice that are deficient in the δ-2 subunit have reduced synapse numbers the δ-2 subunit has also been implicated in synapse formation and maintenance. These knockout mice have also impaired motor learning indicating abnormal synapse formation. The pharmacology of these δ-type receptors are beginning to be discovered. It appears that their endogenous ligand is not glutamate but may be serine or glycine. Emerging evidence indicates that the primary role of δ-type (particularly δ2) iGluRs is not related to their channel activities but rather a structural role in the endocytosis of AMPA receptors (Kakegawa et al., 2009; Yuzaki, 2009). It is known that other members of the iGluR family also have non-ionotropic functions but to a lesser extent. So it maybe that GluD subunits have evolved so that their primary function is not as ion channel.

P2X Receptors

Since their discovery as signalling molecules both purine (ATP, ADP) and pyrimidine (UTP, UDP) nucleotides have been shown to mediate diverse physiological effects through the activation of two major receptor families; ligand-gated P2X receptors and G-protein coupled P2Y receptors. Although not the focus of this section a brief description of the P2Y receptor family is included for completeness. There are eight P2Y receptor subtypes; $P2Y_1$, $P2Y_2$, $P2Y_4$, $P2Y_6$, $P2Y_{11}$, $P2Y_{12}$, $P2Y_{13}$, and $P2Y_{14}$). P2Y receptors can be subdivided pharmacologically into ATP and ADP-preferring receptors (human $P2Y_1$, $P2Y_{11}$, $P2Y_{12}$ and $P2Y_{13}$), those preferring UTP and UDP (human $P2Y_4$ and $P2Y_6$) and receptors of mixed selectivity (human and rodent $P2Y_2$ and rodent $P2Y_4$) that respond to ATP and UTP. The $P2Y_{14}$ receptor is activated by the sugar-nucleotides UDP-glucose, UDP-galactose, UDP-glucuronic acid and UDP-N-acetylglucosamine. At present the $P2Y_{12}$ receptor antagonist clopidogrel (trade name Plavix), which is used as an anti-thrombotic (preventing platelet aggregation), is one of only a few P2Y receptor ligands in clinical use.

P2X receptor structure, signalling and pharmacology

P2X receptors are a family of seven non-selective cation channels, permeable to Na^+, K^+ and Ca^{2+}, that are activated (gated) by extracellular ATP. The P2X receptor family contains seven subunits (P2X1-P2X7) each possessing two TM spanning domains (Figure 4.34). Functional P2X receptors exist as trimers composed of either three identical subunits (homotrimeric channels) or different subunit pairings (heterotrimeric channels). All P2X subunits with the exception of P2X6 form functional homotrimeric channels and to date seven heterotrimeric channels have been identified: P2X1/2, P2X1/4, P2X1/5, P2X2/3, P2X2/6, P2X4/6 and P2X4/7. The trimeric

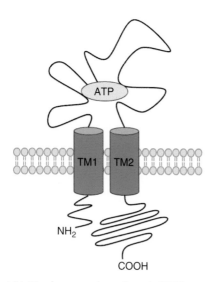

Figure 4.34 Membrane topology of a typical P2X receptor subunit.

subunit arrangement of the P2X receptor differs from other members of the ligand-gated ion channel family which are typically pentameric in structure. In terms of overall size P2X1-6 receptors vary in length between 379–472 amino acids, whereas the P2X7 receptor with its longer COOH-terminus is 595 amino acids in length. The NH_2 and COOH-termini are both located intracellularly and represent important sites for phosphorylation and protein-protein interactions, respectively. The latter are associated with the formation of P2X7 receptor signalling complexes. The large extracellular loop contains the ATP binding site although its precise location is still to be resolved. The publishing in 2009 of the crystal structure of the zebrafish P2X4 receptor confirmed the trimeric arrangement of functional P2X receptors (Kawate et al., 2009). For comprehensive reviews on P2X receptor structure see Young (2009) and Browne et al., (2010).

Detailed pharmacological analysis of concentration-response curves for P2X receptor activation has indicated that three molecules of ATP are required for opening of the ion channel pore. Unfortunately the crystal structure reported by Kawate et al. (2009) was obtained in the absence of ATP (closed state) and as such the precise location of agonist binding site could not be determined. The uncertainty of the location of ATP binding is also partly due to P2X receptors not containing concensus ATP binding site(s) that are characteristic of other ATP-binding proteins. However, as a result of complex mutagenesis experiments the amino acids responsible for ATP binding have been identified and the orthosteric ATP binding pocket appears to be shared between two neighbouring P2X subunits.

As with other members of the ligand-gated ion channel family P2X receptors are subject to allosteric modulation. Examples of allosteric modulators include extracellular Ca^{2+}, Mg^{2+}, H^+ and the trace metals Zn^{2+} and Cu^{2+} (Coddou et al., 2011). In certain cases the allosteric modulation is P2X receptor subtype specific; for example Zn^{2+} potentiates ATP responses mediated via P2X2, P2X3, P2X4 and P2X5 receptors but inhibits responses triggered via P2X1 and P2X7 receptors. The allosteric regulation of P2X receptors may provide an opportunity for the therapeutic development of receptor subtype selective modulators.

When activated P2X receptors regulate numerous cellular processes either through changes in membrane potential or via signalling cascades triggered by Ca^{2+} influx. However, there are some notable differences between the P2X receptor subtypes in terms of ATP sensitivity and desensitisation (Jarvis et al., 2009). For example P2X1 receptors are activated by nanomolar concentrations of ATP and desensitise quickly. In contrast, P2X7 receptors are activated by micromolar concentrations of ATP and are resistant to desensitisation. Sustained activation of the P2X7 receptor also leads to the formation of a large, but reversible, permeability pore in the plasma membrane which allows the influx of hydrophilic solutes into cell. The formation of this permeabilisation pore is a consequence of P2X7 receptor interaction with the transmembrane protein pannexin1 (Panx1). Another distinguishing feature of the P2X7 receptor is its ability form signalling complexes that involve protein-protein interactions with its long C-terminus (Kim et al., 2001). In macrophages the P2X7 receptor/Panx1 complex triggers activation of caspase-1 leading to the cleavage of pro-interleukin-1β (IL-1β) and release of mature inflammatory cytokine IL-1β from the cell (Figure 4.35).

A major obstacle for researchers exploring the physiological and therapeutic potential of P2X receptors has been the lack of subtype selective agonists and antagonists. Studies exploring the physiological role(s) of specific P2X receptor subtypes have used knockout mice. However, in the last few years selective P2X3 and P2X7 receptor antagonists have been produced and other selective P2X ligands are in development. The development of P2X receptor subtype selective ligands is problematic due to structural differences between homotrimers and heterotrimers.

Physiological function of P2X receptors

P2X receptors are widely distributed in mammalian tissue and as such are involved in the regulation and modulation

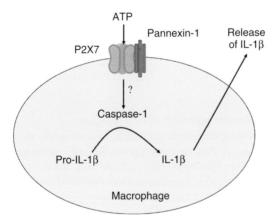

Figure 4.35 P2X7 receptor-mediated release of IL-1β from macrophages. The mechanism(s) linking P2X7/Panx1 to caspase-1 activation are unclear.

of numerous physiological processes (for reviews see Burnstock and Kennedy, 2011; Surprenant and North, 2009). In neuronal tissue P2X receptors are involved in neuromuscular and synaptic neurotransmission mediating both postsynaptic and presynaptic effects. These neuronal effects are a consequence of ATP being an important co-transmitter released from motor nerves, sympathetic nerves and parasympathetic nerves. For example, in the case of sympathetic nerve innervation in vascular smooth muscle, ATP, co-released with noradrenaline, triggers a fast P2X-mediated contraction, whereas noradrenaline is responsible for the slower α-adrenergic receptor mediated response (Figure 4.36a). Likewise the regulation of urinary bladder smooth muscle contraction by the parasympathetic system, following co-release of ATP and acetylcholine, involves fast P2X receptor and slow muscarinic receptor-mediated responses (Figure 4.36b).

P2X receptors are also involved in generating action potentials in afferent sensory neurons (Figure 4.37). These neurons carry nerve impulses to the CNS when activated by transmitters such as ATP released from sensory cells. Evidence suggests various P2X receptor subtypes are involved in afferent neuron activation associated with taste, hearing, pain, bladder distension and carotid bodies (Surprenant and North, 2009).

Besides their functions in neuronal tissue P2X receptors are also expressed in a wide range of non-neuronal cells including astrocytes, endocrine secretory cells, epithelial cells (lung, kidney, trachea, uterus, cornea), fibroblasts, immune cells (macrophages, neutrophils, eosinophils, lymphocytes, mast cells, dendritic cells) and muscle cells (smooth, skeletal and cardiac). Some specific examples of P2X receptor function in the major organ systems relating to non-neuronal cells are briefly discussed below. In the cardiovascular system P2X receptors are involved in the regulation of blood pressure and thrombosis. For example P2X4 receptors expressed on vascular endothelial cells regulate nitric oxide (NO) induced vasodilation of vascular smooth muscle. Whereas activation of P2X1 receptors expressed on platelets appear to mediate thrombosis under conditions of high shear stress. In the respiratory system P2X receptors are expressed on the epithelial cells that line the bronchi and when activated promote the removal of mucus. P2X receptors have also been linked with CO_2-mediated central control of respiration. In the urinary system P2X1 receptors expressed by afferent arteriole smooth muscle cells regulate glomerular filtration rate and in various animals models P2X7 receptor stimulation is linked with renal fibrosis. P2X receptors are also involved in the activation of afferent neurons linked with

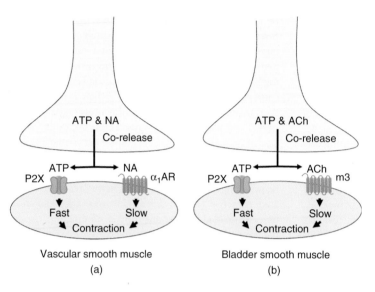

Figure 4.36 Role of P2X receptors in smooth muscle contraction. (a) ATP and noradrenaline (NA) co-released from sympathetic nerves regulate contraction of vascular smooth muscle via P2X and α-adrenergic receptors (α-AR), respectively. (b) ATP and acetylcholine (ACh) co-released from parasympathetic nerves regulate contraction of bladder smooth muscle via P2X and m3 muscarinic receptors (m3), respectively.

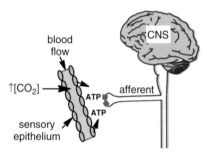

Figure 4.37 Role of P2X receptors in afferent sensory neuron activation. ATP released from sensory cells activates P2X receptors located on afferent sensory nerve terminals. In this example hypoxia-induced release of ATP from glomus cells located in the carotid body (chemoreceptors) activates P2X3 receptors on afferent sensory neurons which relay information to the respiratory centre in the brain.

Table 4.12 The major physiological roles of P2X receptors.

Receptor	Physiological functions
P2X1	Predominant receptor in sympathetic innervated smooth muscle, regulation of glomerular filtration, thrombosis, neutrophil chemotaxis
P2X2, P2X3 or P2X2/3	Inflammatory and neuropathic pain, urinary bladder reflex, chemoreceptor response to hypoxia, taste perception
P2X4	Neuropathic pain, long-term potentiation, vascular smooth muscle tone
P2X7	Cytokine release, inflammatory and neuropathic pain, renal fibrosis, bone remodeling

bladder distension. Finally many of the different cell types associated with the immune system co-express P2X1, P2X4 and P2X7 receptors suggesting a prominent role of P2X receptors in immune control. One major example is P2X7 receptor-mediated release of the pro-inflammatory cytokine IL-1β from macrophages and microglia cells (resident macrophages of the brain and spinal cord). IL-1β is a major player in neurodegeneration (induces cell death in the brain), chronic inflammation and chronic pain. The major physiological functions of P2X receptors are summarised in Table 4.12.

Therapeutic potential of P2X receptors

At present there is considerable interest in the development of P2X receptor ligands for the treatment of numerous conditions that include pain, inflammatory diseases, bladder disorders and irritable bowel syndrome. For example P2X3 and P2X2/3 receptor antagonists such as AF-353 are being developed for the treatment of several pain-related disorders (Gever et al., 2010). The related compound AF-219 is an orally bioavailable P2X3 and P2X2/3 receptor antagonist in Phase II clinical trials for treatment of osteoarthritis, interstitial cystitis/bladder pain syndrome and chronic cough. The involvement of the P2X7 receptor in the release of pro-inflammatory cytokines has led to the development of several selective P2X7 receptor antagonists as potential novel anti-inflammatory agents. For example, the P2X7 antagonist AZD9056 is in phase II clinical trials for the treatment of the inflammatory disorder rheumatoid arthritis. Other potential future therapeutic uses of drugs targeting P2X receptor subtypes include treatment of irritable bowel syndrome, cystic fibrosis and cancer.

4.5 Summary

Ion channels are membrane embedded proteins, which have an intrinsic pore that can facilitate the movement of ions and small molecules between different compartments; organelle/cytosol or extracellular/intracellular. Their opening can be governed by changes in the membrane voltage and/or ligand binding. The voltage-gated ion channels have a basic six-TMS structure; TMS_{1-4} acts as a voltage sensor and TMS_{5-6} forms the pore and selectivity filter. Many members of this family have lost their voltage sensitivity due to either removal of TMS_{1-4} (e.g. K_{2P}) or redundancy within the voltage sensitive domain (e.g. RyR and IP_3 receptors). Conversely a few family members lacking TMS_{1-4} do have a degree of voltage sensitivity (e.g. K_{ir}). The pore forming domain, TMS_{5-6}, shows a high degree of conservation with very precise amino acid sequences conferring ion specificity. Apart from the exception of NMDA receptors, the ligand-gated ion channels have no voltage sensitivity and are purely activated by ligand binding.

Mutation in the genes that encode for ion channels can result in a whole host of pathologies. This is because they perform many cellular functions ranging from electrical and chemical signalling, maintenance of the osmotic composition and the pH of cells and their cellular compartments. The number of disease that are associated with their dysfunction are increasing as we begin to learn about and understand more of their physiology and pharmacology.

The similarity in structure of ion channels has, to a certain extent, hampered drug design due to a lack of specificity that leads to unacceptable side-effects. However, ion channels are a major target of venoms; some of which show astonishing specificity. A chief problem with venoms are that they are short peptides that are prone to degradation due to endogenous peptidase activity. Pharmaceutical companies are currently developing drugs that increase peptide stability or mimic their activity as well as target specific cellular or organ compartments. Another avenue for drug design is naturally occurring ligands such as those found in plant extracts. This explains why drug companies are investing huge amounts of money in the mass screening of various plant species and their extracts in the hope of find naturally occurring ion channel ligands.

References

Accardia A and Picolloa A (2010) CLC channels and transporters: Proteins with borderline personalities. Biochimica et Biophysica Acta (BBA) – Biomembranes 1798:1457–1464.

Ahern CA and Horn R (2004) Stirring up controversy with a voltage sensor paddle. Trends in Neuroscience 27:303–307.

Ashcroft FM and Gribble F (2000) New windows on the mechanism of action of KATP channel openers. Trends Pharmacological Science 21:439–445.

Baenziger JE and Corringer P (2011) 3D structure and allosteric modulation of the transmembrane domain of pentameric ligand-gated ion channels. Neuropharmacology 60:116–125.

Barbe MT, Monyer H and Bruzzone R (2006) Cell-cell communication beyond connexins: the pannexin channels. Physiology 21: 103–114.

Barnard EA, Skolnick P, Olsen RW, Möhler H, Sieghart W, Biggio G, Braestrup C, Bateson AN and Langer SZ (1998) International Union of Pharmacology. XV. Subtypes of gamma-aminobutyric acid A receptors: classification on the basis of subunit structure and receptor function. Pharmacological Reviews 50: 291–313.

Beate N (2011) 5-HT3 receptors: potential of individual isoforms for personalised therapy. Current Opinion in Pharmacology 11:81–86.

Bedner P, Steinhäuser C and Theis M (2012) Functional redundancy and compensation among members of gap junction protein families? Biochimica et Biophysica Acta 1818: 1971–1984.

Ben-Ari Y, Gaiarsa JL, Tyzio R and Khazipov R (2007) GABA: a pioneer transmitter that excites immature neurons and generates primitive oscillations. Physiological Reviews 87: 1215–1284.

Berkefeld H, Fakler B and Schulte U (2010) Ca^{2+}-activated K^+ channels: from protein complexes to function. Physiological Reviews 90:1437–1459.

Biel M (2009) Cyclic nucleotide-regulated cation channels. Journal of Biological Chemistry 284:9017–9021.

Biel M, Wahl-Schott C, Michalakis S, Zong X (2009) Hyperpolarization-activated cation channels: from genes to function. Physiological Reviews 89:847–885.

Bormann J (2000) The 'ABC' of GABA receptors. Trends in Pharmacological Science 21: 16–19.

Bowie D (2008) Ionotropic glutamate receptors & CNS disorders. CNS Neurological Disorders Drug Targets 7:129–143.

Browne LE, Jiang L-H and North RA (2010) New structure enlivens interest in P2X receptors. Trends in Pharmacological Sciences 31: 229–237.

Burnstock G and Kennedy C (2011) P2X receptors in health and disease. Advances in Pharmacology 61: 333–372.

Burra S and Jiang JX (2011) Regulation of cellular function by connexin hemichannels. International Journal of Biochemistry and Molecular Biology 2: 119–128.

Cahalan MD and Chandy KG (2009) The functional network of ion channels in T lymphocytes. Immunological Reviews 231:59–87.

Catterall WA (2010) Ion Channel Voltage Sensors: Structure, Function, and Pathophysiology. Neuron 67:915–928.

Catterall WA (2011) Voltage-gated calcium channels. Cold Spring Harbor Perspectives in Biology 3:a003947.

Choi BH and Hahn SJ (2010) $K_v1.3$: a potential pharmacological target for diabetes. Acta Pharmacology Sin 31:1031–1035.

Coddou C, Yan Z, Obsil T, Huidobro-Toro JP and Stojilkovic SS (2011) Activation and regulation of purinergic P2X receptor channels. Pharmacological Reviews 63: 641–683.

Collingridge GL, Olsen RW, Peters J and Spedding M (2009) A nomenclature for ligand-gated ion channels. Neuropharmacology 56:2–5.

Collinson N, Kuenzi FM, Jarolimek W, Maubach KA, Cothliff R, Sur C, Smith A, Otu FM, Howell O, Atack JR, McKernan RM, Seabrook GR, Dawson GR, Whiting PJ and Rosahl TW (2002) Enhanced learning and memory and altered GABAergic synaptic transmission in mice lacking the alpha 5 subunit of the GABA-A receptor. Journal of Neuroscience 22: 5572–5580.

Cukkemane A, Seifert R and Kaupp UB (2011) Cooperative and uncooperative cyclic-nucleotide-gated ion channels. Trends in Biochemical Sciences 36:55–64.

Darlison MG, Pahal I and Thode C (2005) Consequences of the evolution of the GABA(A) receptor gene family. Cellular Molecular Neurobiology 25: 607–624.

Davies PA, Wang W, Hales TG and Kirkness EF (2003) A novel class of ligand-gated ion channel is activated by Zn^{2+}. Journal of Biological Chemistry 278:712–717.

Deval E, Gasull X, Noël J, Salinas M, Baron A, Diochot S and Lingueglia E (2010) Acid-Sensing Ion Channels (ASICs): Pharmacology and implication in pain. Pharmacology and Therapeutics 128:549–558.

De Vuyst E, Boengler K, Antoons G, Sipido KR, Schulz R and Leybaert L (2011) Pharmacological modulation of connexin-formed channels in cardiac pathophysiology. British Journal of Pharmacology 163: 469–483.

Dutzler R, Campbell EB, Cadene M, Chait BT and MacKinnon R (2002) X-ray structure of a ClC chloride channel at 3.0 A reveals the molecular basis of anion selectivity. Nature 415: 287–294.

Es-Salah-Lamoureux Z, Steele DF and Fedida D (2010) Research into the therapeutic roles of two-pore-domain potassium channels. Trends in Biochemical Sciences 31:587–595.

Evans WH, De Vuyst E and Leybaert L (2006) The gap junction cellular internet: connexin hemichannels enter the signalling limelight. Biochemical Journal 397: 1–14.

Favreau P and Stöcklin R (2009) Marine snail venoms: use and trends in receptor and channel neuropharmacology. Current Opinion in Pharmacology 9:594–601.

Francisco B (2005) The voltage-sensor structure in a voltage-gated channel. Trends in Biochemical Sciences 30:166–168.

Fritschy JM, Benke D, Mertens S, Oertel WH, Bachi T and Möhler H (1992) Five subtypes of type A gamma-aminobutyric acid receptors identified in neurons by double and triple immunofluorescence staining with subunit-specific antibodies. Proceedings of the National Academy of Sciences USA 89: 6726–6730.

Gao L (2010) An update on peptide drugs for voltage-gated calcium channels. Recent Pat CNS Drug Discovery 5:14–22.

Gever JR, Soto R, Henningsen RA, Martin RS, Hackos DH, Panicker S, Rubas W, Oglesby IB, Dillon MP, Milla ME, Burnstock G and Ford APDW (2010) AF-353, a novel, potent and orally bioavailable P2X3/P2X2/3 receptor antagonist. British Journal of Pharmacology 160: 1387–1398.

Gilon P and Rorsman P (2009) NALCN: a regulated leak channel. EMBO Report 10:963–964.

Gonzalez C, Lopez-Rodriguez A, Srikumar D, Rosenthal JJ and Holmgren M (2011) Editing of human K(V)1.1 channel mRNAs disrupts binding of the N-terminus tip at the intracellular cavity. Nature Communications 2:436.

Harvey RJ, Kim H-C and Darlison MG (1993) Molecular cloning reveals the existence of a fourth γ subunit of the vertebrate brain GABA-A receptor. FEBS Letters 331: 211–216.

Harvey RJ, Depner UB, Wässle H, Ahmadi S, Heindl C, Reinold H, Smart TG, Harvey K, Schütz B, Abo-Salem OM, Zimmer A, Poisbeau P, Welzl H, Wolfer DP, Betz H, Zeilhofer HU and Müller U (2004) GlyR alpha3: an essential target for spinal PGE2-mediated inflammatory pain sensitization. Science 304: 884–887.

Hibino H, Inanobe A, Furutani K, Murakami S, Findlay I and Kurachi Y (2010) Inwardly rectifying potassium channels: their structure, function, and physiological roles. Physiological Reviews 90:291–366.

Hofmann F, Biel M and Kaupp UB (2005) International Union of Pharmacology. LI. Nomenclature and structure-function relationships of cyclic nucleotide-regulated channels. Pharmacological Reviews 57:455–462.

Houtani T, Munemoto Y, Kase M, Sakuma S, Tsutsumi T and Sugimoto T (2005) Cloning and expression of ligand-gated ion-channel receptor L2 in central nervous system. Biochemical and Biophysical Research Communications 335:277–285.

Islam MA (2010) Pharmacological modulations of cardiac ultra-rapid and slowly activating delayed rectifier currents: potential antiarrhythmic approaches. Recent Pat Cardiovascular Drug Discovery 5:33–46.

Jarvis MF and Khakh BS (2009) ATP-gated P2X cation-channels. Neuropharmacology 56: 208–215.

Jaskolski F, Coussen F and Mulle C (2005) Subcellular localization and trafficking of kainate receptors. Trends in Biochemical Sciences 26:20–26.

Kakegawa W, Miyazaki T, Kohda K, Matsuda K, Emi K, Motohashi J, Watanabe M and Yuzaki M (2009) The N-terminal domain of GluD2 (GluRdelta2) recruits presynaptic terminals and regulates synaptogenesis in the cerebellum in vivo. Journal of Neuroscience 29:5738–5748.

Kaupp UB and Seifert R (2002) Cyclic nucleotide-gated ion channels. Physiological Reviews 82:769–824.

Kawate T, Michel JC, Birdsong WT and Gouaux E (2009) Crystal structure of the ATP-gated P2X4 ion channel in the closed state. Nature 460: 592–598.

Kim M, Jiang LH, Wilson HL, North RA and Surprenant A (2001) Proteomic and functional evidence for a P2X7 receptor signalling complex. EMBO Journal 20: 6347–6358.

Kunzelmann K, Kongsuphol P, Aldehni F, Tian Y, Ousingsawat J, Warth R and Schreiber R (2009) Bestrophin and TMEM16-Ca(2$^+$) activated Cl($^-$) channels with different functions. Cell Calcium 46: 233–241.

Lasham A, Vreugdenhil E, Bateson AN, Barnard EA and Darlison MG (1991) Conserved organisation of the γ-aminobutyric acidA receptor genes: cloning and analysis of the chicken β4-subunit gene. Journal of Neurochemistry 57: 352–355.

Lesage F, Guillemare E, Fink M, Duprat F, Lazdunski M, Romey G and Barhanin J (1996) A pH-sensitive yeast outward rectifier K+ channel with two pore domains and novel gating properties. Journal of Biological Chemistry 271:4183–4187.

Lewis TM, Schofield PR and McClellan AM (2003) Kinetic determinants of agonist action at the recombinant human glycine receptor. Journal of Physiology 549: 361–374.

Löw K, Crestani F, Keist R, Benke D, Brünig I, Benson JA, Fritschy JM, Rülicke T, Bluethmann H, Möhler H and Rudolph U (2000) Molecular and neuronal substrate for the selective attenuation of anxiety. Science 290: 131–134.

Luscher C and Slesinger PA (2010) Emerging roles for G protein-gated inwardly rectifying potassium (GIRK) channels in health and disease. Nature Reviews Neuroscience 11:301–315.

Lynch JW (2009) Native glycine receptor subtypes and their physiological roles. Neuropharmacology 56: 303–309.

Machu TK (2011) Therapeutics of 5-HT3 receptor antagonists: Current uses and future directions. Pharmacology and Therapeutics 130:338–347.

Macdonald RL, Kang JQ and Gallagher MJ (2010) Mutations in GABA-A receptor subunits associated with genetic epilepsies. Journal of Physiology 588: 1861–1869.

Malosio ML, Marquèze-Pouey B, Kuhse J and Betz H (1991) Widespread expression of glycine receptor subunit mRNAs in the adult and developing rat brain. EMBO Journal 10: 2401–2409.

Mayer ML (2011) Structure and mechanism of glutamate receptor ion channel assembly, activation and modulation. Current Opinions in Neurobiology 21:283–290.

Miceli F, Soldovieri MV, Martire M and Taglialatela M (2008) Molecular pharmacology and therapeutic potential of neuronal Kv7-modulating drugs. Current Opinion in Pharmacology 8:65–74.

Mikoshiba K (2007) IP3 receptor/Ca^{2+} channel: from discovery to new signaling concepts. Journal of Neurochemistry 102:1426–1446.

Mony L, Kew JN, Gunthorpe MJ and Paoletti P (2009) Allosteric modulators of NR2B-containing NMDA receptors: molecular mechanisms and therapeutic potential. British Journal of Pharmacology 157:1301–1317.

Moran MM, McAlexander MA, Biro T and Szallasi A (2011) Transient receptor potential channels as therapeutic targets. Nature Review: Drug Discovery 10:601–620.

Mortensen M, Patel B and Smart TG (2012) GABA potency at GABA(A) receptors found in synaptic and extrasynaptic zones. Frontiers in Cellular Neuroscience 6: 1–10.

Nakagawa T (2010) The biochemistry, ultrastructure, and subunit assembly mechanism of AMPA receptors. Molecular Neurobiology 42:161–184.

Olsen RW and Sieghart W (2009) GABA$_A$ receptors: subtypes provide diversity of function and pharmacology. Neuropharmacology 56: 141–148.

Patel S, Ramakrishnan L, Rahman T, Hamdoun A, Marchant JS, Taylor CW and Brailoiu E (2011) The endo-lysosomal system as an NAADP-sensitive acidic Ca(2+) store: role for the two-pore channels. Cell Calcium 50:157–167.

Payandeh J, Scheuer T, Zheng N and Catterall WA (2011) The crystal structure of a voltage-gated sodium channel. Nature 475:353–358.

Perrais D, Veran J and Mulle C (2010) Gating and permeation of kainate receptors: differences unveiled. Trends in Biochemical Sciences 31:516–522.

Pfenniger A, Wohlwend A and Kwak BR (2011) Mutations in connexin genes and diseases. European Journal of Clinical Investigation 41: 103–116.

Planells-Cases R and Jentsch TJ (2009) Chloride channelopathies. Biochimica et Biophysica Acta 1792:173–189.

Qiu C, Coutinho P, Frank S, Franke S, Law LY, Martin P, Green CR and Becker DL (2003) Targeting connexin43 expression accelerates the rate of wound repair. Current Biology 13: 1697–1703.

Raffa RB (2010) Diselenium, instead of disulfide, bonded analogs of conotoxins: novel synthesis and pharmacotherapeutic potential. Life Sciences 87:451–456.

Remme CA and Bezzina CR (2010) Sodium channel (dys)function and cardiac arrhythmias. Cardiovascular Therapeutics 28:287–294.

Ren D and Xia J (2010) Calcium Signaling Through CatSper Channels in Mammalian Fertilization. Physiology 25:165–175.

Robert BR (2010) Diselenium, instead of disulfide, bonded analogs of conotoxins: novel synthesis and pharmacotherapeutic potential. Life Science 87:451–456.

Rudolph U, Crestani F, Benke D, Brünig I, Benson JA, Fritschy JM, Martin JR, Bluethmann H and Möhler H (1999) Benzodiazepine actions mediated by specific gamma-aminobutyric acid(A) receptor subtypes. Nature 401: 796–800.

Rush AM, Cummins TR and Waxman SG (2007) Multiple sodium channels and their roles in electrogenesis within dorsal root ganglion neurons. Journal of Physiology 579:1–14.

Sáez JC, Berthoud VM, Branes MC, Martinez AD and Beyer EC (2003) Plasma membrane channels formed by connexins: their regulation and functions. Physiological Reviews 83: 1359–1400.

Schild L (2010) The epithelial sodium channel and the control of sodium balance. Biochimica et biophysica acta 1802:1159–1165.

Seeburg PH and Hartner J (2003) Regulation of ion channel/neurotransmitter receptor function by RNA editing. Current Opinions in Neurobiology 13:279–283.

Shiang R, Ryan SG, Zhu YZ, Hahn AF, O'Connell P and Wasmuth JJ (1993) Mutations in the alpha 1 subunit of the inhibitory glycine receptor cause the dominant neurologic disorder, hyperekplexia. Nature Genetics 5: 351–358.

Sieghart W and Karobath M (1980) Molecular heterogeneity of benzodiazepine receptors. Nature 286: 285–287.

Sine SM, Wang HL, Hansen S and Taylor P (2010) On the origin of ion selectivity in the Cys-loop receptor family. Journal of Molecular Neuroscience 40:70–76.

Snyders DJ (1999) Structure and function of cardiac potassium channels. Cardiovascular Research 42:377–390.

Sobolevsky AI, Rosconi MP and Gouaux E (2009) X-ray structure, symmetry and mechanism of an AMPA-subtype glutamate receptor. Nature 462:745–756.

Stewart AP, Haerteis S, Diakov A, Korbmacher C and Edwardson JM (2011) Atomic force microscopy reveals the architecture of the epithelial sodium channel (ENaC). Journal of Biological Chemistry 286:31944–31952.

Striessnig J, Grabner M, Mitterdorfer J, Hering S, Sinnegger MJ and Glossmann H (1998) Structural basis of drug binding to L Ca^{2+} channels. Trends in Biochemical Sciences 19:108–115.

Stühmer W, Alves F, Hartung F, Zientkowska M and Pardo LA (2006) Potassium channels as tumour markers. FEBS Letters 580:2850–2852.

Surprenant A and North RA (2009) Signaling at purinergic P2X receptors. Annual Review of Physiology 71: 333–359.

Swayne LA, Mezghrani A, Lory P, Nargeot J and Monteil A (2010) The NALCN ion channel is a new actor in pancreatic beta-cell physiology. Islets 2:54–56.

Tait MJ, Saadoun S, Bell BA and Papadopoulos MC (2008) Water movements in the brain: role of aquaporins. Trends in Neuroscience 31:37–43.

Taylor CW and Tovey SC (2010) IP(3) receptors: toward understanding their activation. Cold Spring Harbor Perspectives in Biology 2:a004010.

Theile JW and Cummins TR (2011) Recent developments regarding voltage-gated sodium channel blockers for the treatment of inherited and acquired neuropathic pain syndromes. Frontiers in Pharmacology 2:54.

Venault P, Chapouthier G, de Carvalho LP, Simiand J, Morre M, Dodd RH and Rossier J (1986) Benzodiazepine impairs and beta-carboline enhances performance in learning and memory tasks. Nature 321: 864–866.

Waldegger S and Jentsch TJ (2000) Functional and structural analysis of ClC-K chloride channels involved in renal disease. Journal of Biological Chemistry 275: 24527–24533.

Wang, CM, Lincoln J, Cook JE and Becker DL (2007) Abnormal connexin expression underlies delayed wound healing in diabetic skin. Diabetes 56: 2809–2817.

Wesch D, Althaus M, Miranda P, Cruz-Muros I, Fronius M, Gonzalez-Hernandez T, Clauss WG, Alvarez de la Rosa D and Giraldez T (2011) Differential N-termini in epithelial Na^+ channel delta subunit isoforms modulate channel trafficking to the membrane. American Journal of Physiology: Cell Physiolology.

Whiting PJ (2003) GABA-A receptor subtypes in the brain: a paradigm for CNS drug discovery? Drug Discovery Today 8: 445–450.

Wisden W, Laurie DJ, Monyer H and Seeburg PH (1992) The distribution of 13 $GABA_A$ receptor subunit mRNAs in the rat brain. I. Telencephalon, diencephalon, mesencephalon. Journal of Neuroscience 12: 1040–1062.

Wu LJ, Sweet TB and Clapham DE (2010) International Union of Basic and Clinical Pharmacology. LXXVI. Current progress in the mammalian TRP ion channel family. Pharmacological Reviews 62:381–404.

Wollmuth LP and Sobolevsky AI (2004) Structure and gating of the glutamate receptor ion channel. Trends in Neuroscience 27:321–328.

Xiu X, Puskar NL, Shanata JA, Lester HA and Dougherty DA (2009) Nicotine binding to brain receptors requires a strong cation-pi interaction. Nature 458:534–537.

Yang H, Yu Y, Li WG, Yu F, Cao H, Xu TL and Jiang H (2009) Inherent dynamics of the acid-sensing ion channel 1 correlates with the gating mechanism. PLoS Biology 7:e1000151.

Young MT (2009) P2X receptors: dawn of the post-structure era. Trends in Biochemical Sciences 35: 83–90.

Yu FH and Catterall WA (2004) The VGL-chanome: a protein superfamily specialized for electrical signaling and ionic homeostasis. Science's STKE : signal transduction knowledge environment 253:re15.

Yuzaki M (2009) New (but old) molecules regulating synapse integrity and plasticity: Cbln1 and the δ2 glutamate receptor. Neuroscience 162:633–643.

Zhu MX, Evans AM, Ma J, Parrington J and Galione A (2010) Two-pore channels for integrative Ca signaling. Communicative and integrative Biology 3:12–17.

5 Transporter Proteins

5.1 Introduction

Transporters are membrane embedded proteins that facilitate the movement of ions, small molecules and peptides across the lipid bilayer. They can be divided into two groups: channels and carriers. Channels (and pores) facilitate diffusion down the substrate's concentration gradient, whereas carrier-mediated transport involves movement of the transporter and its bound substrate across the membrane.

Carriers can be further divided depending upon whether they use a source of energy for substrate transportation. If energy is derived from a primary source such as a chemical reaction, light adsorption or electron flow then this is known as primarily active transport. However, if a second source of energy is also utilised from, for example, the electrochemical gradient at the expense of the primary energy source, then this is known as secondary active transport; in other words the energy was indirectly provided by a primary active transporter to establish an electrochemical gradient. Tertiary active transport uses energy derived from a secondary active transport-generated gradient. An example of tertiary active transport would be organic anion transporters (OAT) which are involved in maintaining cytosolic organic anion concentrations. They are found in epithelia cells throughout the body and have been studied primarily for their role in urine production in the kidney. OAT use a dicarboxylate gradient to move substrate into the cell; this tertiary gradient is generated by the secondary active transporter, Na^+/dicarboxylate co-transporter and the Na^+ ion gradient is due to the primary active transporter, Na^+/K^+ ATPase which pumps Na^+ ions out of the cell at the expense of ATP hydrolysis (see Figure 5.1).

5.2 Classification

Transporters can be classified in the same way as enzymes, based on their mechanism of action, what they carry and their structure, with the classification continually being updated as more information about transporters emerges (http://www.tcdb.org; Saier et al., 2009). In this chapter we will concentrate on the major groups involved in pathophysiology and drug discovery.

Table 5.1 shows the major classes and their subclasses of transporter. Channels and Pores (Figure 5.2) constitute the first class of transporters and until recently they were not really considered to be transporters because they form an open link between cellular compartments from which

Molecular Pharmacology: From DNA to Drug Discovery, First Edition. John Dickenson, Fiona Freeman, Chris Lloyd Mills, Shiva Sivasubramaniam and Christian Thode.
© 2013 John Wiley & Sons, Ltd. Published 2013 by John Wiley & Sons, Ltd.

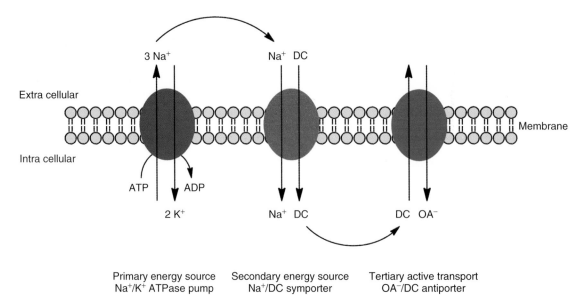

Figure 5.1 Diagram showing how the primary and secondary energy sources are generated for tertiary active transport of organic anions into renal cells. Na^+ ions are pumped out of the cell using the Na^+/K^+ pump with energy derived from the breakdown of ATP (primary active transport). This results in a higher extracellular concentration of Na^+ ions. Dicarboxylate (DC) is transported into the cell via the Na^+/DC symporter using the co-transportation of Na^+ ions down its concentration gradient as the source of energy (secondary active transport). The DC gradient is then used to import organic anions (OA^-) into the cell using the OA^-/DC antiporter.

ions or small molecules can diffuse from a region of high- to one of low- concentration. However, the presence of hydrophobic, hydrophilic and amphipathic groups inside the pore/channel allow them to selectivly facilitate transmembrane ion and small molecule movement which is a characteristic of transporters. Whilst pores are continually open (un-gated channel), channels can be open or closed (gated pore). This is a large family that includes ionotrophic and voltage-gate receptors which have an integral channel that upon activation results in its opening, ion channels that are gated by second messengers (e.g. IP_3, cGMP), as well as porins and gap junctions which allow the transfer of water, signalling molecules and toxins between cells and organisms.

Toxins can cause the formation of pores; some classes of bacteria produce a peptide that forms a channel which allows inorganic ions to flow across the membrane and kill the target organism by destabilising their membrane potential. The antibiotic, gramicidin A, facilitates the movement of K^+, Na^+ and H^+ ions down their concentration gradients. An example of pore-forming toxins that function in mammals are the cardiac glycosides which are produced by foxgloves (*Digitalis*) and related plants. These include digitoxin and digoxin which

were traditionally used to treat heart failure because they increase cytosolic Ca^{2+} levels by inhibiting the Na^+/K^+ pump, reducing the Ca^{2+}/Na^+ exchanger and increasing Ca^{2+} storage within the sarcoplasmic recticulum. But emerging evidence also indicates that these cardiac glycosides can form Ca^{2+} channels (non-ribosomally synthesised channels).

The second class of transporters are the electrochemical potential driven transporters which, as the name implies, utilise the electrochemical gradient to facilitate movement of substrate across membranes. There are three major sub-classes within this group with the largest being porters which can be further divided into three major groupings (see Figure 5.2); uniporters, symporters and antiporters. Uniporters (facilitated diffusion carriers) transport a substrate down its concentration gradient, and hence do not require the co-transport of any other molecules. Porters that translocate substrate across the membrane along with another molecule in the same direction are known as symporters (cotransporters), whereas if movement of substrate and co-transported molecule is in the opposite direction they are referred to as antiporter (counter-transporters). Antiporters are further divided as to whether the co-transported molecule species is the

Table 5.1 Classification of transporters based on their structural homology, what they carry and the source of energy.

Channels & pores
α-type channels
β-barrel porins
Pore-forming toxins (protein & peptides)
Non-ribosomally synthesised channels
Holins
Vesicle fusion pores
Paracellular channels

Electrochemical potential driven transporters
Porters (uniporters, symporters & antiporters)
Non-ribosomally synthesised transporters
Ion gradient-driven energisers

Primary active transporters
Diphosphate bond hydrolysis-driven transporters
Decarboxylation-driven transporters
Methyltransfer-driven transporters
Oxidoreduction-driven transporters
Light absorption-driven transporters

Group translocators
Phosphotransfer-driven group translocators
Nicotinamide Ribonucleoside Uptake Transporters.
Acyl CoA Ligase-Coupled Transporters

Transport Electron Carriers
Transmembrane 2-Electron Transfer Carriers
Transmembrane 1-Electron Transfer Carriers

Accessory factors involved in transport
Auxiliary transport protein
Ribosomally synthesized protein/peptide toxins that target channels and carriers
Non-ribosomally synthesized toxins that target channels and carriers

Incompletely characterised transport systems
Recognised transporters of unknown biochemical mechanism
Putative but uncharacterised transport proteins
Functionally characterised transporters lacking identified sequences

Table reproduced with permission granted from Saier et al., 2009.

same (i.e. solute-solute antiporter) or different (i.e. solute-cation antiporter) to the substrate molecule. Examples of porters include the major facilitator superfamily (MFS; see later).

Another sub-class of the electrochemical potential driven transporters are the non-ribosomally synthesised porters which are derived from non-peptide-like substances or peptides that have had one or more of their amide bonds replaced with ester bonds (depsipeptides). Naturally occurring depsipeptides are produced by some classes of bacteria; inorganic ions bind to these ion carriers (ionophores) so that their charge is shielded and they are ferried across the lipid bilayer by diffusion down their concentration gradient whereby they kill the target organism by destabilising the membrane potential. An example of these bacterial-derived biological weapons is valinomycin which ferries K^+ ions across the membrane. Viruses such as HIV also utilise these non-ribosomally synthesised porters for transfer of DNA and RNA into host cells. They can also translocate drugs and this can be exploited during drug development and specificity. Within this sub-class are members of the cell penetrating peptide (CPP) family which are already being used for drug delivery and targeting.

Finally, the last class of electrochemical potential driven transporters are the ion gradient-driven transporters that are found in some bacteria and use the Na^+ or H^+ gradients as a source of energy to move substrates through channels/pores against their concentration gradients, but how this is achieved is not yet fully understood.

The next major class are the primary active transporters and these use the energy liberated as a consequence of chemical reactions, light absorption or electron flow as their source of energy for substrate translocation. Decarboxylation-, methyltransfer-, oxidoreduction- and light absorption-driven transporters are thought to be restricted to mitochondria, non-eukaryotes and fungi, whereas those driven by the liberation of energy from the breaking of the diphosphate bonds in triphosphate nucleoside (e.g. ATP) are common to both prokaryotes and eukaryotes. Classic examples of primary active transporters are ATPase driven Na^+/K^+ and H^+/K^+ pumps as well as F-type ATPase that synthesise ATP. Also found within this group are the ABC (ATP-binding cassette) transporters, many of which belong to the multidrug resistance (MDR) family of transporters. MDR transporters confer resistance to many drugs including chemotherapeutics and antibiotics and hence they are of considerable interest to the pharmaceutical industry.

The fourth class of transporters are the group translocators which involve the binding of substrate, usually sugars, to the transporter. They chemically modify the substrate by phosphorylation or thioesterification as they

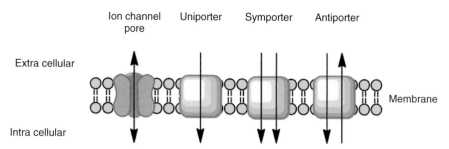

Figure 5.2 The movement of molecules and ions across membranes can be via either ion channels/pores or porters. Porters can ship substrate across the membrane by co-transporting another substrate in the same direction (symporter) or the opposite direction (antiporter) or without a co-transporter molecule/ion (uniporter).

move across the membrane before its subsequent release into the cytoplasm. The only known examples of this class are found in bacteria with none identified in eukaryotes.

In the fifth class are the transport electron carriers that function to contribute or subtract from the membrane potential by moving either a single or two electrons across the membrane. They are mainly found in prokaryotes but cytochrome B_{561} is an example found in mammals, which is located in the membranes of catecholamine and an amidated-peptide containing secretory vesicles and its function is to supply electrons from the cytosol to intra-vesicle enzymes.

Accessory factors are the sixth class of transporters which are not transporters per se but can alter the activity of a transporter system from another class by facilitating trans-membrane movement by stabilising transporter complex formation and/or inhibiting transporter function. For example conotoxins are a family of toxins secreted by the marine cone snail and individual members of this family target different members of the Na^+ channels family and blocking passage of Na^+ or Ca^{2+} across the cell membrane. And finally there are the incompletely characterised transport systems which do not fit easily into any of the major classes of transporters mentioned so far.

It is worthwhile noting that transporters can be described as being importers and exporters; in bacteria, substrates (solutes) can be moved either in or out of the cell. However eukaryotes have organelles like the mitochondria which originate from the phagocytosis of bacteria; so in this case substrates that are exported from the matrix of this compartment into the cytosol are exporters even though the substrate does not leave the cell. For non-bacterial derived organelle such as the endoplasmic reticulum, exporters transport substrates from the cytosol into the organelles matrix.

5.3 Structural analysis of transporters

Transporter structure

Apart from motifs that are characteristic of a particular group of transporters, there appears to be no homology between transporters from different families and even within families when the nucleotide or amino acid sequences are directly compared. However, it is a different story when the 3D structures of these proteins are considered.

Proteins have a primary, secondary, tertiary and quaternary structure which determines how proteins change conformation to suit their different levels of activation and interact with other cellular components to bring about a biological response. In the case of transporters some of these structures are involved in binding and translocation of substrate(s) across membranes. The 3D structure of these proteins, in theory, can be determined by crystallising them and analysing their structure using techniques such as X-ray crystallography or magnetic resonance imaging (MRI). However, membrane embedded proteins contain a number of transmembrane and extra-membrane domains making it difficult (impossible) to maintain both these hydrophobic and hydrophilic regions during crystallisation. Also the different detergents used to isolate these proteins can hinder crystallisation. But the major obstacle in determining the functional structure(s) of transporters is the fact that these proteins exist in different conformational states (active and inactive, and their intermediates) which makes the data derived from X-ray crystallography and similar techniques difficult to interpret. In spite of these difficulties, a number of groups have managed to determine the structures of several different types of transporters by employing substrates/inhibitors that can 'hold' the transporter in a particular conformation during crystallisation. However, most of these studies have been performed on bacterial homologues rather than eukaryote proteins because they can be expressed in large quantities using bacterial host and many of the post-translational modifications found in eukaryotes are absent, making crystallisation easier.

The structure of mammalian transporters can be inferred from bacterial homologues by hydropathy analysis and topology mapping to determine the amino sequences associated with transmembrane regions as well as the intra- and extra-domains and comparing them for similarity from known crystalline transporter sequences. Since it has only been possible to determine the 3D structure of a handful of transporters, biologists have also used the crystalline data from other types of proteins to identify common amino acid sequences and their structural position/role in proteins. These studies have revealed that, like other proteins, transporters contain structural folds that are conserved between families; the name of the fold is ascribed to the first identified example, for example, Glt_{Ph}, $LeuT_{Aa}$ and Nh_{aA} (see Figures 5.3 and 5.7–5.10). This information has shown that whilst the primary structure shows no obvious homology between different classes and subclasses of transporters, there is a degree of conservation at the secondary level and their topology and inferred structural fold(s) (see Figure 5.3) which dictates whether the substrate is taken up or exuded from the cell (compartment) and the mechanisms employed.

Transporters usually have two α-helical transmembrane domains (TMD) with each TMD comprising of 5+1 transmembrane segments (TMS; Figure 5.4b). Typically, five of the TMS in each TMD are virtually identical repeats that can be inverted with the extra TMS being either present or absent (Figure 5.4). This dyad TMD repeat is thought to have arisen from an internal tandem gene duplication / fusion event that occurred within a common ancestor gene. In some instances an extra TMD is present as in the multidrug resistant transporter 1 (MDR1; Figure 5.4a) or, as in the case of the breast cancer resistant protein (BCRP; Figure 5.4c) there is only one TMD present which forms functional homodimers. In the majority of transporters, two TMD should be present so that each TMD can form a 'hinge' that rotates so that the transporter is open to either the cytosolic or extracellular matrix (Figure 5.5b). However, other transporters achieve substrate movement either by the formation of a channel (Figure 5.5c) or via interaction with a trimeric structure that spins around a central axis, which is the case

in F-type ATPase transporters and the ABC transporter, AcrB (Figure 5.5a).

The vast majority of transporters ferry ions across membranes as substrates or co-substrates and analysis of specific structural folding of their TMD have shown that they all share a common feature where the two TMD are involved in forming the substrate pocket and in some cases a physical barrier which prevents the transporter acting like an ion channel/pore (Figure 5.5d). This pair of discontinuous membrane helices either have an extended chain between them as in the P-type ATPases super family (e.g. Na^+/K^+-ATPase, Ca^{2+}-ATPase, H^+-ATPase); they have a short chain between them so that the discontinuous helices span the membrane (e.g. Na^+/H^+ antiporter, Nh_{aA}; Leucine/Na^+ symporter, $LeuT_{Aa}$); or they form an hairpin loop that never completely spans the membrane (e.g. glutamate/Na^+ transporter, Glt_{Ph}) (Sobczak and Lolkema, 2005)(see Figure 5.4). The structures of specific transporters are discussed in subsequent sections.

5.4 Transporter families of pharmacological interest

A complete description of transporters and their role in health and disease is beyond the scope of this book so the following sections will concentrate on types that are of pharmacological interest.

Major facilitator superfamily

The major facilitator superfamily (MFS; also known as the uniporter-symporter-antiporter family) is the largest group of transporters in general, consisting of at least 67 sub-families. These secondary active transporters utilise an electrochemical gradient to move substrate(s) out of or into the cytoplasm with the substrate itself providing the gradient for uniporters, Na^+ or H^+ ions for symporters and H^+ ions or another substrates for antiporters. Individual MFS transporters are specific for only one or two substrates, but the family as a whole transport a diverse range of substrates (Pao, Paulsen and Saier, 1998).

The structural data for a number of bacterial members of this superfamily exist e.g. lactose:H^+ symporter, LacY (Kaback, 2005); the *sn*-glycerol-3-phosphate/phosphate antiporter, GlpT (Huang et al., 2003), the multidrug transporter EmrD that expels amphipathic substrates (Higgins, 2007) and the oxalate:formate antiporter, OxlT (Heymann et al., 2003; Hirai et al., 2002). Even though they differ in amino acid sequence identity their 3D

LeuT$_{Aa}$ Transporter

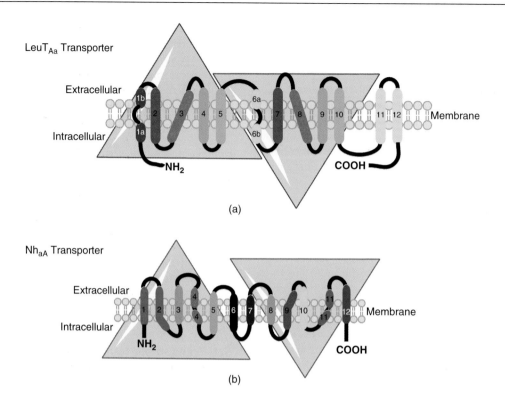

(a)

Nh$_{aA}$ Transporter

(b)

Glt$_{Ph}$ Transporter

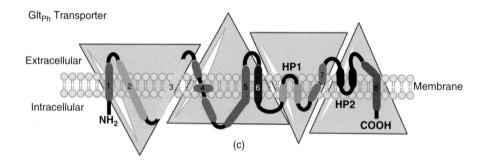

(c)

ACC Transporter

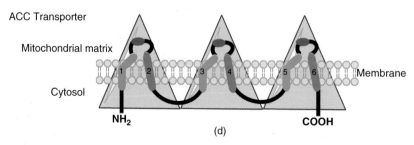

(d)

Figure 5.3 (*Continued on the next page*)

structure is remarkably similar (Chang et al., 2004). MFS are single polypeptides composed of approximately 400–600 amino acids that are highly conserved within single family subtypes. Like transporters in general, the vast majority of MFS family members have 12 TMS (5+1) and when the amino and carboxyl halves are compared it is apparent that TMS_{1-6} are repeats of TMS_{7-12}. There are a few members of the MFS that contain more (14 or 24) or less (6) TMS; how this has occurred is open to speculation but may be due to an insertion of the central cytoplasmic loop into the membrane, gene fusion or a functional homodimer respectively.

Analysis of the primary structure of MFS show that there is low sequence identity or similarity between families, except for a conserved DRXXRR motif in the loops between TMS_2-TMS_3 and TMS_8-TMS_9 which is characteristic of all MSF. It is probably this lack of homology between families that allows this superfamily to be involved in the transport of numerous and diverse compounds such as simple sugars, oligosaccharides, inositols, drugs, amino acids, neurotransmitters, nucleosides, organophosphate esters, tricarboxylic acid cycle metabolites, and a large variety of organic and inorganic anions and cations. Analysis of the substrate-binding pocket of individual MFS transporters indicates that a few amino acid residues are responsible for their ability to differentiate between substrates that are very similar. Interestingly, a point mutation in some MFS can be sufficient to turn a uniporter into a symporter (Law, 2008; Saier et al., 1999).

Since evidence suggests that members of the MFS share a common 3D structure and mechanism for substrate translocation, we shall concentrate on how the bacterial sn-glycerol-3-phosphate/phosphate antiporter (GlpT) transports glucose-3-phosphate (G3P) into, and inorganic phosphate (P_i) out of, E. coli (Figure 5.6). Basically the substrate binding pocket is open to the periplasm and G3P enters and binds between two arginine residues within the pocket that causes a constriction within it resulting in the two TMD moving so that the pocket is now open to the cytoplasm. Since the amino and carboxyl terminals are now closer together G3P's affinity for arginine is reduced and it is released from the binding site, free to diffuse into cytoplasm. G3P's release is probably facilitated by the arginine residues now having a greater affinity for P_i, which moves into the pocket and causes the carboxyl and amino terminals to move away from each other and the TMD to move so that the pocket is now open to the periplasm. The arginine residue's affinity, which is governed by the distance of the carboxyl and amino terminals, is greater for G3P and so P_i is released and another cycle of G3P binding is initiated. MFS also employ salt-bridges to allow the pocket to become open to the internal or external milieu (Lemieux, Huang and Wang, 2004).

MFS in health and disease

The majority of MFS have been indentified in prokaryotes and they are responsible for bacterial cell homeostasis, with a number being associated with protection from

Figure 5.3 (*Continued*) Examples of transporters derived from characteristic structural folds. A fold is a characteristic spatial assembly of secondary protein structures (e.g. α-helices and β-sheets) into a domain-like structure that is common to many different proteins. A particular structural fold is often related to a certain function; in the case of transporters, this is the translocation of substrate(s) across membranes. For this to occur the protein must have two basic conformations where it is either open to the external or internal milieu. Nature has achieved this by duplicating and inverting TMS so that they have the same tertiary fold but opposite orientations in the membrane (indicated by shaded triangles). The figure shows three different structural folds that are based on inverted repeats (LeuT$_{Aa}$, Nh$_{aA}$, and Glt$_{Ph}$). (a) LeuT$_{Aa}$ is an example of a LeuT fold and its name is based on the fact there is a leucine binding site in the middle of the protein, between TMS_6 and TMS_7 which is responsible for Na$^+$ binding and substrate influx/efflux (Khafizov et al., 2010). (b) The Nh$_{aA}$ transporter (sodium hydrogen antiporter (NHA) family fold) like the LeuT$_{Aa}$ transporter has a single inverted repeat but the two TMS that are not duplicated are in the middle of the protein rather than at the carboxyl terminal as in LeuT$_{Aa}$'s case (Boudker and Verdon, 2010). (c) The sodium aspartate symporter (Glt$_{Ph}$) transporter has a Glt$_{Ph}$ fold that arises from a duplication and inversion of TMS in both the carboxyl and amino protein terminus (Faraldo-Gómez and Forrest, 2011). These different structural folds give rise to a structure that transports substrate(s) and gates the 'unopen' conformation slightly differently (see Figure 5.6). (d) A number of transporters like the mitochondrial ADP/ATP carrier (ACC) transporter have been shown to have parallel repeats that have further duplicated to produce three identical TMD repeats (Forrest, Krämer and Ziegler, 2011). This type of fold is an example of a mitochondrial carrier family (MCF) fold. Since this transporter functions as an oligomer (in this case probably a dimer) the different subunits allow it to be 'open' at either the mitochondrial or cytosolic interface. Another example, not shown, is the LacY transporter (major facilitator family–MFS fold) which has the first three TMS duplicated as inverse repeats and these six TMS are replicated again as inverted repeats (Radestock and Forrest, 2011). These different types of structural folds allow transporters to employ diverse mechanisms for substrate translocation.

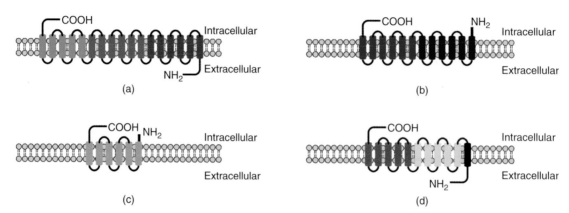

Figure 5.4 Diagram showing typical transporter transmembrane arrangements. Typically there are either five or six transmembrane segments (TMS) per transmembrane domain (TMD; indicated by different colours). However some transporters have an extra TMD whilst others only one TMD. The carboxyl terminus is located intracellular whereas the amino terminus can be either intra- or extra-cellular. (a) The multidrug resistance transporter-1 (MDR-1) has an extra TMD. (b) AcrB, LacY and GlpT transporters contain two TMD with both terminus being cytosolic (c) The breast cancer resistance protein (BCRP) has only one TMD and requires dimerisation for activity. (d) In the ammonium transporter, AmtB, each TMD consist of five TMS and there is an extra TMS.

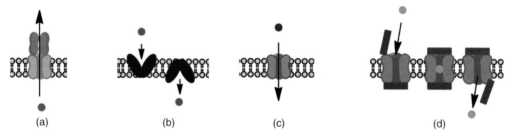

Figure 5.5 Mechanisms used by transporters to translocate substrate across membranes. (a) This type of transporter is found in bacteria or organelles that have a double membrane such as mitochondria. Basically, substrate is actively transported across one membrane and diffuses across the second membrane via a pore (see section on AcrB; Figure 5.20). (b) The transporter's substrate binding pocket is only open to one side of the membrane at a time. Substrate binding triggers a cascade of events that causes a conformational change in the transporter so that it is now open to the other side of the membrane leaving the substrate free to move out (see section on MFS or ABC transporters for examples). (c) The transporter can form a channel so that substrate can move across the membrane. Ionotrophic receptors, pores and some members of the CPP family facilitate substrate movement via this mechanism. (d) Some transporters are essentially channels that are gated on both sides of the membrane so that they are only open to the either the internal or external milieu. The Glt$_{ph}$ transporter is a typical example (adapted with permission from Sobczak and Lolkema, 2005).

xenobiotics as well as drug resistance. In mammals, MFS are expressed all over the body and are involved in a multitude of activities (Saier et al., 1999). They play a major role in neuronal activities including metabolism by supplying nutrients and removing metabolites, maintaining ionic balances across the cell membrane, neurotransmission by packaging of neurotransmitters into synaptic vesicles and protection from potential neurotoxic substances, or uptake of brain-essential substrates through their activity in the blood brain barrier.

Since neuronal tissue cannot store glucose, their metabolic activity is dependent upon the activity of glucose transporters (GLUT) to provide the cell with a constant source of glucose. Any reduction in glucose uptake can have devastating effects on this highly active tissue so it is no surprise that they have been associated with neuronal degeneration. In fact, brain tissue derived from Alzheimer's disease sufferers has a reduced expression of two members of this MFS transporter sub-family, GLUT1 and GLUT3 (Liu et al., 2008). Furthermore, mutations in GLUT1, which is also

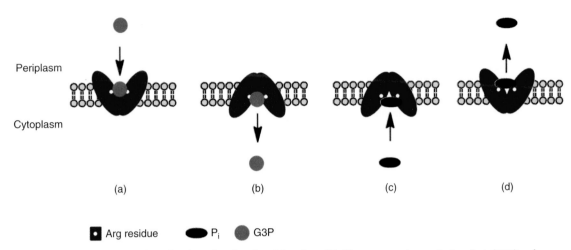

Periplasm

Cytoplasm

(a)   (b)   (c)   (d)

Arg residue P_i G3P

Figure 5.6 Schematic depicting how the glycerol-3-phosphate/phosphate (GlpT) transports glucose-3-phosphate (G3P) and antiporter inorganic phosphate (P_i) across membranes using a 'rocker switch' type mechanism. (a) G3P binds to its pocket which is open to the periplasm, causing the pocket to close and open to the cytoplasm side of the membrane. (b) The substrate binding domain now has a reduced affinity for G3P so it is released, (c) leaving inorganic phosphate (P_i) to bind to this domain. (d) This triggers the pocket to close on the cytoplasmic side and to re-open to the perimplasm and release its P_i cargo. The transporter then enters another cycle of 'rocking' with the associated binding and release of G3P and P_i on opposite sides of the membrane.

expressed in cells of the blood brain barrier, causes the encephalopathy GLUT1, deficiency syndrome (Pascual et al., 2008).

MFS also plays roles in glucose uptake in non-neuronal cells and has been implicated in different forms of diabetes. Until recently mutations in the glucose transporter, GLUT10 (SLC2A10), were associated with type 2 diabetes; however its role may have been indirect. In fact epigenetic analysis has shown it to be a cause of arterial tortuosity syndrome (ATS) where the major arteries are twisted and lengthened, joint hyper-mobility and skin laxity. These phenotypes are believed to be due to two factors. The first is altered glucose uptake resulting in a glucose-dependent increase in transforming growth factor-β (TGFβ) expression which subsequently stimulates vessel wall cell proliferation. The other factor being abnormal collagen and elastin hydroxylases activity compromising the structure of connective tissue; here GLUT10 is thought to co-transport ascorbate which is a cofactor for the aforementioned enzymes (Segade, 2010). Another glucose transporter that is known to cause disease not directly associated with diabetes is GLUT9, which has been reclassified as a uric acid transporter. It is mainly expressed in kidney and liver and mutations in its gene can result in hyperuricemia and gout (Wright et al., 2010).

The vesicular glutamate transporter (vGLUT), which is also a member of the anion-cation subfamily (ACS) concentrates the neurotransmitter glutamate, in synaptic vesicles. The driving force for this is derived from the proton gradient whereby H^+ ions are co-transported out of the vesicle for every molecule of neurotransmitter taken up. A high vesicle proton concentration is achieved through the activity of an ATPase transporter, the vacuolar type ATPases, which is also located in the vesicle membrane and pumps protons into this compartment at the expense of ATP hydrolysis. Malfunction of vesicular transporter proteins results in abnormal neurotransmission, which in turn affects the activity of both local and global neuronal pathways downstream. In addition, since glutamate is the major excitatory neurotransmitter in the central nervous system, vGLUT has the potential to play a role in a whole host of behaviours and pathologies (Takamori, 2006). Three members of this family have so far been identified (vGLUT1-3) and their structure bears remarkable resemblance to the bacterial homologue, GlpT (Figure 5.6), suggesting that vGLUTs employ a similar 'rocking switch' mechanism to transport amino acids across membranes. vGLUTs are also expressed in non-neuronal peripheral organelles such as hormone-containing secretory granules in endocrine cells where they regulate cellular functions (Law, Maloney and Wang, 2008; Almqvist et al., 2007).

Receptors for inositol triphosphate (IP_3) are embedded in the membranes of several organelles, including the endoplasmic reticulum, and activation by IP_3 binding results in the opening of an intrinsic Ca^{2+} ion channel and the efflux of Ca^{2+} ions from its cellular store into the cytosol. This increase in Ca^{2+} ion concentration can activate several secondary messenger pathways as well as trigger neurotransmitter release from pre-synaptic neurones. The H^+/myo-inositol transporter (HMIT) is involved in transporting IP_3 across organelle membranes and since IP_3 plays an important role in neuronal signalling and neurotransmitter release this transporter has been put forward as a potential site of action for mood stabilising drugs (Di Daniel et al., 2009).

The gene, MFSD8, has been implicated in neurodegenerative lysosomal storage disorders. Lysosomes are involved in digestion, sorting and recycling of endocytosed molecules and their membranes contain a similar array of transporters to those seen in synaptic vesicles. Obviously transporters play a significant role in lysosomal function and malfunction can lead to a myriad of pathologies such as neuronal ceroid lipofuscinoses (NCLs) which are characterised by progressive movement abnormalities and seizures. However, the exact substrates and hence function of MFSD8 remains to be determined (Kousi et al., 2009). In the developing brain, thyroid hormones (e.g. T_3 & T_4) have been associated with developmental disorders. These hormones mainly act at neurons with MFS transporters like the mono-carboxylate transporter 8 (MCT8, SLC16A2) used to ferry thyroid hormones in and out of target cells. Mutations in MCT8 result in elevated T_3 serum levels and abnormal brain development and associated human pathologies such as Allan-Herndon-Dudley syndrome which is a severe X-linked condition where neurones involved in intellectual function and movement do not develop properly resulting in psychomotor retardation (Kinne et al., 2010).

Like other transporter families, some MFS have been associated with certain types of cancers. For example, the disruption in renal carcinoma 2 (DIRC2) gene was identified after screening for the causative agent of a familial type of renal cancer, although its substrates remain to be determined (Bodmer et al., 2002). The organic cation/anion transporter (OAT/OCT) subfamilies have also been associated with renal clearance and renal carcinoma. These transporters were originally thought to be primarily involved in the uptake and removal of toxic metabolites and xenobiotics by the liver and kidney as well as maintaining normal brain function through policing of the blood brain barrier and choroid plexus. However, certain members of this superfamily have been shown to be over-expressed in several types of tumours: for example,

OATP1B3 is associated with prostate, colon and liver cancers. So OAT1B3 levels could be used as a possible marker for these cancers as well as a potential therapeutic target.

OAT/OCT are also members of the solute carrier superfamily (SLC; SLC22). They move small charged molecules across membranes using tertiary active transport; Figure 5.1 illustrates how organic anions are transported into renal cells. Whilst they play a major role in hepatic and renal drug uptake and removal they are also found in the brain, heart, lungs, ears, placenta, mammary glands, testes and immune system. Hence a number of pathologies have been associated with these transporters with drugs being developed to exploit their activity. In general, OAT/OCT substrates can be diverse and OAT endogenous compounds include the breakdown products of serotonin and dopamine (5-hydroxy-indoleacetic acid, homovanillic acid), steroid hormones and their metabolites (cortisol, oestrone-3-sulphate), hormones (thyroxine) or exogenous compounds like herbicides (2,4-dichlorophenoxyacetate) and conjugates of mercury or therapeutics such as antibiotics, antineoplastics, antihypertensives and non-steroidal anti-inflammatory drugs (NSAID). OAT are believed to be involved in hepatic uptake and renal elimination of many polar drugs, and they have been associated with drug-related cytotoxicity in the kidney and other tissues after long-term exposure to antivirals (Truong et al., 2008). The endogenous OCT substrates include the neurotransmitters acetylcholine and catecholamines and drugs that utilise OCT include metformin (oral antihyperglycaemic), cimetidine (histamine H_2 receptor antagonist) and acyclovir (antiviral) (Klaassen and Aleksunes, 2010; VanWert, Gionfriddo and Sweet, 2010).

Certain OAT are involved in the transport of sex hormones and the distribution of specific OAT members involved in this process differ between males and females; in the kidney greater expression of OAT1 is found in females whereas OAT2 is more predominate in males. So whilst clinical studies prefer to use male subjects to eliminate possible interactions associated with the oestrus cycle it may not be appropriate to apply inference derived from male subjects to female patients about drugs that act directly or indirectly on steroid carrying OATs (VanWert, Gionfriddo and Sweet, 2010; Klaassen and Aleksunes, 2010).

MFS have also been implicated in drug resistance where they either stop the drug being taken up by the cell or organelle or they exude the drug as soon as it is taken up so that it can never reach therapeutic concentrations at the target site. An example of a MFS sub-family that has been extensively studied is the drug:H^+ antiporter families 1 and 2 (DHA1 and DHA2). These transporters are expressed in lower eukaryotes, particularly yeast and plasmodium, and are associated with homeostasis in response to internal stimuli and to a lesser extent response to physiological and chemical stress. They play a significant role in resistance to the anti-malarial, quinidine. Analysis of these transporters has helped elucidate drug-resistance mechanisms in general (Sa-Correia et al., 2009). Recently the yeast gene TPO1 and its human orthologue, tetracycline transporter-like protein (TETRAN), have been implicated in resistance to NSAID drugs by promoting their efflux. TPO1 was first identified as a polyamine transporter but since it confers resistance to immunosuppressive drugs, herbicides and antimicrobials, it is thought to act as a multidrug efflux pump (Mima et al., 2007; Law, Maloney and Wang, 2008).

Sodium symporter

Sodium symporters, as well as being MFS, are a class of secondary active transporter that co-transport Na^+ ions with sugars, amino acids, ions and other substrate molecules across cytoplasmic and organelle membranes. There are 10 major families in this class including the solute sodium symporter (SSS) and neurotransmitter sodium symporter (NSS), both of which are implicated in brain, intestine, thyroid and kidney function as well as in human disease. The structure of SSS and NSS are very similar (Abramson and Wright, 2009) with slightly different structural folds for example, Leu_{Aa} (leucine transporter), Glt_{ph} (glutamate transporters) or Nh_{aA} (Na^+/H^+ antiporter) which result in the positioning of the TMS that form the substrate binding pocket being different; Glt_{ph} has two re-entrant loops (HP1 and HP2) that never completely transverse the membrane, $LeuT_{Aa}$ has two TMS (1 and 6) whereas TMS_4 and TMS_{11} in Nh_{aA} 'cross over' (see Figure 5.7).

Solute sodium symporter (SSS)

This family of transporters has over 250 members that translocate small molecules such as sugars, amino acids, vitamins, urea, osmolytes and inorganic ions. They also play a role in gluco-sensation and tumour suppression. Pathologies associated with mutations in this family include diabetes, thyroid and bile related problems (Faham et al., 2008; Jung, 2002).

The neurotransmitter: sodium symporter (NSS)

The neurotransmitter: sodium symporter (NSS) family translocate substrates such as biogenic amines (dopamine,

noradrenaline, 5-HT), amino acids (glutamate, GABA, glycine, proline) and osmolytes (betaine, creatine) across membranes. Many of these substrates are associated with terminating the actions of neurotransmitters at the synapse by reuptake into either neurones or glial cells, but they also play roles in maintenance of cellular osmotic pressure and reuptake of small molecules not involved in neurotransmission. Since NSS play such a vital role in neurotransmission, a huge array of diverse neurological pathologies has been associated with NSS dysfunction. This has prompted the pharmaceutical industry to develop drugs that target specific members of the NSS family to treat these disorders. The selective serotonin reuptake inhibitors (SSRI) which are used to treat depression are a prime example.

There are two major NSS sub-classes, solute carrier 1 and 6 (SLC1 and SLC6) with SLC1 involved in glutamate reuptake and SLC6 in biogenic amines and amino acids reuptake. The bacterial homologues, Glt_{ph} and $LeuT_{Aa}$, have been used to study SLC1 and SLC6 transport respectively. Even though they do not co-transport Cl^- and Na^+ ions which is the case in eukaryotes, their structure bears significant resemblance to their mammalian counterparts and inferred mechanism of translocation (Wang and Lewis, 2010).

Glt_{ph} transporters

The major excitatory neurotransmitter found in the brain is glutamate and its concentration at synapses is carefully regulated because too much release can lead to excitotoxicity and neuronal death; many neurodegenerative diseases are associated with excessive glutamate release (see section on excitotoxicity; Figure 5.21). The actions of glutamate at the synapse can be rapidly terminated by uptake into adjacent glial cells or back up into the pre-synaptic neuron via one of the five sub-types of excitatory amino acid transporters ($EAAT_{1-5}$). The EAAT along with the neutral amino acid transporters $ASCT_1$ and $ASCT_2$ are all members of the SLC1 family.

The structure of SLC1 transporters were first studied in a bacterial homologue, Glt_{ph}, which is found in theromophilic archaebacterium *Pyrococcus horikoshii* and transports aspartate or glutamate (although aspartate is its preferred substrate) along with Na^+ ions (Ryan, Compton and Mindell, 2009). Figure 5.7 shows that Glt_{ph} essentially has 10 TMS of which eight transverse the bilipid layer and two are re-entrant loops labelled HP1 and HP2 between TMS_{6-7} and TMS_{7-8} respectively. Careful analysis indicates that Glt_{ph}, like other transporter classes, has two inverted repeats; TMS_{1-3} and

Glt$_{Ph}$ Transporter

Extracellular

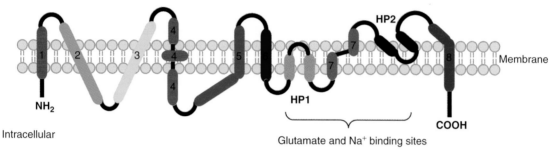

Glutamate and Na$^+$ binding sites

LeuT$_{Aa}$ Transporter

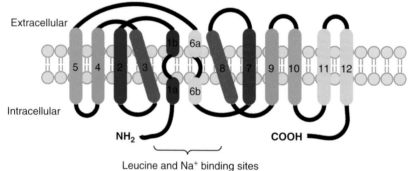

Leucine and Na$^+$ binding sites

Nh$_{aA}$ Transporter

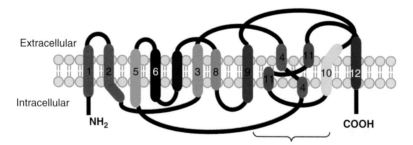

H$^+$ and Na$^+$ binding sites

Figure 5.7 Topolographical comparison of MFS sodium porters. The Glt$_{pH}$ transporter has two re-entrant loops, HP1 and HP2 structure whilst in the LeuT$_{Aa}$ transporter TMS$_1$ and TMS$_6$ have flexible hinges within them so that the substrate binding pocket is exposed to either intra- or extra-cellular. Adapted by permission from Macmillan Publishers Ltd: Nature Yernool et al., copyright (2004). Nh$_{aA}$ has a similar set up to LeuT$_{Aa}$ except the hinge is formed by TMS$_4$ and TMS$_{11}$ crossing over. All three transporters are made up of two TMD that are inverted repeats. Adapted by permission from Macmillan Publishers Ltd: Nature Krishnamurthy et al., copyright (2009).

TMS_{4-6}, and HP1-TMS_7 and HP2-TMS_8 (Yernool et al., 2004). D,L-threo-β-benzloxyaspartate is an inhibitor of Glt_{ph} and hence has helped determine how Glt_{ph} transports substrates. Functionally, TMS_{1-6} form a water-filled 'basin'-like structure which has access to a glutamate and two Na^+ ion binding sites located on TMS_7. The two re-entrant loops, HP1 and HP2, then act as a 'hinge' with only one being open at any one time to either the internal or external milieu, respectively. Initially HP2 is 'open', and glutamate and two Na^+ ions bind within the exposed pocket. This binding actually triggers HP2 to rotate and exposes a further Na^+ ion binding site. The HP2 then enters a 'closed' state where the substrate binding pocket is inaccessible to the extracellular compartment. Substrate and Na^+ ion binding triggers the opening of the pocket to the intracellular compartment as well as reducing the affinity for its cargo so that glutamate and Na^+ ions are free to diffuse into the cytosol. Loss of cargo binding causes HP2 to revert to its original position and closure of the substrate binding pocket at the external interface; the transporter is then ready for a further round of glutamate and Na^+ ions translocation (see Figure 5.8). In reality, a functional transporter consists of three Glt_{ph} subunits so it can transport three glutamate (or aspartate) and nine Na^+ ions during one cycle. This trimeric complex is seen in other types of transporter such as the ABC transporter family (see Figure 5.20; AcrB).

Glt_{ph} has helped elucidate the mechanism of glutamate reuptake via EAATs. However, EAAT differs to Glt_{ph} in that during the reuptake of glutamate it symports three Na^+ ions and one H^+ ion and antiports one K^+ ion. Also both types of transporters activity is influenced by Cl^- by a mechanism not yet fully understood.

$LeuT_{Aa}$

Members of SCL6 are involved in reuptake of neurotransmitters such as dopamine, noradrenaline, serotonin, GABA and glycine. Again the structure of these transporters were initially studied in bacterial homologues such as the leucine transporter of *Aquifex aeolicus* ($LeuT_{Aa}$) which co-transports 2 Na^+ ions along with leucine.

Figure 5.7 shows that $LeuT_{Aa}$ has a dyad fold of symmetry that is typical of the majority of transporters in general. The TMS of $LeuT_{Aa}$ have a α-helical structure with TMS_1 and TMS_6 containing hairpin loops which permit them to rotate approximately 37°, so that in one conformation the transporter is open to the outside of the cell and in the other to the inside of the cell; this is similar to the HP1 and HP2 set up in Glt_{ph} except they are re-entrant loops rather than membrane spanning.

As Figure 5.9 shows functionally leucine and two Na^+ ions move into the substrate pocket and interact with their binding sites. This triggers the formation of a salt bridge between TMS_{1b} and TMS_{10} which prevents the cargo from returning to the extracellular domain.

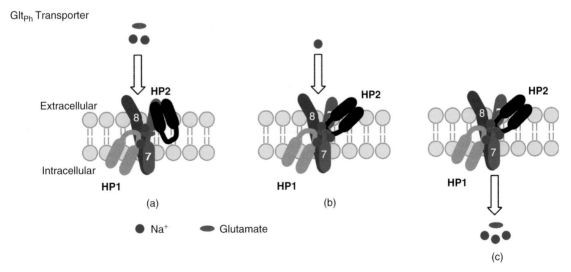

Figure 5.8 Glutamate transporter, Glt_{ph}. (a) Binding of 2 Na^+ ions and glutamate in the substrate binding pocket cause HP2 to rotate. (b) Exposing another Na^+ ion binding site, followed by closure of HP2 and opening of HP1, (c) Where the substrates are released on the other side of the membrane.

LeuT$_{Aa}$ Transporter

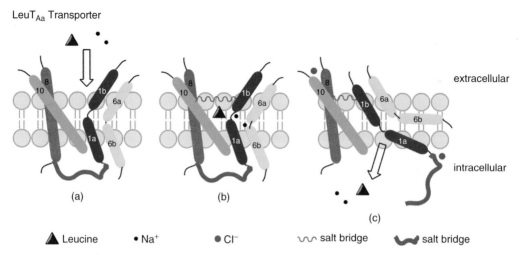

Figure 5.9 Leucine and Na$^+$ transporter, LeuT$_{Aa}$. (a) Leucine and Na$^+$ ions enter the extracellular pocket of LeuT$_{Aa}$ and interact with their binding sites. Exit directly into the cell is prevented by a salt bride between TMS$_8$ and TMS$_{1a}$ and the close proximity of TMS$_{10}$ and TMS$_6$. (b) A salt bridge is formed between TMS$_{10}$ and TMS$_{1b}$ which closed this pocket to the extracellular domain. (c) Substrates are released when the salt bridge between TMS$_8$ and TMS$_{1a}$ is broken and TMS$_{6b}$ moves away from TMS$_{10}$. Cl$^-$ ions binding at both intra- and extra-cellular domains help stabilise this structure and so facilitate release.

In addition, there is a salt bridge already in position between TMS$_{1a}$ and TMS$_8$ and this coupled with the close proximity of TMS$_6$ and TMS$_{10}$ stops the cargo also being released into the cytosol. Next both TSM$_1$ and TSM$_6$ rotate, breaking the salt bridge between TMS$_{1a}$ and TMS$_8$, and leucine and Na$^+$ ions are released into the intracellular compartment. The exact role played by Cl$^-$ ions remains to be elucidated but they are thought to stabilise this conformation by binding to the extracellular and intracellular domains and thereby aid cargo release. This may explain why the activity of these transporters is susceptible to fluctuations in Cl$^-$ concentration.

NSS in health and disease

NSS function to maintain low levels of neurotransmitters at synapses and if their function is compromised then abnormal levels of neurotransmitter will result in either over or under stimulation of adjacent neurones which results in hyper- or hypo-activity of their neuronal pathways leading to cognitive, behavioural and motor abnormalities. In fact a number of neuropathologies are associated with NSS dysfunction and these include depression, obsessive compulsive disorder, epilepsy, autism, orthostatic intolerance, X-linked creatine deficiency syndrome and retinal degeneration.

A mutation in the glutamate transporter, EAAT$_2$, has been related to amyotrophic lateral sclerosis (ALS) which

is characterised by a progressive loss of motor neurones that is probably due to over excitation of these neurones which also have a compromised Ca^{2+} buffering ability, making them more susceptible to the excitotoxic effects of excessive glutamate. Elevated glutamate levels have also been associated with epilepsies and hyperekplexia. Whilst inhibitors of SLC6 transporters have proved to be successful in the treatment of some affective disorders, this has not been the case for SLC1 transporters particularly those specifically targeting EAAT. This is because inhibitors like L-threo-β-benzyloxyaspartate, that have no activity at glutamate receptors, can boost synaptic glutamate levels which lead to excitotoxicity and neuronal death. This has lead to the development of drugs that boost glutamate uptake by increasing the activity of EAAT or their surface expression. In fact, certain β-lactam antibiotics have been shown to increase the surface expression of EAAT$_2$ and hence may be of use in neuroprotection.

A variety of reuptake inhibitors have been developed to target specific SLC6 members. These include a range of drugs to treat depression: such as tri-cyclic antidepressants like imipramine and amitriptyline which are general inhibitors of monoamine reuptake transporters; selective serotonin reuptake inhibitors (SSRI) like fluoxetine (prozac), paroxetine (paxil) and sertraline (Zoloft); serotonin and noradrenaline reuptake inhibitors (SNRI) like venlafaxine; and the noradrenergic and specific serotonergic antidepressants (NaSSA) like mirtazipine. In addition to depression, dysfunctional members of SLC6 have been associated with: severe orthostatic hypotension (noradrenaline transporter); obsessive-compulsive disorder, autism and anorexia (serotonin transporter); and drug addiction and attention deficit hyperactivity disorder (dopamine transporter).

Data from LeuT$_{Aa}$ transporter and the use of SCL6 inhibitors have helped determine the possible conformational states of transporters such as the dopamine transporter. For example tri-cyclic antibiotics are non-competitive inhibitors that can lock the transporter in a conformation where substrate and ions are bound whereas tyrosine can act as a competitive inhibitor, binding to the substrate binding sites and holding the transporter in an open conformation. These inhibitors have been employed to hold the transporter in a specific conformation during crystallisation so that analytical studies can determine their exact structure during cargo binding and prior to their release (Singh et al., 2008).

GABA is the major inhibitory neurotransmitter found in the brain and its primary function is to control excitatory neuronal activity; inhibition of GABA receptor function with pentrazol results in over-excitation of neuronal circuits leading to epileptic seizures. Conversely too much GABA receptor activation within certain neuronal circuits leads to mis-processing of sensory information (hallucinations) and aggressive behaviour. Therefore, synaptic levels of GABA (and glutamate) are strictly controlled with one of the main regulators being GABA transporters (GAT). Glutamine, which plays a role in GABA recycling, is also a substrate of GAT because within astrocytes GABA is converted to glutamine before being released back into the synaptic cleft where it can be taken up by neurones via GAT. In neuronal tissue GAT can also take up GABA as well as glutamine. Once within the neurone glutamine can be converted to glutamate and then GABA (only GABAergic neurones have GABA decarboxylase which catalyses glutamate's conversion to GABA). To date, four GAT have been identified (GAT$_{1-4}$; in some species GAT$_2$ is also known as BGT$_1$) and recent studies suggest that different GAT are located on neurones or astrocytes and that they also have different affinity for GABA or glutamine. Diaminobutyric acid (DABA) is an analogue of GABA and can block neuronal GAT whereas β-alanine can selectively block astrocyte GAT. This selectivity has helped to show that primarily GAT$_1$ is pre-synaptic located, GAT$_3$ is found on astrocytes perisynaptically and that BGT$_1$ is at extrasynaptic

sites. Tiagabine (Gabitril^R) is an inhibitor of GAT$_1$ and is used to treat partial epileptic seizures. Another GAT$_1$ selective inhibitor, LU-32-176B, also shows similar results to tiagabine confirming that GAT$_1$ is targeted. However, since tiagabine has limited use in the treatment of epilepsy and numerous side effects such as agitation, sedation and psychotic episodes it seems unlikely that abnormal GAT$_1$ function is primarily involved in epilepsy. Drugs that target the other members of the GAT family, EF1502 (GAT$_1$/BGT$_1$) and SNAP-5114 (GAT$_{2/3}$), are under investigation to see if they have a better therapeutic outcome for the treatment of epilepsy. In addition, derivatives of muscimol, which is a potent GABA$_A$ receptor agonist and GABA transferase substrate but a poor GAT inhibitor, have helped in our understanding of GABAergic neurotransmission as well as how the different GATs function.

Glycine transporters (GLYT) are an exciting avenue for research because whilst glycine can act at its own receptors to inhibit neuronal activity it is also a co-agonist of the N-methyl-D-aspartate (NMDA) receptors. NMDA receptors are members of the glutamate receptor family and they play an important role in synaptic remodelling which underlies alterations in certain behaviours as well as neurodegenerative diseases. So if GLYT activity can be modulated and hence synaptic glycine levels, then NMDA receptor activity can also be regulated. To date two high-affinity GLYT have been identified; GLYT$_1$ and GLYT$_2$. GLYT$_1$ is associated with astrocytes and control of glycine concentrations at NMDA receptors, whereas GLYT$_2$ is associated with inhibitory glycine receptors. So development of GLYT$_1$ specific drugs may be potential treatments for some behaviour disorders and neurodegenerative diseases.

Sequence comparisons of genes for the SLC6 family reveal relatively low protein identity. However when the comparison is restricted to the transmembrane regions that form the substrates binding pockets the degree of conservation is quite remarkable. In fact mutagenesis studies have revealed that point mutations within the substrate binding pocket can alter what substrate is transported. For example, a creatin SLC6 transporter can successfully be converted to a GABA transporter by altering four key amino acids (Madsen, White and Schousboe, 2010).

Sodium antiporters

These transporters ferry substrates across organelle or cytoplasmic membranes with Na$^+$ ions moving in the opposite direction.

NhaA Na⁺:H⁺ antiporter (Nh$_{aA}$) family

Na⁺/H⁺ antiporters are a sub-class of transporters that belong to the monovalent cation/proton (CPA) antiporter super family. They can be further divided into two sub-families, the Na⁺/H⁺ exchanger (NHE) and the Na⁺/H⁺ antiporters (NHA). Both subfamilies are found in all bacteria and eukaryotes and are important for homeostasis of intracellular Na⁺ ion concentration, pH and cell volume. They also play a role in control of the cell cycle and proliferation, salt tolerance, vesicle trafficking and biogenesis. Within mammals, they have been implicated in hypertension, epilepsy, post-ischaemic myocardial arrhythmia, gastric and kidney disease, diarrhoea, and glaucoma. Drugs have been developed that target specific NHA/NHE antiporters for the treatment of some of these conditions; for example cariporide in the prevention of cardiac ischaemia-reperfusion injury. One of the best characterised members of the NHA family is the bacterial Nh$_{aA}$ antiporter which exchanges one Na⁺ ion (or Li⁺) for two H⁺ ions; human orthologs of these genes, NHA1 and NHA2, have been implicated in hypotension.

In bacteria the Nh$_{aA}$ transporter has been implicated in infection and proliferation of host cells/tissue leading to pathogenicity. Research has focused on the *E. coli* Nh$_{aA}$ antiporter because of its association with mammalian disease. Since it is pH sensitive, the protein can be isolated and crystallised in its inactive (locked) conformation at pH 4 for structural analysis. In addition, this pH sensitivity

has given insight into how antiporters are regulated by pH and how H⁺ ions are counter transported.

Functional Nh$_{aA}$ exist as dimers although exactly how they fit together is as yet unknown. Like other transporters, Nh$_{aA}$ have 12 TMS with a dyad fold of symmetry which is the result of two pairs of discontinuous TMD that span the membrane and are involved in substrate binding/ transduction. However, this structural fold is slightly different to the others in that the chain of amino acids that connect each part of the TMD result in them orientating themselves opposite each other (see Figure 5.7). This structural fold between TMS$_4$ and TMS$_{11}$ forms a barrier between the two halves of the transporter and stop Na⁺ (or Li⁺) from moving straight through the transporter (Figure 5.10).

The substrate binding pore on the cytosolic side is 'V' shaped and only non-hydrated Na⁺ (or Li⁺) ions can physically enter the deepest part of this pore to interact with their binding sites. In acidic conditions (low pH) the high H⁺ ion concentration down-regulates the Nh$_{aA}$ transporter so that it does not bind substrate. However, at physiological pH Na⁺ ions can bind to its substrate binding domain within the TMS$_{4/11}$ pocket due to conformational changes induced by repositioning of TMS$_9$ and TMS$_{10}$. The substrate binding site can now 'invert' so that it is open on the opposite side of the membrane and the Na⁺ ion is released and a H⁺ ion can now bind. Nh$_{aA}$ is 'bi-directional' in that it can transport

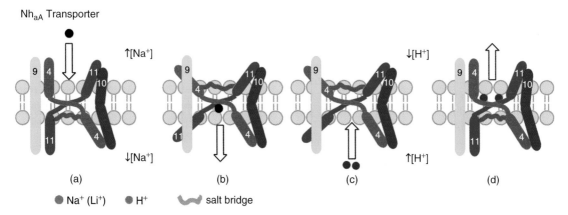

Figure 5.10 Na⁺ and H⁺ ion transporter, Nh$_{aA}$. Na⁺ and H⁺ ions are transported across membranes when the direction of movement is dependent upon the concentration gradients of these ions. (a) Na⁺ ions enters the substrate binding pocket. (b) TMS$_4$ and TMS$_{11}$ rotate so that the pocket is not open to the other side of the membrane and the formation of a salt bridge between TMS$_{4a}$ and TMS$_{11a}$ means that Na⁺ ion can only exit on the opposite side of the membrane. (c) Two H⁺ ions can now enter the pocket. (d) Binding causes TMS$_4$ and TMS$_{11}$ to revert to their original positions and for a salt bridge to form between TMS$_{4b}$ and TMS$_{11b}$, and opening of the pocket on the other side so that the protons can now move out of the pocket.

Na^+ ions in any direction depending upon the H^+ ion concentration and Na^+ ion gradient (Rimon et al., 2008; Padan et al., 2009).

Comparison of several other Na^+ ion coupled transporters has characteristic folds similar to those seen in Glt_{ph}, $LeuT_{Aa}$ and Nh_{aA} (see Krishnamurthy et al., 2009; Krishnamurthy, Piscitelli and Gouaux, 2009). This suggests that these transporters ferry substrate across membranes by either rotating re-entrant loops as in Glt_{ph}, using TMS that contain hairpin loops that rotate against a central axis with no cross-over of these TMS as in $LeuT_{Aa}$, or employing TMS that contain hairpin loops that rotate against a central axis where these TMS cross-over as in Nh_{aA} (Figures 5.8-5.10). Another structural similarity shared by Na^+ ion porters is that the binding sites for substrate and Na^+ ions are in close proximity which ensures that both their movements are thermodynamically tightly coupled.

The cell penetrating peptides (CPP)

The cell penetrating peptides (CPP) are members of non-ribosomally synthesized porters. There is incredible excitement about this family of transporters because of their potential as therapeutic targets for the uptake of pharmaceutical drugs, markers of cell function and gene therapies. CPP, also known as protein transduction domains, are approximately 30 cationic residues long. They were first identified because when certain proteins were added to tissue culture media they were spontaneously taken up into the cell, indicating the involvement of a transporter system. The two best studied proteins were the Tat (trans-activating transcriptional activator) protein from the HIV-1 virus and the Hox gene, antennapedia, which was first identified in fruit flies (drosophila melanogaster). The Tat protein forms part of a complex that is involved in HIV-1 replication (transcription) within host cells. Whilst Hox genes are involved in segmentation and determining the fate of particular cells in early drosophila development; with antennapedia being involved in determining which cells develops into legs. Further analysis of antennapedia showed that only a portion of the protein, a 16 amino acid named penetratin, was required for cell penetration into neuronal cells. Penetratin can be conjugated to a number of different proteins including hydrophobic molecules to aid their cellular uptake and for this reason CPP are also referred to as 'Trojan' peptides. Since the discovery of penetratin and Tat, many more examples of CPP have been identified. CPP

are typically short peptides rich in basic amino acids (lysine and arginine) with some forming amphipathic α-helices CPP; presumably these lipophilic and hydrophilic domains aid translocation of its cargo.

Isolation and fusion of CPP to other molecules facilitates their uptake with no apparent cargo size limit; β-galactosidase has over 1,000 amino acids and CPP-fusion facilitates its cellular uptake. CPP have been shown to transport a number of different types of cargos including small fluorescent probes, drugs, peptides, proteins, liposomes and oligonucleotides, all of which aid our understanding of cellular function. Some CPP work by coating their cargo with polymers or lipids to form a polyplexe or lipoplexe 'micelle' that are then transported into the cell. These 'micelles' can facilitate the uptake of very large cargos; up to 4 μm in diameter (Figure 5.11). The exact method of how CPP transverse the membrane is not well defined and may involve a number of different mechanisms dependent upon the tissue/cell type and individual CPP sequence as well as its cargo. CPP and cargo uptake can be due to endocytosis that is clathrin-dependent, caveolae-mediate or caveolae/clathrin-independent or via macropinocytosis. Heparin sulphate proteoglycans (HSPG) are thought to play a role in CPP internalisation as well as promoting cargo release into the cytosol due to endosomal destabilisation. Several CPP are known to transverse membranes in an endocytosis-independent manner. In the inverted micelles model, CPP is taken up into the lipid bilayer and forms a structure with a lipophilic exterior and hydrophilic interior (reversed micelle); destabilisation of this structure causes its contents (CPP and cargo) to be released into the cytosol. Alternatively the CPP could form a channel that the cargo could pass through to gain entry to the cytoplasm; whether the pore is composed of oligomeric or monomeric CPP remains to be determined. Finally, CPP could transverse the membrane by interacting with the membrane phospholipids resulting in their destabilisation. The subsequent transient lipid bilayer reorganisation provides access for the CPP and cargo and its translocation to the cell's interior. Obviously some mechanism of transportation would be unsuitable for large cargos (Kabouridis, 2003; Trabulo et al., 2010).

CPP in health and disease

Many endogenous proteins with CPP domains have been identified in vertebrates and they play roles in a range of normal cellular functions such as neuronal development, viral infection, prevention of cell death and gene expression. In addition, an array of proteins not

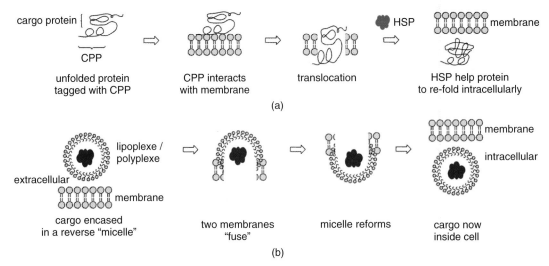

Figure 5.11 Cell penetrating peptides membrane translocation. (a) Unfolded protein is tagged with a cell penetrating peptide (CPP) which allows it to move through the membrane. Heat shock protein (HSP) is also administered to aid reformation of the proteins tertiary structure. (b) Substrate can be encased in carbohydrate or lipid shell (polyplexe or lipoplexe) and move through the membrane utilising the endocytic pathway.

considered to be transporters have been identified that have motifs that correspond to CPP domains which adds a further layer of complexity to their individual function(s) in vivo. Examples include the endogenous neuropeptide, dynorphin, which is considered to only function as an opioid receptor ligand and is important in the treatment of pain. However, it has a number of other actions that appear to be independent of its opioid receptor activity. These include hyperalgesia, apoptosis and altering motor output (Lind, Graslund and Maler, 2006). Another example is cytochrome c which plays a significant role in programmed cell death through activation of pro-apoptopic factors. Analysis of the amino acid sequence of cytochrome c has identified two separate CPP domains which can be manipulated to mediate tumour cell apoptosis (Kagan et al., 2009).

Mass screening of proteins is being conducted to identify novel CPP sequences that may indicate additional roles played by individual proteins with cells. The CPP sequences can also be manipulated and attached to a variety of cargo molecules ranging from nucleotides to nanoparticles for improved drug delivery and tissue targeting. In addition to therapeutic development, they can also be used to study cellular mechanisms like signalling pathways, viral infection or cell viability. Nanoparticles are of extreme interest as they offer the possibility of drug delivery that can evade immuno-surveillance, although this area is controversial because they are relatively large

and the long-period of time between exposure and the development of particulate diseases. Quantum dots are nanoparticles that emit a characteristic wavelength of light and they are used study various aspects of cellular / tissue function.

CPP are being used in clinical trials for drug delivery and gene therapy. Examples include gene silencing, short interfering RNA duplexes and antisense oligonucleotides (See Chapter 8, section 8.9). Multidrug resistance in chemotherapy is a major problem so new delivery strategies are being developed. These include encasing chemotherapeutic drugs with polymers or lipids to form polyplexe or lipoplexe respectively. These can then be injected intravenously, and using ultrasound focused around the tumour site, these complexes can be lysed so that its cargo (drug) is released inside the target cell, thereby reducing drug concentration and side effects due to drug release at other sites (Gao, Fain and Rapoport, 2004; Harasym, Liboiron and Mayer, 2010).

ATPase transporters

These belong to the primary active transporters subgroup, diphosphate bond hydrolysis driven transporters, and there are four main types: P-, V- and F-type, and ABC transporters. The P- and V-type ATPases and ABC transporters using energy derived from the breakdown of ATP for substrate translocation. ABC transporters and P-type ATPases both employ a covalently phosphorylated intermediate for substrate movement, whereas the V-type ATPases are associated with ATP breakdown and the synthesis of an electrochemical (Na^+ or H^+) ion gradient. F-type ATPases work in the 'opposite direction' to V-type ATPases in that they synthesise ATP using energy derived from a Na^+ or H^+ ion gradient and in certain circumstances they can be reversed to form ATP using the eletrogenic gradient (Pedersen, 2007).

Phosphorylation (P)-type ATPase superfamily

The best studied P-type ATPases transport is the Na^+/K^+ ATPase pump. This transporter functions to maintain a low Na^+ ion and high K^+ ion concentrations inside cells. In mammals it plays a significant role in neuronal membrane polarisation and hence action potential propagation. It also helps maintain the osmotic balance within cells. The mechanism underlying this pump was originally investigated using red blood cells (RBC). When RBC are placed in a hypotonic solution they swell and eventually burst due to the movement of water into them via osmosis, whereas in a hypertonic solution water moves out of the RBC and they shrink. Knauf and co-workers (1974) (Knauf, Proverbio and Hoffman, 1974) used resealed RBC ghosts which allow the concentration of ions, ATP and drugs within the RBC to be altered. These studies showed that: (i) Na^+ ions and ATP must be higher inside the RBC and K^+ ions outside for the pump to work; (ii) Na^+ ions and K^+ ion transport was dependent upon ATP hydrolysis; (iii) oubain, which competes with K^+ ions for its binding site, prevents the pump from functioning only when K^+ ions are in the surrounding solution indicating that K^+ ions are transferred from the extracellular fluid to the cytosol; and (iv) the hydrolysis of one ATP resulted in the transport of three Na^+ ions and two K^+ ions. Further studies showed that the pump could be reversed when the concentration gradients of K^+ ions and Na^+ ions were reversed; the ATPase synthesises ATP from ADP.

P-type ATPases can be grouped into five sub-families ($P_I - P_V$), and within these groups there are 10 different distinguishable subtypes, with each subtype being specific for a particular substrate ion (see Table 5.2). The five subfamilies were initially identified after phylogenetic analysis and are thought to have evolved from the P_I family (Kuhlbrandt, 2004). Whilst many P_1 members are found in bacteria and archaea, some are present in humans: for example, the Cu^{2+} ion efflux pumps. Mutations of these genes (e.g. ATP7A or ATP7B) can give rise to fatal hepato-toxic conditions such as Menkes and Wilson disease (Theophilos, Cox and Mercer, 1996; de Bie et al., 2007). Members of the types P_{II} and P_{III} families are amongst the best studied (see Table 5.2) and include: the sarcoplasmic (endoplasmic)-reticulum Ca^{2+}-ATPase (SERCA ;P_{IIa}) which plays a role in skeletal muscle contraction; the Na^+/K^+-ATPase which generates membrane

Table 5.2 Subfamilies of the P-type ATPase with an indication of their specificity and function.

Family	Bacteria/Archaea	Eukaryotes	Specificity	Function
P_{Ia}	*		(K^+)	Turgor pressure regulation
P_{Ib}	*	*	Cu^+, Cu^{2+}, Ag^+, Cd^{2+}, Zn^{2+}, Pb^{2+}, Co^{2+}	Detoxification, trace element homeostasis
P_{IIa}	*	*	Ca^{2+}, Mn^{2+} (incl. SERCA)	Ca^{2+} transport, signalling, muscle relaxation, trace element homeostasis
P_{IIb}		*	Ca^{2+} (incl. PMCA)	Ca^{2+} transport (plasma membrane), signalling
P_{IIc}		*	Na^+/K^+, H^+/K^+	Plasma membrane potential, kidney function, stomach acidification
P_{IId}		*	Na^+, Ca^{2+}	Unknown
P_{IIIa}	*	*[a]	H^+	Plasma membrane potential, pH homeostasis
P_{IIIb}	*		(Mg^{2+})	Unknown
P_{IV}		*	Phospholipids	Lipid transport, lipid-bilayer asymmetry
P_V		*	Unknown	Unknown

Ions in brackets indicate provisional evidence that they are substrates. [a]not found in animals. Taken with permission from Bublitz et al., 2010.

potentials, (P_{IIc}); and the gastric H^+/K^+-ATPase (P_{III}) which acidifies the stomach (Bublitz et al., 2010). P_{IV} transporters have been shown to ferry phospholipids across membranes and hence contribute to establishing lipid bilayer asymmetry. A number of expressed sequence tags (EST) that have characteristics of P-type ATPases have enabled the cloning of several genes that appear to belong to groups P_{IV} and P_V; only eukaryotic members of the P_{IV} and P_V sub-families have so far been identified. So whilst the sequences of these genes are known, their actual substrate remains to be characterised which is the case particularly with P_V members.

Structure and function

In general, P-type ATPases have a catalytic α-subunit which is a single TMD consisting of 10 TMS that complexes with a β-subunit consisting of one TMS which is important for trafficking to, and insertion into the plasma membrane (Figure 5.12). However, there are some instances where either the α-subunit consists of 6 to 12 TMS (which explains why it has a molecular weight ranging from 70 to 150 kDa) or the β-subunit is absent. The catalytic α-subunit has a highly conserved internal amino and carboxyl terminus, a phosphorylation (P) motif (DKTGT[LIVM][TIS]) in which the aspartic (D) residue can be phosphorylated, a nucleotide-binding (N)-domain and an actuator (A)-domain which contains a conserved TEGS motif. The A and P domains are formed by a cytoplasmic loop between TMS_4 and TMS_5 and the A domain between TMS_2 and TMS_3 (see Figure 5.13a).

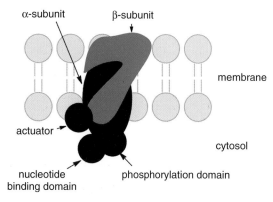

Figure 5.12 General structure of the Na^+/K^+ ATPase pump. P-type ATPase transporters are composed of the catalytic α-subunit composed of 12 TMS with actuator, nucleotide binding and phosphorylation domains, and a β-subunit.

Using the Na^+/K^+ pump as an example of how P-type ATPase transport substrate(s) across membrane has identified two transporter states, E1 and E2 (Figure 5.13b). Basically, unphosphorylated E1 is located on the cytosolic side of the membrane and is 'empty'. When ATP binds to the intracellular domain of the α-subunit, this promotes the movement and binding of three Na^+ ions from the cytoplasm to the substrate binding pocket. This in turn causes an intrinsic ATPase to hydrolyse the ATP molecule resulting in phosphorylation of the α-subunit and its subsequent conformational change (E1-P) which results in a lower affinity of E1 for Na^+ ions and the release of the three Na^+ ions into the extracellular fluid (E2-P). Consequently two K^+ ion binding sites are exposed in the pump so K^+ ions move from the extracellular fluid into the substrate binding pocket. This causes hydrolysis of the phosphorylated aspartic in the P-motif and removal of the phosphate group from the P site (E2) followed by the opening of the pocket to the cytosolic side of the membrane and release of the two K^+ ions into the cytoplasm (E1). The transporter is then ready for another round of Na^+ and K^+ transportation.

There are numerous members of the Na^+/K^+ ATPase transporter because four isoforms of the α-subunit and two of the β-subunit have been identified giving rise to different α– and β-subunit configurations. Other types of P-type ATPase are also composed of similar α– and β-subunits that have multiple isoforms that can transport other ions (e.g. H^+/K^+ and Ca^{2+} pumps).

P-type ATPase transporters in health and disease

Since many of the P-type ATPases play pivotal roles in cell homeostasis any deviation from normal function can result in a myriad of symptoms and diseases. These include the previously mentioned Menkes and Wilsons diseases which are related to abnormal Cu^{2+} ion transport. Three isoforms of the catalytic α-subunit of the Na^+/K^+ ATPase pump (P_{II}) are expressed in neurones and gene mutations result in altered ATPase activity. A mutation in the α-3 subunit is associated with the movement disorder, dystonia Parkinsonism (Blanco-Arias et al., 2009). A mutation in the gene encoding the α-2 subunit (ATP1A2), which is predominately found in neurones (and muscles) can cause a form of migraines (familial hemiplegic migraine type 2) characterised by auras and loss of right or left sided body strength. This α-2 mutation can also indirectly influence the cardio-vascular system due to irregular cardiac Ca^{2+} ion homeostasis since the resultant abnormal Na^+ ion concentration affects the

Ca^{2+}/Na^+ exchanger. Arrhythmias and heart failure due to advanced artherosclerosis can lead to systolic and/or diastolic ventricular dysfunction. Cardiac glycosides such as *Digitalis purpurea* (foxglove plant) have been used for centuries to treat congestive heart failure. Digitalis inhibits the Na^+ pump in the sarcolemma membrane increasing the cytosolic Na^+ concentration and thereby reducing the Na^+ gradient across the membrane. This reduces the activity of the Ca^{2+}/Na^+ pump and hence Ca^{2+} translocation. The higher steady-state level of Ca^{2+} can be used by the muscle's contractile elements to increase the force of contraction to overcome cardiac disturbances (James et al., 1999). Another neuronal expressed transporter that causes a form of Parkinsonism associated with dementia, Kufor-Rakeb syndrome, is ATP13A2 (P_V) which transports inorganic cations and other substrates across lysosomal membranes. It is thought that mutations in this ATP13A2 gene results in decreased lysosomal protein degradation and hence increased aggregation of toxic proteins which leads to degeneration of the neurone (Ramirez et al., 2006).

The sarco(endo)plasmic reticulum Ca^{2+} ATPase transporter (SERCA) SERCA1 gene (ATP2A1) is found in fast-twitch muscle fibres and dysfunction of this gene results in impaired skeletal muscle relaxation and cramping (Brody myopathy; Odermatt et al., 1996). Another isoform of SERCA, SERCA2 (ATP2A2), is highly expressed in keratinocytes and indirectly controls signalling pathways that regulate cell-to-cell adhesion and differentiation of the epidermis by managing Ca^{2+} levels; mutations of the SERCA2 gene results in skin abnormalities associated with Darier-White disease (Sakuntabhai et al., 1999). Isoforms of SERCA are also found on the endoplasmic reticulum and are involved in normal cellular metabolism. However if SERCA is inhibited by compounds such as thapsigargin, then an endoplasmic reticulum (ER) stress response is activated alongside mitochondria-mediated apoptosis. This response can be manipulated to target cancer cells and kill them by coupling the inhibitor to a target peptide to produce a pro-drug that only becomes active at the target tissue; this approach has been used in the treatment of prostate cancer. An H^+/K^+ ATPase is responsible for stomach acid secretions and increased acid secretion is associated with the development of gastric ulcers and drugs that target this transporter (proton-pump blockers) have been employed as a successful therapy.

Immuno-compromised individuals such as those infected with HIV are prone to opportunist fungal infections and are a major cause of morbidity/mortality.

Fungal infections in animals are difficult to treat because the majority of anti-fungal drugs target sites that are found in most eukaryotes and hence toxic to the host mammal. However, fungi use a plasma membrane H^+/K^+ APTase pump, Pma1, to maintain their cytosol pH in neutral / acidic environments such as alveolar spaces or bloodstream or basic locations such as intracellular phagolysomomes of host cells. Since mammalian P-type ATPase only shares approximately 30% sequence identity with Pma1 H^+/K^+ ATPase pumps, they are a potential target for drug development in the treatment of fungal infections in animals. One such candidate is ebselen, which inhibits fungal H^+/K^+ ATPase pump thereby destabilising the plasma membrane potential and cellular homeostasis, and ultimately resulting in cell death (Monk et al., 1995).

F-Type (F_oF_1) ATPases

F-type ATPases are multimeric complexes found in the mitochondria of all eukaryotes and in most bacteria. The numbers of subunits present vary, with prokaryotes members containing eight whereas in mammals there are between 16 and 18. They are involved in the final step of oxidative phosphorylation and the production of ATP. Under normal physiological condition three ATP molecules are synthesised at the expense of $10\,H^+$ ions moving down their concentration gradient into the mitochondrial matrix. A high concentration of H^+ ions within the inner membrane space is achieved by the movement of electrons from the mitochondrial matrix along the electron transport chain which is located in the inner mitochondrial membrane and the subsequent displacement of H^+ by the electron within this chain and its release into the inner membrane space (see section on oxidoreduction transporters; Figure 5.19). Under certain conditions the pump can be reversed so that H^+ ions are transported out of the mitochondrial matrix against its concentration gradient at the expense of ATP. Therefore, ATP synthesis or utilisation is dependent upon the trans-mitochondrial membrane concentration gradient of H^+ ions (Capaldi and Aggeler, 2002).

F-type ATPases are composed of two main complexes that need to be coupled: the membrane bound F_0 and matrix located F_1. F_0 is made up of a single a and two b subunits as well as between 10 to 15 c subunits that form a rotor. These a and b subunits also interact with a d-subunit to form a peripheral stalk that connects the two complexes. Each c-subunit can interact with a single H^+ ion and cross the mitochondrial inner membrane and

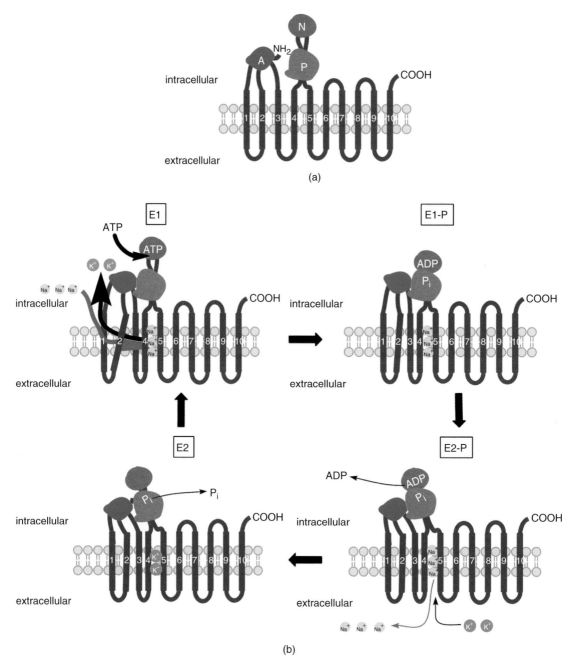

Figure 5.13 (*Continued on the next page*)

cause the rotor to turn relatively to the rigid a-subunit; 36° if it is composed of 10 c-subunits or 24° for a 15 c-subunit structures. The F_1 complex consists of trimeric arrangement of αβ subunits ($α_3β_3$) that can each rotate 120° with each αβ subunit being in a different conformational state at any one time depending upon its proximity to the peripheral stalk. A central stalk which has a ε- and an elongated γ-subunit that is embedded in both the rotor and $α_3β_3$ complex serves to connect and couple the rotation of the c-subunits and the F_1 head. As the $α_3β_3$ complex rotates each β-subunit can manufacture an ATP molecule from ADP and P_i (see Figure 5.14a).

F-type ATPase transporters in health and disease

Mitochondrial F-type ATPases are mainly involved in oxidative phosphorylation and ATP production but during cardiac ischaemia, when oxygen and glucose levels are low, their activity can be reversed so that they hydrolyse ATP in order to maintain the mitochondrial membrane potential. Prolonged ischaemia can have a devastating effect on cardio-myocytes because the Ca^{2+}-dependent ATPase pump is unable to function due to a lack of ATP so that Ca^{2+} accumulates in the cells and mitochondria to such a level that it activates proteases and lipases, and produces reactive oxygen species because the electron transport chain is partially uncoupled, both of which reduce cardiac performance (Morin et al., 2009). Genetic defects in a protein that helps F_1 to assembly correctly, ATP12, (De Meirleir et al., 2004) results in muscle spasticity, renal and hepatic dysfunction as well as elevated lactate levels in urine, plasma, and CSF (De Meirleir et al., 2004). Defects in the gene that encoded for one of the F_1F_0 subunits, ATP synthase 8, results in major defects similar to those seen in patients with ATP12 mutations as well as severe cardiac problems (Ware et al., 2009).

V-Type ATPases

Vacuoular (V) type ATPases are used to generate a high concentration of H^+ or Na^+ ions within cellular compartments, for example vacuoles and vesicles. As Figure 5.14b shows V-type ATPases share a similar organization to F-type ATPases in that they have a membrane-embedded rotor made up of c-subunits and a trimeric (A_3B_3) catalytic head which rotate with the movement of ions (Na^+ or H^+) or ATP hydrolysis respectively. However, the composition of the central stalk (E, d and D) and peripheral stalk (a, E, H and g) are different and may slightly alter the mechanism that enables rotation of the c-subunit oligomer and catalytic head. In addition, V-type ATPase can have up to two peripheral stalks. Whether these differences allow the V_1 and V_0 complexes to uncouple in certain circumstances, such as when ATP hydrolysis has to be stopped during glucose deprivation or moulting of the exocuticle in the larvae stage of some insects, remains to be determined (Beyenbach and Wieczorek, 2006).

V-type ATPase transporters in health and disease

V-type ATPases play important roles in many physiological processes including pH regulation and they are found in a variety of cellular membranes such as endosomes, lysosomes and in some cases the plasma membrane. Within intracellular organelles they aid receptor-mediated endocytosis, protein processing and degradation as well as working in conjunction with other types of transporters to facilitate transmembrane movement of ions and small molecules; they concentrate H^+ ions within synaptic vesicles and it is this driving force which powers the vesicular transporter that moves the neurotransmitter into the vesicle at the expense of an H^+ ion moving out in the opposite direction. Diversity within this family of transporters arises because most of the

Figure 5.13 (*Continued*) Schematic illustrating the topology, functional motifs and how a typical P-type ATPases moves ions across the lipid bilayer. (a) P-type ATPases typically have 10 trans-membrane segments (TMS) and three functional motifs: a nucleotide binding domain (N) where ATP binds, a phosphorylation domain (P) which has ATPase activity for ATP breakdown and an actuator domain (A) that facilitates the formation of various conformations of the transporter. (b) The Na^+/K^+ ATPase pump is used as an example as to how P-type ATPase transporters translocate ions. In the E1 state, ATP binds to the N domain and three Na^+ ions move into between TMS_4 and TMS_5 via a channel formed by TMS_1 and TMS_2. As a result the N and P domains come into close contact so ATP can be broken down into ADP and inorganic phosphate (P_i) by the intrinsic ATPase activity of the P domain and the E1-P configuration is formed. E2-P is formed because ADP dissociates, allowing the three Na^+ ions to move out of and two K^+ ions into the pocket formed by TMS_4 and TMS_5. Finally, the P-domain is dephosphorylated and P_i is released and the transporter enters the E2 conformation. Rotation of the A-domain allows ATP to bind to the N-domain and for two K^+ ions to be released into the cytosol via the channel formed by TMS_1 and TMS_2 and for three Na^+ ions to enter the substrate binding pocket and start the E1, E1-P, E2-P and E2 cycle again.

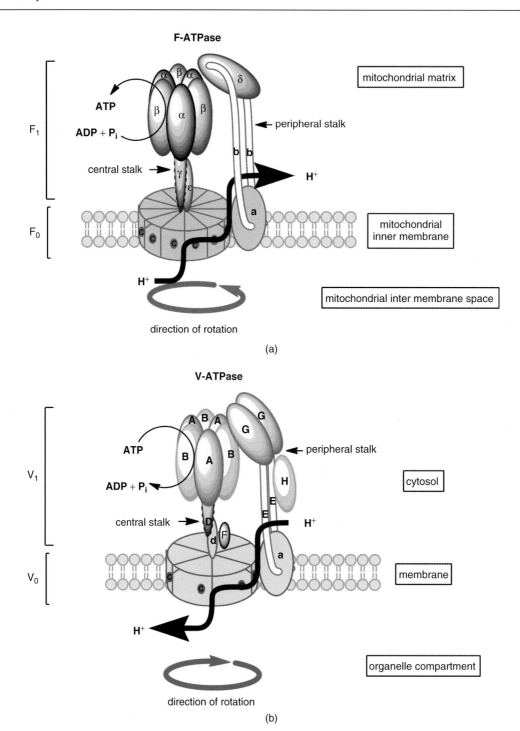

Figure 5.14 (*Continued on the next page*)

V-type ATPase subunits exist in multiple isoforms which are often expressed in a tissue specific manner. Plasma membrane located V-type ATPases are involved in bone resaborption, renal acid secretion, pathogen removal, angiogenesis and sperm processing. In addition, some viruses and bacteria can infect cells via V-type ATPases (Hinton, Bond and Forgac, 2009). Because of their diverse cellular roles they are implicated in a multitude of diseases. Under normal conditions, osteoclasts secrete protons into the extracellular space and this serves to dissolve the adjacent bone matrix and facilitate bone remodelling; defects in the transporter prevent this acidification and which leads to osteopetrosis. When kidney cells are unable to secrete enough acid into the urine, renal tubule acidosis occurs. Sperm cell storage and maturation is dependent upon a low pH environment and problems with these V-type ATPases members can cause male sterility. They have also been implicated in tumour invasion because they provide an acidic extracellular environment that activates mediators involved in metastasis (Toei, Saum and Forgac, 2010; Hinton, Bond and Forgac, 2009).

Mutations in a gene encoding for one of the subunit members of V_1V_0, A2V-ATPase, result in excessive skin wrinkling, connective tissue abnormalities, developmental delay and neurologic problems such as seizures and age-related mental deterioration (Kornak et al., 2008). Defects in the ATP6B1 gene which encoded the B subunit in V_1 produces renal tubular acidosis as well as sensorineural deafness due to abnormal endolymph pH in the cochlea and endolymphatic (Karet et al., 1999).

ABC (ATP-binding cassette) transporters

ABC transporters are generally multi-component primary active transporters, capable of transporting both small molecules and macromolecules in response to ATP hydrolysis. This super family of ATPase transporters have a highly conserved characteristic nucleotide binding domain (NBD) for ATP binding and hydrolysis, and a less conserved transmembrane domain (TMD) that forms the pathway for substrate translocation (Figure 5.15d).

Like other transporters each TMD has six TMS. The vast majority of ABC transporters comprise of two TMD and two NBD (e.g. P-gp; Figure 5.15a), both of which are vital for function. However some have an extra amino TMD (e.g. MRP1; Figure 5.15b) or comprise of only one TMD and one NBD (e.g. BCRP; Figure 5.15c) and in this case they can form a dimer with another hemi-ABC transporter for substrate translocation (Biemans-Oldehinkel, Doeven and Poolman, 2006).

In general, ABC transporters can be divided into three classes based on their topology and phylogeny: Type I and type II are importers whereas type III are exporters. Type I importers utilise a substrate binding protein (SBP) for delivery of ions, amino acids and other small molecules to the transporter. The different conformational structure of this type of transporter has been studied using data derived from the non-eukaryotic molydbate/tungsten (ModBC) and maltose (MalFGK) transporters. Basically, binding of substrate to the TMD results in ATP binding to the NBD and its subsequent hydrolysis, causing the TMD to adopt a new inward facing conformation and the release of substrate into the cytosol (Figure 5.16). Type II importers are similar to type I except their cargo tends to be larger, such as vitamin B_{12} (BtuCD) or heam (HIF; H11470/71). They also have a distinctive 10 TMS in each TMD whereas type I typically only have 5 +1 TMS per TMD. Biochemical studies suggest that unlike type I ABC transporters, NBD activity in type II is independent of TMD conformation. In addition, they are not as promiscuous when it comes to their substrate compared to type I carriers. So far importers (type I and II) have only been identified in prokaryotes whereas the type III ABC transporters are exporters and expressed ubiquitously throughout all phyla. Exporters are involved in homeostasis by removing potentially toxic agents from the cell. However, an undesirable by-product of this function is that they can prevent efficacious levels of a variety of therapeutic drugs from building up by extruding them as soon as they enter the cell. Their structure has been elucidated by studying the bacterial transporter, Sav1866,

Figure 5.14 (*Continued*) Structure of mitochondrial (a) F_0F_1 ATPase and (b) vacuole V_0V_1 ATPase. Both F- and V-type ATPases consist of oligomeric membrane embedded rotor complex (c-subunits) that is coupled to a catalytic head ($\alpha_3\beta_3$ and A_3B_3 respectively) via a central stalk. Binding of an H^+ (or Na^+) ion to each c-subunit and its subsequent release on the other side of the membrane turns the rotor complex a few degrees which in turn rotates the catalytic head. This allows subunits of the peripheral stalk to interact with the β or A catalytic subunit for the synthesis or hydrolyse of ATP respectively. The number of ions (H^+ or Na^+) translocated across the membrane per full rotation is dependent upon the number of c-subunits within the rotor whereas three molecules of ATP are manufactured or broken down per revolution of the trimeric catalytic head ($\alpha_3\beta_3$ or A_3B_3). The main difference between F and ATPases, apart from the direction of rotor rotation, is the subunit composition of the central and peripheral stalks (see text for further details; adapted with permission from Nakanishi-Matsui et al., 2010).

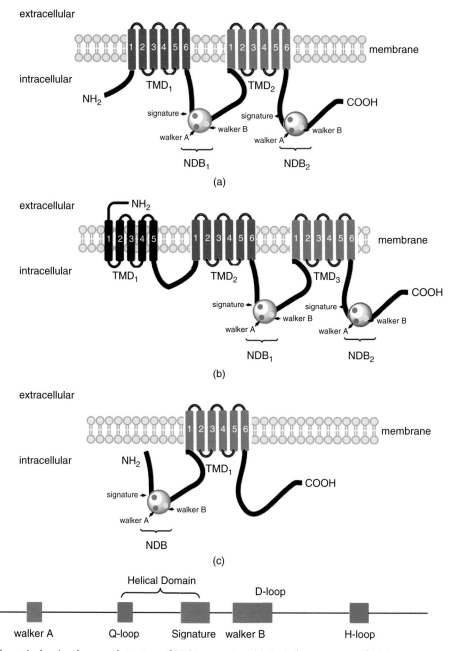

Figure 5.15 Schematic showing the general structure of ABC transporters. (a) Typical arrangement of ABC transporter with two transmembrane domains (TMD) both containing six transmembrane segments (TMS). Each TMD is associated with a nucleotide binding domain (NBD) that has characteristic motifs: signature, Walker A and Walker B. An example of this is the permeability glycoprotein (P-gp). (b) Some ABC transporters contain an extra TMD toward the extracellular NH_2 terminus and an example of this is the multi-drug resistance-protein 1 (MRP1). (c) However, some ABC transporters contain only one TMD and one NBD and an example of this is the breast cancer resistance protein (BCRP). (d) Arrangement of the NBD binding motifs; conserved regions are in red and characteristic motifs are in green. Adapted with permission from Figure 1 of Couture, Nash and Turgeon (2006). The ATP-binding cassette transporters and their implication in drug disposition: a special look at the heart. Pharmacology reviews 58:244–258.

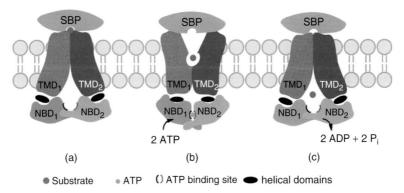

Figure 5.16 Mechanism of substrate uptake by an ABC importer. (a) Substrate binds to the substrate binding protein (SBP) causing the SBP to interact with both TMD_1 and TMD_2. (b) This and the binding of two ATP molecules to their sites between NBD_1 and NBD_2 causes TMD_1 and TMD_2 to rotate along a central axis so that the substrate moves into the binding pocket. (c) Hydrolysis of ATP causes a further rotation so that the transporter binding pocket is now open to the cytosol whereby substrate, ADP and inorganic phosphate (P_i) are released. The SBP moves away from the transporter ready for binding of another substrate molecule and a further round of transporter activity. The ATP binding site consists of p-loops (labelled red) and a signature motifs (labelled black). Some ABCs (e.g. CFRT) only utilise one ATP molecule to energise translocation.

which is a homolog of the human ABC transporter MDR1; MDR1 is associated with multidrug resistance in cancer cells. Like type I importers, exporters can carry a wide range of substrate and they have a two 5+1 helices per TMD but they differ from importers because they do not employ a SBP for substrate delivery and their NBD is fused to their TMDs ((Biemans-Oldehinkel, Doeven and Poolman, 2006; Figure 5.17).

Several ABC transporters have been co-opted for other functions. For example the sulfonylurea receptor is an ABC transporter that can indirectly affect insulin secretion by regulating ATP-sensitive K^+ ion channel activity; mutations in this transporter can lead to hyperinsulinemia. The cystic fibrosis transmembrane regulator (CFTR) is another ABC transporter which acts as a Cl^- channel in epithelia tissue and is involved mucous secretions; mutations in this transporter gives rise to mucoviscidosis (cystic fibrosis; discussed in detail in Chapter 6).

Because of ABC transporter's role in resistance to chemotherapy and antibiotics, as well as the role they play in disease, they are of great interest to the pharmaceutical industry.

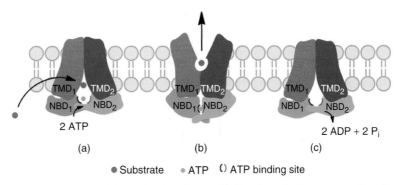

Figure 5.17 Schematic of an ABC exporter. (a) ATP binds to the ATP binding site and substrate moves into the substrate binding pocket. (b) ATP hydrolysis causes the TMD to reconfigure so the pocket is now open to the extracellular domain and the substrate moves out of the cell. The ADP and P_i molecules are released from the interface of NBD_1 and NBD_2. (c) TMD_1 and TMD_2 rotate along their axis so that they are open to the cytosol. The transporter is now ready for another round of substrate and ATP binding.

Structure and function

All ABC transporters have three characteristic motifs (Figure 5.15d): the Walker A (P-loop) and B domains which forms a pocket for nucleotide binding, and the signature motif which is also known as the C-loop (LSGGQ). The Walker domains are not unique to ABC transporters but are found in other ATP-binding proteins; however, it is the presence of the signature motif which identifies a transporter as an ABC member. In addition, ABC transporters also contain Q (glutamine) and H (histidine) loops which interact with the γ-phosphate of ATP. Dimers are formed by the interaction of the D-loop from one NDB with the Walker A domain of another NDB. There is a helical domain between the Q-loop and signature motif which facilitates communication between ABC transporters and their associated proteins within the membrane. In general the difference between importers and exporters is that most importers contain a characteristic EAA motif (L-loop) between TMS_5 and TMS_6 which is absent in exporters, utilise a substrate binding protein (SBP) to deliver the substrate and the NBD subunits are separate from the TMD; whereas exporters do not employ SBP and the NBD and TMD are fused together (Higgins, 1992; Biemans-Oldehinkel, Doeven and Poolman, 2006).

Functionally, two ATP binding pockets are formed by the two NBD lining-up anti-parallel through the interaction of the Walker A and D-loop domains. In ABC importers (see Figure 5.16) the TMD are 'open' to the extracellular space but upon binding of substrate the TMD 'rotate' so that they are now 'open' to cytosol. This conformational change is brought about by the NBD dimers coming closer together in response to substrate binding and the subsequent binding of ATP in the pocket formed by the P-loop and signature motifs followed by its hydrolysis. Substrate is then released into the cytosol along with ADP plus inorganic phosphate (Pi). The SBP moves away from the transporter and awaits the arrival of another substrate molecule bound to SBP and the transporter enters into another cycle of substrate translocation. ABC exporters work in a similar way except they do not employ a SBP and the liberated energy derived from the hydrolysis of ATP causes the TMD to 'open' into the extracellular space and not the cytosol (Figure 5.17).

Bacterial ABC transporters

These transporters play a role in bacterial resistance to antibiotics and hence the treatment of some human pathologies. Since many bacteria have a periplasmic space between the outer and cell membrane, they employ other proteins to help 'funnel' the substrate to a channel for extrusion.

A well-characterised example of a bacterial ABC transporter is the haemolysin (HlyBD-TolC) transporter which is found in *E. coli* and is responsible for removing α-haemolysin from the cell. It has two NBD that bind ATP and two TMD and a HlyB subunit embedded in the cell membrane. Like all ABC transporters the NBD that regulate the relative rotation of the TMD depending upon whether ATP or ADP is bound. Once the substrate is released into the periplasmic space it then has to transverse the bacterial outer membrane. This is achieved by the TolC subunit forming a channel for the substrate to diffuse through. Another subunit, HlyD, which is attached to both TolC and HlyB forms a shield to prevent the substrate from diffusing and accumulating in the periplasmic space (Figure 5.18). A similar set-up is seen in another class of transporters, the resistance-nodulation-cell division (RND), except they use a proton gradient rather than ATP hydrolysis as the driving force for substrate translocation. The RND and their role in drug resistance will be discussed later in this chapter (Thomas, Wagner and Welch, 1992).

ABC transporters in health and disease

To date 49 members of the ABC super-family have been identified in humans and based on their structure (TMD number and combination; see Table 5.3) they have been subdivided into seven groups (A-G; (Klein, Sarkadi and Varadi, 1999). Some ABC transporters are associated with the movement of phospholipids, membrane lipids and cholesterol and are therefore associated with lipid storage diseases. For example, ABCA1 plays a critical role in regulating cholesterol efflux from the plasma membrane to the lipid acceptor protein, apolipoprotein–A1, and mutations in this transporter result in cellular cholesterol accumulation, premature atherosclerosis and peripheral neuropathy which are associated with Tangier disease (Serfaty-Lacrosniere et al., 1994). Over 500 gene mutations have been identified in the phospholipid transporter, ABCA4 (also known as Rim protein), which are associated with a myriad of eye-related disorders such as Stargardt disease. Normally ABCA4 is expressed in rod and cone photoreceptors of the vertebrate retina and is responsible for translocating the phospholipid, retinylidene-phosphatidylethanolamine, which is involved in recycling of the photo-pigment, retinol. So dysfunction of ABCA4 results in early onset macular dystrophy (Molday, Zhong and Quazi, 2009).

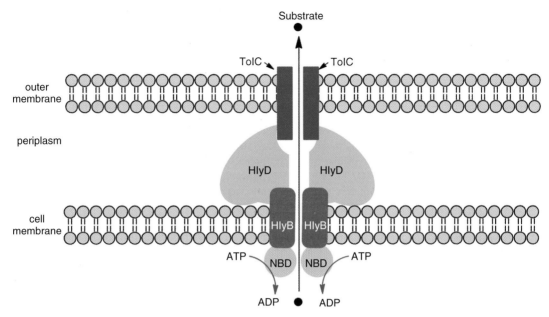

Figure 5.18 Diagram of a bacterial ABC transporter, the haemolysin HlyBD-TolC exporter. Substrate is transferred into the periplasmic space via HlyB which is initially only open to the cytoplasmic side of the membrane. Binding of ATP to NBD causes both HlyBs to rotate so that they are now open to the other side of the membrane. Substrate is released and diffuses out of the periplasmic space via a channel formed by the TolC subunits; HlyD functions to funnel substrate towards this channel.

Table 5.3 ABC transporter genes and their associated monogenetic disorders in humans.

Gene(s)	Disorder	Transporter function and substrate
ABCA1	Tangier disease; Familial hypoapolipoproteinemia	Cholesterol, phospholipids
ABCA3	Respiratory distress syndrome (Neonatal surfactant deficiency)	Phospholipid metabolism?
ABCA4	Stargardt disease; Retinitis pigmentosa 19; Cone rod dystrophy 3; Age-related macular degeneration	Retinoid/phospholipid transporter
ABCA12	Lamellar ichthyosis type 2; Harlequin ichthyosis	Glucosylceramide, other epidermal lipids (?)
ABCB2/B3	ankylosing spondylitis; insulin-dependent diabetes mellitus; celiac disease	Associated with antigen processing Peptide
ABCB4	Progressive familial intrahepatic cholestasis type 3	Bile-acid transport
ABCB7	X-linked sideroblastosis anemia	Mitochondrial iron export
ABCB11	Progressive familial intrahepatic cholestasis type 2	Bile-acid transport
ABCC2	Dubin–Johnson Syndrome	Bile-acid transport
ABCC6	Pseudoxanthoma elasticum	Organic anions (in vitro)
ABCC7	Cystic fibrosis (Mucoviscidosis); Congenital bilateral absence of the vas deferens	Chloride ion channel
ABCC8	Familial persistent hyperinsulinemic hypoglycemia of infancy; AD type 2 diabetes	Sulfonylurea receptor
ABCD1	Adrenoleukodystrophy	Very long chain fatty acids
ABCG5	β-sitosterolemia	Sterols
ABCG8	β-sitosterolemia	Sterols

(Table modification with permission from Kaminski, Piehler and Wenzel, 2006).

ABC transporters are also involved in bile production. The ABCB4 (MDR3) gene encodes for a transporter that is involved in secretion of short chain fatty acids as well as phosphatidylcholine translocase (phospholipid flippase) in to bile and dysfunction of ABCB4 has been shown to cause liver disease due to the gall bladder's inability to secrete bile phospholipids (Smit et al., 1993). Whereas ABCB11 is the major canalicular bile salt export pump (BSEP) found in humans and mutations in this gene are associated with recurrent intra-hepatic cholestasis (Noe et al., 2005). Another example is the canalicular multi-specific organic anion transporter (cMOAT), ABCC2, which is associated with hyper-bilirubinemia and is a characteristic of Dubin-Johnson syndrome (Materna and Lage, 2003). Both of these bile salt exporters (ABCB11 and ABCC2) have also been associated with multi-drug resistance particularly to chemotherapeutics (Evers et al., 1998). Sterols such as cholesterol are excreted into bile via ABCG5 or ABCG8 transporters and impairment of their activity results in the body being unable to respond to daily fluctuations in cholesterol levels resulting in hypercholesterolemia due to more cholesterol being transported across the intestine wall. These genes have been associated with accelerated atherosclerosis and premature coronary artery disease as a consequence of hypercholesterolemia (Small, 2003).

Some transporters are involved in protecting our bodies from the outside world. Skin is the largest organ in the human body and one of its functions is to protect us from infection, UV light and dehydration. The lipid transporter, ABCA12, is found in normal human keratinocytes and plays a role in forming the protective keratin layer of skin. Loss of ABCA12 function leads to a defective lipid barrier resulting in dry, thickened, scaly skin with a range of severities; mild lamellar ichthyosis type 2 to severe Harlequin ichthyosis (Akiyama et al., 2005). The ABCC6 transporter is involved in providing the skin with elasticity and mutations in this gene can lead to a loss of mobility. This gene is also found in other endothelia tissues like the retina and blood vessels and its dysfunction is associated with the condition, pseudoxanthoma elasticum (PXE), which is a systemic connective tissue disorder affecting elastic tissues and is characterised by accumulation of mineralised and fragmented elastic fibres in the aforementioned tissues. How exactly this gene disrupts elastic fibre formation is unclear, but since ABCC6 is highly expressed in the liver and kidney it may play a role in clearance which suggests its dysfunction leads to an excess of its substrate within these tissues which then interacts with the synthesis, turnover, or maintenance of

elastic fibres (Scheffer et al., 2002; Chassaing et al., 2005). This ABC family of transporters also plays an indirect role in gaseous exchange at the lung. The ABCA3 gene encodes for a transporter involved in the production of a mono-layer of lipid-rich mucous that coats the lining of the lungs. One of its functions is to prevent the alveoli from collapsing during expiration by reducing the surface tension at the air-liquid interface. Obviously mutations in this gene can be fatal (Shulenin et al., 2004).

The immune system is able to differentiate between potential pathogens and normal cellular components and transporters play a role in this process. The surface of cells are 'tagged' with a small peptide attached to the class I major histocompatibility complex (MHC); this provides the immune system with information regarding the cell's protein content and its 'health'; cells expressing aberrant proteins will be recognised and targeted for destruction. The ABC transporters associated with antigen processing (TAP; ABCB2 & ABCB3) are found on the endoplasmic reticulum (ER) membrane and are responsible for translocating the tag-peptides into the ER where they are loading onto the MHC. Defects in TAP can cause immunodeficiency related to MHC-associated diseases such as ankylosing spondylitis, insulin-dependent diabetes mellitus, and ceoliac disease (Colonna et al., 1992). Members of the herpes virus family can evade immuno-surveillance by interacting with the TAP transporter to destabilise the MHC (Procko and Gaudet, 2009; Procko et al., 2009; Parcej and Tampe, 2010).

Iron complexes play an important role in many aspects of cellular function including oxidative phosphorylation and delivery of oxygen to respiring tissue. Within the mitochondria, iron forms clusters with sulphur and these clusters interact and are vital for the activity of many mitochondrial enzymes. The ABCB7 transporter is involved in mitochondrial iron homeostasis and several gene mutations are embryonic lethal, mainly due to compromised oxidative phosphorylation. ABCB7 is also involved in haem translocation in the formation of haemoglobin and some mutations are associated with milder symptoms such as anaemia because red blood cells do not form properly (Pondarre et al., 2006). Another transporter that is indirectly involved in metabolism is ABCD1 and dysfunction of this gene can lead to X-linked adrenoleukodystrophy which is characterised by a progressive destruction of myelin and primary adrenocortical insufficiency. ABCD1 is thought to export un-branched saturated very long chain fatty acids out of cells because mutated forms of the gene result in abnormally high levels of this substrate within the cell which impairs peroxisomal β-oxidation (Ho et al., 1995; Kemp and Wanders, 2007).

Some ABC transporters do not employ the same mechanism to transport substrate across the cell membrane as the vast majority of members of this super-family; rather than the substrate binding pocket being open to one side of the membrane at a time, they form a channel for substrate (usually ion) movement. The ABCC7 gene encodes for a transporter that acts as a chloride channel which is involved in the control of mucous secretion as well as vas deferens formation. Mutations in ABCC7 are associated with cystic fibrosis and male sterility (Schinkel et al., 1995; Mickle et al., 2000). Another ABC transporter that functions as an ion channel is ABCC8 which is a K^+-sensitive Ca^{2+} channel (see section 4.3). It is found in pancreatic beta cells and involved in insulin secretion. In fact, it is also known as the sulphonylurea receptor because the

transporter is the site of sulphonylureas action in the treatment of non-insulin-dependent diabetes mellitus. Hence mutations in this gene result in abnormal insulin secretion and altered glucose homeostasis (Aguilar-Bryan et al., 1995; Almqvist et al., 2007)

Oxidoreduction-driven transporters

The best known examples of these primary active transporters are involved in oxidative phosphorylation where they play roles in the progressive movement of electrons down the electron transport chain so that protons are transported across the inner mitochondrial membrane and accumulate in the mitochondria inner membrane space. This proton gradient provides the energy that drives F-ATPase to synthesise ATP (see Figure 5.19). Four complexes are involved in electron transport: complex I (NADH ubiquinone oxidoreductase), complex II

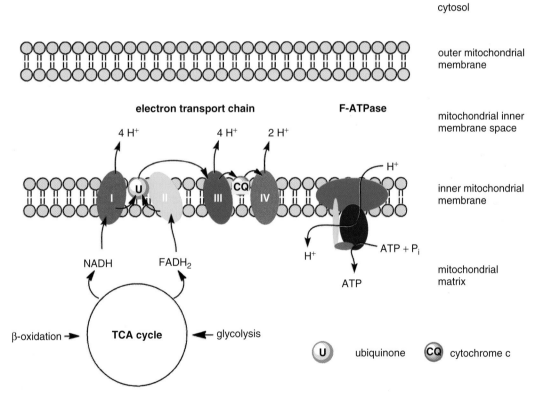

Figure 5.19 Oxidative phosphorylation. Pyruvate from β-oxidation or glycolysis enters the tricarboxylic acid cycle (TCA). NADH or FADH$_2$ provide electrons that enter the electron transport chain via complex I or II. Ubiquinone and cytochrome c transfers the electrons to complexes III and IV respectively. 10 H^+ ions are transferred across the membrane into the inner mitochondrial space for every pair of electrons that move through the four complexes. This provides the H^+ ion gradient essential for F-ATPase activity and ATP synthesis. Dysfunction of any of the complexes within the electron transport chain can have significant consequences on cellular activity.

(succinate ubiquinone oxidoreductase), complex III (cytochrome bc_1 complex) and complex IV (cytochrome c oxidase). Electrons can enter the chain via NADH at complex I or succinate (through $FADH_2$) at complex II and the small carrier molecules, ubiquinone and cytochrome c, transfer electrons to complex III and IV respectively. Two electrons move through this chain and reversibly reduce and oxidise iron-sulphur clusters, ubiquinone, cytochromes and copper ions. This provides enough energy to ferry a total of 10 H^+ ions from the mitochondrial matrix: complex I (4 H^+), complex III (4 H^+), and complex IV (2 H^+).

Apart from complex II, whose subunits are encoded by the nucleus, the electron transport complexes are composed of several subunits derived either from the mitochondrial or nuclear genome. A potential problem with mitochondrial derived subunits is not only are they usually involved in the catalytic activity of the complex, they are also susceptible to misprocessing during translation due to deletions, duplications or mutations in the mitochondrial t-RNA genes. Since the assembly of the complexes are important for their function, this process is tightly coordinated with a number of subunits being involved in assembly and stabilising the complex. Thus abnormal complex assembly as well as the aberrant activity of subunits directly involved in electron transfer can lead to a myriad of pathologies associated with oxidative phosphorylation dysfunction, making it the most common cause of inborn metabolic diseases seen in man. Hence virtually every tissue has the potential to be affected by problems associated with these complexes. It has been estimated that an adult human turns over approximately 65 kg of ATP per day with the brain, heart and skeletal muscle being amongst the most metabolically active tissues, so it is unsurprising that these are the most susceptible to diminished ATP production. Interestingly, dysfunction of a particular complex can lead to different phenotypes/diseases depending upon the individual subunits involved and the tissue type. Since products from different metabolic pathways can feed into various points of the electron transport train some conditions can be due to a build-up of these 'substrates' within the mitochondria and their impact on other pathways. Whilst other diseases are due to a generalised dysfunction of any of the complexes (I-IV) such as a diminished proton gradient and malfunctioning of other mitochondrial transporters that are also dependent upon the proton-motive force (Lazarou et al., 2009; Rutter, Winge and Schiffman, 2010; Benit, 2009).

It should also be noted that in some tissues the partial uncoupling of the electron transport chain is desirable; brown adipose tissue uses the heat generated from this process for non-shivering thermogenesis. It is likely that each complex has multiple family members derived from isoforms of individual subunits which in theory could poise another level of complexity to the electron transport chain.

Information about the structure and order of assembly of complexes I to IV have shown that disruption of any of the complexes can cause similar phenotypes and diseases with varying levels of severity depending upon the tissues/organs affected. These include dysfunction of specific nerves like the optic nerve leading to blindness or generalised neurototoxicity associated with the development of brain lesions and the concomitant loss of cognitive and motor processing. In the periphery they are associated with a range of cardiomyopathies, hypotonias and ataxias. These common phenotypes show how efficiently each complex is coupled and their primary role in formation of a proton gradient. Information regarding the assembly, stability or activity of the complexes I to III is beginning to emerge but they are not as comprehensively understood when compared to complex IV (cytochrome c oxidase), for which there are a number of transgenic animals available to help elucidate the role that some of its subunits play in health and disease.

Cytochrome c oxidase

Cytochrome c oxidase (COX) is the last step in the electron transport chain where molecular oxygen is reduced to water. In mammals COX exists as dimer with each monomer consisting of 13 subunits (Cox_{1-8}). One electron at a time moves from the carrier molecule cytochrome c to a pair of Cu^{2+} ions (Cu_A) located in Cox_2. The electron then moves progressively through three redox sites in Cox_1, onto a haem cluster (cytochrome a), followed by another pair of Cu^{2+} ions (Cu_B) and then to cytochrome a_3 before finally interacting with O_2 to yield H_2O. The progressive movement of the electron provides the energy for an H^+ ion to be translocated by Cox_3. The COX complex also contains binding sites for Zn^{2+} and Mg^{2+} ions which are located on Cox_{5B} and between Cox_1 and Cox_2 respectively. In addition, there are several binding sites for Ca^{2+} and Na^+ ions and these presumably play regulatory roles (Diaz, 2010).

COX in health and disease

COX activity can be regulated in response to different levels of cellular energetic demand by a multitude of factors which include: hormones, nitric oxide, the ratio of ATP:ADP and protein kinases. In addition, there are many tissue-specific subunit isoforms. For example, in the liver, cardiac tissue, testis and lungs, as well as a number of species-specific isoforms. Some isoforms can be induced in response to their environment: for example, Cox_{5b} in normoxic and Cox_{5a} in hypoxic conditions. Cox_4 mRNA is found within axons suggesting that some neurones appear to have the ability to locally translate some subunits in response to local energetic demands such as axonal growth or synapse remodelling.

COX-related pathologies can vary in severity depending upon the subunit involved and the consequences of its malfunction upon assembly, stability or catalytic activity as well as the organ(s) affected (see Table 5.4). Clinically they can be divided into two main groups depending upon whether the symptoms are primarily related to myopathies or brain dysfunction. Since the basic subunit stoichiometry and crystalline structure of COX is known, studies have been conducted to identify their exact role(s) whether it be in assembly, activity or as accessory proteins. This has identified a number of subunits that contribute to the synthesis of the redox clusters such as Cox_{10} and Cox_{15} for heam, and Cox_{11} and the accessory subunits Sco_1 and Sco_2 for Cu_A and Cu_B respectively. Genetic studies in humans, rodents, zebrafish, drosophila and c. elegans have associated specific subunits with a number of conditions which implies that the phenotype is dependent upon the exact mutation. It also illustrates the subtly of COX activity/regulation within different tissues (Diaz, 2010). Table 5.4 indicates Cox genes that have been associated with human pathologies.

Drug resistance

Resistance to therapeutics, for example antibiotics, anti-epileptics and chemotherapy is a major problem in the treatment of a whole host of pathologies. This is because some transporters function to rapidly remove potentially deleterious substance from the cell, whilst others are unintentional substrates for transporters. These transporters are usually involved in cellular homeostasis and/or absorption, distribution, metabolism and elimination of certain substrates.

Multidrug resistance (MDR) transporters

The multi-drug resistance (MDR) transporters were initially investigated in antibiotic-resistant bacteria and subsequently found to be expressed ubiquitously in all organisms. They play roles in preventing the build-up of toxic metabolites, heavy metal or toxins within a cell by promoting their efflux. Typically a single MDR is capable of removing hundreds of different substrates in a non-specific manner. In addition, substrate exposure can induce MDR expression for rapid removal of these potentially harmful compounds. Unfortunately for the pharmaceutical industry and their patients, these transporters can remove drugs such as chemotherapeutics that can kill aberrant host cells or antibiotics used to kill infecting bacteria.

The MDR family is derived from five different transporter families with their grouping based on the energy source used to remove these substances. Primary MDR belong to the ABC (ATP-binding cassette) family which are dependent on ATP for substrate translocation. Secondary MDR derive their energy from either H^+ or Na^+ ion gradients and include the major facilitator superfamily (MFS), the resistance-nodulation-cell division (RND) family, the small multidrug resistance (SMR) superfamily and multidrug and toxic compound extrusion (MATE) superfamily; the first three are drug/H^+ antiporters whereas the latter family is a drug/Na^+ antiporter.

Primary MDR transporters

The structure and function of ABC transporters is discussed earlier in this chapter. The number one disease in the world is malaria because it kills between 1 and 3 million people annually. The causative agent of malaria is the protozoan parasite, *Plasmodium falciparum*, which is carried by mosquitoes who are responsible for infecting humans. Gradually almost all anti-malarial drugs have lost their efficacy due to the development of drug resistance. Chloroquine was successfully used as a treatment for malaria for over 30 years until drug resistant strains of the parasite began to emerge. During erythrocyte infection *P. falciparum* takes up large amounts of heam into its digestive vacuole and chloroquine works by interfering with heam processing so that a toxic metabolite is formed which eventually kills the parasite. The ABC transporter, PfCRT, has been implicated in chloroquine resistance but whether its role is in vacuole uptake or efflux is still being debated. Analysis of the *P. falciparum* genome has identified at least 16 ABC proteins, of which three are thought to be involved in conferring resistance to several anti-malarials (e.g. PfMDR1 and PfMDR2; (Sanchez et al., 2010)).

Three sub-divisions of the human ABC super-family (B, C and G) have members that are associated with multiple resistance to drugs. These include: permeability-glycoprotein (P-gp; MDR1; ABCB1), multi resistance-associated protein (MRP1; ABCC1), and breast cancer resistance protein (BCRP; ABCG2) (for structures see Figure 5.4). Generally, complete transporters containing

Table 5.4 Human diseases associated with COX deficiency.

Gene	Function	Clinical features
mtDNA-encoded subunits		
Cox_1	Catalytic core	Encephalopathy
		Sideroblastic anemia
		Myoglobinuria
		Motor neuron disease
		MELAS-like syndrome
Cox_2	Catalytic core	Myopathy
		Encephalopathy
		Multi systemic disease (bilateral cataracts, sensorineural hearing loss, myopathy, ataxia) and metabolic acidosis
Cox_3	Catalytic core	MELAS
		Encephalopathy
		Leigh-like syndrome
		Exercise intolerance and rhabdomyolysis
Nuclear-encoded subunits		
Cox_{6b1}	Structural subunit	Encephalopathy
Assembly factors		
Surf1	Unknown Assists in early CIV assembly	Leigh syndrome
Cox_{10}	Haeme *a* biosynthesis	Leukodystrophy
		Tubolopathy
		Hypertrophic cardiomyopathy
		Leigh syndrome
		Leigh-like syndrome
Cox_{15}	Haeme *a* biosynthesis	Cardiomyopathy
		Leigh syndrome
Sco_1	Copper delivery and homeostasis	Hepatopathy
		Metabolic acidosis
		Hypertrophic cardiomyopathy
		Encephalopathy
Sco_2	Copper delivery and homeostasis	Hypertrophic cardiomyopathy
		Encephalopathy
LRPPRC	Cox_1 and Cox_3 mRNA stability	French–Canadian Leigh syndrome
$Taco_1$	Cox_1 translational activator	Slowly progressive Leigh syndrome
FASTKD2	unknown	Encephalopathy

These range from myopathies that involve skeletal muscle only as in a particular Cox_2 mutation to those that are primarily brain related such as Leigh syndrome when brain lesion results in death (French–Canadian Leigh syndrome is a less severe phenotype), whilst other myopathies have cardiac and liver involvement. Mitochondrial and nuclear subunits as well COX assembly factors contribute to COX-related disease states. MELAS mitochondrial myopathy, encephalopathy, lactic acidosis and stroke-like episodes. Table taken with permission from Diaz, 2010.

two TMD and NBD are located in the cell plasma membrane (e.g. P-gp and MRP1) whereas those containing only one TMD and NBD are located in intracellular membrane such as the endoplasmic reticulum; BCRP is an exception as it is found in the plasma membrane and not an organelle membrane (Klein, Sarkadi and Varadi, 1999; Kusuhara and Sugiyama, 2007).

Permeability-glycoprotein (P-gp)

The primary function of P-gp is to remove potentially lethal substances from the cytosol; however it cannot differentiate between xenobiotics or therapeutics and so also removes drugs for tissues that target certain cancers, viral infections (e.g. HIV) and psychological conditions. Since P-gp is a major mediator of drug resistance in humans its pharmacology is of great interest. This has led to the development of relatively potent but non-toxic P-gp inhibitors to reverse multidrug resistance

P-gp was first isolated in Chinese hamster ovary cells that developed resistance to the antibiotic, actinomycin D. Subsequent studies also showed that these cells were resistant to unrelated antibiotics that the cells had never been exposed to before (Juliano and Ling, 1976). Later studies showed that cells became resistant to other types of drugs such as chemotherapeutics and that their exposure to these drugs can rapidly induce the expression of P-gp mRNA. In fact P-gp is very promiscuous because a wide range of compounds act as P-gp substrates/inhibitors.

P-gp is expressed in many tissues that influence drug absorption in the intestines, elimination by the kidneys and liver, and access to areas like the brain and immune system via the blood brain barrier and other similar protective borders. Their importance in these processes has been demonstrated using transgenic mice that lack the gene for P-gp. Interestingly under normal conditions these animals do not look any different from wild-type mice but further scrutiny has shown that their blood brain barrier is more permeable and they exhibit drug hypersensitivity (Schinkel et al., 1995). Also there appears to be an age-related decline in P-gp function at the blood brain barrier which can be correlated to the development of several neurodegenerative diseases (Bartels et al., 2010). P-gp has been implicated in the accumulation of β-amyloid proteins which is a characteristic of Alzheimer's disease. Normally P-gp aids the removal of β-amyloid protein but when the action of P-gp in the blood brain barrier is compromised β-amyloid accumulates and aggregates within neurones (Ueno et al., 2010).

In addition to transporting cytotoxoic drugs, such as digoxin, opiates and polycyclic aromatic hydrocarbons,

Pgp can also transport a number of compounds that can be used to assess the structure function and uptake of P-gp inhibitors. These include the single-photon emission computed tomography (SPECT) tracer substrate, technetium (^{99m}Tc) sestamibi, and the florescent dyes calcein-AM and rhodamine 123. Studies have shown that there is an inverse relationship between P-gp expression and ^{99m}Tc sestamibi uptake (Kostakoglu et al., 1997) and increased uptake after treatment with P-gp inhibitors. Interestingly, even though P-gp has the structure of a classic ABC transporter there is much debate as to how it actually removes substrates from cells. Xenobiotics and chemotherapeutic drugs are thought to be removed in an ATP-dependent manner (Gottesman, Fojo and Bates, 2002) whereas there is evidence that P-gp may be acting as a 'flippase' and that the drug never actually entered the cytoplasm but is directly extruded from the lipid milieu: For example, calcein-AM which is a P-gp substrate that does not fluoresce until the AM group is removed by cytoplasmic esterase; however in the absence of P-gp inhibitors no fluorescence is observed even though calcein-AM has interacted with P-gp (Raviv et al., 1990; Higgins and Gottesman, 1992).

Inhibiting the activity of P-gp is one approach that can be employed to overcome P-gp-mediated resistance. However, identifying a suitable compound has been problematic because P-gp can transport over 200 different compounds that either bind to the same residues or different residues within the substrate binding pocket. Despite this a number of first generation P-gp blockers were identified. These include verapamil which prevents L-type voltage operated Ca^{2+} channels from opening primarily in cardiac muscle, which is why it is used in the treatment of cardiac dysrhythmias. Another example was the immunosuppressant, cyclosporin A, which is used to prevent rejection of organ transplants by indirectly preventing activation of a Ca^{2+} sensitive phosphatase (calcineurin) and subsequent T-helper cell activation. However, the concentration of either drug required to inhibit P-gp function sufficiently was far greater than their normal therapeutic range and hence lead to severe non-specific toxicity in clinical trials.

This lead to the development of second generation P-gp inhibitors based on non-toxic derivatives of first generation inhibitors. Since the L-enantiomer of verapamil has a greater affinity for L-Ca^{2+} channels than the D-isomer it was thought that higher concentration of D-verapamil would be less toxic in vivo. This proved to be true in clinical trials since there was a reduction in non-specific toxicity at concentrations that prevented P-gp function.

However, in some cases, the dose of co-administered anti-cancer drugs had to be reduced because of their increased side effects which lead to sub-therapeutic chemotherapy levels. A derivative of cyclosporine, Valspodar (PSC-833), fared a little bit better because it exhibited minimal toxicity at the concentrations required for P-gp inhibition. However, the anticancer drugs were metabolised much more slowly by cytochrome P_{450} 3A4 (CYP3A4; a major player in drug metabolism) because valspodar also acts as a competitive inhibitor of CYP3A4. Phase III clinical studies using a variety of second generation P-gp inhibitors have shown that although the dose of some chemotherapeutics can be reduced, there is little benefit to using these compounds as an 'add-on' therapy in the treatment of different types of cancers (Szakacs et al., 2006). Another factor for consideration is P-gp polymorphisms which influence substrate recognition, transmembrane transport and regulation. To date over 50 single nucleotide polymorphisms have been identified in the P-gp gene and this, coupled with known CYP3A polymorphisms, may explain why some patients require significantly higher or lower doses of the co-administered therapeutic and P-gp inhibitor (Szakacs et al., 2008). The pharmacogenomics of the cytochrome P_{450} and transporter polymorphisms are discussed further in Chapter 7.

Third generation P-gp inhibitors have been developed which bear little structural resemblance to first and second generation inhibitors and do not significantly interact with CYP3A. Hence they do not influence the pharmacokinetic profile of the co-administered therapeutic drugs. These include: elacridar (GF120918), zosuquidar (LY335979) and tariquidar (XR9576). Tariquidar has been shown to have specificity to P-gp and to be approximately 30-fold and 1000-fold more potent than PSC-833 or verapamil respectively. However, phase III clinical trials have failed so far to find any significant increase in benefits from single chemotherapy treatments (Szakacs et al., 2006; Pajeva and Wiese, 2009). Like tariquidar, zosuquidar is a potent and specific P-gp modulator that does not interact with other ABC transporters involved in drug resistance (i.e. BCRP or MRP-1). Whilst zosuquidar has shown promising pre-clinical signs, initial feedback on phase III clinical trials suggest it does not increase the benefits of current single chemotherapy (Cripe et al., 2010; Lee, 2010). A possible complication in these studies may be due to ingestion, by the trial participants, of foods that can inhibit P-gp function such as orange, grapefruit and strawberry juice as well as other unknown modulators of P-gp function. This could at least partially explain why some recipients exhibit signs of toxicity due to a higher bioavailability of chemotherapeutic agents.

A lack of optimism with third generation P-gp inhibitors has lead to different strategies being employed in an attempt to overcome multiple drug resistance. These include screening for natural products that have low non-specific toxicity at concentrations that can modulate P-gp function. One of the most encouraging of these compounds is an extract of turmeric, curcumin, derived from the ginger plant *Curcuma longa* (Lee, 2010). Since curcumin is rapidly digested before it can reach the P-gp transporter, novel mechanisms of delivery have been investigated; including the use of liposomes as cargo carriers (see section on cell penetrating peptides).

An alternative approach is the use of hydrophobic peptides that target the transmembrane segments of P-gp thus preventing proper transporter assembly or function (Sharom et al., 1999). Antibodies targeting extracellular P-gp epitopes as well as immunisation of rodents with corresponding peptides have also been employed with some success as they reduce therapeutic drug extrusion without eliciting an autoimmune response (Mechetner et al., 1997). Another strategy used to treat cancers is to exploit the fact that P-gp is induced by these cells after exposure to chemotherapeutic drugs by employing bi-directional antibodies that recognise P-gp and deliver specific drugs that can be released at the target site thereby reducing chemotherapeutic concentrations as well as non-specific drug effects. Other approaches that have been employed to overcome multi-drug resistance include preventing P-gp translation using a variety of 'knockdown' techniques such as antisense oligonucleotides and RNA interference (see Chapter 8), but results of these studies are very much in their infancy (Lee, 2010; Crooke, 2007).

Secondary MDR transporters

A large number of secondary MDR transporters belong to the RND family and although the best characterised examples are bacterial in origin, there are examples of these transporters being involved in human disease. For example the lipid storage disease, Niemann-Pick C1 (NC-P1), is due to NC-P1 protein within the lysosomal membrane causing an over accumulation of lipids in a number of tissues including the liver. There is a lack of identity between eukaryotic and prokaryotic MDR transporters at the amino acid level and this lack of homology could be advantageous when designing drugs to treat antibiotic-resistant bacterial infections in humans because any potential cytotoxicity due to cross reactions with mammalian counterparts would be minimised.

As stated at the beginning of this chapter, it is easier to crystallise and interpret the data from prokaryotic transporters than eukaryotes and this is one of the reasons why the *E. coli* transporter, acriflavine resistance protein B (ArcB), is the most extensively characterised secondary MDR transporter. ArcB confers resistance to many antibiotics including penicillin G, oxacillin, cloxacillin, nafcillin, macrolides, novobiocin, linezolid, and fusidic acid. It is a member of the RND family and works in combination with TolC and AcrA which are members of the outer membrane factor (OMF) family and the periplasmic membrane fusion protein (MFP) family, respectively (Figure 5.20). In bacteria, the antibiotic moves across the bacterial membrane by diffusion and is then pumped out of the cell via the AcrB/TolC /AcrA complex. Basically AcrB is a homotrimer and each subunit has three main conformations, loose (L; access), tight (T; binding) and open (O; extrusion) which have low, high or no affinity for the substrate. Substrate binds to its pocket in the L form and causes a conformational change so that the substrate moves into a hydrophobic pocket, the T form. This promotes the binding of a proton derived from the periplasma space and binds to the T form, and the opening of the transporter (O form) so that the substrate is released and exits the periplasma space via a channel formed by TolC; the proton is also released into the cytoplasm promoting the formation of the L form of the AcrB protein. The periplasmic protein, AcrA, facilitates the formation of the different conformations of AcrB as well as opening of the AcrA channel. Studies have revealed that all three proteins are essential for drug efflux so the development of compounds that uncouple them would be useful tools with which to overcome drug resistant infections.

It is interesting that when periplasmic domains of ArcB are compared to subunits of the mammalian F-type ATPase transporter, F_0F_1ATP synthase (see Figure 5.14a) they appear to be analogous which is suggestive of a common ancestor. Given the dogma that mitochondria were originally bacteria that entered into a symbiotic relationship, and that F_0F_1ATP synthase is located in the mitochondrial inner membrane that also functions as a homotrimer that derives its energy from a proton gradient, making the common ancestor theory more compelling. Whilst the exact mechanism of how each

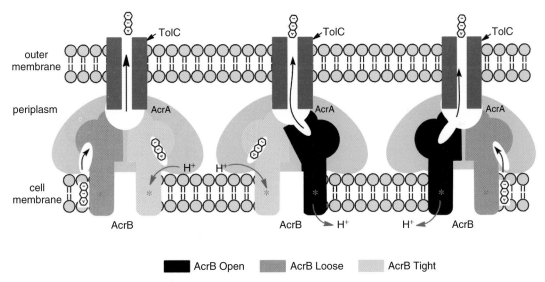

Figure 5.20 Diagram showing how drugs are extruded from cells using the AcrB transporter. Substrate binds to a TMD of AcrB (*) and then moves into the substrate binding pocket in the loose conformation of AcrB. The substrate is now tightly bound to AcrB. An H^+ ion from the periplasm interacts with the transmembrane domain of AcrB (*) which catalyses AcrB's conversion to the open and the release of substrate and its extrusion from the periplasmic space via the channel formed by TolC. The H^+ ion is now released by AcrB into the cytoplasm and another substrate binds and another cycle of substrate translocation and extrusion begins. AcrA functions to help funnel the substrate released from AcrB into the TolC channel. AcrB is a trimer consisting of all three conformations of AcrB (loose, tight and open) at the same time and is believed to spin around a central axis perpendicular to the cell membrane as it transports substrate out of the cell using the energy derived from the movement of H^+ ions from the periplasmic space into the cyctosol. Figure adapted with permission from Macmillan Publishers Ltd: Nature Murakami et al., copyright (2006).

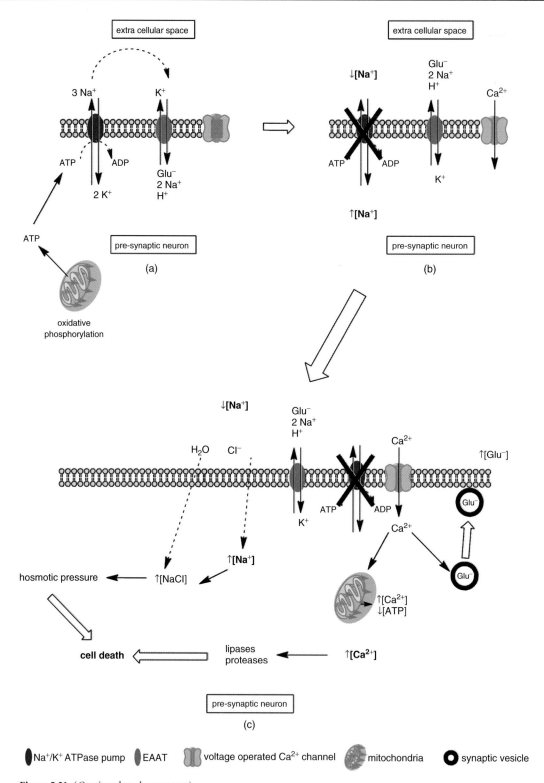

Figure 5.21 (*Continued on the next page*)

substrate moves through AcrB is unknown it is thought that the AcrB homotrimer can rotate around a central core in a similar manner to F_1ATP so that substrate extrusion is achieved in a peristaltic pump-like fashion. However, F_0F_1ATP synthase functions differently to AcrB in that it uses the proton gradient to drive ATP synthesis whereas AcrB uses this gradient to extrude substrates from the cytosol.

Another transporter that bears a resemblance to AcrB (Figure 5.20) is the ABC transporter heamolysisn (HlyBD-TolC; Figure 5.18); both use a funnelling system to shepherd substrate (AcrA or HlyD) towards a channel outer membrane formed by TolC. However HylB is a primary active transporter because it derives its energy from the hydrolysis of ATP whereas AcrB uses the H^+ ion gradient. The resemblance between F_0F_1ATP synthase, AcrB and HlyD suggests that they have evolved independently from a common ancestor.

5.5 Transporters and cellular homeostasis

Drug absorption, distribution, metabolism and elimination

The pharmacokinetic profile of drugs is dependent upon transporters for uptake via the gastro-intestinal tract and liver, delivery to target tissues, removal from the body via the kidneys and liver as well as transportation into cells/compartments that can convert them from a pro-drug to an active one or facilitate their metabolism. Obviously the premature breakdown of a drug or its delivery to an unintended tissue are not desirable effects and they can have quite serious consequences which have to be catered for during drug development. The therapeutic range of a drug can be quite large within a population because of individual variations in response due to genetic and environmental factors that regulate these transporters and hence drug disposition.

The two main groups that are involved in drug uptake and elimination are members of the MFS and ABC transporter families with MFS transporters being primarily involved in absorption and ABC transporters in clearance. In the liver, normally substrates move from the sinusoid blood vessel and are taken up by hepatocytes where they are modified or degraded and then transported out of the hepatocyte into the bile canaliculus and excreted as bile. The major transporters involved in drug uptake at the sinusoidal membrane are: the organic anion transporting proteins (OAT), organic cation transporters (OCT), concentrative nucleoside transporters (CNT), dipeptide transporters (PEPT), and mono carboxylate transporters (MCT); whereas the ABC transporters are involved in drug extrusion across the canalicular membrane. Renal OAT/OCT and ABC transporters also play a role in the removal of drugs and their metabolites in urine although in some cases polar drugs are reabsorbed depending upon the pH of the urine which is dependent to a certain extent on the activity of OAT/OCT; higher urine pHs result in greater aspirin excretion.

Water balance

Aquaporins are channels that control the speed with which water molecules move across cell membranes and to date there are 13 known members of this family expressed in mammals (see section 4.3). They are primarily involved in the water movement but a subset of aquaporins, aquaglyceroporins, also transport glycerol and other small polar molecules. They play important roles in water balance in the kidneys, glandular secretions, brain water balance, cell migration and neuronal activity.

Figure 5.21 (*Continued*) Diagram showing the consequences of ATP depletion on transporter activities and neuronal function. (**a**) Normal conditions. In order for glutamate to be taken up into the cell the excitatory amino acid transporter (EAAT) symports Na^+ ions and uses the Na^+ ion gradient to power glutamate's transportation across the membrane. The Na^+ gradient is generated by the Na^+/K^+ ATPase pump which uses the energy produced by the breakdown of ATP to ADP. ATP is synthesised in the mitochondria using another transporter, the F_0F_1 ATPase pump, using energy from the proton motive force. (**b**) When ATP is in short supply the Na^+ gradient that is vital for glutamate uptake by EAAT is not generated. In fact the intracellular concentration of Na^+ ions soon rises which causes EAAT to reverse and pump glutamate out of the neuron. The reversal of the Na^+ gradient results in membrane depolarisation and activation of voltage operated Ca^{2+} channels. (**c**) Ca^{2+} ion influx triggers synaptic vesicle migration to the synaptic plasma membrane and release of neurotransmitter (glutamate). The mitochondria which also functions as an intracellular Ca^{2+} store becomes gorged with Ca^{2+} ion which further compromises mitochondria function and hence ATP production. High intracellular Ca^{2+} ions concentration activates lipases and proteases which target membranes and protein integrity. High intracellular Na^+ ion concentrations create an electrostatic gradient which attracts Cl^- ions to move into the neuron. The high Na^+ and Cl^- ion concentrations cause water to move in by osmosis thereby increasing the osmotic pressure. The extra pressure on the lipase-weakened membranes causes them to burst resulting in cell death.

The activity of aquaporins can be controlled by many factors such as hormones.

Water concentration and osmotic pressure is tightly controlled because any deviation from normal can be potentially devastating. For example, a typical adult human brain has approximately 150 ml of cerebral spinal fluid (CSF) which is replaced about three times a day. If the rate of CSF production is greater than its reabsorption then intracranial pressure rises and conversely if the rate of secretion is less than reabsorption the intracranial pressure falls. The choroid plexus is thought to be the major producer of CSF, and AQP1 knockout mice have been shown to secrete 25% less CSF and a 50% reduction in intracranial pressure. For this reason drugs that target the AQP1 pore have been proposed as treatment for increased intracranial pressure. AQP1 also plays an important role in controlling ocular pressure through secretions from the ciliary epithelium. As with CSF production secretions from the cilary epithelium are near isomolar and reabsorbed continuously. Inhibition of AQP1 function results in increased ocular pressure leading to retinal damage and glaucoma. AQP1 is also present in other tissues such as lacrimal and sweat glands but abolishment of AQP1 function does not impact significantly on secretion volume or salt concentration. This is because during secretion production salts move from one compartment to another, causing water to move down its osmotic gradient via aquaporins to produce a slightly hyperosmotic secretion. When the aquapores are not functioning, water can only enter the compartment by diffusion, which is not a problem with low secreting tissues/glands because there is enough time for the water molecules to diffuse. However, in high secreting tissues there is insufficient time for water diffusion which results in a low volume hyperosmotic secretion. AQP4, which is the major water channel found in the brain, is involved in water transport across the blood brain barrier and it is expressed in glial cells at the fluid-parenchymal interface. Water intoxication or ischaemic stroke due to trauma or infection results in cytotoxic oedema where water passes through an intact blood brain barrier due to osmotic pull. Studies on mice lacking AQP4 have shown that the intracranial pressure produced by the brain oedema is reduced. In addition, trauma induced spinal oedemas are reduced when AQP4 function is prevented. Both point to a therapeutic role in the early treatment of neuronal trauma and inflammation. Brain oedema due to leaky vessels (vasogenic), brain tumour, abscess or hydrocephalus results from movement of water into the brain through a leaky blood brain barrier, whereas normally AQP4 pores

in the glial limitans which line the ventricles and surface of the brain and functions to remove excess water. So therapies that enhance AQP4 activity will reduce intracranial pressure.

When neuronal cells migrate to form new connections they achieve this via a growth cone which involves an interaction between microbubles (tublins) and microfilaments (actin) within the cell. At the apex the microfilaments are proposed to 'swing back' and generate enough energy for the growth cone to advance a little further. However studies have questioned whether this mechanism would generate the necessary energy for rapid cell migration. APQs are thought to allow the rapid influx of water which increases the local osmotic pressure and provides an additional driving force for membrane protrusion to occur. Cell migration and extension is thought to play a major role in tumour angiogenesis and tumour metastasis. So inhibition of AQP function within these cells may prevent further tumour growth and spread. In fact AQP1 has been proposed as a clinical marker of tumour progress. Glial cells support neurones and participate in neurotransmission and aquaporins are thought to control the size of the extracellular space as a consequence of glial water efflux/influx as well as controlling extracellular K^+ ion concentrations, which will affect neuronal repolarisation and hyperpolarisation characteristics (Verkman, 2009).

pH

Cellular proton concentrations not only provide the driving force for many transporters but they also modulate the activity of many proteins involved in normal cellular function. Therefore pH is tightly regulated using specific transporters which include the Na^+/H^+ antiporter which reduces cellular acidity. In some cells this transporter works in combination with the Na^+-driven Cl^-/HCO_3^- exchanger which couples an influx of Na^+ and HCO_3^- ions with an efflux of Cl^- and H^+ ions. In some cells, such as glial, cellular pH is controlled by the Na^+/HCO_3^- symporter that transports a single Na^+ ion with two or more HCO_3^- ions, which results in a negative charge being brought into the cell and thus lowering the voltage inside the cell making it harder for the symporter to work. So this symporter is sensitive to voltage and is involved in regulating extracellular pH in response to electrical activity, which is very important in brain function. The Na^+-independent Cl^-/HCO_3^- exchanger moves out of the cell and Na^+ in to the cell; this stops the pH becoming too alkali (VanWert, Gionfriddo and Sweet, 2010).

Excitotoxicity and Neuroprotection

Excitotoxicity is the process of neuronal death caused by excessive or prolonged activation of excitatory neurotransmission. A number of transporters can contribute indirectly and directly to neuronal cell death due to over stimulation of excitatory neurotransmitter receptors. Major players in excitotoxicity are glutamate receptors by virtue of the fact that they are the most abundant neurotransmitter found in the brain. N-methyl-D-aspartate (NMDA) receptors are a sub-class of ionotrophic glutamate receptors and they play a pivotal role in excitotoxicity because they are high conductance Ca^{2+} channels. They also require binding of the co-agonist, glycine. Once activated Ca^{2+} and Na^+ move into the cell which initiates activation of certain secondary messenger pathways involved in synapse remodelling. Initially Ca^{2+} binds to Ca^{2+}-dependent calmodulin kinase II (CaMKII), which activates nitric oxide synthetase (NOS) to convert L-arginine into nitric oxide (NO). NO can diffuse back to the pre-synaptic terminal to stimulate further glutamate release (positive feedback).

Glutamate is removed from the synapse via the glutamate transporter (EAAT) which antiports a K^+ ion and symports two Na^+ and one H^+ ions for each glutamate molecule. The Na^+ ion is then removed from the cytosol using the Na^+/K^+ ATPase pump. If the Na^+/K^+ ATPase pump does not function then the concentration of Na^+ ions soon builds up so that it is greater in the pre-synaptic terminal than outside; the Na^+ ion gradient is reversed. The EAAT now works in reverse and pumps glutamate out of the cell into the synaptic cleft. The high intracellular Na^+ ion concentration creates an electrogenic gradient that results in the movement of Cl^- ions into the cell. The osmotic pressure within the neurone increases because of water influx due to the osmotic gradient generated by Na^+ and Cl^- ions. The reversal of the Na^+ ion gradient also depolarises the membrane which leads to opening of the pre-synaptic voltage-dependent Ca^{2+} channels and Ca^{2+} ion influx and further glutamate release from the synaptic vesicles. High Ca^{2+} ion levels also activate Ca^{2+}-dependent proteases and lipases which cause proteins to malfunction and membranes to breakdown. The mitochondria's ability to produce ATP is severely compromised which exacerbates the situation because all transporters that are dependent on ATP can no longer function. This, coupled with the high osmotic pressure of the cell, results in cell swelling and eventual bursting and releasing all of its glutamate which can then start the process again in adjacent neurones.

The consequences in the post synaptic cell are just as devastating due to excessive Ca^{2+} ion influx and the activation of proteases and lipases. In addition, high Ca^{2+} ion concentrations disrupt mitochondria function because more Ca^{2+} ions enter this internal store and this interferes with ATP production due to disruption of the electron transport chain. Again, ATP dependent pumps cannot function (e.g. Na^+/K^+ ATPase pump and Ca^{2+}/Na^+ ATPase pump) and

this prevents many secondary energy sources from being generated. The situation is worsened by production of retrograde secondary messengers like NO causing further glutamate release from the pre-synaptic terminal.

So, excessive NMDA receptor activation and Ca^{2+} influx can cause cell death as well as compromised ATP production. A major cause of reduced ATP production is due to ischaemia because restricted blood flow results in a loss of oxygen and glucose for oxidative phosphorylation and acidosis due to anaerobic oxidation. Acidosis ($\uparrow[H^+]$) can also increase the Ca^{2+} ion conductance of NMDA receptors.

The fact that cell death due to excitotoxicity causes adjacent neurones to die, with the number dying being far greater the further the distance from the epicentre (amplification), is the reason why the prognosis for stroke (cerebrovascular accident) victims is worse the longer the delay in administrating drugs that restore cerebral blood flow.

5.6 Summary

Transporters play a role in every aspect of cellular activity from maintenance of the membrane potential to controlling cell size as well as cellular-, tissue-, organ- and system-homeostasis. Therapeutics have been successfully designed and employed to exploit the action of specific transporters in the treatment of disease. Transporter-mediated drug resistance is a significant problem and a better understanding of how transporters recognise and remove potential xenobiotics is crucial for drug-design.

References

Abramson J and Wright EM (2009) Structure and function of Na(+)-symporters with inverted repeats. Current Opinion in Structural Biology 19:425–432.

Aguilar-Bryan L, Nichols CG, Wechsler SW and Clement JP,4th, Boyd AE, Gonzalez G, Herrera-Sosa H, Nguy K, Bryan J and Nelson DA (1995) Cloning of the beta cell high-affinity sulfonylurea receptor: a regulator of insulin secretion. Science 268:423–426.

Akiyama M, Sugiyama-Nakagiri Y, Sakai K, McMillan JR, Goto M, Arita K, Tsuji-Abe Y, Tabata N, Matsuoka K, Sasaki R, Sawamura D and Shimizu H (2005) Mutations in lipid transporter ABCA12 in harlequin ichthyosis and functional recovery by corrective gene transfer. Journal of Clinical Investigation 115:1777–1784.

Almqvist J, Huang Y, Laaksonen A, Wang DN and Hovmoller S (2007) Docking and homology modeling explain inhibition of the human vesicular glutamate transporters. Protein Science 16:1819–1829.

Bartels AL, de Klerk OL, Kortekaas R, de Vries JJ and Leenders KL (2010) 11C-verapamil to assess P-gp function in human brain during aging, depression and neurodegenerative disease. Current Topic in Medical Chemistry 10:1775–1784.

Beyenbach KW and Wieczorek H (2006) The V-type H+ ATPase: molecular structure and function, physiological roles and regulation. Journal of Experimental Biology 209: 577–589.

Biemans-Oldehinkel E, Doeven MK and Poolman B (2006) ABC transporter architecture and regulatory roles of accessory domains. FEBS Letters 580: 1023–1035.

Blanco-Arias P, Einholm AP, Mamsa H, Concheiro C, Gutierrez-de-Teran H, Romero J, Toustrup-Jensen MS, Carracedo A, Jen JC, Vilsen B and Sobrido MJ (2009) A C-terminal mutation of ATP1A3 underscores the crucial role of sodium affinity in the pathophysiology of rapid-onset dystonia-parkinsonism. Human Molecular Genetics 18: 2370–2377.

Bodmer D, Eleveld M, Kater-Baats E, Janssen I, Janssen B, Weterman M, Schoenmakers E, Nickerson M, Linehan M, Zbar B and van Kessel AG (2002) Disruption of a novel MFS transporter gene, DIRC2, by a familial renal cell carcinoma-associated t(2;3)(q35;q21). Human Molecular Genetics 11:641–649.

Boudker O and Verdon G (2010) Structural perspectives on secondary active transporters. Trends Pharmacological Science 31:418–426.

Bublitz M, Poulsen H, Morth JP and Nissen P (2010) In and out of the cation pumps: P-Type ATPase structure revisited. Current Opinions in Structural Biology 20:431–439.

Capaldi RA and Aggeler R (2002) Mechanism of the F(1)F(0)-type ATP synthase, a biological rotary motor. Trends in Biochemical Sciences 27:154–160.

Chang AB, Lin R, Keith Studley W, Tran CV and Saier MH,Jr (2004) Phylogeny as a guide to structure and function of membrane transport proteins. Molecular Membrane Biology 21:171–181.

Chassaing N, Martin L, Calvas P, Le Bert M and Hovnanian A (2005) Pseudoxanthoma elasticum: a clinical, pathophysiological and genetic update including 11 novel ABCC6 mutations. Journal of Medical Genetics 42:881–892.

Colonna M, Bresnahan M, Bahram S, Strominger JL and Spies T (1992) Allelic variants of the human putative peptide transporter involved in antigen processing. Proceedings of the National Academy of Science U S A 89:3932–3936.

Couture L, Nash JA and Turgeon J (2006) The ATP-binding cassette transporters and their implication in drug disposition: a special look at the heart. Pharmacology Reviews 58:244–258.

Cripe LD, Uno H, Paietta EM, Litzow MR, Ketterling RP, Bennett JM, Rowe JM, Lazarus HM, Luger S and Tallman MS (2010) Zosuquidar, a novel modulator of P-glycoprotein, does not improve the outcome of older patients with newly diagnosed acute myeloid leukemia: a randomized, placebo-controlled, trial of the Eastern Cooperative Oncology Group (ECOG 3999). Blood.

Crooke ST (2007) Antisense Drug Technology: Principles, Strategies, and Applications, Second Edition. CRC Press, USA.

de Bie P, Muller P, Wijmenga C and Klomp LW (2007) Molecular pathogenesis of Wilson and Menkes disease: correlation of mutations with molecular defects and disease phenotypes. Journal of Medical Genetics 44:673–688.

De Meirleir L, Seneca S, Lissens W, De Clercq I, Eyskens F, Gerlo E, Smet J and Van Coster R (2004) Respiratory chain complex V deficiency due to a mutation in the assembly gene ATP12. Journal of Medical Genetics 41:120–124.

Di Daniel E, Mok MH, Mead E, Mutinelli C, Zambello E, Caberlotto LL, Pell TJ, Langmead CJ, Shah AJ, Duddy G, Kew JN and Maycox PR (2009) Evaluation of expression and function of the H+/myo-inositol transporter HMIT. BMC Cell Biology 10:54.

Diaz F (2010) Cytochrome c oxidase deficiency: patients and animal models. Biochimica et Biophysica Acta 1802:100–110.

Evers R, Kool M, van Deemter L, Janssen H, Calafat J, Oomen LC, Paulusma CC, Oude Elferink RP, Baas F, Schinkel AH and Borst P (1998) Drug export activity of the human canalicular multispecific organic anion transporter in polarized kidney MDCK cells expressing cMOAT (MRP2) cDNA. Journal of Clinical Investigation 101:1310–1319.

Faham S, Watanabe A, Besserer GM, Cascio D, Specht A, Hirayama BA, Wright EM and Abramson J (2008) The crystal structure of a sodium galactose transporter reveals mechanistic insights into Na+/sugar symport. Science 321:810–814.

Faraldo-Gómez JD and Forrest LR (2011) Modeling and simulation of ion-coupled and ATP-driven membrane proteins. Current Opinions in Structural Biology 21:173–179.

Forrest LR, Krämer R and Ziegler C (2011) The structural basis of secondary active transport mechanisms. Biochimica et Biophysica Acta (BBA) - Bioenergetics 1807:167–188.

Gao Z, Fain HD and Rapoport N (2004) Ultrasound-enhanced tumor targeting of polymeric micellar drug carriers. Molecular Pharmacology 1:317–330.

Gether U, Andersen PH, Larsson OM and Schousboe A (2006) Neurotransmitter transporters: molecular function of important drug targets. Trends in Pharmacological Science 27:375–383.

Gottesman MM, Fojo T and Bates SE (2002) Multidrug resistance in cancer: role of ATP-dependent transporters. Nature Review Cancer 2:48–58.

Harasym TO, Liboiron BD and Mayer LD (2010) Drug ratio-dependent antagonism: a new category of multidrug resistance and strategies for its circumvention. Methods in Molecular Biology 596:291–323.

Heymann JA, Hirai T, Shi D and Subramaniam S (2003) Projection structure of the bacterial oxalate transporter OxlT at 3.4A resolution. Journal of Structural Biology 144:320–326.

Higgins CF (2007) Multiple molecular mechanisms for multidrug resistance transporters. Nature 446: 749–757.

Higgins CF (1992) ABC transporters: from microorganisms to man. Annual Review of Cell Biology 8: 67–113.

Higgins CF and Gottesman MM (1992) Is the multidrug transporter a flippase? Trends in Biochemical Sciences 17: 18–21.

Hinton A, Bond S and Forgac M (2009) V-ATPase functions in normal and disease processes. Pflugers Archiv : European Journal of Physiology 457: 589–598.

Hirai T, Heymann JA, Shi D, Sarker R, Maloney PC and Subramaniam S (2002) Three-dimensional structure of a bacterial oxalate transporter. Nature Structural Biology 9: 597–600.

Ho JK, Moser H, Kishimoto Y and Hamilton JA (1995) Interactions of a very long chain fatty acid with model membranes and serum albumin. Implications for the pathogenesis of adrenoleukodystrophy. Journal of Clinical Investigation 96: 1455–1463.

Hollenstein K, Dawson RJ and Locher KP (2007) Structure and mechanism of ABC transporter proteins. Current Opinion in Structural Biology 17:412–418.

Huang Y, Lemieux MJ, Song J, Auer M and Wang DN (2003) Structure and mechanism of the glycerol-3-phosphate transporter from Escherichia coli. Science 301:616–620.

James PF, Grupp IL, Grupp G, Woo AL, Askew GR, Croyle ML, Walsh RA and Lingrel JB (1999) Identification of a specific role for the Na,K-ATPase alpha 2 isoform as a regulator of calcium in the heart. Molecular Cell 3:555–563.

Juliano RL and Ling V (1976) A surface glycoprotein modulating drug permeability in Chinese hamster ovary cell mutants. Biochimica et Biophysica Acta 455: 152–162.

Jung H (2002) The sodium/substrate symporter family: structural and functional features. FEBS Letters 529: 73–77.

Kaback HR (2005) Structure and mechanism of the lactose permease. Comptes Rendus Biologies 328:557–567.

Kabouridis PS (2003) Biological applications of protein transduction technology. Trends in Biotechnology 21:498–503.

Kagan VE, Bayir A, Bayir H, Stoyanovsky D, Borisenko GG, Tyurina YY, Wipf P, Atkinson J, Greenberger JS, Chapkin RS and Belikova NA (2009) Mitochondria-targeted disruptors and inhibitors of cytochrome c/cardiolipin peroxidase complexes: a new strategy in anti-apoptotic drug discovery. Molecular Nutrition & Food Research 53:104–114.

Kaminski WE, Piehler A and Wenzel JJ (2006) ABC A-subfamily transporters: structure, function and disease. Biochimica et Biophysica Acta 1762:510–524.

Karet FE, Finberg KE, Nelson RD, Nayir A, Mocan H, Sanjad SA, Rodriguez-Soriano J, Santos F, Cremers CW, Di Pietro A, Hoffbrand BI, Winiarski J, Bakkaloglu A, Ozen S, Dusunsel R, Goodyer P, Hulton SA, Wu DK, Skvorak AB, Morton CC, Cunningham MJ, Jha V and Lifton RP (1999) Mutations in the gene encoding B1 subunit of H+—ATPase cause renal tubular acidosis with sensorineural deafness. Nature Genetics 21: 84–90.

Kemp S and Wanders RJ (2007) X-linked adrenoleukodystrophy: very long-chain fatty acid metabolism, ABC half-transporters and the complicated route to treatment. Molecular Genetics and Metabolism 90: 268–276.

Khafizov K, Staritzbichler R, Stamm M and Forrest LR (2010) A study of the evolution of inverted-topology repeats from LeuT-fold transporters using AlignMe. Biochemistry 49: 10702–10713.

Kinne A, Kleinau G, Hoefig CS, Gruters A, Kohrle J, Krause G and Schweizer U (2010) Essential molecular determinants for thyroid hormone transport and first structural implications for monocarboxylate transporter 8. Journal of Biological Chemistry 285: 28054–28063.

Klaassen CD and Aleksunes LM (2010) Xenobiotic, bile acid, and cholesterol transporters: function and regulation. Pharmacology Reviews 62:1–96.

Klein I, Sarkadi B and Varadi A (1999) An inventory of the human ABC proteins. Biochimica et Biophysica Acta 1461:237–262.

Knauf PA, Proverbio F and Hoffman JF (1974) Chemical characterization and pronase susceptibility of the Na:K pump-associated phosphoprotein of human red blood cells. The Journal of General Physiology 63:305–323.

Kornak U, Reynders E, Dimopoulou A, van Reeuwijk J, Fischer B, Rajab A, Budde B, Nurnberg P, Foulquier F, ARCL Debre-type Study Group, Lefeber D, Urban Z, Gruenewald S, Annaert W, Brunner HG, van Bokhoven H, Wevers R, Morava E, Matthijs G, Van Maldergem L and Mundlos S (2008) Impaired glycosylation and cutis laxa caused by mutations in the vesicular H+—ATPase subunit ATP6V0A2. Nature Genetics 40: 32–34.

Kostakoglu L, Elahi N, Kiratli P, Ruacan S, Sayek I, Baltali E, Sungur A, Hayran M and Bekdik CF (1997) Clinical validation of the influence of P-glycoprotein on technetium-99m-sestamibi uptake in malignant tumors. Journal of Nuclear Medicine 38: 1003–1008.

Kousi M, Siintola E, Dvorakova L, Vlaskova H, Turnbull J, Topcu M, Yuksel D, Gokben S, Minassian BA, Elleder M, Mole SE and Lehesjoki AE (2009) Mutations in CLN7/MFSD8 are a common cause of variant late-infantile neuronal ceroid lipofuscinosis. Brain 132: 810–819.

Krishnamurthy H, Piscitelli CL and Gouaux E (2009) Unlocking the molecular secrets of sodium-coupled transporters. Nature 459: 347–355.

Kuhlbrandt W (2004) Biology, structure and mechanism of P-type ATPases. Nature Review Molecular Cell Biology 5: 282–295.

Kusuhara H and Sugiyama Y (2007) ATP-binding cassette, subfamily G (ABCG family). Pflugers Archiv: European Journal of Physiology 453: 735–744.

Law CJ, Maloney PC and Wang DN (2008) Ins and outs of major facilitator superfamily antiporters. Annual Review of Microbiology 62: 289–305.

Lazarou M, Thorburn DR, Ryan MT and McKenzie M (2009) Assembly of mitochondrial complex I and defects in disease. Biochimica et Biophysica Acta 1793: 78–88.

Lee CH (2010) Reversing agents for ATP-binding cassette drug transporters. Methods Molecular Biology 596: 325–340.

Lemieux MJ, Huang Y and Wang DN (2004) Glycerol-3-phosphate transporter of Escherichia coli: structure, function and regulation. Research in Microbiology 155: 623–629.

Lind J, Graslund A and Maler L (2006) Membrane interactions of dynorphins. Biochemistry 45: 15931–15940.

Liu Y, Liu F, Iqbal K, Grundke-Iqbal I and Gong CX (2008) Decreased glucose transporters correlate to abnormal hyper-phosphorylation of tau in Alzheimer disease. FEBS Letters 582: 359–364.

Madsen KK, White HS and Schousboe A (2010) Neuronal and non-neuronal GABA transporters as targets for antiepileptic drugs. Pharmacology & Therapeutics 125: 394–401.

Materna V and Lage H (2003) Homozygous mutation Arg768Trp in the ABC-transporter encoding gene MRP2/cMOAT/ABCC2 causes Dubin-Johnson syndrome in a Caucasian patient. Journal of Human Genetics 48: 484–486.

Mechetner EB, Schott B, Morse BS, Stein WD, Druley T, Davis KA, Tsuruo T and Roninson IB (1997) P-glycoprotein function involves conformational transitions detectable by differential immunoreactivity. Proceedings of the National Academy of Science U S A 94: 12908–12913.

Mickle JE, Milewski MI, Macek M, Jr and Cutting GR (2000) Effects of cystic fibrosis and congenital bilateral absence of the vas deferens-associated mutations on cystic fibrosis transmembrane conductance regulator-mediated regulation of separate channels. American Journal of Human Genetics 66: 1485–1495.

Mima S, Ushijima H, Hwang HJ, Tsutsumi S, Makise M, Yamaguchi Y, Tsuchiya T, Mizushima H and Mizushima T (2007) Identification of the TPO1 gene in yeast, and its human ortho-logue TETRAN, which cause resistance to NSAIDs. FEBS Letters 581: 1457–1463.

Molday RS, Zhong M and Quazi F (2009) The role of the photoreceptor ABC transporter ABCA4 in lipid transport and Stargardt macular degeneration. Biochimica et Biophysica Acta 1791: 573–583.

Monk BC, Mason AB, Abramochkin G, Haber JE, Seto-Young D and Perlin DS (1995) The yeast plasma membrane proton pumping ATPase is a viable antifungal target. I. Effects of the cysteine-modifying reagent omeprazole. Biochim Biophys Acta 1239: 81–90.

Morin D, Assaly R, Paradis S and Berdeaux A (2009) Inhibition of mitochondrial membrane permeability as a putative phar-macological target for cardioprotection. Current Medicinal Chemistry 16: 4382–4398.

Murakami S, Nakashima R, Yamashita E, Matsumoto T and Yamaguchi A (2006) Crystal structures of a multidrug trans-porter reveal a functionally rotating mechanism. Nature 443: 173–179.

Nakanishi-Matsui M, Sekiya M, Nakamoto RK and Futai M (2010) The mechanism of rotating proton pumping ATPases. Biochimica et Biophysica Acta 1797: 1343–1352.

Noe J, Kullak-Ublick GA, Jochum W, Stieger B, Kerb R, Haberl M, Mullhaupt B, Meier PJ and Pauli-Magnus C (2005) Impaired expression and function of the bile salt export pump due to three novel ABCB11 mutations in intrahepatic cholestasis. Journal of Hepatology 43: 536–543.

Odermatt A, Taschner PE, Khanna VK, Busch HF, Karpati G, Jablecki CK, Breuning MH and MacLennan DH (1996) Mutations in the gene-encoding SERCA1, the fast-twitch skeletal muscle sarcoplasmic reticulum Ca2+ ATPase, are associated with Brody disease. Nature Genetics 14: 191–194.

Padan E, Kozachkov L, Herz K and Rimon A (2009) NhaA crystal structure: functional-structural insights. Journal of Experimental Biology 212: 1593–1603.

Padan E (2008) The enlightening encounter between structure and function in the NhaA Na+−H+ antiporter. Trends in Biochemical Sciences 33: 435–443.

Pajeva IK and Wiese M (2009) Structure-activity relationships of tariquidar analogs as multidrug resistance modulators. The AAPS Journal 11: 435–444.

Pao SS, Paulsen IT and Saier MH, Jr (1998) Major facilitator superfamily. Microbiology Molecular Biology Rev 62: 1–34.

Parcej D and Tampe R (2010) ABC proteins in antigen translo-cation and viral inhibition. Nature Chemistry Biology 6: 572–580.

Pascual JM, Wang D, Yang R, Shi L, Yang H and De Vivo DC (2008) Structural signatures and membrane helix 4 in GLUT1: inferences from human blood–brain glucose transport mutants. Journal of Biological Chemistry 283: 16732–16742.

Pedersen PL (2007) Transport ATPases into the year 2008: a brief overview related to types, structures, functions and roles in health and disease. Journal of Bioenergetics and Biomembranes 39: 349–355.

Pondarre C, Antiochos BB, Campagna DR, Clarke SL, Greer EL, Deck KM, McDonald A, Han AP, Medlock A, Kutok JL, Anderson SA, Eisenstein RS and Fleming MD (2006) The mitochondrial ATP-binding cassette transporter Abcb7 is essential in mice and participates in cytosolic iron-sulfur cluster biogenesis. Human Molecular Genetics 15: 953–964.

Pos KM (2009) Drug transport mechanism of the AcrB efflux pump. Biochimica et Biophysica Acta 1794: 782–793.

Procko E and Gaudet R (2009) Antigen processing and presen-tation: TAPping into ABC transporters. Current Opinions in Immunology 21: 84–91.

Procko E, O'Mara ML, Bennett WF, Tieleman DP and Gaudet R (2009) The mechanism of ABC transporters: general lessons from structural and functional studies of an antigenic peptide transporter. The FASEB Journal 23: 1287–1302.

Radestock S and Forrest LR (2011) The alternating-access mech-anism of MFS transporters arises from inverted-topology repeats. Journal of Molecular Biology 407: 698–715.

Ramirez A, Heimbach A, Grundemann J, Stiller B, Hampshire D, Cid LP, Goebel I, Mubaidin AF, Wriekat AL, Roeper J, Al-Din A, Hillmer AM, Karsak M, Liss B, Woods CG, Behrens MI and Kubisch C (2006) Hereditary parkinsonism with dementia is caused by mutations in ATP13A2, encoding a lysosomal type 5 P-type ATPase. Nature Genetics 38: 1184–1191.

Raviv Y, Pollard HB, Bruggemann EP, Pastan I and Gottesman MM (1990) Photosensitized labeling of a functional multidrug transporter in living drug-resistant tumor cells. Journal of Biological Chemistry 265: 3975–3980.

Rimon A, Hunte C, Michel H and Padan E (2008) Epitope mapping of conformational monoclonal antibodies specific to NhaA Na+/H+ antiporter: structural and functional implications. Journal of Molecular Biology 379: 471–481.

Rutter J, Winge DR and Schiffman JD (2010) Succinate dehydrogenase - Assembly, regulation and role in human disease. Mitochondrion 10: 393–401.

Ryan RM, Compton EL and Mindell JA (2009) Functional characterization of a Na+−dependent aspartate transporter from Pyrococcus horikoshii. Journal of Biological Chemistry 284: 17540–17548.

Sa-Correia I, dos Santos SC, Teixeira MC, Cabrito TR and Mira NP (2009) Drug:H+ antiporters in chemical stress response in yeast. Trends in Microbiology 17: 22–31.

Saier MH, Jr, Yen MR, Noto K, Tamang DG and Elkan C (2009) The Transporter Classification Database: recent advances. Nucleic Acids Research 37: D274-8.

Saier MH, Jr, Beatty JT, Goffeau A, Harley KT, Heijne WH, Huang SC, Jack DL, Jahn PS, Lew K, Liu J, Pao SS, Paulsen IT, Tseng TT and Virk PS (1999) The major facilitator superfamily. J Molecular and Microbiological Biotechnology 1: 257–279.

Sakuntabhai A, Ruiz-Perez V, Carter S, Jacobsen N, Burge S, Monk S, Smith M, Munro CS, O'Donovan M, Craddock N, Kucherlapati R, Rees JL, Owen M, Lathrop GM, Monaco AP, Strachan T and Hovnanian A (1999) Mutations in ATP2A2, encoding a Ca2+ pump, cause Darier disease. Nature Genetics 21: 271–277.

Sanchez CP, Dave A, Stein WD and Lanzer M (2010) Transporters as mediators of drug resistance in Plasmodium falciparum. International Journal for Parasitology 40: 1109–1118.

Scheffer GL, Hu X, Pijnenborg AC, Wijnholds J, Bergen AA and Scheper RJ (2002) MRP6 (ABCC6) detection in normal human tissues and tumors. Laboratory Investigation 82: 515–518.

Schinkel AH, Mol CA, Wagenaar E, van Deemter L, Smit JJ and Borst P (1995) Multidrug resistance and the role of P-glycoprotein knockout mice. European Journal of Cancer 31A: 1295–1298.

Segade F (2010) Glucose transporter 10 and arterial tortuosity syndrome: the vitamin C connection. FEBS Letters 584: 2990–2994.

Serfaty-Lacrosniere C, Civeira F, Lanzberg A, Isaia P, Berg J, Janus ED, Smith MP, Jr, Pritchard PH, Frohlich J and Lees RS (1994) Homozygous Tangier disease and cardiovascular disease. Atherosclerosis 107: 85–98.

Sharom FJ, Yu X, Lu P, Liu R, Chu JW, Szabo K, Muller M, Hose CD, Monks A, Varadi A, Seprodi J and Sarkadi B (1999) Interaction of the P-glycoprotein multidrug transporter (MDR1)

with high affinity peptide chemosensitizers in isolated membranes, reconstituted systems, and intact cells. Biochemical Pharmacology 58: 571–586.

Shulenin S, Nogee LM, Annilo T, Wert SE, Whitsett JA and Dean M (2004) ABCA3 gene mutations in newborns with fatal surfactant deficiency. New England Journal of Medicine 350: 1296–1303.

Singh SK, Piscitelli CL, Yamashita A and Gouaux E (2008) A competitive inhibitor traps LeuT in an open-to-out conformation. Science 322: 1655–1661.

Small DM (2003) Role of ABC transporters in secretion of cholesterol from liver into bile. Proceedings of the National Academy of Science U S A 100: 4–6.

Smit JJ, Schinkel AH, Oude Elferink RP, Groen AK, Wagenaar E, van Deemter L, Mol CA, Ottenhoff R, van der Lugt NM and van Roon MA (1993) Homozygous disruption of the murine mdr2 P-glycoprotein gene leads to a complete absence of phospholipid from bile and to liver disease. Cell 75: 451–462.

Sobczak I and Lolkema JS (2005) Structural and mechanistic diversity of secondary transporters. Current Opinions in Microbiology 8: 161–167.

Szakacs G, Varadi A, Ozvegy-Laczka C and Sarkadi B (2008) The role of ABC transporters in drug absorption, distribution, metabolism, excretion and toxicity (ADME-Tox). Drug Discovery Today 13: 379–393.

Szakacs G, Paterson JK, Ludwig JA, Booth-Genthe C and Gottesman MM (2006) Targeting multidrug resistance in cancer. Nature Reviews Drug Discovery 5: 219–234.

Takamori S (2006) VGLUTs: 'exciting' times for glutamatergic research? Neuroscience Research 55: 343–351.

Theophilos MB, Cox DW and Mercer JF (1996) The toxic milk mouse is a murine model of Wilson disease. Human Molecular Genetics 5: 1619–1624.

Thomas WD, Jr, Wagner SP and Welch RA (1992) A heterologous membrane protein domain fused to the C-terminal ATP-binding domain of HlyB can export Escherichia coli hemolysin. Journal of Bacteriology 174: 6771–6779.

Toei M, Saum R and Forgac M (2010) Regulation and isoform function of the V-ATPases. Biochemistry 49: 4715–4723.

Trabulo S Cardoso AL Mano M and Pedroso de Lima MC (2010) Cell-Penetrating Peptides – Mechanisms of Cellular Uptake and Generation of Delivery Systems. Pharmaceuticals 3: 961–993.

Truong DM, Kaler G, Khandelwal A, Swaan PW and Nigam SK (2008) Multi-level analysis of organic anion transporters 1, 3, and 6 reveals major differences in structural determinants of antiviral discrimination. Journal of Biological Chemistry 283:8654–8663.

Ueno M, Nakagawa T, Wu B, Onodera M, Huang CL, Kusaka T, Araki N and Sakamoto H (2010) Transporters in the brain endothelial barrier. Current Medicinal Chemistry 17:1125–1138.

VanWert AL, Gionfriddo MR and Sweet DH (2010) Organic anion transporters: discovery, pharmacology, regulation and roles in pathophysiology. Biopharmaceutics & Drug Disposition 31:1–71.

Verkman AS (2009) Aquaporins: translating bench research to human disease. Journal of Experimental Biology 212:1707–1715.

Wang CI and Lewis RJ (2010) Emerging structure-function relationships defining monoamine NSS transporter substrate and ligand affinity. Biochemical Pharmacology 79: 1083–1091.

Ware SM, El-Hassan N, Kahler SG, Zhang Q, Ma YW, Miller E, Wong B, Spicer RL, Craigen WJ, Kozel BA, Grange DK and Wong LJ (2009) Infantile cardiomyopathy caused by a mutation in the overlapping region of mitochondrial ATPase 6 and 8 genes. Journal of Medical Genetics 46:308–314.

Wright AF, Rudan I, Hastie ND and Campbell H (2010) A 'complexity' of urate transporters. Kidney International 78:446–452.

Yernool D, Boudker O, Jin Y and Gouaux E (2004) Structure of a glutamate transporter homologue from Pyrococcus horikoshii. Nature 431:811–818.

6 Cystic Fibrosis: Alternative Approaches to the Treatment of a Genetic Disease

6.1 Introduction

It took 50 years from the discovery of the double helix structure of DNA to completion of the human genome project in 2003. Whilst this was remarkable progress it is important to recognise that identification of the gene responsible for a genetic disease is only the start of a long process in developing effective treatments. The discovery of the gene for cystic fibrosis (CF) and the identification of the resultant protein, cystic fibrosis transmembrane conductance regulator (CFTR), was announced in a series of three landmark papers in the 8th September 1989 issue of *Science* (Kerem et al., 1989; Riordan et al., 1989; Rommens et al., 1989). This was the culmination of years of work in the CF scientific community. The euphoria over this key event led to wildly over optimistic predictions in some quarters that gene therapy would be developed for CF within a few years. The rhetoric has sadly not matched the reality and more than 20 years later there are still substantial hurdles to overcome before gene therapy for CF can become an established treatment. This chapter will use CF as a case study to illustrate approaches to the development of treatments for a genetic disease. At the time of writing, whilst clinical trials are currently investigating gene therapy protocols, it is likely to be years before this will lead to effective treatment.

Cystic fibrosis

CF is the commonest lethal genetic disease of Caucasians. It is an autosomal recessive disease that has a carrier frequency of around 1 in 25 of North American and Western European populations. Figure 6.1 illustrates the frequency of CF in children from heterozygous parents.

The heterozygote carrier frequency is around 1 in 25 of the general UK population. This equates to a 1 in 625 chance of both parents being heterozygotes ($1/25 \times 1/25$). Each of their children will have a 1 in 2 chance of being heterozygotes, 1 in 4 of being wild type and a 1 in 4 of

Molecular Pharmacology: From DNA to Drug Discovery, First Edition. John Dickenson, Fiona Freeman, Chris Lloyd Mills, Shiva Sivasubramaniam and Christian Thode.
© 2013 John Wiley & Sons, Ltd. Published 2013 by John Wiley & Sons, Ltd.

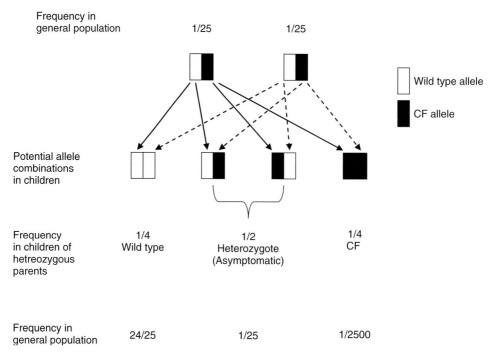

Figure 6.1 Frequency of a CF child with heterozygous parents. Figure adapted from McPherson and Dormer, 1991. Molecular and cellular biology of cystic fibrosis. Molecular Aspects of Medicine 21: 1–81. Elsevier copyright 1991.

being CF. The incidence of CF in the UK is therefore approximately 1 in 2500 live births (1/625 × 1/4).

Clinical features

CF is a disease of exocrine glands and secretory epithelia. The underlying causes of the clinical symptoms are disturbances to electrolyte transport and mucus secretion (McPherson and Dormer, 1991). This then leads to the development of a variety of pathologies (Figure 6.2).

Airways

Whilst CF affects several organs, the predominant cause of premature death is lung disease (Figure 6.2). Lungs of CF patients are normal at birth. Subsequent damage to the airways arises from the increase in viscosity and reduction in depth of the airways surface liquid (ASL). Mucin secretion in CF is stimulated by a variety of inflammatory factors including proteases deriving from bacterial infections, neutrophil recruitment and degranulation, as well as oxidants, cytokines and so on (see Voynow and Rubin, 2009 for a review of airways mucins). These together impair mucociliary clearance and lead to the build up of thick sticky mucus. The concomitant reduction in the antimicrobial defence systems of the lungs paves the way

for recurrent bacterial infections. Generally *Haemophilus influenzae* and *Staphylococcus aureus* are early colonisers. These induce inflammatory processes that initiate lung damage. Later, other bacteria will arrive. Of particular concern is *Psuedomonas aeruginosa* as its arrival tends to lead to an acceleration in airway inflammation, lung damage and decline in lung function (Pilewski and Frizzell, 1999). Once this pathogen has become established it is very difficult to eradicate.

ASL contains a complex cocktail of substances including antibodies, antibiotics, oxidants, antioxidants, proteases and antiproteases, all of which can influence airway inflammation and damage (Wine, 1999). The balance of these can shift in CF airways. For example, the increased neutrophil infiltration of CF airways reflects their enhanced bacterial load. The increased oxidant environment and reduced levels of antioxidants, such as glutathione, in CF airways will contribute to lung damage.

Quorum sensing is a form of bacterial communication whereby gene expression patterns can be altered by certain secreted molecules. As the amount of bacteria build up the concentration of secreted molecules increases. In the case of *P. aeruginosa* this can induce establishment of biofilms and a switch to the mucoid form. Biofilms contain

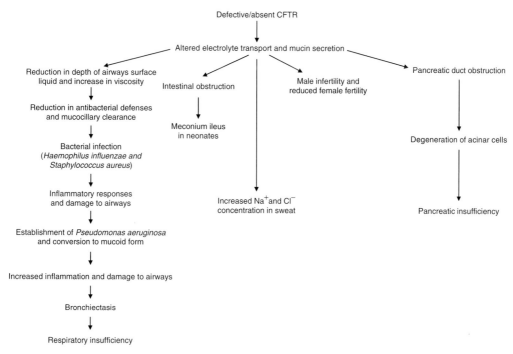

Figure 6.2 CF induced pathology. The defective electrolyte and mucin secretion in CF affects a range of organs. Some pathology is present at birth, whilst others develop gradually. See text for further details. Figure adapted from McPherson and Dormer, 1991; and Amaral and Kunzelmann, 2007.

extracellular matrixes that impede bacterial clearance by phagocytic cells (Buchan et al., 2009). Since the mucoid form is associated with increased lung damage there is interest in quorum sensing inhibitors.

Gastrointestinal tract

Pancreatic insufficiency develops in around 85% of CF patients. This arises due to inadequate bicarbonate (HCO_3^-) and fluid secretion leading to blockage of ducts, atrophy of exocrine acinar cells and subsequent fibrosis of the pancreas. With the degeneration of the acinar cells, pancreatic enzyme secretion is impaired, resulting in inefficient digestion, and hence reduced assimilation of food. Even where pancreatic enzyme secretion is normal, the reduced HCO_3^- secretion may not sufficiently neutralise the gastric juices in the duodenum to allow maximal enzyme activity. Pancreatitis may also develop, whereby autodigestion of the pancreas occurs. This will compound the pancreatic damage. An additional complication is that damage to the pancreatic endocrine functions can lead to failure to adequately control blood glucose concentration. It has been estimated that up to 50% of adult CF patients may develop impaired glucose regulation,

though only around 10% will eventually exhibit diabetes mellitus. Whilst overt CF induced liver disease is only found in a few percent of CF patients, autopsy studies have shown that disorders of the liver and biliary tract such as steatosis (fatty liver) and focal biliary cirrhosis are actually commonplace (Shalon and Adelson, 1996).

Around 15% of CF neonates present with meconium ileus. This is a life threatening blockage of the gut that is usually, but not exclusively, associated with CF. During development in the uterus meconium builds up. Since the foetus imbibes amniotic fluid, the meconium includes the undigested and unabsorbed remnants of sloughed off cellular material (e.g. skin and intestinal epithelial cells, lanugo hair), intestinal secretions, bile and so on. The meconium is a sticky dark coloured material that is passed from the intestine in the first few stools of a neonate. In marked contrast to the much paler stools that arrive later as milk is digested, the meconium is effectively odourless. In CF the meconium is more viscous than normal and may block the intestine. Treatment of meconium ileus can include enemas to soften the blockage or surgery, depending on the severity of the case. Intestinal blockages may also occur later in life, with approximately 15% of

CF patients experiencing recurrent episodes of partial intestinal obstruction (Shalon and Adelson, 1996).

Reproductive tract

More than 95% of males with CF are infertile due to congenital bilateral absence of the vas deferens (CBAVD). Whilst the semen contains no sperm, spermatogenesis is normal so sperm can be harvested and used for ICSI (intra-cytoplasmic sperm injection). This involves the injection of a single sperm into an oocyte in an attempt to fertilise it. Although the success rate is low, with a pregnancy rate of about 30% per attempt, it does offer the opportunity for CF males to father children. CF females have normal anatomy but tend to be less fertile. This is considered to be due to the presence of thick cervical mucus that impedes the transit of sperm. In addition the role of bicarbonate could be important. The female reproductive tract has a high bicarbonate concentration, 35–90 mM, and it may be involved in sperm capacitation (activation of sperm before fertilisation can occur). CFTR appears to have a role in both bicarbonate secretion in the female reproductive tract, and bicarbonate uptake into sperm (Chan et al., 2009). Thus defective CFTR could impact at several levels in reducing fertility (CBAVD in males, mucus impeding sperm in females and faulty bicarbonate transport affecting sperm capacitation in both males and females).

Where one partner has CF it is essential that genetic counselling is given prior to the provision of assisted fertilisation techniques. The risk of a subsequent child having CF varies from 50% for a heterozygote partner to 1 in 50 where the carrier status of the non CF partner is unknown. If the non CF partner is screened and found to lack the common mutations, then the odds of a CF child drops to around 1 in 400.

Sweat glands

In 1948 a heatwave in New York resulted in a much higher incidence of heat prostration in CF patients than the general public. This led di Sant' Agnese to discover that CF patients had abnormally high sodium and chloride concentrations in their sweat. Within five years of his 1953 paper the sweat test was developed and quickly became established as the technique of choice to rapidly and accurately diagnose CF. The test involves iontophoretic application of the non-selective muscarinic agonist pilocarpine to a small area of skin on the arm. The sweat from this area is then analysed. Usually only the chloride concentration is measured, though some centres measure both. An elevated sweat chloride (and sodium)

concentration above 60 mM is indicative of CF. This general rule works well in a paediatric setting, where normal sweat is <40 mM (Quinton, 2007). However with adults there can be some overlap between the low end of the range of CF patients and the high end of the normal range so it is not always a definitive test. In these cases genotyping may be used to confirm CF.

Diagnosis of CF

Although CF was only first recognised as a specific disease in the 1930s, one of its characteristic symptoms of excessively salty sweat had been noticed as early as 1606. The following three lines derive from eighteenth century Swiss-German folklore and refer to the key diagnostic feature of CF and the reduced life expectancy.

> Woe to that child,
> which when kissed on the forehead tastes salty.
> He is bewitched and soon must die.

Screening for CF in neonates is not routine in most countries. Where it does occur it tends to measures the level of immunoreactive trypsinogen (IRT) in heel prick blood samples. This is only a primary screen, where elevated levels of IRT indicate an increased risk of CF and must be followed up by further diagnostic tests to confirm CF. IRT only suggests pancreatic damage. This may not be caused by CF but could be due to other causes such as pancreatitis, or even be a false positive. Hence positive IRT tests are usually repeated after a month.

If routine neonatal screening does not occur and meconium ileus is not present, CF is usually determined in the first few years of life following investigation for a range of conditions such as gastrointestinal problems (e.g. steatorrhea), recurrent chest infections, failure to thrive etc. It should however be noted that in some cases CF may not be diagnosed until adolescence in patients where the disease is very mild.

The normal criteria used to diagnose CF is that there would be an indication of possible CF together with a diagnostic tests to confirm CF. Indicators of possible CF include family history, clinical history suggestive of CF such as meconium ileus, recurrent chest infections, steatorrhea, or a positive neonatal IRT test. Diagnostic tests used to confirm CF include genetic analysis, which must demonstrate two CF alleles (as one normal allele is sufficient to maintain function), sweat sodium and/or chloride >60 mM, or a nasal potential difference more negative than −32 mv, though this latter test is restricted in availability (Hudson and Guill, 1998). It should however be noted that failure to find two CF alleles does not rule out CF. There are >1900 mutations and screening tends to only look at the most common mutations. For some ethnic groups with well characterised mutations, a screen of common mutations can pick up around 90% of cases, whilst in other ethnic groups it is substantially lower.

6.2 Cystic fibrosis transmembrane conductance regulator

The CF gene is located on chromosome 7 and consists of ≈250,000 base pairs of genomic DNA. This contains 27 exons and gives rise to an mRNA transcript ≈6,500 nucleotides long, which in turn is translated into the cystic fibrosis transmembrane conductance regulator protein (CFTR) of 1480 amino acids. The protein has several domains that contribute to its function (Figure 6.3).

CFTR has two membrane-spanning domains (MSD1 and 2) that each consist of six transmembrane segments. These MSD together form a Cl⁻ channel. At the end of each MSD is a nucleotide binding domain (NBD1 and 2) that can bind ATP. Between the first NBD and the second MSD in the R domain. The first extracellular loop of MSD2 is glycosylated.

CFTR Cl⁻ channel activity is regulated by the balance between phosphorylation and dephosphorylation. There are several protein kinase A (PKA) phosphorylation sites on the regulatory R domain, and some of them are also capable of phosphorylation by protein kinase C (PKC). By itself, PKC phosphorylation has little effect on CFTR Cl⁻ channel activity. However, PKC phosphorylation does potentiate the effect of subsequent PKA phosphorylation events (Gadsby and Nairn, 1999).

CFTR has chloride channel activity

Before CFTR was discovered it was already known that the cyclic adenosine 3′, 5′ monophosphate (cAMP) activated Cl⁻ conductance of several epithelia was defective in CF (Sheppard and Welsh, 1999). This might arise due to CFTR regulating a Cl⁻ channel, or alternatively CFTR itself forming a Cl⁻ channel. Within a short time after the publication of the CFTR gene sequence it was demonstrated that CFTR was a cAMP activated Cl⁻ channel. The key experiments found that:

i) Introducing CFTR into cells that do not have cAMP regulated Cl⁻ channels induces a cAMP regulated Cl⁻ conductance. This was further strengthened by the observation that different CF mutations alter the conductance to varying extents (e.g. Drumm et al., 1991).

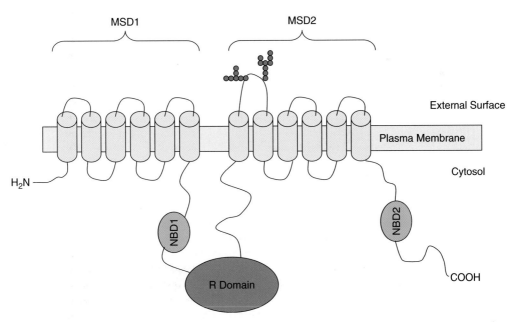

Figure 6.3 Model of CFTR. Adapted by permission from Macmillan Publishers Ltd [Nature] Wine JJ 1993. Indictment of pore behaviour, Nature 366: 18–19 copyright 1993.

ii) Incorporating purified CFTR into an artificial lipid membrane produces a cAMP activated Cl^- conductance with the biophysical and regulatory properties identical to CFTR expressing epithelia (Bear et al., 1992).

iii) Mutation of a single amino acid within the first MSD of CFTR could alter the anion selectivity of the Cl^- channel. The normal conductivity sequence of the wild type CFTR Cl^- channel is $Br^- \geq Cl^- > I^- > F^-$. Andersen et al. (1991) showed that the mutation of the basic amino acid lysine at position 95 or 335 to acidic amino acids (aspartate and glutamate respectively) changed the conductivity sequence to $I^- > Br^- > Cl^- > F^-$.

Taken together, these experiments are strong evidence the CFTR is a cAMP regulated Cl^- channel.

CFTR chloride channel regulation

Initially the CFTR Cl^- channel is in a quiescent state. Phosphorylation of the R domain is required for channel opening. However, the roles of the various phosphorylation sites on the R domain is not fully understood (Hwang and Sheppard, 2009). The two nucleotide binding domains (NBD) can each bind one ATP and this induces the formation of a dimer between the two NBDs. The two ATP binding sites are located at the junction between the NBDs and one NBD has a Walker A and B consensus sequence, with a corresponding LSGGQ amino acid sequence on the other. For site 1 the Walker A and B sequence is on NBD1, with the LSGGQ on NBD2, whilst for site 2 the opposite is present (Hwang and Shepard, 2009). Initially one ATP binds to each NBD, which induces a conformational change resulting in NBD1 and NBD2 dimer formation. This causes opening of the CFTR Cl^- channel. Subsequent ATP hydrolysis at site 2 produces a rapid cessation of the ATP induced Cl^- channel activity. Whilst NBD ATP binding is required for maximal CFTR Cl^- channel activity, a low rate of ATP independent Cl^- channel activity can also occur.

Various models have been proposed to account for the experimental observations on Cl^- channel activity of CFTR. Although none of these can fully explain the results, this approach has derived a useful conceptual framework. The model based on scheme B from Bompadre et al. (2007) includes both ATP dependant Cl^- channel opening events and spontaneous ATP independent opening events. The differences in opening and closing rates, and interconversion between different sub-states, result in a complex model that can explain many of the observations in the literature. Initially the CFTR has a low rate of spontaneous opening. If the first NBD of CFTR binds ATP,

the rate of spontaneous opening changes. Binding of ATP to the 2nd NBD increases the open channel probability. Removal of ATP at one, or both NBDs will then alter the open channel probability. See Bompadre et al. (2007) for a full discussion of this model.

CFTR is monomeric

It has been suggested that CFTR may form dimers. To investigate this possibility CFTR was labelled with green fluorescent protein (GFP) and expressed in COS and CHO cell lines (Haggie and Verkman, 2008). Total internal reflection fluorescence imaging (TIRF) can detect single fluorescent molecules. The analysis of fluorescence intensity distributions demonstrated a single peak, indicating that CFTR-GFP is present as a monomer. This was confirmed with photobleaching studies, where only single step photobleaching was observed. Dual labelling of CFTR with two GFPs demonstrated that the test system could have detected CFTR dimers as fluorescence intensity was approximately double. In addition, two-step photobleaching (i.e. one for each GFP) was observed (Haggie and Verkman, 2008). It was therefore concluded that CFTR is monomeric in plasma membranes, though it should be noted that NBD1 and 2 from the same CFTR protein do form dimers.

Role of CFTR in the airways

The epithelia of the tracheobronchial region of the lungs are mainly composed of ciliated cells together with some goblet cells and submucosal glands (McPherson and Dormer, 1991). On the surface of airways epithelial cells is the airways surface liquid (ASL). The goblet cells and submucosal glands produce mucus which traps particles such as dust and bacteria. These foreign particles are then removed by the mucociliary escalator, which is an important component of the airways antibacterial defence system.

CFTR has now been implicated in a range of functions in the airways. These include:

1. Acting as a cAMP regulated chloride channel (section 6.2).

2. Regulating the activity of the outwardly rectifying chloride channel (Egan et al., 1992).

3. Inhibiting the activity of the epithelial sodium channel (ENaC) (Scwiebert et al., 1999).

In the airways epithelia chloride secretion induces fluid secretion, whilst sodium absorption causes fluid resorption. It is the balance between these that determines the constitution of the ASL. CF causes an alteration in the composition, reduction in depth and increase in viscosity of ASL (Song et al., 2009). This is accompanied by a reduction in mucociliary clearance and bacterial defences. Cathelicidins and β defensins are small antimicrobial peptides present in ASL. Smith et al. (1996) suggested that CF caused an abnormally high sodium and chloride concentration of ASL, which in turn brought about a decrease in the antimicrobial activity of ASL. Although the antimicrobial activity of CF ASL is reduced (Bals et al., 2001), the ASL is not excessively salty when compared to normal. Indeed, in both CF and wild type the ASL is almost isotonic (Knowles et al., 1997, Song et al., 2009). An alternative hypothesis suggests that CF airways have an abnormally high rate of absorption of ASL and this accounts for the reduced thickness of the ASL (Matsui et al., 1998). This is known as the low volume hypothesis and is the most widely accepted model (Song et al., 2009). Direct measurement of ASL depth in explants of human and porcine trachea demonstrated that inhibition of ENaC increased ASL depth. It also demonstrated agonists which raised intracellular cAMP increased ASL depth beyond the normal value (Song et al., 2009).

ENaC has a major influence on ASL. Proteolytic cleavage of extracellular site(s) of ENaC subunit(s) causes its constitutive activation (Lazarowski and Boucher, 2009). This will result in sodium hyperabsorption from the ASL leading to impairment of mucociliary clearance, if the activity of ENaC is left unchecked by faulty CFTR.

The importance of ENaC regulation in airways function is supported by the observation that mice overexpressing ENaC exhibit several features of lung disease that are similar to CF. The enhanced sodium absorption gives rise to airways mucus plugging, reduction in depth of ASL, and impaired mucociliary clearance (Mall, 2009). This leads to an enhanced susceptibility to allergens and inflammation.

Although reduced mucociliary clearance would increase the risk of airways bacterial colonisation, it is not sufficient on its own to explain the characteristic colonisation by *P. aeruginosa* evident in CF (Poschet et al., 2001). Barash et al. (1991) found that CF caused the defective acidification of the TGN. This led to the suggestion that the observed alkalinisation might lead to a reduction in the sialyltransferase activity and deficient sialylation of membrane glycolipids and glycoproteins. These could then act as attachment sites for *P. aeruginosa*. The proposed influx of Cl^-, via CFTR, into the lumen of the acidifying organelle, would help to restrict the developing membrane potential due to H^+ influx. CF would then lead to the failure of CFTR to allow Cl^- influx into the lumen. This in turn would lead to a rise

in membrane potential that would inhibit further H^+ influx, thereby producing the defective acidification observed. Since then, some groups have reported that the pH of some endomembrane compartments is altered in CF, whilst other groups have failed to find this. The review by Haggie and Verkman (2009) addressed this controversial area and mostly attributed the discrepancies between groups to methodological concerns. In particular the early data tended to use single wavelength optical probes to determine compartmental pH, which are more susceptible to artifacts than ratiometric probes (see Chapter 9 for a discussion of this). Also there was concern as to how robust the targeting of optical probes to organelles was. Their conclusion was that the evidence does not support an alkalinisation of endomembrane compartments due to CF. Since other, non CFTR, Cl^- channels appear to be involved in organelle acidification, it does seem that on balance, there is insufficient evidence to support the hypothesis of defective acidification of organelles in CF. Poschet et al. (2001 and 2007) reported that the CF induced defective acidification of organelles was not actually alkalinisation, but rather hyper-acidification. CFTR has been linked to inhibition of ENaC. In their scheme, ENaC would permit the enhanced efflux of Na^+ from organelles, thereby dissipating the developing positive charge due to H^+ influx. Thus in CF, overactive ENaC would allow increased organelle H^+ uptake to occur without excessive build up of membrane potential, which would otherwise inhibit H^+ uptake. This results in organelle hyper-acidification. Although these workers did use a ratiometric optical probe, the small difference in signal observed between normal and CF organelles may simply be sample noise rather than reflect an actual difference in pH (Haggie and Verkman, 2009).

In normal airways epithelial cells basolaterally located Na^+/K^+-ATPase provides the driving force for transmembrane Na^+ movement (Figure 6.4). Its activity aids basolateral Cl^- entry via the sodium potassium 2 chloride (NKCC) cotransporter. The Na^+ arriving through the NKCC cotransporter is removed via Na^+/K^+-ATPase, preserving a low intracellular Na^+ and thereby maintaining Cl^- entry into the cell. ENaC activity in the luminal membrane is inhibited by CFTR. This ensures that the correct concentration of Na^+ is retained in the ASL. The Cl^- content of the ASL is due to CFTR, both via its intrinsic Cl^- channel activity, and its regulation of the outwardly rectifying chloride channel (ORCC) activity. The regulated ion content of the ASL causes water movement, via osmosis, through

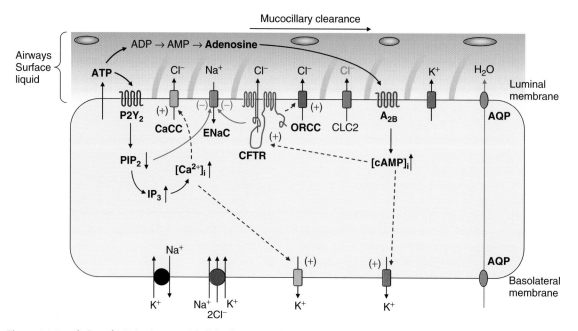

Figure 6.4 Regulation of ASL in airways epithelial cells. See text for details. This model was adapted from Amaral and Kunzelmann, 2007; Clunes and Boucher, 2008; and Zeitlin, 2008.

aquaporins (AQP) in the cell membranes, thus ensuring the correct hydration of the ASL, and aiding mucociliary clearance.

Airways epithelial cells release ATP and UTP to the extracellular environment. Although the resting level of ATP release for airways epithelia is low, mechanical stress induced by breathing movements substantially increases ATP release (Lazarowski and Boucher, 2009). This results in a sufficiently high concentration in the ASL to stimulate the P2Y$_2$ receptors. These purinergic agonists stimulate the luminal P2Y$_2$ G protein coupled receptor (GPCR), leading to the hydrolysis of phosphatidylinositol 4,5-bisphosphate (PIP$_2$) into inositol 1,4,5-trisphosphate (IP$_3$) and diacylglycerol (DAG). The subsequent rise in cytosolic IP$_3$ concentration causes an increase in [Ca^{2+}]$_i$, which stimulates the Ca^{2+} activated chloride channels (CaCC) in the luminal membrane and the Ca^{2+} activated K$^+$ channels in the basolateral membranes. The basolateral K$^+$ efflux helps to hyperpolarise the cell, increasing the electrical driving force for Cl$^-$ movement into the ASL via luminal Cl$^-$ channels (CFTR, ORCC, and CaCC). The fall in PIP$_2$ further inhibits ENaC activity. The positively charged N terminal amino acids of ENaC normally bind PIP$_2$, which help regulate its open channel probability. Binding of PIP$_2$ is thought to stabilise ENaC in the open

state, in a manner analogous to how PIP$_2$ activates some K$^+$ channels (Kunzelmann et al., 2005). Hence a fall in PIP$_2$ binding will reduce ENaCs activity.

The ATP in the ASL is degraded by ecto-nucleotidases that generate free adenosine, which can then act as an agonist at the A$_{2B}$ adenosine receptor GPCR. Stimulating this receptor leads to an increase in adenylate cyclase activity and a rise in intracellular cAMP concentration. This in turn induces K$^+$ efflux via cAMP stimulated K$^+$ channels, indirectly stimulating Cl$^-$ movement via hyperpolarisation. It also causes an increased CFTR Cl$^-$ channel activity due to a rise in PKA activity induced by cAMP. The net effect of purinergic stimulation of airways epithelial cells is that luminal Cl$^-$ fluxes are increased and luminal Na$^+$ absorption is reduced, maintaining the ASL volume and mucociliary clearance.

In CF, the activity of CFTR is diminished or absent (Figure 6.5). Thus Cl$^-$ movement via the CFTR Cl$^-$ channels and the ORCC are reduced. In addition the inhibitory effect on CFTR on ENaC is eased. The influence of extracellular ATP is also lessened as the ecto-nucleotidase content of ASL is increased due to bacterial infection (Tarran et al., 2005). This fall in ATP reduces P2Y$_2$ receptor activation, causing a decrease in Cl$^-$ movement via CaCC, and allows PIP$_2$ to stimulate ENaC. In addition,

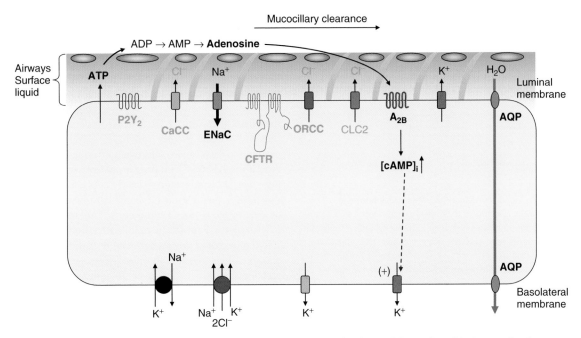

Figure 6.5 Failure of ASL regulation in CF airways epithelia. See text for details. This model was adapted from Amaral and Kunzelmann, 2007; Clunes and Boucher, 2008; and Zeitlin, 2008.

adenosine now stimulates ENaC activity as the inhibitory effect of CFTR has been lifted (Tarran et al., 2006). This results in reduced Na^+ and Cl^- content of the ASL and a decrease in its depth. Submucosal gland hypertrophy and goblet cell hyperplasia leads to enhanced mucin release. Combined with the changes in the ASL, this causes impaired mucociliary clearance.

Faulty HCO_3^- transport may contribute to CF pathology

Defective HCO_3^- transport has been implicated in reduction in fertility (Chan et al., 2009), see section 6.1. It has also been suggested that this may contribute to the characteristic defects in mucins in CF airways and GI tract. Bicarbonate transport has been proposed to occur either via CFTR, and/or a CFTR influenced Cl^-/HCO_3^- exchanger. Where insufficient HCO_3^- is released, the mucins aggregate (Garcia et al., 2009). Mucins are tightly packed into secretory vesicles that also contain high levels of Ca^{2+} and H^+. Upon exocytosis, removal of the Ca^{2+} and H^+ from the mucins allows rapid expansion via electrostatic interactions between the large number of negative charges on the oligosaccharide side chains (Garcia et al., 2009). A reduction in HCO_3^- transport would therefore be less effective at removal of the Ca^{2+}

and H^+ ions, leaving the mucins in a condensed state that is more difficult to clear. There is some evidence to support this view as increases in medium Ca^{2+} and/or H^+ significantly reduces the rate of mucin swelling, and the observation that secreted CF mucins contain more Ca^{2+} than wild type (Garcia et al., 2009).

6.3 Mutations in CFTR

Although there are >1900 mutations, the commonest mutation, $\Delta F508$, alone accounts for around 70% of North American and Northern European CF alleles. This mutation is due to a deletion of phenylalanine at position 508 (Figure 6.6).

Classes of mutation

Class I mutations give rise to failure to produce full length CFTR (Figure 6.7). This could be due to the presence of premature stop codons (e.g. G542X, R553X or W1282X), or unstable mRNA. The resultant CFTR protein is truncated and liable to be degraded by the ubiquitin proteasome system. These mutations are characterised by an absence of functional CFTR in the apical membrane and therefore the mutations are severe.

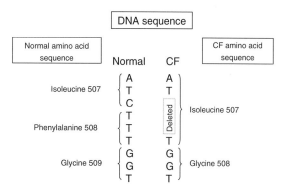

Figure 6.6 The ΔF508 mutation is due to deletion of a phenylalanine. The loss of the three deoxynucleotides CTT, and the corresponding base pairs, is an in frame deletion. Whilst the last deoxynucleotide has been changed from C to T, due to the degenerate nature of the triplet code, it still codes for isoleucine and position 507. The net result is a loss of phenylalanine at position 508, the code for the remaining amino acids is still in frame. Modified from McPherson and Dormer 1991. Molecular and cellular biology of cystic fibrosis. Molecular Aspects of Medicine 21: 1–81. Elsevier copyright 1991.

Class II mutations are trafficking defects. The mutant CFTR is produced but the protein does not traffic to the correct locations. The commonest mutation, ΔF508, interferes with the folding of CFTR. The ER quality control system recognises this, prevents the movement of ΔF508-CFTR to the Golgi and degrades the protein. Although most of the mutant CFTR is destroyed, some may still manage to correctly locate. However, the mutated protein is less efficient than the wild type and the large reduction in amount at the correct cellular locations means that these mutations are severe.

Class III mutations exhibit defective activation and regulation of CFTR. The mutant protein correctly locates but some aspect of ATP binding, hydrolysis, phosphorylation by protein kinases and dephosphorylation by phosphatases is disturbed. This then affects CFTR function, though the degree of disturbance differs between mutations. For example, G551D is located in the first NBD and is a severe mutation.

Class IV mutations have defective Cl⁻ conductance or channel gating. The protein correctly locates, but the mutation affects the gating and/or the conductance on chloride channels. This results in less transit of Cl⁻ ions into the extracellular environment. Since there is some residual Cl⁻ current these mutations tend to be milder (e.g. R117H).

Class V mutations give rise to partial reduction in amount of CFTR. This can arise due to alteration in the promoter sequence or mRNA splicing. Since normal and abnormally spliced transcripts can be produced, the severity of the disease will depend on the balance between the normal and abnormal transcripts. This balance may also vary between tissue types in the same individual. Hence these mutations occupy a range from mild to severe.

The classification scheme outlined above is based on the effect it has on CFTR. Not all mutations fit easily into this scheme as they can have several effects. For example, ΔF508 causes defective trafficking (class II) but even if the ΔF508-CFTR does locate correctly it still has defective Cl⁻ conductance (class IV). As CF is a recessive disease it is possible for CF patients to be homozygous or heterozygous for CF mutations. This means that in heterozygote CF mutations, a mild mutation can ameliorate the degree of a severe mutation in the other allele. However it is important to recognise that environmental and background genetic factors also influence the severity of the disease.

6.4 Why is cystic fibrosis so common?

It is thought that ΔF508, the commonest mutation of CFTR arose over 11,000 years ago (Wiuf, 2001). Since CF severely reduces life expectancy and impairs fertility it is striking that the carrier frequency is so high. This led to the suggestion that there may be a heterozygote advantage analogous to that proposed for sickle cell trait in red blood cells and resistance to malaria. Where adequate sewage disposal systems are not present faecal contamination of water supplies results in frequent outbreaks of diarrhoeal diseases. The bacteria *Vibrio cholerae*, which causes cholera and some forms of *Escherichia coli* can colonise the intestine and induce diarrhoea. Both *V. cholerae* and enterotoxigenic *E. coli* secrete toxins that enter intestinal epithelial cells and cause the ADP ribosylation of the Gsα subunit of the Gs heterotrimeric G protein. This inhibits the intrinsic Gsα GTPase activity forcing the subunit to remain in the active state. Since Gsα activates adenylate cyclase, this results in an increase in intracellular cAMP. The rise in cAMP in turn activates the cAMP activated Cl⁻ channel and causes excessive Cl⁻ loss from intestinal cells (Quinton, 1994). This is followed by water via osmosis and results in life threatening secretory diarrhoea. In addition enterotoxigenic *E. coli* also secretes another toxin that is heat stable and activates guanylate cyclase via an extracellular receptor that directly couples to the enzyme. This causes an increase in intracellular cyclic guanosine 3′, 5′ monophosphate (cGMP), which

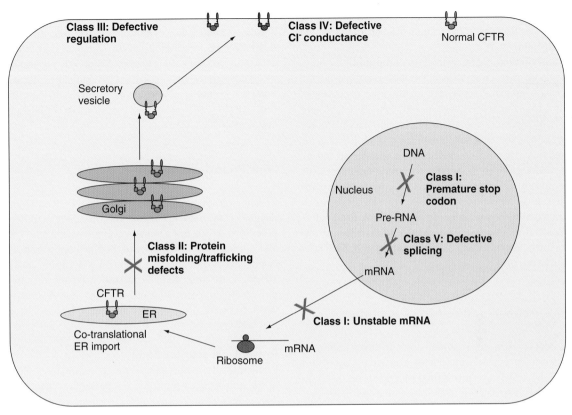

Figure 6.7 Mutations to CFTR can be grouped into five classes. Class I fail to produce full length CFTR, class II cause misfolding and trafficking defects, class III affect regulation of CFTR, class IV result in defective Cl⁻ conductance and class V gives rise to abnormal splicing. Adapted by permission from Macmillan Publishers Ltd [Nature Medicine] Delaney SJ and Wainwright BJ 1996. New pharmaceutical approaches to the treatment of cystic fibrosis, Nature Medicine 2: 392–393, copyright 1996. Also adapted from Amaral and Kunzelmann, 2007. Molecular targeting of CFTR as a therapeutic approach to cystic fibrosis. Trends in Pharmacological Sciences 28: 334–341. Elsevier copyright 2007.

in turn activates protein kinase G and inhibits Na⁺ and Cl⁻ absorption into intestinal epithelial cells. High concentrations of cGMP may also activate protein kinase A, which could result in activation of CFTR Cl⁻ channels (Quinton, 1994) and exacerbate Cl⁻ loss. This results in increased salt content on the gut lumen and water follows via osmosis, enhancing the diarrhoea. In the case of CF the defective cAMP regulated Cl⁻ channel in the intestinal epithelium has been proposed to protect against cholera and *E. coli* enterotoxins (Quinton, 1994) by leading to lower Cl⁻ loss into the gut lumen, less water follows by osmosis and hence less severe diarrhoea occurs. There is some evidence to support this hypothesis. When a CF mouse model was exposed to cholera toxin, the CF homozygote had the lowest fluid loss, the normal genotype (non CF) had the highest and the CF heterozygote

was approximately halfway between the CF and normal mouse (Gabriel et al., 1994). This was not due to differences in the ability of cholera toxin to induce a rise in intracellular cAMP suggesting a downstream event consistent with differences in the ability to activate a cAMP activated Cl⁻ channel.

Salmonella typhi bacteria can invade intestinal epithelial cells leading to damage to the integrity of the epithelium (Jones et al., 1994). Subsequent spread of *S. typhi* from the intestine to the bloodstream and the reticuloendothelial system leads to the development of typhoid fever. Experiments have demonstrated that *S. typhi* uses CFTR as a receptor for internalisation into intestinal epithelial cells. For a set dose of *S. typhi* the epithelial cells of ΔF508 mice had only a small fraction of the internalised bacterial load of wild type mice (Pier et al., 1998). This suggests that the CF gene may confer resistance to typhoid as it reduces bacterial translocation through the intestinal epithelium.

Since cholera did not impact on Europe until the nineteenth century it is unlikely that this disease underlies the selective pressure responsible for the high incidence of the ΔF508 mutation (Quinton, 1994). Hence *S. typhi* and enterotoxigenic *E. coli* are more plausible candidates for the driving forces of selection in the case of the CF gene. If CF heterozygotes do indeed have a selective advantage in resistance to some diarrhoeal causing organisms, the question then arises as to why CF is much more common in cooler climates such as Northern Europe, when compared to hotter climates such as Africa. Presumably the selective advantage in resistance to diarrhoea is offset by the increased salt loss in sweating in hot climates (Quinton, 1994).

6.5 Animal models of Cystic fibrosis

Animal models are important tools to investigate how a defect in a gene can lead to a genetic disease and help determine which potential treatments are likely to be of benefit. Since mice are easy to keep in the lab and relatively amenable to genetic manipulation they are commonly used as genetic models of human diseases. Within three years of the discovery of the CF gene a mouse model was produced. Since then several others have been generated (Guilbault et al., 2007). Unfortunately it soon became clear that mice do not make a good model system for CF. Most murine models exhibit a relatively severe gastrointestinal pathology with abnormal Cl^- electrophysiology. They also have ion transport abnormalities in nasal epithelia. However, Cl^- transport appears normal in the CF mouse lung (Griesenbach and Alton, 2009ba). It has been suggested that this might be due to the presence of additional Cl^- channel(s) in mouse lung such as non CFTR cAMP activated Cl^- channels or Ca^{2+} regulated Cl^- channels, though this remains to be confirmed. Since most cases of premature death in CF are due to pathological changes in the lung, it casts doubt on the utility on murine CF model systems. In 2008 pig and ferret CF models were produced. They represent important advances over murine models as the structure of pig and ferret lungs are much more similar to humans than mice (Griesenbach and Alton, 2009ba). Since ferrets and pigs live longer than mice, there is also a greater potential for lung disease to develop in

these CF models. Caution is still warranted in the use of animal models as species differences in sensitivity to different transport inhibitors are apparent (Liu et al., 2007). In addition the porcine ΔF508 CF pig model has a milder CF phenotype than the equivalent human mutation (Liu et al., 2008). This suggests that species differences in processing and trafficking of CFTR may also be present.

6.6 Pharmacotherapy

To date over 1900 mutations are listed in the CF mutation database (http://www.genet.sickkids.on.ca/cftr). Of these mutations ΔF508 has a frequency of approximately 70% and around 90% of CF patients of Northern European origin have at least one copy (Gelman and Kopito, 2002). Hence, apart from ΔF508, the vast majority of mutations are too infrequent for pharmaceutical companies to develop specific drugs for each mutation. Instead, drugs that target specific types of mutation are more practical.

Premature stop codons

Premature stop codons account for approximately 5–70% of the mutations of most genetic diseases (Welch et al., 2007). In CF they cause the formation of truncated non-functional CFTR. Although this class of mutation is relatively infrequent, in some populations it can be the predominate form. For example W1282X is found in approximately 60% of CF patients of Ashkenazi Jewish origin. This mutation alters the sequence from tryptophan to a stop codon (UGG to UGA). Some aminoglycoside antibiotics such as G418 and gentamicin have the ability to override premature stop codons causing the insertion of an amino acid. Howard et al. (1996) demonstrated the potential for this type for drug in HeLa cells transfected with cDNA coding for mutated CFTR, namely G542X or R553X, both in frame premature stop codons. However, the process is inefficient with both full length and truncated versions of CFTR produced. The rescued full length CFTR protein sequence may also differ to the wild type at the place of amino acid substitution for the mutant stop codon. This in turn may affect CFTR function. Whilst aminoglycoside antibiotics are already used to treat lung infections, the high concentrations needed for readthrough of premature stop codons are likely to induce unacceptable side effects such as nephrotoxicity and ototoxicity. This will severely limit their clinical use. Newer, non-aminoglycoside based compounds, are currently being tested. It is critical that these only override premature stop codons and are without effect on normal (native) stop codons. Ataluren (formerly PTC124), being developed by PTC Therapeutics, appears to be very selective for premature stop codons over native stop codons and does not seem to disrupt nonsense mediated mRNA decay (Welch et al., 2007; Hyde and Gill, 2008). Ataluren is currently undergoing Phase 3 clinical trials in CF. It is also being considered as a treatment for some forms of haemophilia A and B and Duchene/Becker muscular dystrophy that derive from premature stop codons. Ataluren was identified by high throughput screens as it promotes readthrough of UGA and UAG stop codons in the range 0.01–10μM, with a maximum effect around 3 μM (Welch et al., 2007). UGA had the highest amount of readthrough with ataluren, followed by UAG, whilst UAA was little different to control. This corresponds to the intrinsic termination efficiencies of these codons, where UGA is more leaky, UAA has least readthrough and UAG is intermediate (Du et al., 2009). There are also differences in efficiency in overriding the same premature stop codon depending on which nucleotide follows it on the mRNA. For example, readthrough of UGA-G (e.g. G542X) with ataluren is greater than that achieved with UGA-A (e.g. W1281X) (Linde and Kerm, 2008).

Defective trafficking

In some mutations CFTR fails to become fully glycosylated. This indicates that the mutated CFTR did not exit the endoplasmic reticulum (ER) and traffic to the Golgi. The underlying cause is assumed to be deletion of an amino acid (e.g. ΔF508), or substitution of an inappropriate amino acid that leads to misfolding. The importance of the correct folding of proteins is emphasised by the observation that even in wild type CFTR, 75% fails to exit the ER and be transported to the Golgi. This failure rate increases greatly in ΔF508 CFTR, though some differences between tissues with respect to their CFTR protein expression are apparent. In essence ΔF508 becomes degraded in the ER, thereby preventing trafficking to the Golgi and beyond. Early studies were contradictory; in *Xenopus* oocytes ΔF508 CFTR did correctly locate to the plasma membrane (Drumm et al., 1991), in contrast this was very much reduced in mammalian cell lines. This led to the observation that reducing the incubation temperature to below 29°C could restore the trafficking of ΔF508 CFTR to the Golgi and therefore the amount at the plasma membrane (Denning et al., 1992). This created interest in the possibility of using

chemical chaperones to correct the cellular location of mistrafficked CFTR.

Natural chemical chaperones help organisms cope with situations that would otherwise lead to denaturation of proteins (Welch and Brown, 1996). For example, to cope with hyperosmotic stress cells can take up low molecular weight compounds such as carbohydrates (e.g. glycerol), free amino acids and methylamines (e.g. trimethylamine N-oxide, TMAO). These alter the cellular osmotic balance without disrupting protein function (Welch and Brown, 1996). One well known example is in salt water elasmobranchs, such as sharks, where the blood is almost isosomotic to sea water due to the high concentration of urea in the blood. In this case TMAO is also present to counteract the negative effect of urea on proteins.

Wild type CFTR matures to a correctly folded proteasome resistant state (Zeitlin, 1999). This process involves chaperones such as calnexin and the heat shock protein Hsp70. The failure of most ΔF508 CFTR to exit the ER could be due to prolonged interaction with chaperones or the involvement of the ubiquitin-proteasome degradation pathway (Gelman and Kopito, 2002). Since blocking the proteasome pathway did not allow more ΔF508 CFTR to reach the plasma membrane, efforts to correct the trafficking defect are now focused towards chemical chaperones. This is also a preferred target as proteasome inhibition has the potential to cause intracellular protein aggregations reminiscent of those observed in some neurodegenerative disease. Given the lifelong treatment that would be necessary, the risk of delayed toxic side effects is considerable and may not be detectable for decades (Gelman and Kopito, 2002). The use of chemical chaperones is however also not without risk as they may enable other, non-target, defective proteins to escape the ER quality control checkpoint with unknown consequences.

Over-expression studies have found that increased levels of ΔF508 occur at the plasma membrane. This could be due to saturation of the quality control checkpoint in the ER and the subsequent overspill evading this machinery (Gelman and Kopito, 2002). However even if ΔF508 CFTR is delivered to the plasma membrane, its cell surface half-life and Cl⁻ channel activity are still less than wild type CFTR. The reduced plasma membrane residence time of ΔF508 CFTR, compared to wild type CFTR, raises the possibility that if chemical chaperones help ΔF508 CFTR exit the ER, they may also stabilise its presence at the cell surface (Gelman and Kopito, 2002).

Initial experiments with chemical chaperones used glycerol, dueterated water or TMAO (Brown et al., 1996). Although they did substantially correct ΔF508 CFTR Cl⁻

channel activity in the NIH 3T3 fibroblast cell line, the high concentrations used render them inappropriate for clinical use. Subsequently butyrate and 4–phenyl butyrate (4PB) have also been used. Unfortunately due to the short plasma half-life of butyrate it would need to be administered as an intravenous drip (Zeitlin, 1999). Whilst butyrate and 4PB did cause an increase in the amount of ΔF508 CFTR at the cell surface, these compounds have been reported to inhibit CFTR Cl⁻ channel activity and may also inhibit other ion transporting proteins. Sildenafil (Viagra) and a related phosphodiesterase (PDE) 5 inhibitor, KM11060, appear to be able to cause much more rapid increase in plasma membrane localisation of ΔF508 CFTR than butyrate or 4PB (Dormer et al., 2005; Robert et al., 2008). KM11060 is particularly promising as it rescued ΔF508 plasma membrane localisation at 10 nM, whilst sildenafil required 1 μM to significantly increase plasma membrane localisation (Robert et al., 2008). VX-809 (Vertex Pharmaceuticals), another chemical chaperone, was found to have lowered sweat chloride by a small, but significant, amount (6–8 mM) in ΔF508 homozygous CF patients in a phase 2a clinical trial.

Activating cAMP regulated Cl⁻ channel activity

Although mutant CFTR may correctly locate to the plasma membrane, it might still have defective cAMP activated Cl⁻ channel activity (e.g. G551D, which is carried by approximately 4% of CF patients). The attempts to increase ΔF508-CFTR expression at the cell surface using chemical chaperones also fall into this category. Whilst ΔF508-CFTR does have some Cl⁻ channel activity, it is less than the wild type. The reduction in Cl⁻ channel activity could arise from a direct defect in the channel *per se*, or altered interactions with regulatory kinases and phosphatases (Gelman and Kopito, 2002).

Genistein has been shown to increase G551D chloride channel activity. This does not appear to be related to its ability to inhibit tyrosine kinases, as some other tyrosine kinase inhibitors are without effect (Zeitlin, 1999). Genistein is an isoflavone phytoestrogen found in legumes such as soya beans and is therefore a common component of the diet. However, it is not considered suitable for clinical use due to its very low bioavailability when delivered via the oral route (Clunes and Boucher, 2008).

Phosphodiesterase (PDE) inhibitors will reduce the breakdown of cAMP and/or cGMP. Early work demonstrated that the non-selective PDE inhibitor, 3-isobutyl-1-methylxanthine (IBMX), in conjunction with a β adrenergic agonist could partially restore mucin secretion in the submandibular salivary gland in human CF tissue (McPherson et al., 1986), a CFTR antibody induced CF phenotype (Lloyd Mills et al., 1992) and a CF mouse model (Lloyd Mills et al., 1995). IBMX also stimulated Cl⁻ secretion in CF cells (Becq et al., 1994). Since then work has focused on selective PDE inhibitors. Milrinone, a PDE III inhibitor reduces the breakdown of cAMP. When this is combined with a β agonist it has been shown to increase cAMP activated Cl⁻ secretion in CF-T43, a human nasal epithelial cell line derived from a homozygous ΔF508 CF patient (Kelley et al., 1996). However, milrinone in combination with a β agonist failed to alter the nasal potential difference (PD) of either CF human subjects or CF mice (Smith et al., 1999).

VX-770 (Vertex Pharmaceuticals) completed a phase 2a clinical trial in 2008. In a 14-day period this compound reduced sweat chloride from a mean of 95.5 mM to 53.2 mM in CF patients with the G551D mutation. In addition this was accompanied by a mean increase of FEV_1 (forced expiratory volume in 1 second) of 10% (0.22 L). These encouraging results were confirmed in a 48-week phase 3 trial, where it was also shown that VX-770 caused a significant reduction in the risk of pulmonary exacerbations (Ramsey et al., 2011). Subsequently in January 2012 the U.S. Food and Drug Administration approved Kalydeco™ (formerly VX-770) for CF patients over six years old with the G551D mutation. This is the first mutation specific CF treatment to reach the market and is an example of the developing trend for personalised medicines. However, it should be noted that only around 4% of North American CF patients have at least one allele of this mutation. However, there is the possibility that VX-770 may be suitable for the treatment of other CFTR Cl⁻ channel gating defect mutations. Yu et al. (2012) found that VX-770 increased the open channel probability of the CFTR Cl⁻ channel in a variety of CF gating defect mutations including G178R, S549N, S549R, G551D, G551S, G970R, G1244E, S1251N, S1255P and G1349D. Consideration is also being given to dual VX-770 and VX-809 therapy. This may be of particular benefit to mutations that have both trafficking and Cl⁻ channel defects (e.g. ΔF508). VX-809 would aim to deliver the mutant CFTR to the cell surface (section 6.3) whilst VX-770 would aim to activate it. Both these compounds were developed in collaboration with the Cystic Fibrosis Foundation Therapeutics Inc, which is a non-profit affiliate of the Cystic Fibrosis Foundation.

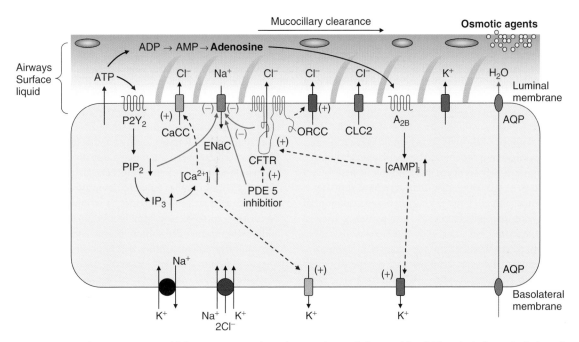

Figure 6.8 General non CFTR potential drug targets. A variety of approaches are being considered. These include manipulation of the osmotic environment of the ASL via hypertonic saline, stimulation of the $P2Y_2$ receptors, activation of alternate Cl^- channels, and inactivation of ENaC. See text for further details. This model was adapted from Amaral and Kunzelmann, 2007; Clunes and Boucher, 2008; Thelin and Boucher, 2007; and Zeitlin, 2008.

Mutation independent amelioration of CF

The strategies mentionned above, namely overriding premature stop codons, correcting trafficking defects and activating the cAMP activated Cl^- channels are directed at specific types of mutation. An alternative approach is to manipulate non CFTR targets that have the potential to benefit all CF patients regardless of the type of mutation. Increasing Cl^- secretion or reducing Na^+ absorption in the airways will increase the water content of the ASL and thereby aid mucociliary clearance.

Hypertonic saline

Nebulised hypertonic saline treatment is now clinically available to certain categories of CF patients and research is ongoing to determine which groups would most benefit. The hypertonic NaCl draws water into the ASL and rehydrates it, increasing the depth of ASL and facilitating mucociliary clearance. Inhaled mannitol (Bronchitol) is also being considered as an agent to manipulate the water content of airways surface layers. Whilst its high molecular weight may prolong the osmotic effect, relatively large amounts of mannitol need to be inhaled (Clunes and Boucher, 2008).

Activation of alternative chloride channels

Agonists binding to $P2Y_2$ or A_{2B} receptors stimulate ciliary beating and therefore mucociliary clearance (Lazarowski and Boucher, 2009). Hence agonists directed at these GPCRs may be of benefit to CF airways (Figure 6.8). Adenosine in the ASL is degraded by extracellular adenosine deaminase (converts adenosine to inosine). There is also a cellular uptake pathway via the concentrative nucleoside transporter (CNT) (Hirsh et al., 2007). Potential mechanisms of raising the extracellular adenosine concentration of ASL could be via blocking adenosine deaminase reducing its breakdown, inhibiting the CNTs, lessening removal, and/or application of exogenous adenosine. However, the use of adenosine, and by extension ATP, which breaks down to adenosine due to ecto-nucleotidases, is not recommended. Adenosine has been linked to airways inflammation. UTP is therefore preferred for activation of the $P2Y_2$ receptors.

Airways epithelial cells contain calcium activated chloride channels (CaCC) that are activated by $P2Y_2$ purinergic receptor agonists such as ATP and UTP (see section 6.2). Currently some potential treatments are directed towards stimulating the luminal $P2Y_2$

purinergic receptors in an attempt to maintain the Cl^- content of the ASL. The UTP analogue Denufosol (Inspire Pharmaceuticals) is resistant to extracellular ATPases, thereby enabling longer airways availability between aerosolised doses. A phase 3 trial that ended in 2008 reported a small (45 ml/sec) significant increase in FEV_1. A second phase 3 trial is currently underway.

However, whilst application of agonists to the $P2Y_2$ receptor may be of short-term benefit, longer term amelioration might be best achieved by use of inverse agonists. This approach may seem counter intuitive at first. Initial application of inverse agonists may even have short-term detrimental effects. Thus a gradual dose escalation of inverse agonists needs to occur over a period of time to ensure the adverse effects are minimised. Previous studies with β blockers acting as inverse agonists in congestive heart failure (CHF) has demonstrated a large sustained increase in receptor number (Helibrunn et al., 1989). This upregulation will lead to a rise in second messenger production due to constitutive activity of the receptors. Large scale trails of β blocker inverse agonist treatment for CHF have been so successful that they are now part of the standard treatment, though not all patients can tolerate them. In contrast, continual treatment with agonists is likely to cause receptor downregulation and reduction of stimulatory effect. Hence, agonists will have short-term benefit, but reduced efficacy over the longer term, whilst for inverse agonists there is potential for short-term adverse effects, but longer term benefit. This manifests as a significantly greater five-year survival rate for CHF patients with inverse agonist treatment when compared to β agonists (see section 3.4 to 3.5 for a fuller consideration of GPCR constitutive activity and desensitisation). However, it remains to be demonstrated whether an inverse agonist to the $P2Y_2$ receptor will be of benefit.

An alternative approach is to target downstream intracellular events, thereby negating the influence of agonist induced alteration in GPCR expression. Moli 1901 (Lantbio Inc) also targets CaCC. This small polypeptide releases calcium from the ER which then activates the CaCC directly. A phase 2 study reported a statistically significant increase in FEV_1 in CF patients on a daily aerosolised dose of 2.5 mg of Moli 1901 for 28 days. A further follow on trial is underway (Clunes and Boucher, 2008).

An alternative non CFTR Cl^- channel to CaCC is the ClC-2 chloride channel, whose gating is influenced by Cl^- concentration, membrane voltage, pH and tonicity (Bao et al., 2008). Prostones, which are a new class of compound derived from fatty acids, have been shown to activate ClC-2 chloride channels. Lubiprostone has already been

approved for chronic constipation, where it increases the Cl^- content of the gut lumen via ClC-2, promoting water movement and softening of the stools. This class of compounds may also be of benefit in modifying the ASL in CF.

Inhibition of epithelial sodium channels

The hyperabsorption of sodium from ASL in CF is due to the inappropriately high activity of ENaC. This is due to a failure of CFTR to negatively regulate ENaC activity. Hence, there have been attempts to directly inhibit ENaC via nebulised sodium channel blockers such as amiloride. However, amiloride has failed to demonstrate consistent improvements in lung function. It is rapidly absorbed by airways epithelia and also blocks an aquaporin, in addition to the intended sodium channel, thereby impeding water movement (Clunes and Boucher, 2008). Work on newer sodium channel blockers is continuing, with the most promising having greater effectiveness and selectivity when compared to amiloride.

An alternative approach to regulate ENaC allows a dual target approach (Figure 6.8). Purinergic $P2Y_2$ agonists activate PLC, which in turn cleaves PIP_2 into IP_3 and DAG. The IP_3 will then mobilise Ca^{2+} from intracellular stores such as the ER. The rise in $[Ca^{2+}]_i$ will then open calcium activated chloride channels and aid ASL rehydration (section 6.2). PIP_2 also regulates the activity of ENaC by binding to the N-terminal region of the β subunit of ENaC via the positive charges of the N-terminal amino acids. This helps to maintain channel activity. Hence, when PIP_2 is cleaved into IP_3 and DAG, the loss of PIP_2 at the N-terminal region of β ENaC reduces its sodium channel activity (Kunzelman et al., 2005). This reduction in sodium absorption retains more sodium in the ASL, thereby increasing water content and aiding mucociliary clearance. Although this approach might initially appear promising, it is important to recognise the problem of receptor downregulation.

Inhibition of PDE 5

PDE 5 inhibitors, which reduce the breakdown of cGMP, partially correct defective mucin secretion in the CFTR antibody induced CF phenotype (McPherson et al., 1999) and Cl^- secretion in the nasal epithelia of $\Delta F508$ mice (Lumba et al., 2008). Sildenafil (Viagra) and the structurally related KM11060, both PDE 5 inhibitors, increased the trafficking of $\Delta F508$-CFTR to the apical membrane. Nitric oxide (NO) levels in the CF airways are lower than normal. This may contribute towards the chronic infections in CF as NO is a potent antimicrobial (Hassett et al., 2009). NO also activates guanylate cyclase.

The fall in airways NO in CF will lead to a reduced intracellular cGMP concentration when compared to normal airways. Sildenafil increases intracellular cGMP and inhibits ENaC, thereby helping to correct the sodium hyperabsorption defect in CF (Poschet et al., 2007). In addition, in CF lung epithelial cells, sildenafil corrected the enhanced inflammatory responses of proinflammatory factors derived from *P. aeruginosa* (Poschet et al., 2007) and lipopolysaccharide (LPS) induced inflammation in normal guinea pig lung (Toward et al., 2004). The multifactorial potential of PDE 5 inhibitors towards correcting the CF defects, namely restoring CFTR trafficking, stimulating secretion of Cl^- and mucins, inhibiting ENaC, and reduction in inflammatory responses are therefore of considerable interest (Figure 6.8).

6.7 Gene therapy

The discovery of the CF gene in 1989 introduced the possibility of correcting the genetic defect using gene therapy. The potential of this technique was quickly demonstrated in both cell lines and mouse models. These initial encouraging results lead to intensive research effort in this area. In 1993 the first human CF gene therapy trial was started. Unfortunately, it soon became clear that there are substantial hurdles to overcome before gene therapy can become a viable treatment option. Apart from the considerable technical difficulties, gene therapy raises ethical issues. CF affects a range of tissues including the reproductive system. It is essential that the genetic code of the germ line is not altered as these changes will then be inherited by the next generation. This restricts the use of gene therapy to specific tissues, which in the case of CF is focused on the lungs. In contrast, pharmacotherapy has the potential to treat all affected tissues. In order to be of maximum benefit, it is important that treatment starts as soon as CF is diagnosed.

Control of expression

A major confounding factor is the heterogeneous nature of CFTR expression in the lung. CFTR expression is greatest in the submucosal glands, though some surface epithelial non-ciliated cells at the ductal openings of glands also have high levels (Jiang and Engelhardt, 1998). Even within submucosal glands CFTR expression is highly variable. Elsewhere, low level CFTR expression is observed. This creates difficulties in using gene therapy to deliver the correct degree of CFTR expression in different cell types, which depends not only on the cell type, but also on its location in the airways.

Matching the natural CFTR expression patterns in the airways is impractical. Even if the different cell types could be individually targeted, control of CFTR expression to the correct level in each is likely to be problematic. Also, a gene therapy vehicle delivered via the airways will have considerable difficulty reaching the submucosal glands. It is hoped that failure to replicate the natural heterologous CFTR expression patterns will not prevent significant improvement in the underlying pathology.

Care is needed to ensure overexpression of CFTR does not occur. The endogenous CFTR promoters are very weak and strong viral promoters run the risk of producing basolateral localisation of CFTR in addition to the normal apical and intracellular sites (Farmen et al., 2005). Inappropriately located CFTR will have a functional implication. In order to allow transepithelial movement of Cl^- across airways epithelia, Cl^- must first cross the basolateral membranes. This is primarily due to the NKCC transporter (Figure 6.4) If CFTR is present in the basolateral membranes it will provide an alternative route for Cl^- movement. Farmen et al. (2005) showed that basolateral CFTR reduces transepithelial Cl^- movements, presumably by acting as a Cl^- shunt pathway. Thus, some of the Cl^- cross the basolateral membranes by the NKCC exits via basolateral CFTR before it can traverse the cell.

What % of cells need to be corrected?

It is unlikely that 100% of cells can be corrected by gene therapy. Indeed, since heterozygotes appear normal, there is not a linear relationship between gene expression and CFTR function. The central question is therefore what proportion of cells in CF airways are required to express the corrected gene in order to substantially ameliorate the underlying genetic defect and resultant pathophysiology. This has been investigated with both cell lines and mouse models. Johnson et al. (1992) used a CF airways cell line that exhibited the characteristic Cl^- transport defect. They found that as few as 6% corrected cells in an epithelial sheet converted the CF epithelium into a normal phenotype with respect to indicators such as forskolin stimulation of short circuit current (an indicator of cAMP activated Cl^- movement). An alternative approach was adopted by Dorin et al. (1996). They cross-bred wild type mice and 2 CF homozygote mouse models, m1UNC which produces no CFTR, and m1HGU which produces 10% of wild type CFTR levels. This breeding programme

Table 6.1 Generation of different CFTR expression levels by cross breeding wild type and CF mouse models. A large reduction in CFTR expression is required before the 35 day survival rate falls. Adapted by permission from Macmillan Publishers Ltd [Gene Therapy] Dorin et al. (1996). A demonstration using mouse models that successful gene therapy for cystic fibrosis requires only partial gene correction. Gene Therapy 3: 797–801. Copyright 1996.

Mouse genotype	% of wild type CFTR level	% survival to 35 days
+/+ (wild type)	100	100
+/m1HGU	55	100
+/m1UNC	50	100
m1HGU/m1HGU	10	93
m1HGU/m1UNC	5	93
m1UNC/m1UNC	0	7

produced six different levels of CFTR expression in the offspring (Table 6.1).

It was found that 93% of the m1UNC homozygote mice, which have no functional CFTR, died within 35 days. However in m1HCU/m1UNC heterozygote mice, which have only 5% of the CFTR of wild type, more than 90% survived to adulthood. These early results were highly encouraging, suggesting that only a small proportion of cells (Johnson et al., 1992) need to be fully corrected, or a large number of cells require only low level partial correction (Dorin et al., 1996) for there to be significant benefit to patients. Presumably the surprisingly low level of correction needed arises from functional coupling of epithelial cells via gap junctions. This would then allow Cl^- ions to move from the uncorrected to the corrected cells, where they could then be transported across the apical membrane (Johnson et al., 1992). A note of caution is however needed. These studies have concentrated on correction of the Cl^- transport defect and have not considered Na^+. It is therefore conceivable that a higher degree of correction is needed to restore the normal level of Na^+ absorption from the ASL (Boucher, 1999).

General approaches

Gene therapy protocols can be split into *ex vivo* and *in vivo* strategies. *Ex vivo* gene transfer involves removing stem cells from the body, introducing the corrected gene, and returning the cells to the body. Whilst this approach is feasible for some diseases (e.g. genetic blood disorders,

where bone marrow stem cells could be manipulated), it is not practical for airways epithelia. *In vivo* techniques have to deliver the corrected gene to the airways *in situ*. Although it is relatively easy to correct CF cell lines, transfection of CF airways is much more difficult. There are several barriers to successful gene therapy in the airways, some of which are illustrated in Figure 6.9.

The viscous mucus characteristic of CF severely impedes vector transit. This is likely to require pre administration of mucolytics such as Pulmozyme®, which is a recombinant human DNase (rhDNase) that degrades DNA. This reduces the viscosity of the sputum aiding mucociliary clearance. It has already become an established part of CF treatment plans and has the added benefit of improving access for therapeutic gene delivery vectors. However, rhDNase may also affect the plasmid DNA in transit to the cell. The degree of degradation will depend on the vehicle used, with viruses being the most resistant. Non-viral vectors such as liposomes enter the airways cells via the apical (luminal) cell membrane. Whilst CF sputum impedes both viral and non-viral vectors, normal airways mucus is much more of a barrier to liposomes than viruses. This is probably due to cationic lipid interaction with the negatively charged mucus. Since adenoviruses are negatively charged, this may partially explain the difference in transport efficiency to the cell surface (Kitson et al., 1999). The glycocalyx may also bind gene delivery vectors, thereby reducing delivery to cell surface receptors. In addition, mucociliary clearance is likely to reduce the effectiveness of transfection, as it will lessen the time that vectors have to access the cell membrane (Griesenbach and Alton, 2009b). Most vectors target receptors that are on the basolateral membranes of the airways cells (Boucher, 1999). If cells could be made more leaky by disruption of the tight junctions it might allow more efficient uptake. This was demonstrated by Kitson et al. (1999) with sheep tracheal explants. They found that increasing the paracellular permeability, via calcium free media, caused a 60% fall in transepithelial resistance. This induced a 5-fold increase in adenovirus driven gene expression, but only a 1.5-fold increase in liposome mediated gene expression. These results suggest that increased access to the basolateral membranes would particularly benefit viral vectors. However, it is doubtful that this approach is practical. Even if transient and reversible increases in paracellular permeability could be achieved, it would lead to pathogen access to normally inaccessible sub-epithelial tissue. Instead it might be possible to target luminal cell surface receptors such as the $P2Y_2$ and A_{2B} GPCRs. The

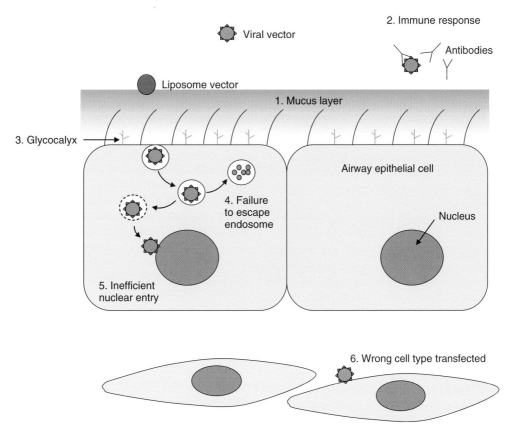

Figure 6.9 Extracellular and intracellular barriers to CFTR gene therapy in the airways. These barriers include: 1. the mucus layer impedes transit of viral and non viral vectors, 2. immune responses target viral vectors, 3. the glycocalyx can bind some viral vectors, 4 endocytosed vectors need to escape the endosmome, 5. cryptozoic vectors may have restricted nuclear entry, 6. the wrong cell type may be transfected. Figure adapted from Davies et al., 1998. Prospects for gene therapy for cystic fibrosis. Molecular Medicine Today 4: 292–299. Elsevier copyright 1998.

$P2Y_2$ receptor is internalised via the clathrin coated pits. Since many viruses can escape from these, it makes this route a potentially viable target (Boucher, 1999).

Techniques used to increase the efficiency of gene expression in the laboratory include electroporation, magnetofection and ultrasound. Although there has been some limited success in mouse models, these techniques are unlikely to result in clinical application. This is due in part to the technical difficulties in upscaling to humans, and the physical damage to the lung epithelia induced by these techniques (Griesenbach and Alton, 2009b).

Most CF gene therapy trials to date have used alteration of nasal PD as an indicator of success. This is a questionable surrogate of likely improvement in lung function. The nasal epithelium is easily accessible, safer, allows local application of gene therapy agents, and is easy to assess via

nasal PD measurements. However, the nasal epithelium is not a clinically significant tissue in CF. It also has a simpler structure than the deeper respiratory epithelia. Unfortunately, clinical measurements of improvements in lung bioelectrics and function will require much more invasive techniques such as bronchoscopic sampling.

After the gene delivery vehicle has been endocytosed it needs to escape the endosome, as otherwise it will be acidified and subject to lysosomal digestion. Viruses have a natural endosomolytic ability, so can overcome this barrier. Cytoplasmic end nucleases will limit the time genetic material has to reach the nucleus, thereby restricting nuclear entry. This will particularly affect liposomes and viruses that uncoat at the plasma membrane, or in the cytosol. Adenoviruses however deliver their DNA direct to the nucleus, via a capsid that docks with the nuclear pore. Viral vectors are likely to provoke immune responses. Even if the first dose does not, the repeat dosing necessary will induce immune responses such as antibody production. This is likely to reduce transfection efficiency.

Viral vectors

Viral vectors make use of the natural ability of viruses to enter cells and deliver genetic material. However, there are substantial safety concerns about using this approach for gene therapy. For example, if viral DNA integrates into the genome it risks insertional mutagenesis by stimulating oncogenes and/or inhibiting tumour suppressor genes (Rosenecker et al., 1998). Retroviruses used in some gene therapy protocols are not a suitable vector for CF as they only target actively dividing cells and randomly insert into the genome. Initial work concentrated on adenovirus (AV) vectors which only cause transient expression of the engineered gene as it does not integrate into the genome. This type of double stranded DNA virus is trophic for the airways and commonly causes respiratory illness in man. This virus has a sufficiently large capacity to easily accommodate the CFTR construct. A $5'$ upstream promoter region is needed to regulate expression of the CFTR gene, and a downstream $3'$ region to influence post transcriptional events such as RNA splicing and polyadenylation. Viruses gain entry into cells via components of their surface coat interacting with receptors on cell membranes. It is therefore possible to strip out several viral coding regions, but still allow the virus to invade a cell. The first attempts removed the E1a and 1b coding regions to make the AV replicant deficient. However, it is still possible that the engineered AV could recombine with a wild type virus, producing a hybrid strain that can reproduce (Davies et al., 1998). Whilst early results in rodents were encouraging, it soon became clear that AV vectors could only induce limited expression and were inefficient. This was primarily due to differences in cell surface receptor expression, with the human airways lacking the apical (luminal) expression of the coxsackie-adenovirus receptor that is present in the rodent models (Griesenbach and Alton, 2009b). Repeat administration of AV caused increasing immune responses with a fall in transfection efficiency. This is a particular concern since expression of the transfected gene is transient, requiring periodic re-exposure to the AV vector. Attempts have been made to suppress the immune system prior to AV treatment, but repeat dosing still caused a rapid fall in transfection efficiency. Alternative strategies to increase

transfection include covering the virus with a polyethylene glycol derivative (PEGylation) to mask the viral coat, or 'gutting' the vector of all AV genes (Greisenbach and Alton, 2009b). Despite some improvements in transfection efficiency with repeat dosing, AV vectors are not yet sufficiently developed to be a viable treatment option.

An alternative to AV is the adeno-associated virus (AAV). This provokes less of an immune response than AV, but is still trophic for the target tissue (Rosenecker et al., 1998). As these integrate into the genome it has the potential for much longer expression than AV, though with the attendant risk of insertional mutagenesis. The small capacity of AAV does severely limit the size of the CFTR construct. Attempts have been made to allocate the required full length sequence between two different types of AAV vector. Co-administration of both types of vector has resulted in recombination and expression in the target tissue (Griesenbach and Alton, 2009). An alternative approach is to design an AAV that only codes for a truncated version of CFTR. Partial deletion of the R domain did give some restoration of Cl^- channel activity (Griesenbach and Alton, 2009b). However, this is an intrinsically less attractive option as the function(s) of each region of CFTR is not yet fully understood.

An intriguing approach is the use of AAV vectors to tone down the inflammatory response in the lungs. In a mouse model an AAV5 vector designed to induce the expression of interleukin 10 (IL-10) was found to reduce the inflammatory response to *P. aeruginosa* (Buff et al., 2010). Elevated levels of IL-10, significantly above control values, were maintained for at least 6 weeks post exposure to the AVV5 vector. The concentration of proinflammatory cytokines (IL-1β and KC) and the chemokine, macrophage inhibitory protein-1α, were also significantly reduced. This suggests that it might be feasible to manipulate the immune response to viral vectors, thereby allowing a rise in transfection efficiency. However, suppression of immune responses does risk systemic infection as the activity of macrophages will be reduced.

At present other types of viruses are also being considered for CF gene therapy. It is not yet clear which type offers the best combination of efficacy and safety. The DNA for some viruses can integrate into the genome, potentially allowing expression for the lifetime of the cell. Whilst this increases the time between treatments, it does risk insertional mutagenesis. Others do not integrate, but the transient expression requires more frequent re-exposure to the vector. A major problem is combating the immune response which increasingly reduces transfection efficiency with each subsequent dose of a vector.

Non-viral vectors

In order to negate some of the safety concerns over viral vectors, other non-viral gene delivery systems (NVGDS) have been considered, whilst they are less likely to provoke immune responses, they suffer from reduced efficiency. Alternative NVGDS include DNA nanoparticles and cationic liposomes. Work on DNA nanoparticles is at an early stage. The nanoparticle is designed to hold a single copy of the plasmid and be small enough to enter the nucleus via the nuclear pore complex. Initial trials produced changes in the nasal epithelium of CF patients, though this remains to be demonstrated in the lungs.

Liposomes are further along the development pipeline. In a preclinical trial of three types of NVGDS, it was found that cationic lipid DNA complexes were slightly better than DNA nanoparticles or polyethlenimine DNA complexes (Ziady and Davis, 2006). The cationic liposomes consist of a cationic lipid DNA complex in an attempt to restrict degradation by nucleases, and improve transfection of cells, when compared to naked DNA plasmids. Early studies were limited due to immune responses triggered by the presence of cytosine-phosphate-guanine (CpG) nucleotide sequences in the DNA plasmid (Zaidy and Davis, 2006). These have subsequently been reduced and were found to be less immunogenic. A plasmid that is completely free of CpG sequences has now been produced by the UK CF Gene Therapy Consortium (Griesenbach and Alton, 2009b). A clinical trial to assess whether this cationic lipid DNA complex can produce clinical benefit is in progress.

Gene silencing

An alternative to inducing expression of corrected CFTR is to inhibit expression of other genes that contribute to the pathology of CF. Potential candidates include genes involved in ion transport, inflammation, and protein folding and trafficking. Of these, manipulating the defective ion transport is probably the most attractive as it directly addresses the fundamental defects in CF. As previously discussed, overactive ENaC accounts for much of the disregulation of ASL observed in CF airways. Caci et al. (2009) demonstrated that short interfering RNA (siRNA) could down regulate ENaC expression. They found that all three ENaC subunits, α, β and γ could be down regulated by the siRNA approach, but that silencing of the β subunit was more effective than either the α or γ in reducing amiloride sensitive short circuit current (I_{sc}) (70%, 53% and 43% inhibition respectively). Since ENaC consists of a heterotrimer of the α, β and γ

subunits, it would be expected that knockdown of one of these subunits would reduce the amiloride sensitive I_{sc}. However, expression of the subunit isoforms is not uniform, with increased levels of the α subunit present in the airways compared to the other subunits. Caci et al. (2009) suggested that this may be due to the α subunit either being able to form a (semi) functioning ENaC, with possibly reduced Na^+ flux and/or forming part of the non-selective cation channel. This was in part based on the experiments of Jain et al. (1999), who found that down regulation of the α ENaC subunit in rat alveolar cells caused a fall in the abundance of non-selective cation channels. Gene silencing of ENaC is an innovative approach that might bring clinical benefit in the future. However, there is likely to be significant difficulties in achieving delivery of the expression vector to the target airways cells.

Artificial chromosomes

An interesting approach to provide extended expression, but without the risk of insertional mutagenesis is the artificial chromosome. These currently consist of bacterial artificial chromosomes, yeast artificial chromosomes, and human artificial chromosomes. Whilst they have the advantage of sufficient capacity to allow both coding and regulatory regions to be included, they are fragile and unlikely to survive aerosolisation in the current generation of nebulisers used to deliver drugs to the airways (Macnab and Whitehouse, 2009). Even if the artificial chromosome arrives at the target tissue intact, the delivery across the cell membrane is still problematic. Using infectious transfer (viral delivery) or liposomes will encounter the same problems as previously discussed. Although bacterial artificial chromosome have been used in a proof of principle study for CF gene therapy in a cell line, this technology is still at an early stage and unlikely to be a serious contender for CF gene therapy for some time.

6.8 Conclusion

The early optimism for the rapid development of a gene therapy cure for CF was misplaced. Indeed, it has now been recognised that the initial concentration of resources on gene therapy following the discovery of the CF gene was probably a mistake (Couzin-Frankel, 2009). Over the years the number of groups working on this aspect of CF has dwindled as the problems with this approach became apparent. Whilst there are at present considerable technical difficulties to overcome, it is anticipated that CF gene therapy will become a viable treatment option in the future. Issues that still require resolution include which vehicle is the best choice, avoiding or minimising immune responses, maintaining transfection efficiency with repeated dosing, targeting of cells and so on. At present it is likely that pharmacotherapy will have a large clinical impact before CF gene therapy can deliver its promise. The realisation that the discovery of the gene responsible for a genetic disease is only the first step along the long road towards a cure has been a salutary lesson.

References

Amaral MD and Kunzelmann K (2007). Molecular targeting of CFTR as a therapeutic approach to cystic fibrosis. Trends in Pharmacological Sciences 28: 334–341.

Anderson MP, Gregory RJ, Thompson S, Souza DW, Paul S, Mulligan RC, Smith AE and Welsh MJ (1991). Demonstration that CFTR is a chloride channel by alteration of its anion selectivity. Science 253: 202–207.

Bals R, Weiner DJ, Meegla RL, Accurso F, and Wilson JM (2001). Salt-independent abnormality of antimicrobial activity in cystic fibrosis airway surface fluid. American Journal of Respiratory Cell Molecular Biology 25: 21–25.

Barasch J, Kiss B, Prince a, Saiman L, Grunenert D and Al-Awqati Q (1991). Defective acidification of intracellular organelles in cystic fibrosis. Nature 352: 70–73.

Bao HF, Liu L, Self J, Duke BJ Ueno R and Eaton DC (2008). A synthetic prostone activates apical chloride channels in A6 epithelial cells. American Journal of Physiology 295: G234–G251.

Bear CE, Li C, Kartner N, Bridges RJ, Jensen TJ, Ramjameesingh M and Riordan R (1992). Purification and functional reconstitution of the cystic fibrosis transmembrane conductance regulator (CFTR). Cell 68: 809–818.

Becq F, Jensen TJ, Chang X-B, Savoia A, Rommens JM, Tusi L-C, Buchwald M, Riordan JR and Hanrahan JW (1994) Phosphatase inhibitors activate normal and defective CFTR chloride channels. Proceedings of the National Academy of Sciences USA 91: 9160–9164.

Boucher RC (1999). Status of gene therapy for cystic fibrosis lung disease. Journal of Clinical Investigation 103: 441–445.

Bompadre SG, Sohma Y, Li M, Hwang T-C (2007). G551D and G1349D, two CF-associated mutations in the signature sequences of CFTR, exhibit distinct gating defects. Journal of General Physiology 129: 285–298.

Brown CR, Hong-Brown LQ, Biwersi J, Verkman AS and Welch WJ (1996). Chemical chaperones correct the mutant phenotype of the ΔF508 cystic fibrosis transmembrane conductance regulator protein. Cell Stress and Chaperones 1: 117–125.

Buchanan PJ, Ernst RK, Elborn S and Schock B (2009). Role of CFTR, *Psuedomonas aeruginosa* and toll-like receptors in cystic

fibrosis lung inflammation. Biochemical Society Transactions 37: 863–867.

Buff SM, Yu H, McCall JN, Caldwell SM, Ferkol TW, Flotte TR and Virella-Lowell IL (2010). IL-10 delivery by AAV5 vector attenuates inflammation in mice with Psuedomonas pneumonia. Gene Therapy 17: 567–576.

Caci E, Melani R, Pdemonte N, Yueksekdag G, Ravazzolo R, Rosenecker J, Galietta LJV and Zegarra-Morgan O (2009). Epithelial sodium channel inhibition in primary human bronchial epithelia by transfected siRNA. American Journal of Respiratory Cell and Molecular Biology 40: 211–216.

Chan HC, Ruan TC, He Q, Chen MH, Xu WM, Chen WY, Xie C, Zhang XH and Zhou Z (2009). The cystic fibrosis transmembrane conductance regulator in reproductive health and disease. Journal of Physiology 587: 2187-2195.

Clunes MT and Boucher RC (2008). Front-runners for pharmacotherapeutic correction of the airway ion transport defect in cystic fibrosis. Current Opinion in Pharmacology 8: 292–299.

Davies JC, Geddes DM and Alton EWFW (1998). Prospects for gene therapy for cystic fibrosis. Molecular Medicine Today 4: 292–299.

Couzin-Frankel, J (2009). The promise of a cure: 20 years and counting. Science 324: 1504–1507.

Davies JC, Gedes DM and Alton EWFW (1998). Prospects for gene therapy for cystic fibrosis. Molecular Medicine Today 4: 292–299.

Delaney SJ and Wainwright BJ (1996). New pharmaceutical approaches to the treatment of cystic fibrosis. Nature Medicine 2: 392–393.

Denning Gm, Anderson MP, Amara JF, Marshall J, Smith AE and Welsh MJ (1992). Processing of mutant cystic fibrosis transmembrane conductance regulator is temperature-sensitive. Nature 358: 761–764.

Dormer RL, Haris CM, Clark Z, Pereira MMC, Doull IJM, Norez C, Becq F and McPherson MA (2005). Sildenafil (Viagra) corrects ΔF508-CFTR location in nasal epithelial cells from patients with cystic fibrosis. Thorax 60: 55–59.

Dorin JR, Farley R, Webb S, Smith SN, Farini E, Delaney SJ, Wainwright BJ, Alton EWFW and Porteous DJ (1996). A demonstration using mouse models that successful gene therapy for cystic fibrosis requires only partial gene correction. Gene Therapy 3: 797–801.

Drumm ML, Wilkinson DJ, Smit LS, Worrell RT, Strong TV, Frizzell RA, Dawson DC and Collins FS (1991). Chloride conductance expressed by ΔF508 and other mutant CFTRs in *Xenopus* oocytes. Science 254: 1797–1799.

Du L, Damoiseaux R, Nahas S, Gao K, Hu H, Pollard JM, Goldstine J, Jung ME, Henning SM, Bertoni C and Gatti RA (2009). Nonaminoglycoside compounds induce readthrough of nonsense mutations. Journal of Experimental Medicine 206: 2285–2297.

Elferink RO and Beuers U (2009). Are pigs more human than mice? Journal of Hepatology 50: 836–841.

Egan M, Flotte T, Afino S, Solow R, Zeitlin PL, Carter BJ and Guggino WB (1992). Defective regulation of outwardly rectifying Cl⁻ channels by protein kinase A corrected by insertion of CFTR. Nature 358: 581–584.

Farmen SL, Karp PH, Ng P, Palmer DJ, Koehler DR, Hu J, Beaudet AL, Zabner J and Welsh MJ (2005). Gene transfer of CFTR airway epithelia: low levels of expression are sufficient to correct Cl⁻ transport and overexpression can generate basolateral CFTR. American Journal of Physiology – Lung Cell and Molecular Physiology 289: L1123–L1130.

Gabriel SE, Brigman KH, Koller BH, Boucher RC, Stutts MJ (1994). Cystic fibrosis heterozygote resistance to cholera toxin in the cystic fibrosis mouse model. Science 266: 107–109.

Gadsby DC and Nairn AC (1999). Control of CFTR channel gating by phosphorylation and nucleotide hydrolysis. Physiological Reviews 79: S77–S107.

Garcia MA, Yang N and Quinton PM (2009). Normal mouse intestinal mucus release requires cystic fibrosis transmembrane regulator-dependant bicarbonate secretion. Journal of Clinical Investigation 119: 2613–2622.

Gelman MS and Kopito RR (2002). Rescuing protein conformation: prospects for pharmacological therapy in cystic fibrosis. Journal of Clinical Investigation 110: 1591–1597.

Griesenbach U and Alton EWFW (2009a). Ferreting with fibroblasts for cystic fibrosis. Gene Therapy 16: 1–2.

Griesenbach U and Alton EWFW (2009b). Gene transfer to the lungs: lessons learned from more than 2 decades of CF gene therapy. Advanced Drug Delivery Reviews 61: 128–139.

Guilbault C, Saeed Z, Downey GP and Radzioch D (2007). Cystic fibrosis mouse models. American Journal of Respiratory Cell and Molecular Biology 36: 1–7.

Haggie PM and Verkman AS (2008). Monomeric CFTR in plasma membranes in live cells revealed by single molecule fluorescence imaging. Journal of Biological Chemistry 35: 23510–23513.

Haggie PM and Verkman AS (2009). Defective organellar acidification as a cause of cystic fibrosis lung disease: re-examination of a recurring hypothesis. American Journal of Physiology Lung Cell and Molecular Physiology 296: L859–L867.

Hassett DJ, Sutton MD, Schurr MJ, Herr AB, Caldwell CC and Matu JO (2009). *Pseudomonas aeruginosa* hypoxic or anaerobic biofilm infections within cystic fibrosis airways. Trends in Microbiology 17: 130–138.

Hellibrunn SM, Shah P, Bristow MR, Valentine HA, Ginsburg R and Fowler MB (1989). Increased β-receptor density and improved hemodynamic response to catecholamine stimulation during long-term metoprolol therapy in heart failure from dilated cardiomyopathy. Circulation 79: 483–490.

Hirsh AJ, Stonebraker JR, van Heusden CA, Lazarowski ER, Boucher RC and Picher M (2007). Adenosine deaminase 1 and concentrative nucleoside transporters 2 and 3 regulate adenosine on the apical surface of human airway epithelia: implications for inflammatory lung diseases. Biochemistry 46: 10373–10383.

Howard M, Frizzell RA and Bedwell DM (1996). Aminoglycoside antibiotics restore CFTR function by overcomming premature stop mutations. Nature Medicine 2: 467–9.

Hudson VL and Guill MF (1998). New developments in cystic fibrosis. Pediatric Annals 27: 515–520.

Hyde SC and Gill DR (2008). Ignoring the nonsense: a phase II trial in cystic fibrosis. Lancet. 372: 691–692.

Hwang T-C and Sheppard DN (2009). Gating of the CFTR Cl⁻ channel by ATP-driven nucleotide-binding domain dimerisation. Journal of Physiology 587: 2151–2161.

Jain L, Chen X-J, Malik B, Al-Khali O and Eaton DC (1999). Antisense oligonucleotides against the α-subunit of ENaC decreases lung epithelial cation-channel activity. American Journal of Physiology: Lung Cellular and Molecular Physiology 276: L1046–L1051.

Jiang Q and Engelhardt JF (1998). Cellular heterogeneity of CFTR expression and function in the lung: implications for gene therapy for cystic fibrosis. European Journal of Human Genetics 6: 12–31.

Johnson LG, Olsen JC, Sarkadi B, Moore KL, Swanstrom R and Boucher RC (1992). Efficiency of gene transfer for restoration of normal airway epithelial function in cystic fibrosis. Nature Genetics 2: 21–25.

Jones BD, Ghori N and Falkow S (1994). *Salmonella typhimurium* initiates murine infection by penetrating and destroying the specialised epithelial m cells of the Peyer's patches. Journal of Experimental Medicine 180: 15–23.

Kelley TJ, Al-Nakkash L, Cotton CU, and Drumm ML (1996). Activation of endogenous ΔF508 cystic fibrosis transmembrane conductance regulator by phosphodiesterase inhibition. Journal of Clinical Investigation 98: 513–520.

Kerem B, Rommens JM, Buchanan JA, Markiewicz D, Cox TK, Chakravarti A, Buchwald M and Tusi L-C (1989). Identification of the cystic fibrosis gene: genetic analysis. Science 245: 1073–1080.

Kitson C, Angel B, Judd D, Rothery S, Severs NJ, Dewar A, Huang L, Wadsworth SC, Cheng SH, Geddes DM and Alton EWFW (1999). The extra- and intracellular barriers to lipid and adenovirus-mediated pulmonary gene transfer in native sheep airway epithelium. Gene Therapy 6: 534–546.

Knowles MR, Robinson JM, Wood RE, Pue CA, Mentz WM, Wager GC, Gatzy JT and Boucher RC (1997). Ion composition of airways surface liquid of patients with cystic fibrosis as compared with normal and disease-control subjects. Journal of Clinical Investigation 100: 2588–2597.

Kunzelmann K, Bachhuber T, Regger R, Markovich D, Sun J and Schreiber R (2005). Purinergic inhibition of epithelial Na⁺ transport via hydrolysis of PIP₂. FASEB Journal 19: 142–143.

Lazarowski ER and Boucher RC (2009). Purinergic receptors in airways epithelia. Current Opinion in Pharmacology 9: 262–267.

Linde L and Kerem B (2008). Introducing sense into nonsense in treatments of human genetic diseases. Trends in Genetics 24: 552–563.

Liu X, luo M, Zhang L, Ding W, Yan Z, Engelhardt JF (2007). Bioelectric properties of chloride channels in human, pig, ferret and mouse airway epithelium. American Journal of Respiratory Cell and Molecular Biology 36: 313–323.

Liu Y, Wang Y, Jiang Y, Zhu N, Liang H, Xu L, Feng X, Yang H. and Ma T (2008). Mild processing defect of porcine ΔF508-CFTR suggests that ΔF508 pigs may not develop cystic fibrosis disease. Biochemical and Biophysical Research Communications 373: 113–118.

Lloyd Mills C, Pereira MMC, Dormer RL and McPherson MA (1992). An antibody against a CFTR-derived synthetic peptide, incorporated into living submandibular cells, inhibits beta-adrenergic stimulation of mucin secretion. Biochemical and Biophysical Research Communications 188: 1146–1152.

Lloyd Mills C, Dorin JR, Davidson DJ, Porteus DJ, Alton EWFW, Dormer RL and McPherson MA (1995). Decreased β adrenergic stimulation of glycoprotein secretion in CF mice submandibular glands: reversal by the methylxanthine, IBMX. Biochemical and Biophysical Research Communications 215: 674–681.

Lubamba B, Lecourt H, Lebacq J, Lebecque P, De Jonge H, Wallemacq P and Leal T (2008). Preclinical evidence that sildenafil and vardenafil activate chloride transport in cystic fibrosis. American Journal of Respiratory and Critical Care Medicine 177: 506–515.

Macnab S and Whitehouse A (2009). Progress and prospects: human artificial chromosomes. Gene Therapy 16: 1180–1185.

Mall MA (2009). Role of amiloride-sensitive Na$^+$ channel in the pathogenesis and as a therapeutic target for cystic fibrosis lung disease. Experimental Physiology 94: 171–174.

Matsui H, Grubb BR, Tarran R, Randell SH, Gatzy JT, Davis CW and Boucher RC (1998). Evidence for periciliary layer depletion, not abnormal ion composition, in the pathogenesis of cystic fibrosis airways disease. Cell 95: 1005–1015.

McPherson MA and Dormer RL (1991). Molecular and cellular biology of cystic fibrosis. Molecular Aspects of Medicine 21: 1–81.

McPherson MA, Dormer RL, Bradbury NA, Dodge JA and Goodchild MC (1986). Defective β-adrenergic secretory responses in submandibular acinar cells from cystic fibrosis patients. Lancet 328: 1007–1008.

McPherson MA, Piera MMC, Lloyd Mills C, Murray KJ and Dormer RL (1999). A cyclic nucleotide PDE5 inhibitor corrects defective mucin secretion in submandibular cells containing antibody directed against the cystic fibrosis transmembrane conductance regulator protein. FEBS Letters 464: 48–52.

Moreau-Marquis S, Stanton BA and O'Toole George A (2008). Psuedomonas aeruginosa biofilm formation in cystic fibrosis airway. Pulmonary Pharmacology and Therapeutics 21: 595–599.

Pier GB (2000). Role of cystic fibrosis transmembrane conductance regulator in innate immunity to Pseudomonas aeruginosa infections. Proceeding of the National Academy of Sciences USA 97: 8822–8828.

Pier GB, Grout M, Zaidi T, Meluleni G, Mueschenbor SS, Banting G, Ratcliff R, Evans MJ and Colledge WH (1998). Salmonella typhi uses CFTR to enter intestinal epithelial cells. Nature 393: 79–82.

Pilewski JM and Frizzell RA 1999. Role of CFTR in airway disease. Physiological Reviews 79: S216–S255.

Poschet JF, Boucher JC, Tatterson L, Skidmore J, Van Dyke RW and Deretic V (2001). Molecular basis for defective glycosylation and Pseudomonas pathogenesis in cystic fibrosis lung. Proceedings of the National Academy of Sciences USA, 98: 13972–13977.

Poschet JF, Timmins GS, Taylor-Coussar JL, Ornatowski W, Fazio JF, Perkett E, Wilson KR, Yu HD, de Jonge HR and Deretic V (2007). Pharmacological modulation of cGMP levels by phosphodiesterase 5 inhibitors as a therapeutic strategy for treatment of respiratory pathology in cystic fibrosis. American Journal of Physiology - Lung Cellular and Molecular Physiology 293: L712–L719.

Quinton PM (1994). What is good about cystic fibrosis? Human Genetics 4: 742–743.

Quinton PM (2007). Cystic fibrosis: lessons from the sweat gland. Physiology 22: 212–225.

Ramsey BW, Davies J, McElvaney NG, Tullis E, Bell SC, Dřevínek P, Griese M, McKone EF, Wainwright CE, Konstan MW, Moss R, Ratjen F, Sermet-Gaudelus I, Rowe SM, Dong Q, Rodriguez S, Yen K, Ordoňez C,Elborn JS. (2011). A CFTR potentiator in patients with cystic fibrosis and the G551D mutation. New England Journal of Medicine 365: 1663–1672.

Riordan JR, Rommens JM, Kerem B, Aslon N, Rozmahel R, Grzelczak Z, Zielnski J, Lok S, Plavsic N, Chou J-L, Drumm ML, Iannuzzi MC, Collins FS and Tsui L-C. (1989). Identification of the cystic fibrosis gene: cloning and characterization of complementary DNA. Science 245: 1066- 1073.

Robert R, Carlile GW, Pavel C, Anjos SM, Liao J, Luo Y, Zhang D, Thomas DY, and Hanrahan JW (2008). Structural analog of sildenafil identified as a novel corrector of the F508del-CFTR trafficking defect. Molecular Pharmacology 73: 478–489.

Rommens JM, Iannuzzi MC, Kerem B, Drumm ML, Melmer G, Dean M, Rozmahel R, Cole JL, Kennedy D, Hidaka N, Zsiga M, Buchwald M, Riordan JR, Tusi L-C and Collins FS (1989). Identification of the cystic fibrosis gene: chromosome walking and jumping. Science 245: 1059-1065.

Rosenecker J, Schmalix WA, Schidelhauer D, Plank C and Reinhardt D (1998). Towards gene therapy of cystic fibrosis. European Journal of Medical Research 3: 149–156.

Schwiebert EM, Benos DJ, Egan ME, Stutts MJ and Guggino WB (1999). CFTR is a conductance regulator as well as a chloride channel. Physiological Reviews 79: S145–S166.

Shalon LB and Adelson JW (1996). Cystic fibrosis. Gastrointestinal complications and gene therapy. Pediatric Clinics of North America 43: 157–196.

Sheppard DN and Welsh MJ (1999). Structure and function of the CFTR chloride channel. Physiological Reviews 79: S23–S45.

Smith SN, Middleton PG, Chadwick S, Jaffe A, Bush KA, Rolleston S, Farley R, Delaney SJ, Wainwright B, Geddes DM and Alton EWFW (1999). The in vivo effects of milrinone on the airways of cystic fibrosis mice and human subjects. American Journal of Respiratory Cell and Molecular biology 20: 129–134.

Smith JJ, Travis SM, Greenberg EP and Welsh MJ (1996). Cystic fibrosis airways epithelia fail to kill bacteria because of abnormal airway surface fluid. Cell 85: 229–236.

Song Y, Namkung W, Nielson DW, Lee J-W, Finkbeiner WE and Verkman AS (2009). Airway surface liquid depth measured in ex vivo fragments of pig and human trachea: dependence on Na^+ and Cl^- channel function. American Journal of Physiology – Lung Cellular and Molecular Physiology 297: L1131–L1140.

Tarran R, Button B, Picher M, Paradiso AM, Ribeiro CM, Lazarowski ER, Zhang L, Collins PI, Pickles RJ, Fredberg JJ and Boucher RC (2005). Normal and cystic fibrosis airway surface liquid homeostasis: the effects of phasic shear stress and viral infections. Journal of Biological Chemistry 280: 35751–35759.

Tarran R, Trout L, Donaldson SH and Boucher RC (2006). Soluble mediators, not cilia, determine airways surface liquid volume in normal and cystic fibrosis superficial airway epithelia. Journal of General Physiology 127: 591–604.

Thelin WR and Boucher RC (2007). The epithelium as a target for therapy in cystic fibrosis. Current Opinion in Pharmacology 7: 290–295.

Toward TJ, Smith N and Broadley KJ (2004). Effect of phosphodiesterase-5 inhibitor sildenafil (viagra), in animal models of airways disease. American Journal of Respiratory and Critical Care and Medicine 169: 227–234.

Voynow JA and Rubin BK (2009). Mucins, mucus and sputum. Chest 135: 505–512.

Welch WJ and Brown CR (1996). Influence of molecular and chemical chaperones on protein folding. Cell Stress and Chaperones 1: 109–115.

Welch EM, Barton ER, Zhou J et al. (2007). PTC124 targets genetic disorders caused by nonsense mutations. Nature 447: 87–91.

Wine JW (1993). Indictment of pore behaviour. Nature 366: 18–19.

Wine JW (1999). The genesis of cystic fibrosis lung disease. The Journal of Clinical Investigation 103: 309–312.

Wiuf C (2001). Do ΔF508 heterozygotes have a selective advantage? Genetical Research 78: 41–47.

Yu H, Burton B, Huang C-J, Worley J, Cao D, Johnson JP, Urrutia A, Joubran J, Seepersaud S, Sussky K, Hoffman BJ and Van Goor F (2012). Ivacaftor potentiation of multiple CFTR channels with gating mutations. Journal of Cystic Fibrosis 11: 237–245.

Zaidy AG and Davis PB (2006). Current prospects for gene therapy of cystic fibrosis. Current Opinion in Pharmacology 6: 515–521.

Zeitlin L (1999). Novel pharmacologic therapies for cystic fibrosis. Journal of Clinical Investigation 103: 447–452.

Zeitlin L (2008). Cystic fibrosis and estrogens: a perfect storm. Journal of Clinical Investigation 118: 3841–3844.

7 Pharmacogenomics

Individual variation in the human genome is recognised as the main cause of variable response to prescribed drugs and other xenobiotics. In recent years the field of pharmacogenomics has developed rapidly. This is the study of how an individual's genetic makeup affects their response to therapeutic drugs. Pharmacogenetic tests are already in use for some disease conditions (Table 7.1) and it is predicted that personalised medicines will become the norm in the future. For background reviews on the topic of pharmacogenomics see Brockmöller and Tzvetkov (2008), Shastry (2006) and Pfost et al. (2000). In this chapter we will discuss how genetic variations in drug metabolising enzymes, drug transporters and G-protein coupled receptors influence therapeutic response and in some cases disease progression. The concept that individual genetic variability can result in life-threatening adverse drug reactions is illustrated by polymorphisms in thiopurine S-methyltransferase and cardiac K^+ channels (see section 7.2).

7.1 Types of genetic variation in the human genome

The inherited variation in the human genome has only just become apparent since the completion of the human genome project. The different categories or types of genetic variation are summarised in Table 7.2.

Single nucleotide polymorphisms (SNPs; pronounced snips) are naturally occurring variations within the genome involving single nucleotide differences between the same species. It is estimated that the human genome contains 10 million SNPs, which equates to one SNP approximately every 1200 bases. The International HapMap project is currently working to document all common genetic variants of the human genome (see http://hapmap.ncbi.nlm.nih.gov/). This does not mean that a SNP appears every 1200 bases; some areas of genome may be SNP 'rich' whereas others may SNP

Molecular Pharmacology: From DNA to Drug Discovery, First Edition. John Dickenson, Fiona Freeman, Chris Lloyd Mills, Shiva Sivasubramaniam and Christian Thode.
© 2013 John Wiley & Sons, Ltd. Published 2013 by John Wiley & Sons, Ltd.

Table 7.1 Pharmacogenetic tests.

Disease	Test	Advice if the test is positive
Venous thrombosis	Mutated factor V Leiden gene	Avoid oral contraceptives since they may trigger venous thrombosis.
HIV	Variations in *HLA-B*5701* and *Hsp70-Hom* genes	Increased hypersensitivity reactions when using abacavir.
Maturity-onset diabetes of the young	Altered *Kir6.2* gene	Prescribe sulphonylurea instead of insulin.

Table 7.2 Types of variation in the human genome.

Genetic Variation	Abbreviation	Description	Frequency in human genome
Single nucleotide polymorphism	SNP	Variation in a DNA sequence that occurs when a single nucleotide is altered	12,000,000
Deletions/ Insertions		Deletion or insertion of between 1 to 1000 nucleotides	>1,000,000
Tandem repeats	TR	Microsatellites: tandem repeats of between 2 and 10 nucleotides.	>500,000
		Minisatellites: 10–100 nucleotides repeated.	
		Satellites: 100–1000 nucleotides repeated.	
Copy number variation	CNV	Deletion or multiplication of DNA segments larger than 1 kb	>1500 loci covering ~12% of the genome

'deserts'. SNPs account for approximately 80% of all genetic variation and two out of three SNPs involve substitution of cytosine with thymine.

Since approximately 95% of the human genome is classified as non-coding DNA, which includes 5' untranslated regions, promoters, 3' untranslated regions and introns, the vast majority of SNPs do not occur within coding regions. However, non-coding SNPs may influence gene splicing or the binding of transcription factors. When occurring within coding regions SNPs may alter the amino acid code (termed non-synonymous polymorphisms) or due to the redundancy of the genetic code have no effect on the encoded amino acid (synonymous or silent polymorphisms). Changes in amino acid are classified as conservative (minimal effect on protein structure or function) or non-conservative (dramatic effects on protein structure and function). Some SNPs result in a premature stop codon and are referred to as nonsense. Figure 7.1 illustrates two sequenced DNA fragments of the same gene from different individuals containing two

SNPs. In this case the C/T polymorphism (change from cytosine to thymine), produces a change in amino acid (in this case threonine to isoleucine), whereas the A/G SNP (adenine to guanine) is synonymous and has no effect on the encoded amino acid. In this chapter non-synonymous SNPs will be denoted as Thr3Ile where 3 is the amino acid number in the protein, Thr the 'wild-type' amino acid at that position, and Ile the amino acid variant produced by the SNP. Other forms of genetic variation include nucleotide deletions and insertions, tandem repeats and variable copy number (for more detail see Table 7.2).

7.2 Thiopurine S-methyltransferase and K⁺ channel polymorphisms

Thiopurine S-methyltransferase (TPMT) is a cytoplasmic enzyme which catalyses the S-methylation of thiopurine drugs such as 6-mercaptopurine and azathioprine.

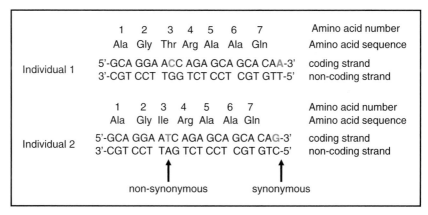

Figure 7.1 Single nucleotide polymorphisms.

These drugs, which are important in the treatment of childhood leukaemia and autoimmune diseases, have a narrow therapeutic range with elevated levels producing life-threatening toxicity. Two common non-synonymous single nucleotide polymorphisms (Ala154Thr and Tyr240Cys) have been identified within the TPMT gene leading to reduced levels of active TPMT protein. Patients who are homozygous for Thr[154] experience severe thiopurine toxicity and are generally prescribed much lower doses than patients with wild-type alleles. TPMT genetic variants represent a key example of how pharmacogenetics can be used to improve clinical treatment and as such genetic testing for TPMT polymorphisms is routine for patients taking thiopurine medication.

Cardiac K⁺ channel polymorphisms

The cardiac action potential involves an array of different ion channels which generate the inward and outward currents that are associated with the depolarising and repolarising phases, respectively. A variety of K⁺ channel proteins are responsible for the outward repolarising currents and any delay in repolarisation prolongs the cardiac action potential resulting in an increase in the QT interval observed in an ECG trace. Prolonging the action potential in this way can lead to life threatening arrhythmias.

Inherited long QT syndrome (LQTS) is an uncommon cardiac disorder associated with ventricular arrhythmias resulting from mutations in ion channel genes such as *HERG, KCNE1, KCNE2, KCNQ1 and SCN5A* (see Chapter 4). In contrast, acquired LQTS is a common disorder triggered by drugs and metabolic abnormalities. A wide variety of frequently prescribed drugs including antihistamines, antibiotics, antiarrhythmics and anticancer

drugs may trigger life-threatening arrhythmias by inhibiting cardiac potassium channels. It is now recognised that certain single nucleotide polymorphisms within cardiac ion channel genes increase an individual's susceptibility to drug-induced arrhythmias (see Table 7.3). For example the anti-bacterial drug sulphamethoxazole induces LQTS in patients who have the Thr8Ala SNP within the K⁺ channel subunit MiRP1 (Sesti et al., 2000). For reviews

Table 7.3 Polymorphisms in ion channels associated with cardiac arrhythmias.

Gene	Gene product	Polymorphisms
SCN5A (Na$_V$1.5)	Na⁺ channel, α subunit	Ser1102Tyr and His558Arg
HERG (K$_V$11.1)	K⁺ channel, α subunit[a]	Lys897Thr
KCNE2 (K$_V$β)	K⁺ channel, β subunit[a] (MiRP1)	Thr8Ala
KCNQ1 (K$_V$7.1)	K⁺ channel, α subunit[b] (KvLQT1)	Gly643Ser
KCNE1 ((K$_V$β)	K⁺ channel, β subunit[b] (mink)	Asp85Asn and Gly38Ser

[a]Assemble to form rapid delayed rectifier I$_{Kr}$ potassium channel.
[b]Assemble to form the slow delayed rectifier I$_{Ks}$ potassium channel. Ala: alanine, Arg: arginine, Asn: asparagine, Asp: aspartate, Gly: glycine, His: histidine, Lys: lysine, Ser: serine, Thr: threonine, Tyr: tyrosine

on the pharmacogenetics of cardiac potassium channels see Firouzi and Groenewegen (2003) and Escande (2000).

7.3 Polymorphisms affecting drug metabolism

The human genome project has resulted in increasing amounts of information becoming available on the existence of polymorphisms within human genes that encode for drug metabolising enzymes. These enzymes have evolved to help eliminate and detoxify xenobiotics such as prescribed drugs and toxins. However, before studying genetic polymorphisms in drug metabolising enzymes it is important to remember the key steps associated with drug metabolism. These are summarised in Figure 7.2.

Many drugs are metabolised either by Phase I, Phase II or both and therefore there are overlaps between the phases. Furthermore, some drugs are converted directly into non-toxic metabolites and because most of these inactive metabolites are water soluble they are eliminated

easily from the body. Depending on their chemical nature, metabolites are excreted via urine (predominant route), bile, breath or sweat. On other hand, some drugs are converted into intermediate metabolites which may be active or toxic to the body. Some of these intermediate metabolites are eventually converted into water soluble non-toxic metabolites which can easily be eliminated from the body, whereas others can be excreted as toxic metabolites. Overall, drug metabolism increases drug water solubility to aid renal excretion. Since the enzymes responsible for drug metabolism (mostly the CYP450 group) are proteins, they are potentially affected by genetic polymorphisms. In this section we will focus on the influence of CYP450 polymorphisms on drug metabolism.

As indicated above the CYP450s are the largest group of enzymes associated with drug metabolism accounting for 75-80% of total metabolism (Ingelman-Sundberg, 2004). The human genome project identified 57 genes encoding for CYP450 enzymes which have the following nomenclature; CYP followed by an Arabic number to indicate the gene family, a capital letter signifying the

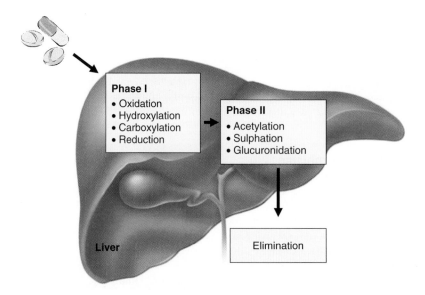

Figure 7.2 Principle steps involved in drug metabolism. Drug metabolism is predominantly carried out in the liver and involves two different types of chemical reaction called Phase I and Phase II. Phase I reactions generally involve the introduction of reactive groups into the target substrate via oxidation, reduction, carboxylation, and hydroxylation. The addition of hydroxyl groups catalysed by the cytochrome P450 (CYP450) family of enzymes is the most common form of Phase I modification. In Phase II the activated xenobiotics are conjugated to larger chemical groups to increase their water solubility and aid elimination. Such reactions include sulphation, methylation, acetylation, glucuronidation, glutathione and amino acid conjugation. Enzymes carrying out Phase II reactions include glutathione S-transferases (GSTs), N-acetyltransferases (NATs), UDP-glucuronosyltransferases (UGTs), sulfotransfereases (SULTs), and methyltransferases such as thiopurine S-methyltransferase (TPMT) and catechol O-methyl transferase (COMT). Genetic polymorphisms are found within enzymes associated with both Phase I and Phase II chemical reactions.

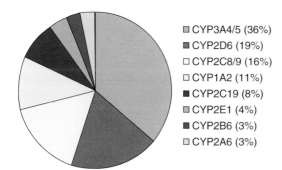

Figure 7.3 Percentage share of drugs metabolised by CYP450 isoenzymes.

subfamily and finally another number for the individual gene (e.g. CYP2D6). Three CYP families (namely CYP1, CYP2, and CYP3) are responsible for the majority of drug metabolism. The proportion of drugs metabolised by the various CYP450 isoenzymes is summarised in Figure 7.3.

Drugs can influence the activity of CYP450s either by inducing the biosynthesis of a particular isozyme or by directly inhibiting the activity of the enzyme. This can be a major cause of adverse drug reaction since if one drug inhibits CYP450 activity then a second drug may accumulate to toxic levels as a consequence of this. In fact, almost all inherited variability in pharmacokinetics is exclusively restricted to drug metabolism. Although it is well established that the variability in drug action is mainly due to the influence of polymorphisms, the understanding of how these genetic polymorphisms affect drug metabolism has only been made recently (see Chapter 8 regarding metabolism of drugs that target P-glycoprotein transporters).

Most drugs are usually metabolised in three main ways which are summarised in Figure 7.4. Drugs such as aspirin (acetylsalicylic acid) are initially converted to an active metabolite (salicylic acid) by hydrolysis (route 1). Salicylic acid is converted into several forms of inactive metabolite such as salicylglucuronide, salicyluricacid, and gentisic acid by conjugation (route 3). These inactive metabolites are eventually excreted. On the other hand, drugs such as phenytoin (an anti-convulsant drug) are converted directly into an inactive metabolite by reduction (route 2).

Most of the phase I and II enzymes fall in route 2, metabolising drugs into inactive metabolites that can be excreted. However, some CYP450 enzymes produce an active or toxic metabolite which can then be converted into inactive metabolites by route 3.

Interestingly, the enzymes (CYP450 group) that are involved in all three routes are subject to genetic polymorphisms with resultant variability in drug response (Lin and Lu, 2001). However it should be noted that there are considerable overlaps between different CYP450 groups of enzymes (see below); and therefore the effects of polymorphism may be masked by other enzymes compensating for the defect. Therefore, any clinical implications of changes in drug metabolism depend on (a) whether the biological effects (i.e. the activity of the drug or metabolite) lies with the affected drug or metabolite; (b) the importance of the pathway in overall activation/elimination; and (c) whether there is any overlapping substrate specificity of CYP450 groups of enzymes. Some examples of these are discussed below.

Scenario 1: Route 1 is the major pathway for drug elimination and it is affected by a polymorphism that results in **less active enzyme**.

In this scenario, the effects of genetic polymorphism would be dependent on whether the drug or its metabolite is active. If the drug is active and because it uses route 1 as the main pathway for elimination, it cannot be converted to a metabolite. Therefore drug will accumulate in the body resulting in toxic activity. A good example for this is metoprolol, a selective β_1 adrenergic receptor blocker used in the treatment of hypertension. The major route for metabolising this drug is by CYP2D6 (route 1). It has been found that poor metabolisers have a 5-fold higher risk of developing adverse effects during metoprolol treatment than patients who are not poor metabolisers (Chen et al., 2007).

On the other hand, if the metabolite produced from route 1 is active, then there will be diminished response, in other words, therapeutic failure. Proguanil is a biguanide derivative used in prophylactic anti-malarial treatment. This pro-drug is converted by the route 1 enzyme CYP2C19 to an active metabolite, cycloguanil pamoate. This active metabolite acts by preventing malaria parasites from reproducing once inside red blood cells. The genetic polymorphism of CYP2C19 would result in poor metabolisers of proguanil not responding to malaria prophylaxis or treatment.

Scenario 2: Routes 2 and 3 are the major pathways for drug elimination and they are affected by polymorphisms that result in **less active enzymes**.

In the above scenario, one would expect accumulation of the drug since route 2 is one of the major pathways of metabolism. However, this would not be the case because, although route 1 is the minor pathway in this scenario, the enzymes of route 1 would compensate for the affected pathway (route 2). Therefore, the drug would still be converted to an inactive metabolite. As explained before,

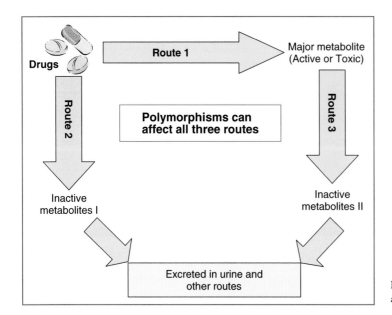

Figure 7.4 Routes in metabolism that are affected by genetic polymorphisms.

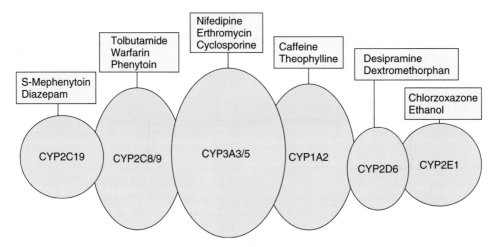

Figure 7.5 Schematic representation of overlapping substrate specificities amongst different CYP450 isoenzymes. Representative substrates for each CYP450 isoenzyme are listed above the respective circles. Due to the overlap between enzymes, the true effects of genetic polymorphisms are not phenotypically shown.

there is considerable overlap in the structural specificity of some of these enzymes amongst different routes. In other words, a drug may be a substrate for more than one enzyme in the various pathways. Figure 7.5 illustrates the overlap between CYP450 isoenzyme substrate specificity in humans. In scenario 2, if the metabolite is active then there would be exaggerated response due to the accumulation of active metabolite.

Scenario 3: Route 1 is the minor pathway for drug metabolism and it is affected by a polymorphism that results in a **less active enzyme**.

In this scenario, as route 1 is a minor pathway for drug elimination, there is less chance of drug accumulation as the enzymes in route 2 would compensate for the less active enzyme. Therefore, in the case of the drug being active the genetic polymorphism will not show any effects on drug metabolism e.g. the drug dapsone used in combination with rifampicin to treat leprosy. In contrast, in a situation where the metabolite is active there will be diminished drug response. A good example is the analgesic codeine. Since codeine is a pro-drug and dependant on route 1 for conversion into the metabolite morphine, genetic polymorphisms affecting route 1 would result in therapeutic failure of this drug.

Scenario 4: Route 1 is the minor pathway and route 3 is the major pathway for drug elimination. **Route 3 enzymes are affected by polymorphisms that result in poor metabolism**.

In this scenario, drug accumulation would not happen as route 1 is only a minor pathway for metabolism and is not affected by polymorphisms. A good example is caffeine, which is metabolised into various active intermediate metabolites such as paraxanthines, dimethyl and monomethyl uric acids, trimethyl- and dimethylallantoin, and uracil derivatives. Paraxanthines are produced via route 1 and they have marked pharmacological activity. Although further metabolism of paraxanthine is affected by genetic polymorphisms affecting the route 2 enzyme CYP1A2, this would not produce any adverse effects in individuals taking the therapeutic dose of caffeine, as paraxanthines only form a small fraction of all the metabolites of caffeine. However, in a situation where successful therapy depends upon the active metabolite of a pro-drug, genetic polymorphisms affecting route 2 would result in accumulation of an active metabolite and therefore has the potential to produce toxic effects.

These are some of the examples showing different scenarios of genetic polymorphisms and how they affect the pathways and result in poor metabolism. However, genetic polymorphisms do not always result in poor metabolism. In fact, there are four different types of

drug responders in the general population; (a) normal metabolisers (NM), those who are not affected by polymorphisms, and therefore respond to the therapeutic dose; (b) poor metabolisers (PM; generally lack the functional enzyme) for whom therapeutic dose will not produce expected results; (c) ultra-fast metabolisers (UM; generally have multiple gene copies) for whom the therapeutic dose would result in toxic effects; and (d) intermediate metabolisers (IM; either heterozygous for one deficient allele or carry two copies of the gene with reduced activity), although these individuals respond to therapeutic dose, any increase in dosage frequency would result in toxic effects. Therefore as mentioned previously, the clinical effects of altered metabolism are not only dependant on the enzymes affected by polymorphism but also dependant on whether the effects lie with the affected drug or the metabolite and the importance of the pathway in overall activation/elimination. Figure 7.6 shows the clinical implications of polymorphisms affecting drug metabolism.

The following are two examples (see Tables 7.4 and 7.5) to show how the clinical outcomes of drugs would be affected in different types of metabolisers. Table 7.4 shows the effects of nortriptyline, a second-generation tricyclic antidepressant, which is metabolised in the liver by CYP2D6 into an inactive metabolite hydroxy-nortriptyline. Approximately 6-10% of Caucasians are poor metabolisers and might experience more adverse effects than normal metabolisers. In these individuals the normal dosage regimen would result in drug accumulation. Therefore, a lower dosage is often necessary in these individuals. Likewise, extensive metabolisers of nortriptyline inactivate the drug faster than usual and this therefore results in therapeutic failure (Table 7.4).

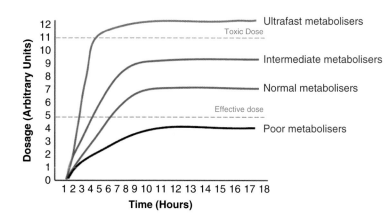

Figure 7.6 Therapeutic implications of polymorphisms affecting drug metabolism. PM; poor metabolisers, Metabolisers, NM; normal metabolisers, IM; intermediate metabolisers, UM; ultra-fast.

Table 7.4 Clinical effects of CYP2D6 genetic polymorphisms where the drug is active (e.g. nortriptyline).

CYP2D6 status	Relief of depression	Adverse reactions	Overall response
Normal metaboliser	Yes	No	Therapeutic success
Extensive Metaboliser	No	No	Therapeutic failure due to reduced efficacy
Poor Metaboliser	Yes	Yes	Therapeutic failure due to toxic effects

Table 7.5 Clinical effects of CYP2D6 genetic polymorphisms where the metabolite is active (e.g. codeine).

CYP2D6 status	Pain relief	Adverse reactions	Overall response
Normal metaboliser	Yes	No	Therapeutic success
Extensive Metaboliser	Yes	Yes	Therapeutic failure due to toxic effects
Poor Metaboliser	No	No	Therapeutic failure due to reduced efficacy

On the other hand, codeine, an analgesic, is considered as a pro-drug which depends on CYP2D6 activity to be converted to the active metabolite morphine for it to be effective. Approximately 6-10% of the Caucasian population, 2% of Asians, and 1% of Arabs are poor metabolisers and therefore codeine is less effective as an analgesic in these patients. Conversely, the extensive metabolisers will produce morphine from codeine at faster rates than in normal metabolisers and this produces toxic effects (Table 7.5).

The examples illustrated in Tables 7.4 and 7.5 show the clinical implications of genetic polymorphism depend mainly on whether the drug or the metabolite is active as well as the importance of the respective metabolic pathway. Some other examples of polymorphism affecting different CYP450 enzymes and their clinical outcomes are given in Table 7.6.

It should be noted that genetic polymorphisms in drug metabolising enzymes are not exclusive to the hepatic CYP450 family of enzymes. Other important drug metabolising enzymes display polymorphisms. A good example is plasma cholinesterase which is a non-specific enzyme found in the plasma. It is responsible for the metabolism by acetylation of the depolarising muscle relaxant, suxamethonium (Lockridge, 1990). Certain individuals have a single amino acid substitution due to a SNP. This results in altered enzyme activity, with significantly slower metabolism of the drug and prolonged neuromuscular blockade. These patients may remain paralysed for many hours after a standard dose of suxamethonium, and must be kept anaesthetised and ventilated until the suxamethonium has been eliminated by other, slower methods.

In summary genetic polymorphisms in drug metabolising enzymes can have dramatic affects on the therapeutic regimen. That is, given different drug metabolism genotypes, the same dose of a drug can lead to variable results in patients. Compared with most other genes, the extent of polymorphism is higher in genes encoding for enzymes that metabolise drugs and other xenobiotics. Therefore an understanding of the functional significance of these polymorphisms is essential in formulating drug therapy. This would enhance the transition from evidenced-based prescribing to an individual-based approach. Indeed, clinical trials researchers use genetic tests for variations in CYP450 genes to screen and

Table 7.6 Polymorphism affecting different CYP450 enzymes and their clinical outcomes.

CYP450 Enzyme	Drug type	Adverse reaction	
		In slow metabolisers	In fast metabolisers
CYP1A2	Clozapine (atypical anti-psychotic)		Tardive dyskinesia (a slow progressing disorder resulting in involuntary, repetitive body movements)
CYP2C9	Warfarin (anti-coagulant)	Haemorrhage	
	Tolbutamide (K^+ channel blocker used to treat type II diabetes)	Hypoglycaemia	
	Phenytoin (anti-epileptic)	Phenytoin toxicity	
	Losartan (AT_1 receptor antagonist)	Decreased anti-hypertensive effect	
	Gilipizide (K^+ channel blocker used to treat type II diabetes)	Hypoglycaemia	
CYP2C19	Diazepam	Prolonged sedation	
	Anti-arrhythmics	Arrhythmias	
	β-adrenergic receptor antagonists (beta-blockers)	Bradycardia	
	Tricyclic anti-depressants	Toxicity	Loss of efficacy
	Codeine	In-efficacy of codeine as an analgesic	Narcotic side-effects, dependence

monitor patients. In addition, many pharmaceutical companies screen their chemical compounds to see how well they are metabolised by variant forms of CYP450 enzymes (see Chapter 8 regarding metabolism of drugs that target P-glycoprotein transporters).

7.4 Methods for detecting genetic polymorphisms

As we have seen already in this chapter genetic polymorphisms are a major cause of individual differences in drug response. The effects of other factors such as age, gender, weight and race related physiological functioning and concomitant disease on pharmacokinetics have been well established. Although it is estimated that 20 to 95% of individual variability is genetic-based, until now, the genotype of the patient has been the major unknown factor in clinical practice. This section summarises different methods that are currently available to detect genetic polymorphisms.

Genetic polymorphisms can be detected either by: (a) functional (or metabolic) phenotyping or (b) genotyping.

Functional phenotyping is carried out by administering a probe drug or substrate and measuring the metabolites and/or clinical outcomes. The principal steps of functional phenotyping are illustrated in Figure 7.7.

Functional phenotyping is only suitable for detecting polymorphisms within drug metabolising enzymes and for those polymorphisms which have measurable functional consequences. Other limitations of this approach are (a) it requires repeated sample collection from the individual being tested and is therefore labour intensive; (b) it involves the risk of developing undesirable effects to the directly administered drug (in case of poor metabolisers); and (c) it is difficult to detect and locate the drug and its metabolite, if there is a simultaneous administration of other drugs.

In contrast, genotyping involves the determination of individual DNA sequence differences for a particular trait. Commonly used genotyping methods are gel electrophoresis-based techniques such as polymerase chain reaction (PCR) coupled with restriction fragment length polymorphism analysis (RFLP), multiplex PCR, and allele-specific amplification. These are direct approaches for phenotype prediction, allowing, at the

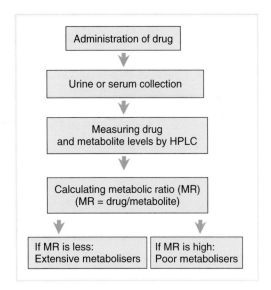

Figure 7.7 Functional phenotyping to detect genetic polymorphisms. Functional phenotyping is mainly useful for detecting polymorphisms in drug metabolism; where accumulation of the drug or metabolite indicates whether the affected individuals are poor or extensive metabolisers.

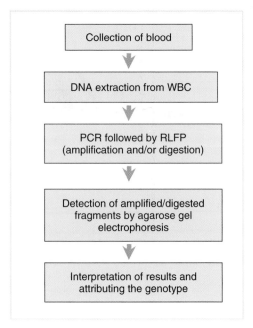

Figure 7.8 Genotyping using PCR coupled with RFLP. PCR-based genotyping would identify whether the affected individuals are homozygous or heterozygous for the polymorphism.

same time, the identification of heterozygote mutant alleles and the detection of 95% of the poor metabolisers. Some of these methods are explained below.

PCR-RFLP analysis

Traditional genotyping methods involve PCR-based analysis combined with restriction fragment length polymorphism (RFLP); the main steps of which are summarised in Figure 7.8. This method is simple to use in any laboratory. For example PCR-RFLP analysis of the $5HT_{2A}$ receptor is shown in Figure 7.9. In this case a SNP occurs at position 102 within the $5\text{-}HT_{2A}$ receptor gene resulting in cytosine being replaced with thymine (102T/C polymorphism). Genotyping of the $5\text{-}HT_{2A}$ receptor 102T/C polymorphism can be carried out by PCR followed by *MspI* restriction enzyme digestion since the polymorphism results in the formation of a restriction site at position 102 (102C; see Figure 7.9a). This site is absent in the wild-type $5\text{-}HT_{2A}$ receptor (102T).

In order to identify the polymorphism, DNA is isolated from peripheral blood lymphocytes and the region of interest, a 342 base pair (bp) genomic fragment that corresponds to nucleotides −24 to +318 of the $5\text{-}HT_{2A}$ receptor gene, is amplified by PCR. The PCR product (342 bp fragment) is then subjected to restriction digest using the *Msp I* enzyme and the fragments analysed by

agarose gel electrophoresis. After gel electrophoresis an uncut fragment of 342 bp would represent the wild type $5HT_{2A}$ receptor. On the other hand, the presence of digested products of 216 bp and 126 bp would show the existence of the $5\text{-}HT_{2A}$ receptor polymorphism.

As shown in Figure 7.9b, the results would not only show the presence of an SNP but also reveal information about the genetic trait. For instance, if the individual is homozygous for 102C, two products of 126 and 216 bps would be evident (lane 1). The RFLP of a heterozygous individual would show all three (342, 216 and 126 bps) products (lane 2). Likewise, the RFLP of a wild type individual would only show a 342 bp product. Although PCR-RFLP analysis is considered as a traditional method, it is still used to detect known polymorphisms even in clinical studies. The major disadvantage of PCR-RFLP is that it is only useful for detecting one polymorphism per assay.

Large-scale SNP analysis

Most of the large-scale SNP analyses are carried out by fluorescent dye-based high-throughput genotyping procedures. A variety of methods including oligonucleotide ligation assay, direct heterozygote sequencing, and TaqMan® allelic discrimination have been used to detect

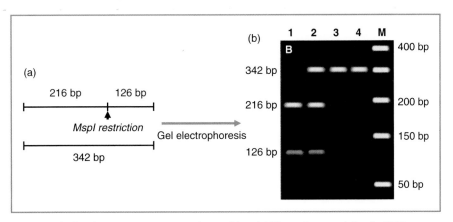

Figure 7.9 PCR-RLFP method to detect $5HT_{2A}$ receptor polymorphism. (a) The region containing the $5HT_{2A}$ receptor polymorphism (342 bp fragment) is shown. This region is amplified by PCR. The existence of an SNP would produce a restriction site for Msp I enzyme and therefore produce two shorter fragments (216 and 126 bps). (b) Typical RFLP patterns for Msp I restriction enzyme treated PCR products analysed by agarose gel electrophoresis. Lane 1: homozygous $5HT_{2A}$ SNP (102C +/+); Lane 2: heterozygous $5HT_{2A}$ (102T/C); Lane 3: homozygous $5HT_{2A}$ wild-type (102T +/+); Lane 4: Positive control (not treated with MsP I; Lane M = DNA ladder.

SNP. High-density chip array and mass spectrometry technologies are the newest advances in the genotyping field, but their wide application is yet to be developed. Novel mutations/polymorphisms also can be identified by conformation-based mutation screening.

A brief explanation of the basic principles behind allele specific primer extension (ASPE) assay to detect polymorphisms is described below. ASPE is carried out by converging techniques such as DNA denaturation, PCR, hybridisation, and fluorescent emission analysis. In ASPE, the SNP (or point mutation) in the DNA sequence is used as the marker for allele-specific gene expression analysis. Initially, genomic DNA is denatured and subject to PCR with specific primers incorporating the SNP (step 1; Figure 7.10). Two probes are designed for each SNP. Each is a perfect match to one of the expected SNP alleles, with the nucleotide matching the polymorphic base at the 3' end. The 5' end of each probe carries a unique tag (step 2; Figure 7.10). The PCR products are then incubated with specific anti-tags corresponding to respective tags that are incorporated into each SNP (step 3; Figure 7.10). After several stringent washes, the mean fluorescent intensities are analysed by a detection system which is designed to identify each PCR product by its fluorescent emission. The intensity detected for a pair of SNP probes is used to calculate an 'allele ratio' and interpreted as a genotype (step 4; Figure 7.10).

7.5 Genetic variation in drug transporters

Drug transporters are predominantly expressed in the intestine, liver, kidney and brain, and as such are extremely important players in drug pharmacokinetics influencing absorption, distribution and elimination. Drug transporters work in conjunction with enzyme-based detoxification systems to remove xenobiotics. The completion of the human genome project resulted in the identification of a large number of membrane-spanning proteins involved in endogenous compound and drug transport which can be divided into two major groups. The first group includes members of the solute carrier (SLC) transporter superfamily, which facilitate the influx or efflux of a wide range of compounds without the use of ATP. The second major group of transporters are the multi-drug resistance (MDR) ATP binding cassette (ABC) proteins which carry out ATP-dependent drug efflux. Table 7.7 shows the main drug transporter families highlighting their distribution and example drug substrates. It is now recognised that genetic polymorphisms within drug transporters can contribute to individual variability in drug response. This section will highlight some examples of drug transporter pharmacogenomics. For comprehensive reviews on this topic see Kerb (2006) and Mizuno et al. (2003).

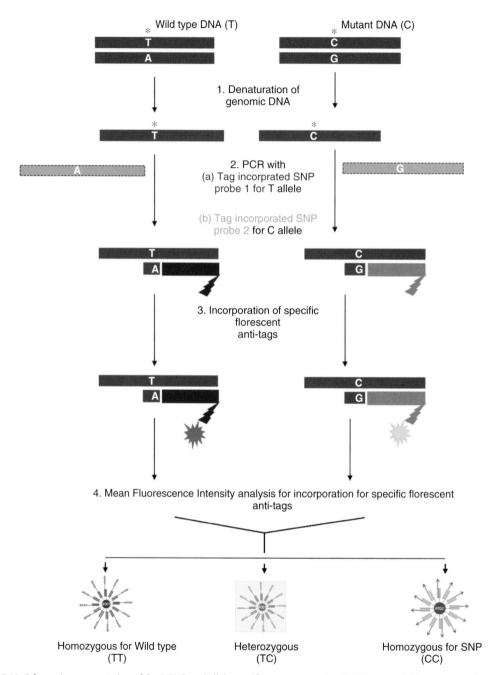

Figure 7.10 Schematic representation of the PCR-based allele specific primer extension (ASPE) assay. This scheme explains the basic concepts behind ASPE. Step 1 and 2: Genomic DNA is denatured and subject to PCR with two specific primers incorporating the two SNP alleles at the 3' end. These primers contain specific tags at the 5' end. Step 3: PCR products are then incubated with specific anti-tags corresponding to respective tags Step 4: mean fluorescent intensities are analysed by a detection system.

Table 7.7 Human drug transporter families.

Transporter family	Protein members	Distribution	Example of drug substrate
Multi-drug Resistance Transporter (MDR1) (*P*-glycoprotein)	MDR1	Liver, Kidney, Intestine, Blood–brain barrier, Lymphocytes, Placenta	See Table 7.8.
Multi-drug Resistance Associated Proteins (MRP)	MRP1	Ubiquitous	Methotrexate
	MRP2	Liver, Kidney, Intestine,	Glibenclamide
	MRP3	Liver, Kidney, Intestine,	Etoposide
	MRP4	Ubiquitous	Methotrexate
	MRP5	Ubiquitous	Adefovir
Organic Anion Transporters (OAT)	OAT1	Kidney, Brain, Placenta	Methotrexate
	OAT2	Kidney, Liver	Tetracyclines
	OAT3	Kidney, Brain, Muscle	Cimetidine
	OAT4	Kidney, Placenta	Aspirin
Organic Cation Transporter (OCT)	OCT1	Liver	Verapamil
	OCT2	Kidney	Cimetidine
	OCT3	Liver, Kidney, Heart	Catecholamines
Organic Anion Transporting Polypeptide (OATP)[a]	OATP1A2	Brain, Liver, Kidney	Oubain
	OATP1B1	Liver	Statins
	OATP1B3	Liver	Digoxin
	OATP2B1	Ubiquitous	Benzylpenicillin

[a]The human genome contains 11 OATP genes.

Multi-drug resistance protein MDR1 (*P*-glycoprotein)

Multi-drug resistance protein MDR1 (*P*-glycoprotein) is the most widely studied drug efflux transporter. It displays broad substrate specificity and is responsible for the development of resistance to anti-cancer drugs due to decreased drug accumulation within the target tissue as a consequence of increased *P*-glycoprotein expression (Table 7.8). To combat drug resistance there is considerable interest in the development of *P*-glycoprotein transporter inhibitors to combat drug resistance in cancer patients. Although several compounds have undergone clinical trials none are in current clinical use.

Genetic variability of the MDR1 transporter (*P*-glycoprotein)

At present more than 50 single nucleotide polymorphisms have been reported for the MDR1 gene. The three most common MDR1 SNPs and their frequency in different ethnic groups are detailed in Table 7.9. The synonymous polymorphism in exon 26 (C3435T) is in linkage

Table 7.8 Some key drug substrates of the *P*-glycoprotein.

Category	Drug substrates
Anti-cancer drugs	Daunorubicin, Doxorubicin, Vinblastine, Vincristine
Antibiotics	Cefazolin, Cefoperazon, Erythromycin, Levofloxacin
Ca^{2+} channel blockers	Diltiazem, Mibefradil, Nicardipine, Verapamil
β_1-blockers	Bunitrolol, Celiprolol, Talinolol
Anti-histamines	Terfenidine, Cimetidine, Ranitidine
Lipid-lowering drugs	Atorvastatin, Lovastatin, Simvastatin
Steroids	Aldesterone, Dexamethasone, Hydrocortisone

disequilibrium (a measure of how often alleles are inherited together) with the other two common SNPs C1236T and G2677T and together they form a common haplotype.

Table 7.9 Common exon-located MDR1 (*P*-glycoprotein) variants.

Nucleotide Position	Location	Effect	Allelic frequency (%)		
			Ca	As	AA
C1236T	Exon 12	Synonymous	45	69	26
G2677T/A	Exon 21	Ala893Ser/Thr	46/2	45/7	>1
C3435T	Exon 26	Synonymous	56	40	10

Abbreviations: AA; African Americans, As; Asians, Ca; Caucasians, A; adenine, C; cytosine, G; guanine, T; thymine, Ala; alanine, Ser; serine, Thr; threonine. Data from Kerb (2006) Cancer Letters 234: 4–33.

Although synonymous SNPs are generally considered to be 'silent' there is evidence that they may influence protein translation and folding. This may be the case with the C3435T variant which appears to influence protein conformation and hence substrate interactions (Kimchi-Sarfaty et al., 2007). Many studies have investigated the clinical influence of the C3435T and G2677T/A variants on *P*-glycoprotein expression levels and drug disposition. Although, much of the data is inconclusive there are some interesting and important examples illustrating how *P*-glycoprotein SNPs can influence clinical outcome to drug therapy (see Table 7.10). For a comprehensive review on the pharmacogenetics of the *P*-glycoprotein transporter see Kerb (2006).

Multi-drug resistance associated protein (MRP) transporters

This family of membrane transporters, which mediate the ATP-dependent drug efflux, contains several members which differ in their substrate specificity, tissue distribution and cellular location (see Table 7.7). MRP1 is expressed in many cell types and is associated with resistance to anti-cancer drugs due to over-expression of the protein in cancer cells resulting in increased drug efflux.

MRP2 has a more limited tissue distribution and is found on the apical membrane of hepatocytes and epithelial cells of the renal proximal tubule and intestine. As such MRP2 is associated with drug elimination from the body. To date more than 50 SNPs have been reported for the MRP2 transporter including the -24C/T variant which occurs within the 5'-UTR and appears to influence MRP2 expression levels. Pharmacogenetic studies indicate that the -24C/T variant is associated with higher methotrexate plasma levels and liver toxicity in patients treated for acute lymphoblastic leukaemia (Gradland and Kim, 2008).

Organic anion-transporting polypeptide (OATP) transporters

One of the most widely studied members of the organic anion-transporting polypeptide transporter family is the liver-specific OATP1B1 transporter (alias OATP-C). This

Table 7.10 Clinical impact of *P*-glycoprotein variants.

Drug Response	Associated Polymorphism	Ethnic group (study size)
Anti-epileptic therapy: drug resistance	3435C	CA (315)
Drug toxicity: cyclosporine nephrotoxicity	3435TT	CA (97)
AML treatment: decreased survival rate	1236C/2677G/3435C	CA (405)
HIV treatment: better recovery after anti-retroviral therapy	3435T	CA (123)

Abbreviations: AML; acute myeloblastic leukaemia, CA; Caucasian, 3435TT; genotype containing two 3435T alleles.

transporter is involved in the uptake into the liver of a wide variety of clinically important therapeutics including pravastatin, a member of the statin family of cholesterol-lowering compounds. Statins reduce cholesterol levels by inhibiting HMG-CoA reductase, which is the rate limiting enzyme in cholesterol biosynthesis in the liver. Although very successful and widely prescribed (4 million adults take statins in the UK alone!) there are a number of serious side effects associated with statins including neuropathy, muscle weakness and memory loss.

Several functionally relevant SNPs within the OATP1B1 gene have been identified that influence substrate specificity and transporter protein expression levels (for a comprehensive review see Ieiri et al., 2009). One notable SNP occurs at nucleotide position 521 (T/C) and produces a switch in amino acid at position 174 from valine (wild-type) to alanine with the functional consequence of reduced transporter activity. Several studies have examined the influence of OATP1B1 transporter SNPs on statin responses. For example, following a single oral dose of pravastatin, patients with alanine at position 174 in OATP1B1 displayed a reduced clearance rate (and hence higher serum-concentration) compared to patients with the valine[174] allele (Nishizato et al., 2003). Hence SNPs within the OATP1B1 gene may account in part for the individual variability in the therapeutic effects of pravastatin and related compounds.

7.6 Genetic variation in G protein coupled receptors

Polymorphisms have been identified in both the coding and non-coding regions of many GPCR genes. Given the prominent clinical role of GPCR based pharmaceuticals there is considerable interest in understanding how genetic variants of GPCRs modify receptor pharmacology, expression, desensitisation and signal transduction. In this section we will illustrate how SNPs can influence clinically important GPCR targets with particular emphasis on the adrenergic receptor family. Examples of SNPs modifying GPCR function are listed in Table 7.11. For comprehensive reviews on GPCR polymorphisms and their influence on human disease and therapeutic drug response see Insel et al. (2007) and Rana et al. (2001).

Genetic variation within the adrenergic receptor family

Adrenergic receptors (AR) are the protein targets for adrenaline and noradrenaline released either from adrenal glands or following activation of the sympathetic nervous system. There are nine subtypes of human adrenergic receptors which are classified into three main groups; the α_1-ARs, α_2-ARs and the β-ARs with each group containing three subtypes. The nine subtypes being as follows; α_{1A}-, α_{1B}-, α_{1D}-, α_{2A}-, α_{2B}-, α_{2C}-, β_1-, β_2-, and β_3-AR. The classification of adrenergic receptors was summarised in

Table 7.11 Examples of single nucleotide polymorphisms influencing GPCR function.

GPCR	Polymorphism (location)	Effect on receptor function
5-HT_{2C}	Cys23Ser (N)	Ser[23] variant has a lower affinity for agonists compared to wild-type Cys[23]. Schizophrenic patients with Ser[23] respond less well to the antagonist clozapine.
5-HT_{1A}	Gly22Ser (N)	Decreased receptor down-regulation
MOR	Asn40Asp (N)	Increased agonist-binding affinity
P2Y_2	Arg334Cys (C)	Extra palmitoylation site
CCR2	Val64Ile (N)	Decrease in AIDS progression
D4	Val194Gly (TM)	Decreased agonist binding
D4	−521 (Promoter)*	Decreased transcriptional activity

Abbreviations: Arg; arginine, Asn; asparagine; Asp; aspartate, Cys; cysteine, Gly; glycine, Gln; glutamine, Glu; glutamate, Ile; isoleucine, Ser; serine, Val; valine. CCR2; chemokine receptor 2, D4; dopamine D4 receptor, MOR; μ-opioid receptor. N = amino-terminus, C = caroboxyl terminus, TM = transmembrane domain. * Nucleotide position within the gene and is based on the first nucleotide of the starting codon being +1.

Table 7.12 Clinical use of adrenergic receptor ligands.

Receptor	Use
α_1 antagonists	Symptomatic treatment of Benign prostatic hyperplasia and hypertension
α_1 agonists	Shock, hypotension and nasal congestion
α_2 agonists	Anaesthesia and pain, hypertension
β_1 antagonists	Heart failure and hypertension
β_2 agonists	Asthma
β_3 agonists	Overactive bladder syndrome

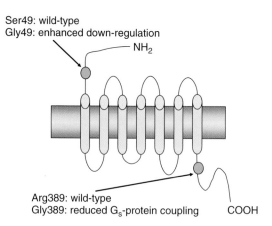

Figure 7.11 Functional β_1-adrenergic receptor single nucleotide polymorphisms.

Table 3.2 (Chapter 3). Virtually every cell type in the body expresses one or more adrenergic receptor subtype and they represent important therapeutic targets for a range of diseases. For example, the β_2AR agonists are commonly used to treat asthma, whereas β_1AR antagonists or 'β-blockers' are frequently used to treat chronic heart disease and hypertension. There is also considerable interest in the development of selective β_3AR agonists for the treatment of overactive bladder syndrome. The clinical use of adrenergic receptor ligands is summarised in Table 7.12.

β_1-adrenergic receptor single nucleotide polymorphisms

β_1ARs are abundantly expressed in the heart where they mediate increases in heart rate and contractility in response to the endogenous catecholamines noradrenaline and adrenaline. Given their prominent role in regulating cardiovascular function there is considerable interest in understanding how β_1AR SNPs influence the clinical response to β_1AR antagonists. Two major non-synonymous SNPs have been identified within the coding region of the β_1AR; one within the amino terminus of the receptor at amino acid number 49 which changes the major allele serine to glycine (Ser49Gly) and the other located within the carboxyl terminus at amino acid 389 which changes arginine to glycine (Arg389Gly). There is a strong linkage disequilibrium (a measure of how often alleles are inherited together) between these two sites which generates a set of defined haplotypes. Gly^{49} is always linked with Arg^{389}, whereas Ser^{49} is always associated with Gly^{389}. There are 11 other non-synonymous SNP changes within the β_1AR coding region and three SNP in the 5'-promoter region but the functional significance of these

are not known. β_1AR SNPs are summarised in Figure 7.11 and Table 7.13. It is important to remember that there are marked variations in the frequency of SNPs between different ethnic groups of the human population. This is particularly relevant when investigating clinical responses in specific patient groups.

The consequences of the Ser49Gly and Arg389Gly variants on β_1AR function have been explored in transfected cell systems using recombinant 'wild-type' and variant receptors generated by site-directed mutagenesis. However because of the strong linkage disequilibrium between these two sites results from studies exploring one SNP site *in vitro* are sometimes difficult to compare to results obtained *in vivo* or *ex vivo*. The Arg^{389} β_1AR variant is associated with a greater activation of adenylyl cyclase (presumably via enhanced G_s-protein coupling) and hence cAMP production compared to the Gly^{389} variant. The Arg^{389} variant also displays greater short-term agonist-induced desensitisation compared to the Gly^{389} form. Both the Ser^{49} and Gly^{49} alleles display comparable agonist and antagonist binding affinities together with similar activation of adenylyl cyclase. However, the Gly^{49} variant is down-regulated by prolonged agonist activation (24 h exposure) significantly more than the Ser^{49} variant. Similar functional studies have also been performed using recombinant β_1AR haplotypes (Ser^{49}Arg^{389}, Gly^{49}Arg^{389}, Ser^{49}Gly^{389}, and Gly^{49}Gly^{389}). As may be expected the Gly^{49}Arg^{389} variant desensitised the greatest, whereas the Ser^{49}Gly^{389} desensitised the least.

Given the prominent role of the β_1AR in regulating heart rate and cardiac muscle contractility several studies have used transgenic mice to explore the cardiovascular

Table 7.13 Functional β_1-adrenergic single nucleotide polymorphisms.

SNP	Amino acid position	Common → minor allele	Frequencies of the minor allele			
			Caucasians	African-Americans	Asians	Latino-Hispanics
A145G	49	Ser → Gly	0.12–0.16	0.13–0.15	0.15	0.20–0.21
C1165G	389	Arg → Gly	0.24–0.34	0.39–0.46	0.20–0.30	0.31–0.33

SNP; single nucleotide polymorphism (position of nucleotide within the gene), Arg; arginine, Gly; glycine, Ser; serine. A; adenine, C; cytosine, G; guanine. Data from Leineweber and Heusch (2009) British Journal of Pharmacology 158: 61–69.

consequences of the Arg[389] and Gly[389] variants *in vivo*. Mialet Perez et al. (2003) generated transgenic mice that specifically over-expressed homozygous Arg[389] or Gly[389] β_1AR variants in the heart. Mice expressing the Arg[389] β_1AR developed a complete loss of heart muscle contractile response to the β_1AR agonist dobutamine at 6 months of age compared to non-transgenic and Gly[389] β_1AR mice. This is notable since the loss of β_1AR-induced inotropic response is a recognised hall-mark of heart failure and validates the use of transgenic animal models to study *in vivo* the potential consequences of β_1ARs SNPs.

Whilst of great interest studies using transgenic animals do not answer the important question of whether β_1AR SNPs influence cardiac responses to β-agonists/antagonists in humans? To address this several approaches have been used including the use of *ex vivo* human heart tissue obtained from patients having coronary artery bypass grafting surgery. Such studies have shown enhanced ionotropic responses to β_1AR agonists in heart tissue obtained from patients with the Arg[389] β_1AR variant. The effect of β_1AR SNPs on cardiovascular responses *in vivo* have also been explored and significantly greater increases in heart rate and contractility in response to the β_1-AR agonist dobutamine have been reported in subjects homozygous for Arg[389] β_1AR (Figure 7.12).

Are β_1AR SNPs risk factors for heart failure?

Several studies have explored whether β_1AR SNPs are risk factors for heart failure. During chronic heart failure there is increased noradrenaline release from sympathetic nerve terminals in an attempt to improve heart rate and cardiac muscle contractility. Paradoxically, the increase in noradrenaline release exacerbates the situation by causing further down-regulation of β_1AR expression. Remember

when GPCRs are activated for prolonged periods of time they become down-regulated (see Chapter 3). Hence, it is conceivable that the presence of the Arg[389] β_1AR variant may make the situation even worse due to the enhanced signalling and down-regulation associated with the Arg[389] β_1AR. However, studies to date indicate that there is no association between Arg389Gly and/or Ser49Gly β_1AR polymorphisms and the risk of developing heart failure or the clinical outcome of heart failure.

β_1AR SNPs and response to β-blockers

Since β_1AR antagonists are widely used for the treatment of hypertension and chronic heart failure several studies have investigated whether the Arg389Gly and/or Ser49Gly β_1AR SNPs influence the clinical response to β-blockers. Such studies have produced conflicting results. One study explored the relationship between β_1-AR SNPs and the anti-hypertensive response to the β-blocker metoprolol (Johnson et al., 2003). Patients who were homozygous for the Ser[49]Gly[389] haplotype responded significantly better than patients who carried the haplotype pair Gly[49]Arg[389]/Ser[49]Gly[389]. These differences may in part explain the marked variation in hypertensive patient response to 'β-blockers' with between 30-60% of patients not responding adequately to the treatment. A number of studies have also reported beneficial effects of the Arg[389] and Ser[49] β_1AR variants on the clinical response to chronic β-blocker therapy in chronic heart failure patients.

Studies have also been performed to determine if Arg389Gly and/or Ser49Gly β_1AR SNPs modify the long-term survival rates of chronic heart failure patients treated with β-blockers. One study has indicated that patients with Gly[49] have better five-year survival rate compared to patients who are homozygous for Ser[49]. Overall it would appear that β_1AR SNPs are not risk factors for

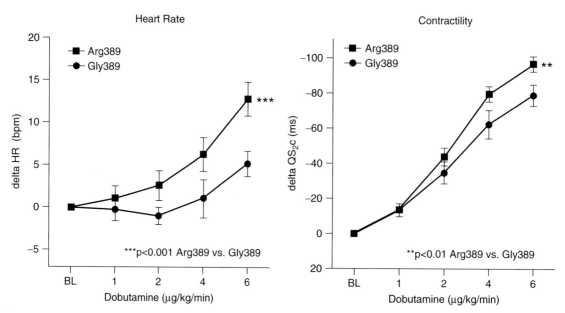

Figure 7.12 Dobutamine infusion-induced changes in heart rate and cardiac muscle contractility in male subjects homozygous for Arg[389] or Gly[389] β_1AR. Reprinted from Pharmacology and Therapeutics 117: Brodde O-E, β_1 and β_2 adrenoceptor polymorphisms: functional importance, impact on cardiovascular diseases and drug responses, 1–29 (2008) with permission from Elsevier.

developing chronic heart failure but they may influence treatment with β-blockers and long-term survival rates following therapy. In the future genotyping of the β_1AR may represent a useful method of predicting responses to β-blockers in patients with chronic heart failure and hypertension.

β_2-adrenergic receptor single nucleotide polymorphisms

To date more than 80 SNPs have been reported for the human β_2AR gene of which four have been extensively studied (Figure 7.13 and Table 7.14). There is strong linkage disequilibrium between the four prominent β_2AR SNPs. For example, Arg[-19] usually occurs with Gly[16], Cys[-19] with either Arg[16] or Gly[16], Glu[27] usually with Gly[16], Gln[27] with either Arg[16] or Gly[16], and finally Ile[164] with Gly[16] and Gln[27].

β_2AR SNPs within the coding region

The Arg16Gly and Gln27Glu single nucleotide polymorphisms which are located within the amino-terminus of the β_2AR do not influence agonist/antagonist binding or adenylyl cyclase activation. However, they do show marked differences in their propensity to undergo agonist-induced receptor down-regulation. The presence

of glycine at position 16 appears to enhance β_2AR down-regulation compared to arginine at this position. In contrast the Glu[27] polymorphism is resistant to agonist-induced receptor down-regulation. What about β_2ARs containing the haplotype pair Gly[16]Glu[27]? These receptors also undergo agonist-induced down-regulation suggesting that Gly[16] is dominant over Glu[27].

The Thr164Ile polymorphism which is located in the fourth transmembrane spanning domain (TMIV) of the receptor reduces agonist binding affinity. This is not surprising given the location of the Thr164Ile SNP within TMIV, a region of the receptor involved in ligand binding. The Ile[164] variant activates adenylyl cyclase less effectively than Thr[164] due to reduced G_s-protein coupling. The rare Val34Met SNP does not appear to modify receptor function and at present the Ser220Cys SNP has not been explored.

β_2AR SNPs within the non-coding region

Of the eight β_2AR SNPs identified within the 5' UTR region the variant at position −47 has received the most attention. Interestingly this SNP is located within a short reading frame sequence found in the 5' region of the β_2AR gene which encodes for the *Beta Upstream Peptide* (BUP; 19 amino acids in length). The thymine to cytosine switch at position −47 results in the carboxyl-terminal

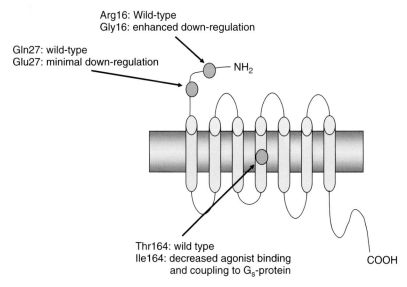

Arg16: Wild-type
Gly16: enhanced down-regulation

Gln27: wild-type
Glu27: minimal down-regulation

NH$_2$

Thr164: wild type
Ile164: decreased agonist binding
and coupling to G$_s$-protein

COOH

Figure 7.13 β_2-adrenergic receptor single nucleotide polymorphisms.

Table 7.14 Functional β_2-adrenergic receptor polymorphisms.

SNP	Amino acid position	Common → minor allele	Frequencies of the minor allele (%)			
			Caucasians	African-Americans	Asians	Latino-Hispanics
C-47T	−19	Cys → Arg	0.35	0.21	0.08–0.12	n.d.
A46G	16	Gly → Arg[a]	0.38–0.46	0.49–0.51	0.54–0.59	n.d.
C79G	27	Gln → Glu	0.35–0.46	0.20–0.27	0.07–0.20	n.d.
C491T	164	Thr → Ile	0.02–0.04	0.02–0.04	0–0.01	0.3

[a]In African-Americans and Asians, Arg is the major allele. SNP; single nucleotide polymorphism (position of nucleotide within the gene), Arg; arginine, Cys; cysteine, Gln; glutamine, Glu; glutamate, Gly; glycine, Thr; threonine, and Ile; isoleucine. A; adenine, C; cytosine, G; guanine, T; thymine, n.d. not determined. Data from Leineweber and Heusch (2009) British Journal of Pharmacology 158: 61–69.

cysteine^{-19} being replaced with arginine. The BUP regulates the cellular expression of the β_2AR by controlling mRNA translation and the Arg^{-19} variant results in lower levels of receptor expression (see McGraw et al., 1998).

Several studies have also explored whether 5' UTR promoter region haplotypes influence transcription of the human β_2AR gene, which is controlled by a 550 base pair sequence immediately 5' to the start of translation. This region includes the following four SNPs: – 468 (C to G), -367 (T to C), −47 (T to C), and −20 (T to C). Johnatty et al., 2002 used luciferase-based reporter gene assays to investigate the influence of these promoter

region SNPs on β_2AR gene expression. Using *in vitro* site-directed mutagenesis all 16 possible combinations (2^4) of the four SNPs were generated from a recombinant 570 base pair fragment of the β_2AR gene promoter. The possible combinations being: CTTT, CTCT, CCTT, CTTC, CCCT, CCTC, CTCC, CCCC, GTTT, GTCT, GCTT, GTTC, GCCT, GCTC, GTCC, and GCCC. The recombinant human β_2AR gene promoter haplotypes were each cloned into a luciferase reporter gene plasmid and expressed in HEK293 cells (Figure 7.14).

Two of the haplotype constructs, CTCT (−468C, −367T, −47C, −20T) and GCCT (−468G, −367C, −47C, −20T), reduced luciferase expression compared

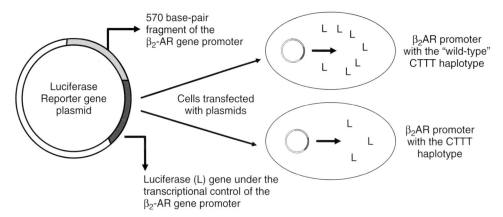

Figure 7.14 Single nucleotide polymorphisms within the promoter region of the β_2AR gene influence transcription. Luciferase-based reporter gene plasmids containing different β_2AR gene promoter haplotypes were generated using *in vitro* site-directed mutagenesis. Expression of luciferase (L) activity was monitored following transfection of cells with the reporter gene plasmids. High levels of luciferase activity were detected in cells expressing the 'wild-type' CTTT haplotype, whereas lower levels of luciferase activity were measured in cells expressing the CTCT β_2AR gene promoter haplotype.

to the 'wildtype' haplotype CTTT. Both of these contained the -47C SNP (see above) and in addition the GCCT haplotype included the -367G SNP which is located within a possible glucocortocoid response element (GRE). This is notable since glucocorticoids are known to increase the rate of β_2AR gene transcription. Two haplotypes studied (CTTC and CCTC) elicited an increase in luciferase expression. These interesting studies indicate that SNPs located within the promoter region of the β_2AR do influence receptor expression.

Reporter gene assays

A reporter gene is simply a gene whose protein product can easily be detected and measured once expressed in the cell of interest. Commonly used reporter genes include the luminescent enzyme luciferase, which catalyses the production of light using the substrate luciferin, and green fluorescent protein (GFP) which glows green when cells are exposed to blue light. Absorbance based reporter genes include β-galactosidase and secreted placental alkaline phosphatase, both of which are detected using colourimetric substrates. The DNA plasmid containing the reporter gene, which is under the transcriptional control of a suitable promoter, needs to be expressed in the cell of interest prior to experimentation. The transfection of cells with plasmid DNA was described in Chapter 2.

Molecular pharmacologists often use reporter gene assays as an alternative method for assessing GPCR activation. This is easily achieved if transcription of the reporter gene is controlled by a promoter responsive

to second messenger-dependent signalling. Widely used promoters include the c-fos promoter and the cyclic AMP response element (CRE) promoter which is activated by the transcription factor CREB (cyclic AMP response element binding protein); see Figure 7.15). Many reporter gene based assays are being developed for use in high-throughput screening of GPCR drug libraries (Figure 7.16).

Reporter genes also provide a convenient way of assessing promoter activity in a cell. The expression of the reporter gene is simply under the control of the promoter under investigation as illustrated in Figure 7.16.

Consequences of β_2AR SNPs: in vivo and ex-vivo

The functional consequences of coding region β_2AR SNPs observed in transfected cell systems (namely desensitisation and second messenger responses) have been confirmed in many *ex vivo* studies using either human tissue or human primary cell lines which express the β_2AR such as lymphocytes and airway smooth muscle. The *in vivo* consequences of β_2AR SNPs have also been explored by measuring cardiac or vasodilatory responses to β_2 agonists and are summarised in Table 7.15.

β_2AR SNPs and asthma

β_2AR agonists are widely used as bronchodilators in the treatment of asthma and their clinical response shows marked individual variation. β_2AR agonists are divided into two types: short-acting and long-acting.

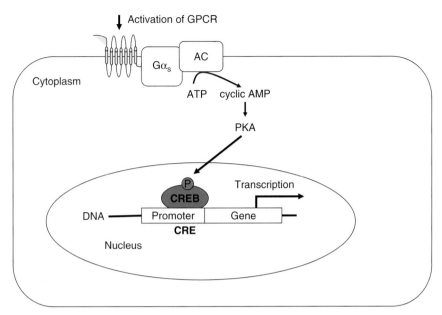

Figure 7.15 G protein coupled receptors activate gene transcription via CREB. When phosphorylated at serine[133] the transcription factor CREB (cyclic AMP response element binding protein) triggers gene transcription via binding to the cyclic AMP response element (CRE) within the promoter region of a gene. A variety of protein kinases including protein kinase A (PKA), Ca^{2+}/calmodulin-depedent protein kinases IV and II, and ribosomal S6 kinase are capable of phosphorylating CREB at serine[133]. Classically CREB activation is associated with GPCRs coupled to G_s protein (via the cyclic AMP/PKA pathway) but both G_i- and G_q-protein coupled receptors may also activate CREB via increases in intracellular Ca^{2+} concentration and/or stimulation of mitogen-activated protein kinase signalling cascades.

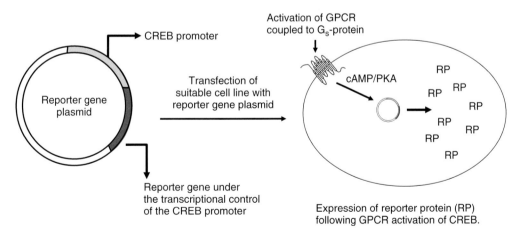

Figure 7.16 GPCR-induced reporter gene expression. Reporter gene assays represent a simple and sensitive method for assessing GPCR activation. A cell line expressing the GPCR of interest is transfected with the reporter gene plasmid which is under the transcriptional control of a suitable promoter such as CREB. Following GPCR activation the reporter gene protein product (RP; for example luciferase or green fluorescent protein) is expressed and detected using an appropriate assay.

Table 7.15 *In vivo* consequences of β_2AR polymorphisms.

β_2AR SNP	Cardiac response	Vasodilatory response to systemic infusion of β_2-agonists
Gly[16]	No difference in contractile response to β_2AR agonists	Contradictory results
Glu[27]	No difference in contractile response to β_2AR agonists	Contradictory results
Ile[164]	Decreased contractile and heart rate responses to infused β_2AR agonists	Evidence of reduced vasodilatory responses to β_2AR agonists

The therapeutic effect of long-acting β_2 agonists such as salmeterol lasts for up to 12 hours, whereas short-acting β_2 agonists (for example salbutamol) last between 4–6 hours. Long-acting β_2AR agonists are usually prescribed in conjunction with corticosteroids to patients with severe persistent asthma who have previously been using short-acting β_2 agonists.

As you would expect many studies have investigated whether there are any associations between β_2AR SNPs and asthma. The outcome of these studies has shown that Gly16Arg and Gln27Glu SNPs are not associated with asthma, that is, they are not disease causing and do not occur with increased frequency in asthmatic patients.

A major problem associated with β_2AR agonist therapy is that patients often develop tachyphylaxis following repeated use of the drug. As covered in Chapter 3 the continuous or repeated stimulation of a GPCR reduces subsequent responsiveness to an agonist via a process termed desensitisation. Since Gly16Arg and Gln27Glu SNPs influence agonist-induced receptor down-regulation they may influence the clinical response to β_2AR agonist asthma therapy. The majority of pharmacogenomic studies have revealed that asthma patients who are homozygous for Gly[16] (Gly[16]/Gly[16]) were less responsive to acute short-acting β_2AR agonist therapy than heterozygotes (Gly[16]/Arg[16]) or homozygotes for Arg[16]. At present there is very little information concerning the influence of the Thr164Ile SNP on the clinical response to β_2AR agonists.

Many studies investigating GPCR pharmacogenomics have explored the consequences of individual SNPs rather than specific haplotypes. An intriguing study by Drysdale et al. (2000) explored how promoter and coding region β_2AR haplotypes influenced receptor expression and drug response in asthmatic patients. Analysis of 13 β_2AR SNPs

amongst asthmatic patients revealed that they are organised into just 12 haplotypes out of the 8,192 possible combinations (2^{13})! The three most common β_2AR haplotypes and their distribution amongst different ethnic groups are detailed in Table 7.16.

Having identified the three most common β_2AR haplotypes the next logical step was to assess the *in vivo* functional consequences of these haplotypes on the bronchodilatory response to the short-acting β_2AR agonist albuterol. This was achieved using spirometry by measuring forced expiratory volume in 1 sec (FEV$_1$) before and after inhalation of albuterol. Figure 7.16 shows the changes in FEV$_1$ following albuterol inhalation determined in the five most common haplotype pairs amongst the asthmatic cohort studied by Drysdale et al. (2000). Remember for each gene you will have two possibly different haplotypes, one on the chromosome inherited from your mother and the other on the chromosome inherited from your father. Asmatic patients with the haplotype pair 4/4 did not respond as well to β_2AR agonist therapy (Figure 7.17).

β_2AR haplotype also determines the level of receptor transcript (mRNA) and protein expression with haplotype 2 displaying higher levels of expression than haplotype 4. These findings correlate nicely with the *in vivo* data, since asthma patients with the haplotype pair 2/2 responded 50% better than those with the haplotype pair 4/4 (Figure 7.17). The observation that β_2AR haplotypes influence the clinical effectiveness of β_2AR agonist therapy for asthma highlights the potential of pharmacogenomics and the development of personalised medicine. For comprehensive reviews on the pharmacogenomics and pharmacogenetics of common drugs used in the treatment of asthma see Kazani et al. (2010) and Lima et al. (2009).

Table 7.16 The three most common β_2AR haplotypes are their distribution amongst ethnic groups.

Nucleotide	−1023	−709	−654	−468	−406	−367	−47 (AA19 BUP)	−20	46 (AA16)	79 (AA27)	252 (Syn)	491 (AA164)	523 (Syn)	Ethnic Groups			
Alleles	G/A	C/A	G/A	C/G	C/T	T/C	T/C	T/C	G/A	C/G	G/A	C/T	C/A	Ca	AA	As	LH
Haplotype														Frequency (%)			
2	**A**	C	G	**G**	C	**C**	**C**	**C**	G	**G**	G	C	C	48	6	10	27
4	G	C	A	C	C	T	T	T	A	C	G	C	C	33	30	45	40
6	G	C	G	C	C	T	T	T	G	C	A	C	A	13	31	30	13
Location	5'	5'	5'	5'	5'	5'	5'	5'	3'	3'	3'	3'	3'				

Abbreviations: AA; African Americans, As; Asians, Ca; Caucasians, LH; Latino-Hispanics. AA; amino acid; A; adenine, C; cytosine, G; guanine, T; thymine, BUP; beta upstream peptide, Syn; synonymous. Nucleotide number is based on the first nucleotide of the starting codon being +1 and nucleotide changes from 'wild-type' are in bold. Data from Drysdale CM et al. (2000) Proceedings of the National Academy of Science 97: 10483–10488.

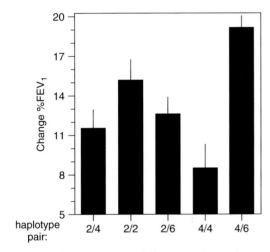

Figure 7.17 *In vivo* response to β_2AR agonist therapy in asthmatics with different β_2AR haplotype pairs. The data is from 121 asthmatic subjects whose FEV_1 was measured before and after inhalation of the β_2AR agonist albuterol. The results are expressed as the percentage change in FEV_1. Reprinted from Drysdale CM et al. (2000) Proceedings of the National Academy of Science 97: 10483–10488 with permission. Copyright (2000) National Academy of Sciences, USA.

β_2AR SNPs and cardiovascular function

Although the predominant β-AR subtype in the mammalian heart is the β_1AR (approximately 70%), the β_2AR is also expressed (30%) and plays a role in the regulation of heart rate and contraction of cardiac muscle. β_1 and β_2AR-induced cardiac muscle contraction involves PKA-dependent phosphorylation of proteins involved in the regulation of intracellular calcium levels. The levels β_2AR become more prominent and functionally important during chronic heart failure due to down-regulation of the β_1AR. Although several studies have explored the association of β_2AR SNPs and heart failure the results are inconclusive. It does appear that patients with the $Arg^{16}Gln^{27}$ haplotype have a higher risk of heart failure and hence this may be of use as a predictive marker.

Studies have been conducted to determine whether the Ile164 β_2AR phenotype influences the survival rates of patients with congestive heart disease. For example Liggett et al. (1998) discovered that the one-year survival rate for patients with Ile164 β_2AR was 42% whereas for patients with the Thr164 β_2AR the survival rate was 76%. Several follow-up studies have failed to confirm this initial and intriguing observation.

α_{2C}-adrenergic receptor polymorphisms

One polymorphic form of the α_{2C}AR has been reported which involves deletion of four amino acids (numbers 322–325; Gly-Ala-Gly-Pro) within the third intracellular loop. This particular polymorphism is common in African-Americans (approx. 40%) but is rare in Caucasians with a frequency of only approximately 4%. What are the consequences of the Del322-325 α_{2C}AR polymorphism on receptor function? The α_{2C}AR couples to

$G_{i/o}$-proteins and when activated triggers the inhibition of adenylyl cyclase activity. Studies have shown that the Del322-325 α_{2C}-AR variant does not inhibit adenylyl cyclase as effectively as the wild-type receptor suggesting reduced activation of $G_{i/o}$-proteins. Interestingly, the α_{2C}AR (along with the α_{2A}AR) is located on cardiac pre-synaptic sympathetic nerve terminals and is involved in the auto-inhibition of noradrenaline release. These pre-synaptic $G_{i/o}$-protein-linked receptors attenuate neurotransmitter release through the activation of potassium channels. Potassium channel activation causes the pre-synaptic membrane to hyperpolarise, which blocks neurotransmitter release. Thus a reduced α_{2C}AR function may cause increased noradrenaline release and predispose individuals to heart failure especially in subjects with Arg[389] β_1AR. Indeed, one study using African American patients suggested that the α_{2C}AR Del322-325 is a risk factor for developing heart failure and that this is enhanced when combined with the β_1AR Arg389 variant.

β_3-adrenergic receptor single nucleotide polymorphisms

The β_3AR was first reported to be expressed on adipocytes where it plays an important role in regulating metabolic processes such as lipolysis and thermogenesis in white and brown adipose tissue, respectively. As a consequence of these initial findings there was considerable interest in use of β_3AR agonists for the treatment of obesity and diabetes which unfortunately have failed following Phase

II clinical trials. The β_3AR is also expressed in the urinary bladder where it mediates relaxation of the detrusor smooth muscle. β_3AR agonists are being developed for the treatment of overactive bladder syndrome with drugs already in Phase III clinical trials. For a comprehensive review on the β_3AR as a therapeutic target see Ursino et al., (2009).

At present three non-synonymous SNPs have been identified within the coding region of the β_3AR; with the Trp64Arg variant located within TM1 attracting the most attention (Figure 7.18). The β_3AR gene also contains two non-coding region SNPs; one located within an intron (G1856T) the other at the three' non-coding regions (G3139C).

Functional consequences of the Trp64Arg SNP

The exact functional consequence of the Trp64Arg SNP is a controversial area. Several *in vitro* studies, using cells transfected with site-directed mutagenesis generated variants, suggest that the Arg[64] polymorphism is hypofunctional with respect to cyclic AMP accumulation. Furthermore, β_3AR agonist-induced lipolysis (which is mediated via cyclic AMP) is reduced in human fat cells expressing the Arg[64]β_3AR variant. Interestingly the Arg[64] variant, which is present in approximately 10% of Caucasians, is apparently associated with overactive bladder syndrome. All of the above support the notion that the Arg[64] variant is hypofunctional. However, there are a

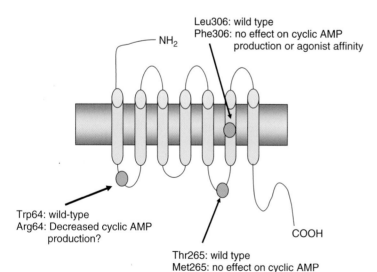

Leu306: wild type
Phe306: no effect on cyclic AMP production or agonist affinity

NH₂

Trp64: wild-type
Arg64: Decreased cyclic AMP production?

Thr265: wild type
Met265: no effect on cyclic AMP production or agonist affinity

COOH

Figure 7.18 β_3-adrenergic receptor single nucleotide polymorphisms.

number of studies which have not shown any functional difference between the Trp[64] and Arg[64] variants (e.g. no differences in cyclic AMP accumulation). The reasons for these differences are not clear but may relate to the use of different cell lines (human versus non-human), the use of different agonists or interactions of the Trp64Arg polymorphism with other coding/non-coding region SNPs present in the β_3AR. In a recent comprehensive study it was shown that none of the three SNPs within the coding region of the β_3AR (Trp64Arg, Thr265Met, Leu306Phe) either alone or in combination altered agonist-induced cyclic AMP accumulation or agonist-induced desensitisation when measured in a transfected human cell line (Vrydag et al., 2009).

β_3AR Trp64Arg SNP: disease associations

There has been considerable interest in the possible association of the Trp64Arg β_3AR polymorphism with obesity and type 2 diabetes mellitus (Liu et al., 2007). For example one study has shown that morbidly obese patients with the Arg64 β_3-AR variant have a significantly higher body weight compared to patients with the Trp64 variant. Although the Arg64 β_3-AR polymorphism is not found at higher frequencies in obese individuals its presence is likely to lead to greater increases in weight gain and thus maybe a risk factor. However a large number of studies have also reported no association between the Trp64Arg β_3AR polymorphism and obesity.

7.7 Summary

Individual variation to drug response is a well known phenomenon amongst clinical patients. In the United States more than 2 million cases of adverse drug reaction are recorded annually including 100,000 deaths! It is now recognised that inherited genetic variability in the human genome can dramatically influence a patients' response to drug therapy. In this chapter we covered how genetic polymorphisms in drug metabolising enzymes, drug transporters and drug targets (in particular G protein-coupled receptors) influence response to drug treatment. There are already several pharmacogenetic tests in use and many commercial companies offer genetic testing for cytochrome P_{450} variants to improve clinical treatment. Certainly in the not too distant future the concept of personalised medicine may become the norm.

References

Brockmöller J and Tzvetkov MV (2008) Pharmacogenetics: data, concepts and tools to improve drug discovery and drug treatment. European Journal of Clinical Pharmacology 64: 133–157.

Brodde O-E (2008) β-1 and β-2 adrenoceptor polymorphisms: Functional importance, impact on cardiovascular diseases and drug responses. Pharmacology and Therapeutics 117: 1–29.

Drysdale CM, McGraw DW, Stack CB, Stephens JC, Judson RS, Nandabalan K, Arnold K, Ruano G and Liggett SB (2000) Complex promoter and coding region β_2-adrenergic receptor haplotypes alter receptor expression and predict *in vivo* responsiveness. Proceedings of the National Academy of Science 97: 10483–10488.

Escande D (2000) Pharmacogenetics of cardiac K^+ channels. European Journal of Pharmacology 410: 281–287.

Firouzi M and Groenewegen WA (2003) Gene polymorphisms and cardiac arrhythmias. Europace 5: 235–242.

Gradland U and Kim RB (2008) Pharmacogenomics of MRP transporters (ABCC1-5) and BCRP (ABCG2). Drug Metabolism Review 40: 317–354.

Ieiri I, Higuchi S and Sugiyama Y (2009) Genetic polymorphisms of uptake (OATP1B1, 1B3) and efflux (MRP2, BCRP) transporters: implications for inter-individual differences in the pharmacokinetics and pharmacodynamics of statins and other clinically relevant drugs. Expert Opinion in Drug Metabolism and Toxicology 5: 703–729.

Ingelman-Sundberg M (2004) Pharmacogenetics of cytochrome P450 and its applications in drug therapy: the past, present and future. Trends in Pharmacological Sciences 25: 193–200.

Insel PA, Tang C-M, Hahntow I and Michel MC (2007) Impact of GPCRs in clinical medicine: genetic variants and drug targets. Biochim Biophys Acta 1768: 994–1005.

Johnatty SE, Abdellatif M, Shimmin L, Clark RB and Boerwinkle E (2002) β_2 adrenergic receptor 5' haplotypes influence promoter activity. British Journal of Pharmacology 137: 1213–1216.

Johnson JA, Zineh I, Puckett BJ, McGorray SP, Yarandi HN and Pauly DF (2003) β_1-adrenergic receptor polymorphisms and antihypertensive response to metoprolol. Clinical Pharmacology and Therapeutics 74: 44–52.

Kazani S, Wechsler ME and Israel E (2010) The role of pharmacogenomics in improving the management of asthma. Journal of Allergy and Clinical Immunology 125: 295–302.

Kerb R (2006) Implications of genetic polymorphisms in drug transporters for pharmacotherapy. Cancer Letters 234: 4–33.

Kimchi-Sarfaty C, Mi Oh J, Kim I-W, Sauna ZE, Calcagno AM, Ambudkar SV and Gottesman MM (2007) A 'silent' polymorphism in the *MDR1* gene changes substrate specificity. Science 315: 525–528.

Kwok PY (2001) Methods for genotyping single nucleotide polymorphisms. Annual Review. Genomics and Human Genetics 2: 235–258.

Leineweber K and Heusch G (2009) β_1- and β_2-adrenoceptor polymorphisms and cardiovascular diseases. British Journal of Pharmacology 158: 61–69.

Liggett SB, Wagnoor LE, Craft LL, Hornung RW, Hoit BD, McIntosh TC and Walsh RA (1998) The Ile164 β_2-adrenergic receptor polymorphism adversely affects the outcome of congestive heart failure. Journal of Clinical Investigation 102: 1534–1539.

Lima JJ, Blake KV, Tantisira KG and Weiss ST (2009) Pharmacogenetics of asthma. Current Opinion in Pulmonary Medicine 15: 57–62.

Lin JH and Lu AYH (2001) Interindividual variability in inhibition and induction of cytochrome P450 enzymes. Annual Review of Pharmacology and Toxicology 41: 535–567.

Liu Z, Mo W, Huang Q and Zhou H (2007) Genetic polymorphisms of human β-adrenergic receptor genes and their association with obesity. Zhong Nan Da Xue Xue Bao Yi Xue Ban 32: 359–367.

Lockridge O (1990) Genetic variants of human serum cholinesterase influence metabolism of muscle relaxant succinylcholine. Pharmacology and Therapeutics 47: 35–60.

McGraw DW, Forbes SL, Kramer LA and Liggett SB (1998) Polymorphisms of the 5' leader cistron of the human β_2-adrenergic receptor regulate receptor expression. Journal of Clinical Investigation 102: 1927–1932.

Mialet Perez J, Rathz DA, Petrashevskaya NN, Hahn HS, Wagoner LE, Schwartz A, Dorn GW and Liggett SB (2003) β_1-adrenergic receptor polymorphisms confer differential function and predisposition to heart failure. Nature Medicine 9: 1300–1305.

Mizuno N, Niwa T, Yotsumoto Y and Sugiyama Y (2003) Impact of drug transporter studies on drug discovery and development. Pharmacological Reviews 55: 425–461.

Nishizato Y, Ieiri I, Suzuki H, Kimura M, Kawabata K, Hirota T, Takane H et al. (2003) Polymorphisms of OATP-C (SLC21A6) and OAT3 (SLC22A8) genes: consequences for pravastatin pharmacokinetics. Clinical Pharmacology and Therapeutics 73: 554–565.

Pfost DR, Boyce-Jacino MT and Grant DM (2000) A SNPshot: pharmacogenetics and the future of drug therapy. Trends in Biotechnology 18: 334–338.

Rana BK, Shiina T and Insel PA (2001) Genetic variations and polymorphisms of G protein-coupled receptors: functional and therapeutic implications. Annual Review Pharmacology and Toxicology 41: 593–624.

Rowland M and Tozer TN (2010) Clinical Pharmacokinetics and Pharmacodynamics: Concepts and Applications (4th edition). Lippincott Williams & Watkins, USA.

Sesti F, Abbott GW, Wei J, Murray KT, Saksena S, Schwartz PJ, Priori SG, Roden DM, George, Jr, AL and Goldstein SAN (2000) A common polymorphism associated with antibiotic-induced cardiac arrhythmia. Proceedings of the National Academy of Science 97: 10613–10618.

Shastry BS (2006) Pharmacogenetics and the concept of individualized medicine. The Pharmacogenomics Journal 6: 16–21.

Shen H, He MM, Liu H, Wrighton SA, Wang L, Guo B and Li C (2007) Comparative Metabolic Capabilities and Inhibitory Profiles of CYP2D6.1, CYP2D6.10, and CYP2D6.17 Drug Metabolism and Disposition 35: 1292–1300.

Shi MM, Michael R, Bleavins xx and Felix A. de la, Iglesia (1999) Technologies for detecting genetic polymorphisms in pharmacogenomics Molecular Diagnosis 4: 343–351.

Small KM, McGraw DW and Liggett SB (2003) Pharmacology and physiology of human adrenergic receptor polymorphisms. Annual Review of Pharmacology and Toxicology 43: 381–411.

Ursino MG, Vasina V, Raschi E, Crema F and De Ponti F (2009) The β_3-adrenoceptor as a therapeutic target: current perspectives. Pharmacological Research 59: 221–234.

Wuttke H, Rau T, Heide R, Bergmann K, Böhm M, Weil J, Werner D and Eschenhagen T (2002) Increased frequency of cytochrome P450 2D6 poor metabolizers among patients with metoprolol-associated adverse effects. Clinical Pharmacology and Therapeutics 72: 429–437.

Vrydag W, Alewijinse AE and Michel MC (2009) Do gene polymorphisms alone or in combination affect the function of human β_3-adrenoceptors? British Journal of Pharmacology 156: 127–134.

Useful Web sites

The International HapMap project: http://hapmap.ncbi.nlm.nih.gov/ This is the database of the single nucleotide polymorphism consortium which catalogues sequence variation among individuals. It allows you to search for genetic polymorphisms associated with human disease.

The Human Genome Variation database of Genotype-to-Phenotype project: http://www.hgvbaseg2p.org/index This website allows you to search genetic association studies.

8 Transcription Factors and Gene Expression

8.1 Control of gene expression

The central dogma regarding gene expression is that DNA is transcribed to mRNA which is then translated into a protein. There are several steps in this cascade where gene expression can be controlled. For example, DNA can be tightly packed into nucleosomes to form chromatin. Each nucleosome consists of a histone with DNA wrapped around this protein core which condenses and gives rise to chromatin. This supercoiled structure prohibits molecules involved in transcription from accessing the gene. Partial chromatin unwinding can be achieved through acetylation by enzymes such as histone acetyltransferases (HATs), whereas tighter binding between histones and DNA is achieved through removal of acetyl groups using histone deacetylases (HDAs). Other factors, such as SW1/SNF (switching mating type/sucrose non-fermenting) proteins which destabilise the interaction between histones and DNA can also remodel chromatin.

DNA methylation can also reduce its affinity for histones and thereby promote chromatin unwinding.

Genes contain a promoter region of DNA which is not translated and is upstream of the encoding sequence. The promoter is responsible for initiating and determining the direction of transcription. Transcription factors (trans-acting factors) interact with specific DNA sequences called regulatory elements (cis-acting factors) within the promoter region of genes to regulate their transcription, with a particular transcription factor being able to promote or repress the expression of multiple gene targets. The activity of transcription factors can be regulated by their nuclear abundance and DNA binding activities, whereas the activity of the regulatory elements are influenced by chromatin structure and DNA modifications such as methylation.

RNA polymerases (RNA pol) recognise specific sequences within the promoter region and are responsible for gene transcription. Unlike DNA polymerases they do not need a primer to initiate RNA synthesis

Molecular Pharmacology: From DNA to Drug Discovery, First Edition. John Dickenson, Fiona Freeman, Chris Lloyd Mills, Shiva Sivasubramaniam and Christian Thode.
© 2013 John Wiley & Sons, Ltd. Published 2013 by John Wiley & Sons, Ltd.

or possess proofreading ability. There are three types of RNA pol: I transcribes genes encoding the 28S, 18S and 5.8S ribosomal RNAs; II transcribes genes encoding for messenger RNA (proteins) and small nuclear RNAs involved in splicing and; III transcribes genes encoding transfer RNA and 5S ribosomal RNA genes. General (basal) transcription factors (e.g. TFIIA, TFIIB etc.) interact with RNA pol II to form a holoenzyme complex and are required before RNA pol can initiate transcription. The TATA box is a target of RNA pol II and general transcription factors and its sequence is found in approximately 20% of human gene promoters. Many genes including housekeeping genes (e.g. β-actin) do not contain a TATA box and in these cases they employ a different initiator of transcription (e.g. initiator, GC

box, CCAAT box, CACCC box and octamer motif) (see Figure 8.1).

Genes also contain regulatory elements that serve to enhance or repress gene expression. They are usually located upstream of the promoter but in some cases they are found within introns. The interaction of transcription factors with these regulatory elements can significantly influence the activity of the general transcription factors found in RNA pol holoenzyme. Transcription factors and regulatory elements are thought to hinder or promote the interaction of RNA pol holoenzyme sterically, by the formation of a hairpin loop where the distance between promoter and regulatory elements is large.

As we will see later in this chapter, gene expression can also be controlled at the mRNA level by altering mRNA

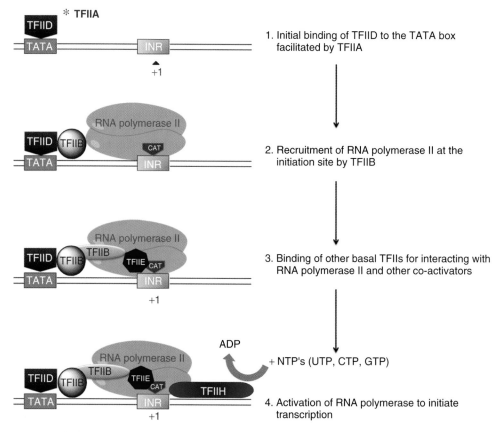

Figure 8.1 Steps involved in the initiation phase of transcription by basal transcription factors. Initially TFIID binds to the TATA-box (or another initiator of transcription site) after which different members of TFII family are recruited and transcription commences. INR = initiator element (or transcription initiator – an element that overlaps a transcription start site); +1 = refers to the transcription start site.

stability, expression of splice variants and production of antisense transcripts to prevent translation (Sakabe and Nobrega, 2010; Carroll, 2008; Wray et al., 2003).

8.2 Transcription factors

Transcription factors are involved in the initiation of mRNA production. Basically they interact with the DNA helix to either facilitate or hinder access of the RNA holoenzyme; DNA must be 'unwound' so that RNA pol II can act to express that gene. They have two functional components; (a) a DNA-binding domain (DBD), which binds to highly conserved sequence in the DNA strand with high affinity, and (b) a trans-activation domain (TAD), where modulatory proteins (including other transcription factors) can interact and thus influence gene expression. There are hundreds

of different types of transcription factors that can be allocated to one of five superfamilies according to their DBD structure: basic domains; zinc-coordinating DNA-binding domains; helix-turn-helix; β-scaffold factors with minor groove contacts and other transcription factors (see Table 8.1). The helix-turn-helix group have a characteristic three α-helix structure, with two running antiparallel and a third adjacent to them so that they can bind to their cognate sequence within the major and minor grooves of DNA. The β-scaffold factors have a similar antiparallel structure except they have two β-sheets that interact with minor groove contacts. Members of the basic element family have two α-helixes that interact with DNA to form a 'scissor' like structure. Interactions of repeat leucines in the carboxyl portion allows the two helixes to form a zip-fastener like structure; hence the name leucine zipper. Transcription factors with a helix-loop-helix have a similar structure to leucine zippers except

Table 8.1 Classification of transcription factors according to their DNA binding structural motif.

Structural domain	DNA interaction	Examples
Helix-turn-helix (HTH)	 helix-turn-helix	Homeodomain proteins POU factors (Oct-1, Oct-2, Pit-1, Unc-86)

Zinc finger
  Cys-His Zn finger
  Cys-Cys Zn finger
	
	zinc finger
		Developmental/cell cycle regulators, viral regulators (TFIIIA, Kruppel, SP1)
		Steroid hormone receptors, thyroid hormone receptor-like factors, GATA-factors

Basic element
  Leucine zipper (bZIP)
  Helix-loop-helix (bHLH)
  bHTH + bZIP
	
	leucine zipper
	helix-loop-helix
		C/EBP, Fos, Jun, CREB, bZIP/PAR,
		Myogenic transcription factors (MyoD1, E12, E47)
		Cell-cycle controlling factors (Myc family, heat shock factor)

β-scaffold factor	 β-scaffold factor	Rel proteins, NF-κB

Transcription factors facilitate gene expression by interacting with the minor and major grooves of DNA and thereby allowing RNA pol II access. There are four major classes of transcription factors based upon their DNA binding structural folds and hence interaction with DNA. Transcriptions factors can act as either monomer (e.g. Sp-1 and Oct-1), dimers (e.g. CREB) or trimers (e.g. heat shock factor). A number of transcription factors do not contain any of these characteristic folds and are assigned to the 'other transcription factor' superfamily (not shown).

dimerisation occurs via additional carboxyl α-helixes that are separated by loops. Finally, members of the zinc finger transcription factor family contain loops that are formed due to Zn^{2+} ions stabilising the interaction of cysteine-cysteine or cysteine-histidine residues. These loops enable the proteins' three α-helixes to interact with their DNA sequences within the grooves. Members of this family can be classified further depending upon the number of zinc finger loops present.

A further superclass of transcription factors has been identified as the high mobility group (HMG). Members of this group are involved in the complex of proteins that regulate gene expression and they can directly initiate transcription. However, their main function is in the remodelling of chromatin (e.g. bending and wrapping) so that the transcriptional complex can gain access. This is independent of histones which are involved in chromatin formation through DNA supercoiling and unwinding (Adcock et al., 2006).

The number of transcription factors found within an organism is dependent on their genome size, with larger genomes tending to have more transcription factors. In humans approximately 10 transcription factors can bind to their target sequence within a single gene. Transcription factor binding sites can occur at several sites adjacent to a gene as illustrated in Figure 8.2 whether a gene is expressed or repressed depends upon the individual transcription factor and specific members of its transcription complex (Glass and Rosenfeld, 2000). Since there are so many different types of transcription factors, in this chapter we will focus on those that are of pharmacological interest.

Types of transcription factors

Transcription factors can be grouped as either basal (general) or modulatory. Basal transcription factors (BTFs) are involved in constitutive gene expression in a fashion that is similar in all cells, whilst modulatory transcription factors (MTFs) can regulate gene expression depending upon the cell type and its requirements (Gill, 2001; Müller and Helin, 2000).

Regulation of transcription by basal transcription factors

The term basal transcription factors is preferred to 'general' because every transcription factor within this class does not utilise the same repertoire of proteins in the pre-initiation complex nor do they have the same DNA recognition sequence (binding elements). Hence there is nothing general about them. BTFs mediate unwinding of the target DNA gene as well as recognising the gene's promoter. They achieve this by participating in a pre-initiation complex that comprises of RNA pol II plus the BTFs: TFIIA, TFIIB, TFIID, TFIIE, TFIIF, and TFIIH. Different basally expressed genes can utilise other BTFs that are in addition to the aforementioned BTFs. The best studied BTF DNA binding element is the TATA box which is recognised by the TATA-binding protein (TBP). This TBP is a part of TFIID. Other BTF binding elements have been identified since not all genes have a TATA box. These include the downstream promoter element (DPE), TFIIB recognition elements (BREs), and the initiator element (INR). The pre-initiation complex is also associated with a multitude of co-activators and chromatin-modifying proteins.

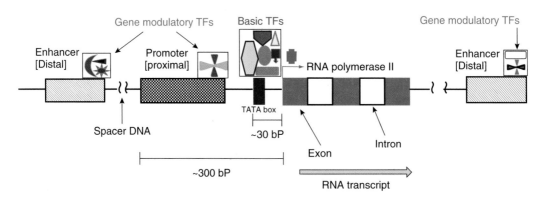

Figure 8.2 Potential transcription factor target sites. Gene regulatory (modulatory) transcription factors can bind at distal and proximal sites up- or down-stream of a gene to regulate gene expression in response to cellular demands. While the majority of the basal (general) transcription factors bind within the promoter region to ameliorate RNA pol II activity and constitutive gene expression. In some genes a TATA box is found around 15–30 base pairs upstream of the initiation site.

Polymorphisms in the TATA box have been associated with a variety of conditions due to the altered expression of some genes. For example, problems with β-globin lead to β-thalassemia or superoxide dismutase 1 have been associated with lateral sclerosis. Whereas defects in some BTF like TFIID has no consequences due to it only playing a modulatory role in the pre-initiation complex (Savinkova et al., 2009).

Regulation of transcription by modulatory transcription factors

Unlike BTFs, MTFs regulate the expression of a gene, or a set of genes depending on the need of the cells. They are vital for multicellular organisms as they allow the body to differentially express genes in both a temporally and spatially manner. This enables the body to produce many different types of cells, tissues and organs. As Figure 8.2 shows, they differentially regulate the expression of various genes by binding to enhancer regions of DNA that are adjacent to regulated genes. That is, they have the ability

of 'reciprocal repression' whereby MTFs can repress one set of genes to accommodate the activation of genes that have an antagonistic physiological function. This reciprocal repression can play a part in minimising the energy expenditure at the gene-transcriptional level.

Since a single cell can express several different types of transcription factors at any one time that target the same gene, its expression will be depend upon several aspects. This includes whether the facilitatory or repressive transcription factors have greater affinity for their DBD, the types of modulatory factors bound to the TAD and/or the exact components of the RNA holoenzyme complex. Therefore the functions of MTFs can differ between cells, be it development, control of the cell cycle, pathogenesis or enhancing intra-cellular signals in response to hormones and neurotransmitters.

MTFs can control and regulate the organised spatial distribution of cells during embryonic development. These include gene clusters such as homeobox (*Hox*), paired box (*Pax*), fibroblast growth factor (*fGF*), and

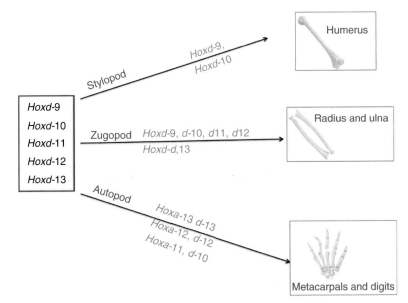

Figure 8.3 Involvement of MTFs from the *HOX* gene cluster in limb development of lower vertebrates. The pattern of *Hox* expression changes along the proximo-distal axis of the limb to produce different bone parts (Metcalfe, 2007). The upper arm consists of one bone (the humerus). In embryological terms, this region is called the stylopod and its development is mainly determined by *Hoxd-9* and *10*. Next the region immediately distal to this is called the zugopod. Here, in addition to *Hoxd-9* and 10, other *Hox* MTFs such as d11, d12 and d13 are recruited to produce the radius and the ulna. In contrast, the autopod which is the most distal element utilises entirely different Hox MTFs (such as Hoxa-13, -d13, -d10) to form the metacarpals and the digits. Due to the coordinated control of MTFs, both upper- and lower- limbs develop in stages from proximal to distal such that the stylopod develop first followed by the zugopod and the sudopod. Thus MTFs play an important role in morphogenesis. Similar patterns are also observed during lower limb formation.

Sonic hedgehog homolog (*Shh*); all of which are believed to be involved in organogenesis (Mundlos and Olsen, 1997). They can either switch on (or off) the transcription of genes that are responsible for cell morphology and differentiation. Figure 8.3 depicts how various members of the *Hox* family interact in different cells to determine which bones are expressed in the arm (Glass and Rosenfeld, 2000; Olsen et al., 2000). Mutations in these MTF gene families have been associated with developmental disorders and anomalies including dwarfism.

MTFs are also involved in determining which sex organs are expressed. Development of the penis and testicles can be attributed to the presence of a MTF that is produced by the Y-chromosomal testis-determining gene; *Sry* (sex-determining region on the chromosome Y). Since females do not have a Y-chromosome they cannot produce this MTF so the ovaries and uterus develop using a different array of MTFs. (Brenan and Capel, 2004). This is outlined in Figure 8.4. There is an important balance between the MTFs, DAX1/WNT4 and Sry/SOX9 MTF in gender determination of the growing foetus: both groups of MTFs have the ability to repress each other. Over-expression of DAX1/WNT4 results in repression of Sry/SOX9 and therefore results in female gonad formation. Whereas the over-expression of Sry/SOX9 results in repression of the DAX1/WNT4 and therefore results in male gonad formation. Furthermore, absence of WNT4 leads to testis-like development within the ovary and conversely, over-expression of WNT4 in the male leads to female sex reversal. RSPO1 is another gene essential in gender determination responsible for the protein RSPO1, which plays an important role in suppression of the SOX9 gene (Parma et al., 2006; Biason-Lauber, 2010). Loss of function mutations in RSPO1 gene in mice may result in the formation of ovo-testes in the XX chromosome foetus.

MTFs also play a role in downstream signalling cascades involved in responses to environmental stimuli. These include hypoxia inducible factor (HIF) that responds to low levels of oxygen, heat shock factor (HSF), which helps cell survival at high temperatures and sterol regulatory element binding protein (SREBP), which helps maintain proper lipid levels in the cell.

Different phases of the cell cycle involve several MTFs. These include determining cell size and the timing of mitosis. Some of these MTFs are also proto-oncogenes, oncogenes and tumour suppressor-gene products, which have been implicated in both normal and abnormal cell growth and apoptosis (Bartek and Lukas, 2001). An exhaustive review of all these factors and their functional

activities is beyond the scope of this book. So we will concentrate on those implicated in the transition of the cell from the growth (G1) to the synthesis (S) phase. This is an important transitional phase where the cell goes from preparing for DNA synthesis to DNA replication. Hence it is equally important in both mitosis and meiosis and thus proliferation.

Normally within the G1 phase the transcription initiator E2F is locked by several chromatin-remodelling complexes like pRb (retinoblastoma protein) and MTFs such as Brm and Brg1 (helicase-like proteins similar to SW1 and SNF in *Saccharomyces cerevisiae*; Harbour and Dean, 2000; Muchardt and Yaniv, 2001). These chromatin-remodelling complexes are involved in both activation and repression of a variety of genes. The main function of pRb is to prevent excessive cell growth by inhibiting cell cycle progression until a cell is ready to divide. Since pRb activity can be controlled by phosphorylation, so can cell proliferation. Various cyclin/cdk enzyme complexes (Nakayama et al., 2001) can phosphorylate pRb and thereby reduce its affinity for EF2 as well as the MTFs Brm/Brg1. This enables proteins involved in DNA replication to become active.

The role of MTFs in hormonal-activated transcription regulation is a complex phenomenon. This can be seen in nuclear receptor (NR) activation. NR comprises a family of transcription factors that regulate gene expression in a ligand dependent manner. Members of the NR superfamily include receptors for steroid hormones (e.g. oestrogens and glucocorticoids receptors); and non-steroidal ligands, such as thyroid hormones and retinoic acid (Glass and Rosenfeld, 2000). Interestingly, oestrogen receptors (ERs) themselves can act as transcription factors, either by activating or inhibiting the expression of a wide array of genes.

Role of MTFs in pathogenesis and pharmacotherapy

As seen in the previous section transcription factors play a major role in the regulation of gene expression which underlies human development, and physiology. Therefore, solutions for many pathological processes might be found by simply turning genes on or off by manipulating the functions of transcriptional factors (both BTFs and MTFs). Apparently there is growing interest in studying the involvement of specific transcription factors in the pathophysiology of many diseases (Landles and Bates, 2004; Harjes and Wanker, 2003). Some of these are summarised in Table 8.2.

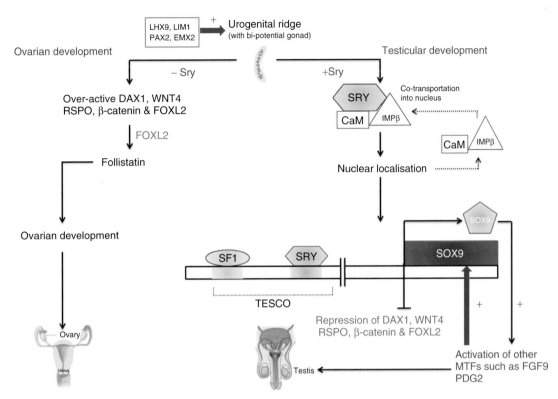

Figure 8.4 The role of MTFs in gender determination during development. The DAX1 (dosage-sensitive sex reversal) gene is necessary for gonadal development in both genders (Houmart et al., 2009; MacLauglin and Donahoe, 2004); with levels of DAX1 expression determining the gender of the developing foetus. Its over-expression prevents testis formation, instead favouring female sex organ development. In females, the DAX1 and/or WNT4 (wingless-type MMTV [mouse mammary tumour virus] integration site family), RSPO1 (R-spondin-1), and β-catenin genes are over-expressed leading to gonad differentiation into granulosa cells and the activation of yet another MTF, fork-head box protein L2 (FOXL2). Ultimately, FOXL2 causes the formation of the fallopian tubes, uterus and the upper two-thirds of the vagina. Whereas in males the Y-chromosome produces the MTF, SRY, approximately six weeks into gestation. SRY ameliorates the activity of several other downstream regulation sex-determining MTFs. These include activation of a 'testis-forming' pathway by up-regulating testis-specific enhancer of Sox9 (TESCO) to produce SOX9 (SRY-related HMG box-9) which in turn activates PGD2 and FGF9 genes. The MTFs produced by the latter (i.e. PGD2 [prostaglandin G2] and FGF9 [fibroblast growth factor 9]) forms a positive feed-forward loop to maintain SOX9 expression. It is also believed several autosomal genes may contribute to MTF activity in the process of testis formation (Houmart et al., 2009). The second step in male sex differentiation is a more straightforward hormone-dependent process. Testosterone produced by the developing testis induces the formation of epididymis, deferent ducts and seminal vesicles. The Leydig cells also produce insulin-like factor 3 (INSL3) and relaxin-like factor (RLF), which causes the testes to descend to the scrotum. CaM (calmodulin) & IMPβ (myo-inositol monophosphatase) are needed for transportation of SRY into nucleus. SF1 = Steroidogenic Factor-1.

8.3 CREB

One of the best known transcription factors is the cAMP responsive element binding protein (CREB). CREB is of considerable interest because of its involvement in a whole host of cellular functions including homeostasis, glucose metabolism, neuronal plasticity and cancer. (Phu

et al., 2011). Like many responsive elements (e.g. Ca^{2+} responsive element, serum responsive element), its name is based on the fact that a particular substance, which in the case of CREB is cAMP, leads to expression of a repertoire of certain genes. Sequencing of the promoter regions of these cAMP-induced genes and DNA-foot printing has identified a sequence common to these genes

Table 8.2 Some examples of disease associated with mutations transcription factors.

Disease	Transcription factor involved
Autoimmune disease	FOXP3; mutations in IPX and/or in proto-oncogene (van der Vilet and Nieuwenhuis, 2007)
Multiple Cancers	HOX family; up-regulations of many proto-oncogenes and/or down-regulation of tumour suppressor genes. (Shah and Sukumar, 2010)
Li-Fraumeni syndrome (wide range of malignancies)	Germ line mutations of the p53 tumour suppressor gene. (Iwakuma, et al, 2005)
Breast Cancer	STAT (Signal Transducer and Activator of Transcription) family genes and/or oestrogen receptor (Momand et al, 2006; Parma et al, 2006)
Maturity onset diabetes mellitus	Hepatocyte nuclear factor(HNF); functional mutations in insulin promoter; LPK (liver pyruvate kinase)(Lennon et al, 207; Al-Quobaili and Montenarg, 2008)
Developmental vertebrate dyspraxia	FOXP-3
Hypoplastic left heart syndrome	TBX (T-Box) genes (Wang et al, 2009)
Hashimoto's Thyroiditis	Up-regulation of thyroid TF-1
COPD (Chronic obstructive pulmonary disease)	AP-1 and NFκB (Brown et al, 2009)
Parkinson's Disease	GATA-1 and/or α-synuclin (Lee and Lupski, 2006)
Hypoparathyroidism-deafness-renal (HDR) syndrome	GATA-3 (Ali, et al, 2007)
Familial platelet disorder with myeloid malignancy Arthritis and inflammatory arthropathies	CBFA-2 (Co-binding factor-2) (Engelkamp and van Hetnigen, 1996) STAT/NF-κB pathways and NFAT (nuclear factor of activated T cells' family of transcription factors (Pessler et al, 2006)

that is inaccessible during cellular exposure to cAMP. This domain was called the cAMP responsive element (CRE). Since cAMP can induce the expression of a number of genes its cytosolic concentration is tightly regulated, with adenylyl cyclase (AC) and phosphodiesterase (PDE) being the main enzymes involved in its synthesis and breakdown respectively. Activation of GCPRs coupled to G_s or G_i protein result in either AC being stimulated or inhibiting the production of cAMP respectively (see Chapter 3). Up to four cAMP can then bind to a single protein kinase A (PKA) to stimulate PKA catalytic subunits dissociation which are then free to diffuse through nuclear pores into the nucleus to phosphorylate CREB and thus promote target gene expression (see Figure 8.5) (Altarejos and Montminy, 2011).

Subsequent studies have identified the CRE sequence in the promoter region of over 5,000 genes. However, only 100 genes are up regulated when cytosolic cAMP is elevated suggesting a complex array of transcription factors and co-factors are involved in regulating gene expression in those genes whose expression/repression appear to be independent of cAMP levels. One such factor that is known to ameliorate gene expression that is independent of cAMP is Ca^{2+}. Calmodulin is a Ca^{2+} substrate that has four Ca^{2+} ions bind sites and occupation of these binding sites allows it to interact with other proteins, such as calcium-dependent calmodulin kinase (CaMK) II or IV, to regulate their activity. These kinases can then alter gene expression via CRE by phosphorylating proteins involved in CRE activation. Within neurones, CaMKII has been shown to inhibit CRE-mediated gene

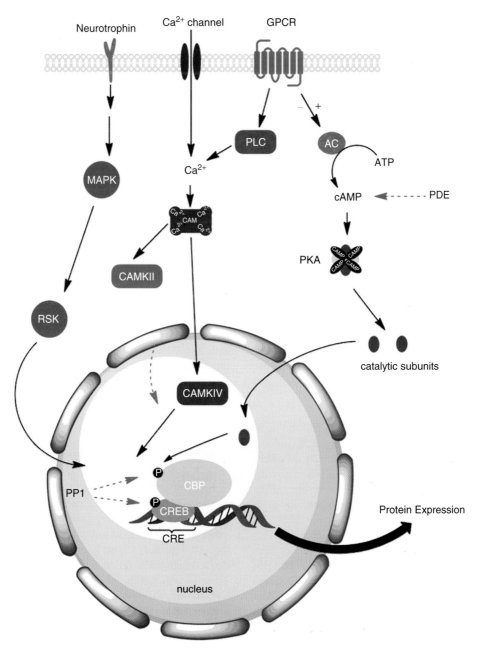

Figure 8.5 Different signal transduction pathways can lead to gene expression by phosphorylation of cAMP responsive element binding protein (CREB) and/or CREB binding protein (CBP). For clarity only one CREB protein is shown. (i) Activation of tyrosine kinase receptors can lead to the recruitment of mitogen-activated protein kinase (MAPK) signalling pathways; (ii) cytosolic Ca^{2+} concentrations can increase by influx via Ca^{2+} channels or release from internal stores due to GPCR coupled to PLC and IP_3 production. Ca^{2+} can activate calcium-dependent calmodulin (CAM) which in turn can activate CAMKII and CAMKIV and induce or repress CRE-mediated gene expression respectively; (iii) ligand binding to GPCRs coupled to adenylyl cyclase (AC) can stimulate (or repress) this enzyme to produce cAMP from ATP. cAMP can release the catalytic subunits of PKA so that they are now free to enter the nucleus and phosphorylate CREB/CBP. MAPK-activated ribosomal S6 kinases (RSK) pathway phosphorylate CREB at Ser 133. Protein phosphatase 1 (PP1 and PP2) can dephosphorylate CREB/CBP and phosphodiesterase (PDE) can breakdown cAMP and hence regulate the activity of PKA. (Adapted from Carlezon, Duman and Nestler, 2005).

expression whereas CaMKIV promotes CRE-mediated gene expression (Carlezon, Duman and Nestler, 2005). Figure 8.5 illustrates how cytosolic Ca^{2+} levels can be elevated due to influx through Ca^{2+} channels or release from internal stores. In the latter case activation of GCPRs coupled to phospholipase C (PLC) stimulates the breakdown of phosphatidyl-inostitol biphosphate (PIP_2) to inositol triphosphate (IP_3) which in turn promotes release of Ca^{2+} via its receptor channel located in the membranes of organelles such as the endoplasmic reticulum.

The mitogen-activated protein kinases (MAPK) signalling pathways are also known to regulate expression of genes that contain a CRE by phosphorylating CREB. This pathway can be activated by growth factors and neurotrophins via tyrosine kinase receptors (Trk) and growth factor receptors. The picture is further complicated by the fact that there is considerable cross-talk between the different signalling pathways. For example, diacylglycerol (DAG) is also released after PIP_2 breakdown by PLC. DAG can activate protein kinase C (PKC) which phosphorylate proteins involved in MAPK signalling. Trk receptor activation can inhibit PLC activity and CAM can inhibit the activity of AC. Since protein phosphatase 1 (PP1) can dephosphorylate CREB, PP1 activity can also control CRE-mediated gene expression (Figure 8.5).

Structure

Like many other transcription factors, CREB needs to form a dimer before it can interact with its CRE and this is achieved through a leucine zipper. Basically within the carboxyl region there are heptad repeats which give the protein an α-helix structure with a leucine every seven amino acids. The leucines can interact with those in the other CREBs to form a zipper structure. CREB also contains a basic-region at the proteins amino terminus that can then interact with CRE sequence in the target gene. Following dimerisation, these two major domains produce a structure that resembles a pair of scissors (Figure 8.6). In addition to these major domains, CREB can have a number of characteristic motifs at the amino terminal; glutamine-rich 1 (Q1), kinase-inducible (KID) and Q2 domains. The Q1 and Q2 domains can interact with TATA-binding protein factor II (TBF-2) for recruitment of RNA pol II holoenzyme. The KID contains a serine at position 133 (Ser 133) and this is a target of various protein kinases (e.g. CaMKII, CaMKIV, PKA, PKC, MAPK, casein kinases, glycogen synthase kinase-3 etc.) that are known to induce CREB-mediated gene expression (see Figure 8.5). Another potential phosphorylation site is found at serine 142 and its phosphorylation causes CREB

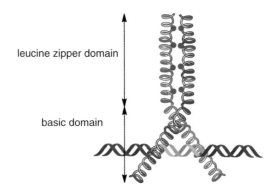

● leucine 〰〰 CRE ⋘b-zip protein A ⋘b-zip protein B

Figure 8.6 The interaction of two b-zip proteins to form a functional transcription factor. CREB can interact with another b-zip protein (e.g. CREM) and aid transcription at the CRE site. Each b-zip protein has a leucine binding domain where leucines from both proteins can align to form a 'zipper'. The basic domain facilitates interaction with the CRE regulatory site.

to de-dimerise as well as preventing it from interacting with its associated factor, CREB-binding protein (CBP), thus repressing target gene expression. Since CaMKIV acts at Ser 133 and CaMKII at Ser 142 this explains why CaMIV promotes whilst CaMII represses target gene expression. The phosphorylation status of other serines within the KID also influences CREB activity. For example glycogen synthase kinase-3β has been shown to act at Ser 129 to both repress and induce CRE-mediated gene expression. However, the role of other serines in this region is less defined when compared to Ser 133 and Ser 142.

The basic-region/leucine zipper (b-zip) domains are common to a number of transcription factors and CREB is a member of this b-zip superfamily. This means that whilst the CREB prefers to form homodimers it can also form heterodimers with certain members of the b-zip family. These include CRE modulator (CREM) and activation transcription factor 1 (ATF1). However, heterodimers are less stable and have a reduced CRE binding affinity. These dimers can bind to the palindromic CRE sequence, TGACGTCA (or hemi-sites; TGACG or CGTCA), within target genes to induce their transcription. For efficient initiation of transcription the CRE sequence usually lies within 250 base pairs of the TATA box. And although over 5,000 different genes contain a CRE sequence many are silent because either one or two cysteines located within the DNA binding domain of CREB is methylated which prevents CREB (and other b-zips) from interacting with CRE.

Dimerisation of CREB leads to the recruitment of the transcriptional co-activators CBP and p300. The CBP/p300 complex can directly interact with TBP, TBF2 and RNA pol II to stimulate gene transcription or indirectly due to CBP/p300 intrinsic HAT activity which promotes chromatin unfolding thereby allowing the aforementioned proteins to gain access to the transcriptional start of the target gene.

CREB target genes

CREB's role in learning and memory as well as psychiatric disorders has been studied extensively. It is known to alter the expression of glutamate receptors (AMPA; GluA1), transcription factors and co-activators (Fos, CREM), enzymes involved in neurotransmitter synthesis (tyrosine hydroxylase; TH), neuropeptides (corticotropin releasing factor; CRF, brain-derived neurotrophic factor; BDNF) and intracellular signalling enzymes (AC8) within neurones.

Glutamate receptors (see Chapter 4), especially the ionotrophic N-methyl-D aspartate (NMDA) receptors, play an important role in synaptic plasticity. These receptors can control the amount of Ca^{2+} influx and hence the activity of signalling pathways and gene expression via CRE (see Figure 8.5) and the calcium responsive element (CaRE; see Chapter 9). During normal neurotransmission NMDAR are inactive because a Mg^{2+} ion sits inside its channel. However, during synapse remodelling there is a prolonged and sustained release of glutamate and NMDAR become active because this Mg^{2+} block is removed due to local membrane depolarisation which is mainly achieved by activation of another class of ionotrophic glutamate receptors – AMPAR. AMPAR are predominantly Na^+/K^+ channels but one of its subunits, GluA2, does permit Ca^{2+} influx. The cytosolic concentration of Ca^{2+} is tightly controlled because at high levels it can cause excitotoxicity and neuronal death (see Figure 5.21). In addition, during synapse remodelling the number of AMPAR found at the post synaptic membrane needs to be reduced. Since CREB can control the expression of another AMPAR subunit, GluA1, perturbations in its level of expression can have many consequences ranging from neurodegeneration and impaired memory formation to enhanced cognition.

There are 10 AC isoforms (AC1-10) and a number of these isoforms have been linked to particular cells and signal transduction. Whilst all isoforms can be controlled by the α-subunit of GPCR there are subtle differences in the regulation of AC by other factors, for example the βγ-GPCR subunit can interact with AC8 to alter its activity and even override the inhibiting effects of α_i. AC8 had been associated with neuronal plasticity, in particular memory formation. In addition to being controlled by CREB, its promoter region also has a CaRE which can regulate its expression. Elevated Ca^{2+} levels can therefore affect the induction of this enzyme especially in neuronal tissue to affect synaptic plasticity.

Tyrosine hydroxylase (TH) is the enzyme responsible for converting tyrosine in DOPA which is a precursor of both noradrenaline and dopamine. The expression of neuropeptides, especially neurotrophins like CRF and BDNF, are under the control of CREB. All of these neurotransmitters/neuropeptides have been implicated in depression, drug addiction, learning and memory and other disorders of cognition. So alteration in the level of TH expression can result in the development of numerous neuropsychiatric disorders.

Peroxisome proliferator-activated receptor α, co-activator 1α (PGC-1α) is the master regulator of lipid metabolism and metabolic control and the expression of this gene can be regulated by CREB. As we see in the next section of this chapter, alterations in the level of expression of this gene expression can have profound effects on metabolism and cell function in general. In addition, CREB and its associated factors like cAMP-regulated transcriptional co-activator family (CRTC) have been implicated in a number of metabolic functions within tissue ranging from expression of metabolic enzymes such as glucose-6-phosphatase in the liver to the expression of peptides in the hypothalamus that are responsible for altering appetite.

Drugs that target specific moieties on transcription factors such as phosphorylation sites, nuclear localisation domains, DNA binding sites, or co-activator(s) interaction sites have been developed for the treatment of tumourgenesis. However, this approach can lead to the development of drugs that target regions that could be conserved in other proteins. So unless compartment specific therapies can be developed the side effects of these drugs would be unacceptable. This has led researchers to develop strategies that determine which genes are regulated by these 'transcription factor-mediating' drugs. Employment of reporter gene assays (e.g. green fluorescent protein; GFP) would create large libraries that can be analysed to determine which transcription factor(s) are affected by these drugs. This would allow the development of transcription factor specific agonists and antagonists. In fact this approach has led to development of an inhibitor of a transcription factor STAT1 (signal transducer and activator of transcription 1); 2-(1,8-naphthyridin-2-yl)phenol (2-NP). This transcription factor is implicated in cancer formation and 2-NP has been shown to reduce proliferation in breast cancer studies (Lynch et al., 2007). Nifuroxazide is another anti-cancer drug that has been shown to be a potent inhibitor of the transcription factor, STAT3 function as well as possessing anti-proliferation activity (Nelson et al., 2008).

8.4 Nuclear receptors

Nuclear receptors (NR) are transcription factors that can facilitate or repress gene expression. Ligands or metabolic factors can enter the cell and either activate NRs in the cytoplasm so that they enter the nucleus or activate nuclear located NRs. Once activated the NR can alter gene expression as monomers, homodimers or as heterodimers with, for example, the retinoic acid receptor

(RAR). There is considerable debate in the literature as to how NRs evolved. The current view is that they evolved from environmental sensors where extracellular factors enter the cell enabling the cell to adapt to changing environments. This theory is compelling because in animals NRs play an important role in homeostasis, development and growth. In addition, NRs can be activated by ligand binding or their activity can be modulated by the activity of signalling pathways within the cell.

In man NRs function to regulate gene expression in response to small lipophilic molecules that include hormones such as steroids (oestrogens and glucocorticoids) and non-steroids (thyroid hormones), morphogens (retinoic acid) and dietary factors (fatty acids) (Markov and Laudet, 2011). They have a zinc-finger structure (see Table 8.1 and Figure 8.7) which allows the transcriptional machinery access. NRs have a typical gene structure, consisting of a ligand-binding domain (LBD), DNA-binding domain (DBD) and ligand-independent transcriptional activating function

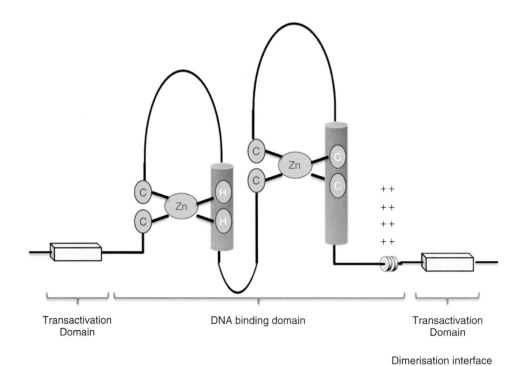

Figure 8.7 Structure of a typical nuclear receptor. Loops are formed in the DNA binding domain due to the interaction of a Zn^{2+} ion with two cysteine and two histidine (or cysteine) residues on opposite sides of the loop. Formation of these 'zinc fingers' helps the transcriptional machinery gain access to the DNA and hence facilitate (or repress) gene expression.

(AF-1) at the amino terminus and a ligand-dependent transcriptional activating function (AF-2) at the carboxyl terminal (see the gene structure of PPAR, Figure 8.11). The LBD is a major site of modulation since it can bind regulatory factors/complexes and therefore it is a target of allosteric modulating drugs. Binding of ligand promotes a conformational change in the receptor so that it can either recruit the binding or dissociation of proteins to the transcriptional complex and hence alter target gene expression.

Even though NRs have a broad common structure their biochemistry and pharmacology is very complex. NRs do not work in isolation but as a huge protein complex that can contain a multitude of proteins such as co-activators, co-repressors, other transcription factors, signalling molecules. In addition, they can be activated either by ligand binding or in a ligand-independent manner. Figure 8.8 illustrates this complexity using the glucocorticoid receptor (GR) as an example.

To date 48 NRs have been identified in the human genome and phylogenetic analysis has identified six major evolutionary groups; NR1-6 (Table 8.3). The endogenous ligands for half of the NRs are unknown and are therefore referred to as orphan receptors. Recently it was discovered

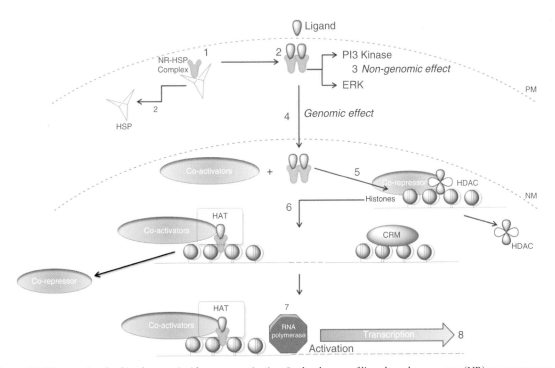

Figure 8.8 The steps involved in glucocorticoid receptor activation. In the absence of ligand, nuclear receptor (NR) monomers are bound to heat shock proteins (HSP) to form an NR-HSP complex (1). As the ligand diffuses through the plasma membrane (PM), HSP is released from the NR-HSP complex. The ligand then binds to its NR enabling it to dimerise with another NR monomer (2). Depending on the type of cell, the ligand-receptor complex can either produce non-genomic effects by activating for example the PI3 kinase and ERK pathways (3), have a genomic effect (4) or both. The usual cellular functions such as cell growth, proliferation, differentiation, motility, survival and intracellular trafficking, can be achieved via the PI3 and ERK pathways. Conformational changes within the NR dimer produces genomic effects by inducing the recruitment of other MTFs [such as activator protein 1 (AP-1); and specificity protein 1 (SP-1)] and co-activator proteins including the steroid receptor coactivator-1 (SRC-1) and cAMP responsive element binding protein (CBP), to enhance ligand-dependent steroid receptor transcriptional activity (6). These proteins have an intrinsic histone acetyltransferases (HAT) which facilitates DNA unwinding, enabling RNA pol II access (7) and therefore promotes gene transcription (8). Co-repressors can modify chromatin structure by recruiting histone deacetylase (HDAC) or a chromatin remodelling complex to prevent DNA unwinding and hence repress gene expression (5). (Molenda-Figueira et al., 2006) Key PI3 = Phosphatidylinositol 3-kinases; ERK = extracellular-signal-regulated kinases; PM = plasma membrane; NM = Nuclear membrane.

Table 8.3 Types of nuclear receptors.

Receptor	Nomenclature	Ligands
TRα/β	NR1A1-2	Thyroid hormones
RARα/β/γ	NR1B1-3	Retinoic acid
PPARα/β/γ	NR1C1-3	Fatty acids, leukotriene B_4, fibrates, prostaglandin J_2, thiazolidinediones
Rev-erbα/β	NR1D1-3	Haem?
RORα/β/γ	NR1F1-3	Cholesterol, cholesteryl sulphate, retinoic acid
LXRα/β	NR1H2-3	Oxysterols, T0901317, GW3965
FXRα/β	NR1H4-5	Bile acids, fexaramine, lanosterol
VDR	NR1I1	Vitamin D, 1,25-dihydroxyvitamin D3
PXR	NR1I2	Xenobiotics, 16α-cyanopregnenolone
CAR	NR1I3	Xenobiotics, phenobarbital
HNF4α/γ	NR2A1-2	Linoleic acid?
RXRα/β/γ	NR2B1-3	Retinoic acid
TR2/4	NR2C1-2	Retinoic acid?
TLL / PNR	NR2E2-3	Orphan
COUP-TFI/II	NR2F1-2	Orphan
EAR2	NR2F6	Orphan
ERα/β	NR3A1-2	Oestradiol-17β, tamoxifen, raloxifene
ERRα/β/γ	NR3B1-3	DES, 4-OH tamoxifen
GR	NR3C1	Cortisol, dexamethasone, RU486
MR	NR3C2	Aldosterone, spirolactone
PR	NR3C3	Progesterone, medroxyprogesterone acetate, RU486
AR	NR3C4	Testosterone, flutamide
NGFI-B / NURR1/ NOR1	NR4A1-3	Orphan
SF1 / LRH-1	NR5A1-2	Orphan
GCNF	NR6A1	Orphan
DAX-1 / SHP	NR0B1-2	Orphan

Nuclear receptors are classed according to their phylogeny and assigned to one of six families. The identity of the ligand for a number of NRs is unknown and hence they are referred to as orphan receptors. Ligands followed by a ? mean that only preliminary data exists (Adapted from Germain et al., 2006).

that haems can activate Rev-erb receptors allowing these NRs to be deorphanised. In addition, in some cases, the same ligand has the ability to activate several different NRs, for example, retinoic acid. Here retinoic acid and its derivatives can be used to treat a number of diseases including leukaemia and skin disorders. Over 10% of the most commonly prescribed medicines target NRs. Tamoxifen blocks the ERα receptor and is effective in the treatment of breast cancer. Dexamethasone acts at the GR and is an effective anti-inflammatory and immunosuppressant. As we shall see in the next section, thiazolidinediones exert their action via the PPARγ receptor and are commonly used to treat type II diabetes as well as inflammatory diseases.

8.5 Peroxisome proliferator-activated receptors

Peroxisome proliferator-activated receptors (PPAR) are ligand-dependent transcription factors. This superfamily of nuclear hormone receptors of which there are three main groupings: PPARα (NR1C1), PPARβ/δ (NR1C2; NUC1; fatty-acid-activated receptor) and PPARγ (NR1C3), are involved in regulating gene expression. The first members to be identified, PPARα, were shown to respond to compounds that induce peroxisomal proliferation and hence their name. However this property is unique to PPARα and subsequent studies show that PPAR plays a major role in lipid metabolism and metabolic control by regulating the expression of key factors involved in lipid and glucose metabolism. In fact, PPARγ has attracted a lot of attention because of its role in type 2 diabetes.

Regulation of metabolic homeostasis

Before we discuss how PPAR regulates gene expression we must first appreciate the relationship between metabolism, stress and the cardiovascular system because problems with metabolism rarely manifest themselves as a single disease/phenotype. In fact they tend to be part of a number of diseases and these groups are often referred to as metabolic syndrome. In other words conditions such as diabetes, hypertension and obesity usually accompany each other. PPAR play a central role in metabolic syndrome and Table 8.4 shows a variety of metabolic

intermediates can act as PPAR ligands for the expression of target genes.

Diet plays a role in normal cellular and body functions. Carbohydrates in the form of glucose can be stored as glycogen or metabolised to produce ATP. As Figure 8.9 shows an important intermediate in metabolism is acetyl CoA because it can enter the tricarboxylic acid (TCA) cycle for energy production or the fatty acid synthesis pathway for lipid storage. Acetyl CoA is also involved in the synthesis of cholesterol which is the precursor for steroid hormones and vitamin D and in Chapter 11 we will see how important cholesterol is for membrane structure and function. When food is plentiful the body stores energy in the form of fat (triacylglycerol) derived from dietary glucose and fatty acids. During fasting-states these fats can be broken down by lipolysis to glycerol and fatty acids and released into the blood supply. Glycerol is take up

Table 8.4 Partial list of endogenous and synthetic ligands for PPARs.

Receptor	Endogenous ligands	Synthetic ligands
PPARγ	Unsaturated fatty acids 15-HETE 9- and 13-HODE 15-deoxy-$\Delta^{12,14}$-PGJ$_2$ oxLDL	**Thiazolidinediones** Rosiglitazone Pioglitazone Troglitazone Ciglitazone **Tyrosine derivatives** Farglitazar GW7845
PPARα	Unsaturated fatty acids Saturated fatty acids (weak) Leukotriene B4 8-HETE	Fibrates Fenofibrate Clofibrate Gemfibrozil GW7647 Wy14643
PPARβ/δ	Unsaturated fatty acids Saturated fatty acids (very weak) Carbaprostacyclin (cPGI$_2$) Components of vLDL	GW501516 L-165041
PPARα/γ (dual agonists)	None selective for PPARα and PPARγ only	Muraglitazar Tesaglitazar Ragaglitazar

Carbaprostacyclin (cPGI2) is a synthetic, long-lived analogue of the presumed endogenous ligand PGI$_2$. Components of oxidised, low-density lipoprotein (oxLDL) that bind to PPARγ with high affinity include hexadecyl azelaoyl phosphatidylcholine. Other abbreviations: HETE, hydroxyeicosatetraenoic acid; HODE, hydroxyoctadecadienoic acid; vLDL, very low-density lipoprotein (Taken with permission from Straus and Glass, 2007).

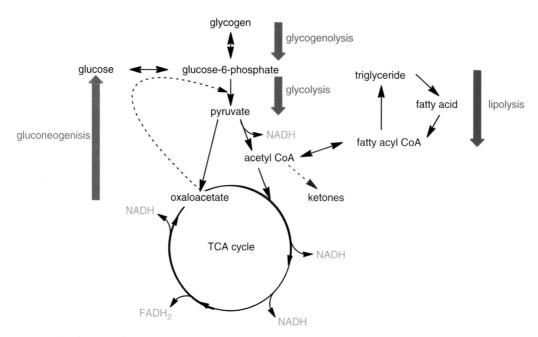

Figure 8.9 Highly schematised flow chart illustrating the relationship between glucose and lipid metabolism. Dietary carbohydrates such as glucose are taken up by cells and converted to glycogen for storage (glycogenesis) or broken down into pyruvate for entry into the tricarboxlyic acid (TCA) cycle and ATP production via the intermediates, NADH and FADH$_2$. Alternatively, pyruvate can be converted to acetyl CoA before it enters the TCA or it can be converted to fatty acyl CoA for lipogenesis and storage as lipids in adipose tissue. During periods of high ATP production not only can pyruvate enter the fatty acid synthesis pathway, the TCA intermediate, oxaloacetate, can be converted back to glucose-6 phosphate for gluconeogenesis. During fasting, fatty acids are released for conversion into acetyl CoA and entry into the TCA. If the rate of acetyl CoA synthesis is greater than the rate at which it enters the TCA the formation of ketones is favoured.

by the liver and metabolised to glucose, whereas the fatty acids are oxidised (β-oxidation) to acetyl CoA for entry into the TCA cycle and subsequent ATP production. This process can occur in most tissues, with the exception of the brain because the blood brain barrier is impermeable to fatty acids. When the rate of β-oxidation is very high then there is a build-up of acetyl CoA because it cannot be utilised by the TCA cycle fast enough. The excess acetyl CoA is converted to ketone bodies which are then released into the blood supply because the liver is unable to metabolise them. This gives the characteristic smell of pear drops in the breath of people who have excessive β-oxidation due to starvation or when the ability to store energy via glycogenesis is compromised as is seen in diabetes mellitus.

Glycerol is hydrophilic and hence does not need a plasma carrier to move between tissues via the blood. However, hydrophobic substances such as free fatty acids require the carrier plasma albumin, for transportation. Lipids are transported in the blood using a hydrophilic carrier protein of which there are four main types: chylomicrons, very low density lipoprotein (VLDL), low density lipoprotein (LDL) and high density lipoprotein (HDL). Chylomicrons which are the least dense lipoproteins are mainly associated with triglyceride and cholesterol transport from the intestines to adipose tissue during non-fasting conditions, whereas VLDL are involved in the transport of endogenous triglycerides primarily from the liver to adipocytes during fasting conditions. LDL are thought to be metabolites of VLDL and are mainly involved in cholesterol transport from the liver. HDL are believed to be involved in the removal of cholesterol by transporting it to the liver for degradation and excretion. Diet can alter the normal balance of these lipoproteins. High cholesterol and saturated fats increases LDL whereas high carbohydrate intake (including alcohol) enhances VLDL levels. Three apolipoproteins are also associated with lipid transport: apo-A for HDL, apo-B for LDL, VLDL and chylomicrons, apo-C for HDL, VLDL and chylomicrons. Defects in any one of these apolipoproteins have been associated with lipid storage diseases.

Atherosclerosis is the build-up of substances such as fats and cholesterol within blood vessels, particularly medium and large arteries. As these deposits thicken they become hardened and start to calcify to form plaques that can obstruct blood flow. Decreased blood flow into coronary blood vessels results in the heart not receiving enough oxygen and nutrients thereby reducing its ability to pump blood around the body. This can manifest itself as chest pains as in angina or a heart attack. Pieces of plaques can also break away and obstruct blood flow in smaller blood vessels like the lungs (pulmonary embolism) or brain. Blood clots can also form around plaque tears to reduce blood flow. The clot can also dissociate from the plaque and block smaller vessels. In some cases atherosclerotic plaques have also been associated with the development aneurisms due to weakening of the arterial wall.

The build-up of deposits on the arterial wall is due to oxidised LDL, which can be formed after attack by reactive oxygen species (ROS), interacting with and damaging the wall. In response to this, the body releases macrophages and T-lymphocytes to remove the oxidised LDL. This gives rise to characteristic foam cells that can be seen under the microscope. Unfortunately the white blood cells cannot breakdown the oxidised LDL and the complex continues to grow until it ruptures. Since the main cargo of LDL is cholesterol, when the foam cells rupture cholesterol is deposited onto the atrial wall. This vicious cycle continues with more macrophages and T-lymphocytes attacking the wall until either the blood vessel is completely occluded or bits of the plaques break off to block smaller blood vessels.

Inflammation is also associated with other cardiovascular pathologies. These include hypertension due to stenosis of blood vessels, cardiac hypertrophy as the heart tries to compensate for an increase in blood pressure and peripheral vascular disease where reduced blood flow to tissues at extremities cause cellular death; necrosis of fingers and toes are a problem associated with poorly managed diabetes.

Insulin is the hormone involved in glucose tissue uptake and glycogenesis. Insufficient insulin expression leads to diabetes of which there are two main types. Type 1 occurs due to destruction of the pancreatic β-cells that produce insulin and type 2 is due to insufficient insulin being produced by these cells. If there is an excess of glucose it can be fatal because glucose starts to be excreted in the urine causing osmotic diuresis leading to dehydration. But because the body relies on β-oxidation for energy,

the development of ketoacidosis can be more serious. Conversely hypoglycaemia caused by too much insulin secretion (or administration) can give rise to diabetic coma because the brain relies on glucose as its main source of energy; fatty acids cannot transverse the blood brain barrier. So glucose levels are closely regulated by the body.

Stress can influence metabolism by activating the inflammatory response. Whilst stress can play a role in normal physiological responses such as infection and maintenance of circadian rhythms, excessive/inappropriate stress can have pathophysiological consequences. The hypothalamus, pituitary, adrenal axis (HPA) plays a major role in the stress response. The HPA is also involved in control of metabolism and PPAR expression. Stress causes the adrenal glands to release glucocorticoids which indirectly increase the expression of hepatic enzymes involved in β-oxidation and other metabolic pathways. Catecholamines, such as adrenaline, are also released and act as adipocytes to stimulate free fatty acid release.

A consequence of metabolism is the production of ATP via the generation of intermediates of the electron transport chain (FADH$_2$ and NADH; Figure 8.9). In brown adipose tissue an uncoupling protein allows some of the energy produced during electron transport to be released as heat rather than production of a H$^+$ ion gradient within the mitochondrial inner membrane (see Chapter 5; Figure 5.19). This uncoupling is important for non-shivering thermogenesis and thermoregulation. So with white adipose tissue acting as a lipid store and brown adipose tissue as a heat generator, abnormal lipolysis or lipogenesis can result in obesity, malnutrition or hypothermia.

So as you can see perturbations of gluconeogenesis, glycogenolysis, glycolysis and lipolysis have profound effects on each other leading to a number of pathologies including cardiovascular disease, chronic inflammatory disease and obesity.

Regulation of gene expression by PPAR

PPAR become active upon heterodimerisation with the 9-cis-retinoic acid receptor (RXR)(Kliewer et al., 1992). They influence gene expression via their regulatory element, the PPAR response element (PPRE), which is present in a number of genes. However, gene regulation via PPRE is far more complicated than simple binding of these factors to PPRE. In fact a myriad of co-factors, kinases and other factors can alter the activity of this complex giving rise to tissue and cellular specific regulation of target gene expression. This is probably the reason why PPARs have been implicated in cellular growth and development, inflammation, wound healing, as well as diverse human diseases such diabetes, cancer and atherosclerosis (Tontonoz and Spiegelman, 2008).

The PPAR/RXR dimer can interact with its PPRE, however gene expression is determined by the presence or absence of interacting ligand(s). When no ligand is attached, then binding of a co-repressor complex is favoured, whereas the presence of activating ligands results in a higher affinity for a co-activator complex (Figure 8.10). Basically, co-repressors cause de-acetylation of histones or DNA de-methylation both of which cause tight binding between histones and DNA and thus prevent access of general and specific

transcription factors. On the other hand, co-activators have the opposite effect and facilitate chromatin remodelling and access of RNA pol II to its sequence within the promoter to initiate transcription. The composition of either co-repressor or co-activator can be extensive and varied. Examples of co-activator and associated proteins are given in Table 8.5 (Viswakarma et al., 2010; Chandra et al., 2008). A more detailed review of PPAR transcriptional co-activators can be found in Yu and Reddy, 2007 (Yu and Reddy, 2007).

Expression of PPARs follows a circadian rhythm in white and brown adipose tissue. This is to be expected as during periods of fasting when food intake is low PPARs are expressed abundantly, but at night time after a large meal PPAR expression is repressed because glucose

Repression of Gene Expression

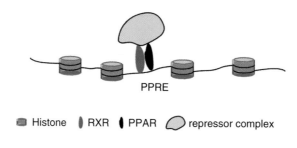

Induction of Gene Expression

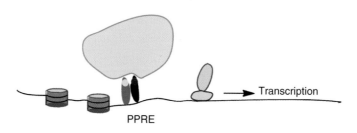

Figure 8.10 The PPAR/RXR heterodimer can repress or induce expression of target gene depending upon whether an activating ligand is bound. During repression, binding of a co-repressor complex to RXR/PPAR prevents chromatin unwinding. This co-repressor complex can contain many different proteins, including HDACs which de-acetylate histones and thus prevents DNA from dissociating. Binding of a ligand to RXR and/or PPAR causes dissociation of the co-repressor complex. The heterodimer is now free to associate with a co-activator complex which contains factors that facilitate chromatin unwinding and histone release. RNA pol II and associated transcription factors (TF) can now interact with the DNA and begin transcribing. Adapted from (Viswakarma et al., 2010).

Table 8.5 Showing examples of some known co-activator and co-activator associated proteins that regulate PPAR function.

Co-activator proteins	Enzyme activity	Function
SRC-1/NCoA-1	HAT	Histone acetylation
SRC-2/TIF2/GRIP1	HAT	Histone acetylation
SRC3/pCIP/AIB1	HAT	Histone acetylation
CBP/p300	HAT	Histone acetylation followed by recruitment of p160/SRCs
MED1/TRAP220/PBP	None	Anchor for Mediator complex
PGC-1α	None	Recruit co-activator with HAT activities
PGC-1β/PERC	None	Recruit co-activator with HAT activities
PRIP/NCoA6	None	Recruit ASC complex
PRIC285	Helicase	Chromatin remodelling by histone displacement and nucleosomal sliding
PRIC320/CHD9	Helicase	Chromatin remodelling by histone displacement and nucleosomal sliding
SWI/SNF	ATPase	ATP dependent mobilization of nucleosome
BAF60a/SMARCD1	None	Recruit SWI/SNF complex
BAF60c/SMARCD3	None	Recruit SWI/SNF complex
Co-activator-associated proteins		
PIMT/NCoA6IP	Methyltransferase	Methylation of caps of snRNAs and snoRNAs
CARM1/PRMT4	Methyltransferase	Potentiate SRCs by methylation of Histone H3
CoAA	None	RNA splicing

Taken from (Viswakarma et al., 2010).

now becomes the main source of energy (Yu and Reddy, 2007). Figure 8.9 shows the fine balance between lipid and glucose metabolism. Hence, giving us an insight into how PPARs could interrelate to control various aspects of metabolism.

RXR provides PPAR with a further level of regulation because so far three isoforms, α, β and γ, have been identified with variable tissue distribution. They can act as RXR-homodimers or bind with other members of the nuclear receptor superfamily. This gives rise to greater diversity in PPAR/RXR dimer expression and function and the genes whose activity they regulate.

PPARα

Homozygous PPARα$^{-/-}$ knockouts have helped elucidate the role of PPARα. These mice exhibit phenotypes with heightened inflammatory responses and associated diseases as well as autoimmune problems. During fasting conditions they also exhibit severe metabolic imbalances such as low glucose and ketones levels as well as hypothermia. PPARα plays a role in placental development by controlling the expression of various enzymes involved in metabolism as well as hormone production (e.g. human chorionic gonadotrophin and progesterone).

PPARα is expressed in tissue with high fatty acid β-oxidation activity and plays a vital role in regulating lipid catabolism. Since PPARα is a target for peroxisomal proliferators, some fatty acids and their metabolites play a major role in regulating key enzymes involved in mitochondrial peroxisomal and microsomal fatty acid oxidation systems within organs such as the liver and kidneys, as well as smooth, cardiac and skeletal muscle. This is particularly evident during conditions when fatty acid levels are high such as during starvation/fasting; high fatty acid concentrations positively feedback to induce enzymes involved in β-oxidation. Fasting or stress also activates the HPA axis causing the adrenal glands to release (i) glucocorticoids which increases the expression of PPARα in the liver and (ii) catecholamine, such as adrenaline, which act as adipocytes to stimulate free fatty acid release. Drugs such as hypolipidemic-fibrate drugs and some xenobiotics which are used to treat hypertriglyceridemia are known to act via PPARα (see Table 8.4).

Cytochrome P$_{450}$ is a major enzyme found in the liver and is responsible for metabolising steroids, fatty acids and other drugs. 7α-hydroxylase P$_{450-b1}$ (CYP7b1) is an isoform that is highly expressed in males compared to females. This enzyme is involved in the metabolism of a metabolite that can activate hepatic oestrogen receptors to such a level that it causes inflammation or hepatotoxicity. As a result its level in women is tightly controlled. However, oestrogen induces CYP7b1 expression, therefore in situations where levels of this hormone are high (for example, during pregnancy or when taking oral contraceptives/hormone replacement therapies that contain oestrogen) this can result in hepatitis/hepatotoxicity. Since CYP7b1 expression can be repressed by PPARα it is a potential target for the treatment or prevention of oestrogen-induced inflammation and hepatotoxicity. During the acute phase of inflammation PPAR ligands have been shown to prevent the expression of pro-inflammatory proteins in hepatocytes and dendritic cells (Yessoufou and Wahli, 2010).

PPARβ/δ

PPARβ/δ is expressed ubiquitously throughout the body, but it is found in high levels in the skin, brain and adipose tissue. It controls the expression of genes involved in β-oxidation as well as controlling lipid levels that if left unregulated would contribute to obese phenotypes. Like PPARα, PPARβ/δ activity can be regulated by high levels of fatty acids that are seen as a result of fasting but PPARβ/γ is more responsive to extra-hepatic plasma levels rather than hepatic plasma levels.

PPARβ/δ plays a role in skin wound healing. Immediately after skin damage the PPARβ/δ ligands, TNF-α and AP-1 are released, which induce PPARβ/δ expression. This activates pathways involved in re-epithelialisation of the keratinocytes. Once healing is complete TGFβ-1 expression is induced which prevents AP-1 from interacting with its regulatory element in PPARβ/δ thus preventing its further expression. Development of ligands that target PPARβ/δ could treat a host of inflammatory-related skin diseases such as psoriasis, benign epidermal tumours and papillomas. PPARβ/δ also plays a role in thermogenesis, embryo placenta implantation, bone reabsorption and myelination of CNS neurones. Within the liver, PPARβ/δ is thought to suppress the expression of some genes involved in inflammation. PPARβ/δ can increase the expression of repressor proteins (e.g. BCL-6 or TGFβ) and proteins with anti-oxidant properties (e.g. superoxide dismutase) or suppress genes usually expressed during the acute phase of inflammation (e.g. NF-κB, ERK1/2 and cell adhesion molecules) (Yessoufou and Wahli, 2010).

In humans, several polymorphisms have been identified in PPARβ/δ that are associated with tumourigenesis and atherosclerosis. In fact sulindac, which is a chemo-preventive non-steroidal anti-inflammatory drug (NSAID), prevents target genes that contain the PPARβ/δ responsive element from being expressed thereby reducing tumour related angiogenesis and preventing atherosclerotic lesions from forming. (Yessoufou and Wahli, 2010). So targeting of PPARβ/δ expression may be an avenue for drug development to treat these various pathologies. In fact, amelioration of PPARβ/δ activity has been shown to suppress weight gain and autoimmune-mediated inflammation.

PPARγ

Whereas PPARα and PPARβ/δ are involved in energy catabolism, PPARγ is more concerned with adipocyte differentiation and energy anabolism. (Viswakarma et al., 2010). PPARγ achieves this by regulating the expression of several genes involved in these two processes within adipocytes. This PPARγ 'master gene' can control sensitivity to insulin, lower glucose levels, and stimulate lipid uptake for storage in tissues such as skeletal muscle, liver and adipocytes. Emerging evidence indicates that PPARγ also has vascular and immunological properties by playing a role in reducing both inflammation and atherosclerosis.

Activation of PPARγ results in the expression of insulin; the hormone involved in glucose tissue uptake and glycogenesis. Insufficient insulin expression leads to diabetes of which there are two main types. Type 1 occurs due to destruction of the pancreatic β-cells that produce insulin and type 2 is due to insufficient insulin being produced by these cells or insensitivity to insulin. The development of exogenous ligands that target PPARγ and hence enhance insulin production have transformed the treatment of type 2 diabetes. Whilst the endogenous ligand(s) of PPARγ is still unknown a number of exogenous ligands have been developed. These include thiazolidinediones (TZDs; e.g. rosiglitazone) which act as PPARγ's ligand binding site and are the major class of drugs used to treat type 2 diabetes. TZDs have also been shown to cause differentiation of adipocytes as well as having anti-inflammatory and anti-atherosclerotic properties.

Since PPARγ has a role in cell differentiation and metabolism it has been suggested that PPARγ activity could be manipulated in cancer cells to prevent tumourigenesis. In fact TZDs have been used in animal models to successfully treat a variety of cancers. However, these initially promising findings have not been replicated in human clinical trials. This lack of TZD efficacy and the fact that PPARγ transcripts are not elevated in cancerous cells indicates that PPARγ may not be as important as initially thought in tumorigenesis and raises the possibility that TZD is acting to supress neoplastic changes via a PPARγ-independent mechanism. Since TZDs can bind to the metabotropic receptor, GPR40, resulting in release of calcium from internal stores into the cytoplasm this probably is the case (Luconi, Cantini and Serio, 2010).

Interestingly, PPARγ can repress the expression of certain genes by either preventing other transcription factors from binding directly to their sites or by interfering with the activity of proteins that modulate other transcription factor's activity. For example it can inhibit the activity of NF-κB and AP-1 and so repress the expression of genes involved in inflammation which would explain PPARγ's anti-inflammatory properties (Yessoufou and Wahli, 2010).

Two splice variants are produced by the human PPARγ gene with the amino terminal exon being either spliced in (PPARγ2) or out (PPARγ1). The expression of each transcript is controlled by different promoters, with PPARγ1 being expressed ubiquitously in nearly every tissue type with the exception of muscle and PPAR-γ2 expressed mainly in adipose and intestinal tissues. As Figure 8.11 shows, there are four main structural motifs found in the protein. The A/B region has a ligand-independent transcriptional activating function (AF1) and may confer less ligand-dependant binding activity on the longer PPARγ2 form. The C motif contains the PPRE which has a two-folded zinc finger-like motif for PPAR/RXR binding. Section D encodes for the hinge region that enables the protein to adopt different conformations depending upon whether the co-activator or co-repressor complexes are bound. And finally the E/F region contains the ligand binding site as well as the ligand-dependent transcriptional activating function (AF2).

It has been suggested that post-translational modifications of PPARγ may alter its activity and give some 'fine tuning' of its activity that may be important/applicable to the treatment of human diseases. However, given the overlapping of secondary signalling pathways and the downstream consequences of manipulating the phosphorylation, summoylation, ubiquination and/or nitration

status of PPARγ, this may be too costly. An alternative could be the development of antisense oligonucleotides that prevent the expression of certain splice variants of this gene (PPARγ2 or PPARγ1; see Section 8.8).

8.6 Growth factors

As we saw in the previous section, growth factors can alter gene expression by recruitment of secondary messenger pathways such as MAPK leading to phosphorylation of transcription factors such as CREB. In Chapter 11, we saw that growth factors like BDNF bound to its receptor can act as a signalling endosomes (Figure 11.24). Here the entire complex is internalised and the complex, with its associated signalling factors, such as those in the mitogen-activated protein kinase (MAPK) pathway, the phosphoinositol-3-kinase (PI-3K) pathway and the phospholipase C-gamma (PLCγ) pathway can be activated depending upon the signalling complexes associated with the endosome. This in turn, through phosphorylation, can activate transcription factors like CREB to alter gene expression. In fact, there is evidence that rather than the signalling endosome activating nuclear-located CREB, that CREB actually joins the signalling endosome in the cytoplasm and is transported to the nucleus (Sadowski, Pilecka and Miaczynska, 2009). Whether CREB in combination with its regulatory protein, CBP, is transported as well is unknown, but since CBP has intrinsic HAT activity it is tempting to speculate as to whether this signalling endosome can influence transcription by acetylation of histones to promote chromatin unwinding and subsequent interaction of transcription factors (Wang et al., 2011).

8.7 Alternative splicing

Most genes are composed of exons that are separated by introns. Initially a gene is transcribed into pre-mRNA which contains both exons and introns. The introns are then spliced out to produce a mature mRNA transcript that is ready for translation into a protein. In certain circumstances some exons can also be removed during this process. This means that by alternative splicing of exons a single gene can produce multiple transcripts that have different translated characteristics, thus adding a further level of genomic diversity to an organism.

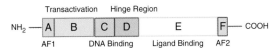

Figure 8.11 Showing the gene structure of PPARγ. The length of AF1 is greater in PPARγ2 than PPARγ1. Since this region can, to a certain extent, mediate ligand-independent PPARγ activity it may confer PPARγ2 with a degree of activity that is less dependent on ligand binding.

Epigenetics and alternative splicing

There are a number of mechanisms that an organism can employ to alter the phenotype of many genes without changing the genotype (epigenetics). These include DNA methylation, histone acetylation and post-translational modification of transcription factors to induce or repress expression of certain genes at critical times such as during development. In addition, a single gene can express a variety of different transcripts due to alternative splicing of exons and in some cases, introns. As Figure 8.12 shows alternative splicing can result in a single gene expressing a number of proteins with slightly different properties. Basically during RNA processing, the gene is first transcribed as a pre-mRNA which retains both introns and exons. Next introns are removed and exons are ligated together to form mature mRNA. In practice whole or partial exons can be spliced in or out to give truncated proteins with different transcriptional start sites, or introns can be retained so that protein translation is prematurely halted or the pre-mRNA transcript contains further information that aids cellular compartment specific translation.

In addition, retention of non-coding sequences can have an effect on the level of protein expression due to the presence of alternative regulatory elements which can enhance translation or increase mRNA stability. This complicated process of splicing and ligation is controlled by a ribonucleoprotein complex called a spliceosome. The presence of consensus nucleotide sequences between introns and exons that are recognised by proteins within the spliceosome (see Figure 8.13), allows exons/introns to be spliced in or out of the mRNA giving rise to a number of differently spliced transcripts. Spliceosomal activity can be influenced by signalling cascades which can therefore control RNA splicing and hence which transcripts are expressed. However, the activity of some members of this complex may be ameliorated by mutations or polymorphisms (e.g. single nucleotide polymorphisms; SNP) within their own genes resulting in altered splice variant expression. Finally mutations and SNP within or near splicing sites or regulatory elements could have a profound effect on splicing/ligation and hence which transcripts are expressed in response to a specific signal

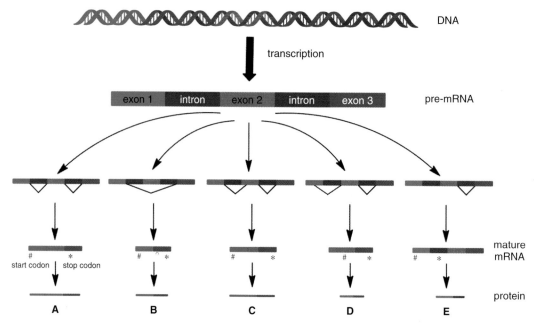

Figure 8.12 The effect of alternative splicing events on expressed protein. A single gene can be transcribed to pre-mRNA that undergoes a number of splicing events to give rise to a variety of transcripts that can be translated. (a) both introns are excised to give the full length transcript and protein. (b) the second exon is spliced out and gives rise to a truncated protein, (c) an alternative site splicing site located in exon 2 removes part of the 5′ sequence of exon 2 and since the reading frame is not moved the resultant protein is shorter than that seen with the full length transcript. (d) an alternative splicing site in exon removes the start codon, however there is another start codon in exon 2 so a very short protein lacking exon 1 is produced. (E) the first intron is not spliced out and it contains a stop codon so translation of the transcript is prematurely terminated.

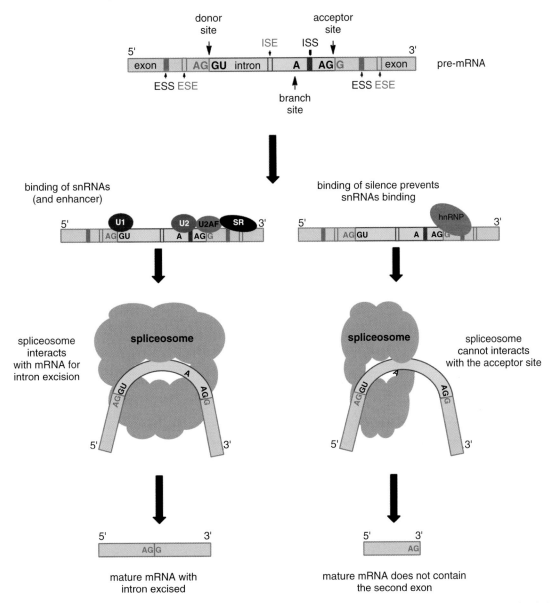

Figure 8.13 Spliceosomal excision of introns. Introns contain characteristic dinucleotides at the donor (GU) and acceptor (AG) sites as well as a branch site which has a conserved A between 20–50 nucleotides from the acceptor site. Within introns and exons there are intron splicing enhancer (ISE), intron splicing silencer (ISS), exon splicing enhancer (ESE) and exon splicing silencer (ESS) sites. Binding of enhancers such as serine/arginine-rich proteins (SR) to an ESE promotes interaction with the spliceosome. In contrast, binding of repressors like heterogeneous nuclear ribonucleoproteins (hnRNP) to ESS prevents splicing at the acceptor site (but not at the donor site) so that the proceeding exon is not spliced into the mature mRNA transcript. Poly adenylation tail in mature transcript is not shown for clarity.

(Bracco and Kearsey, 2003). Dysregulation of alternative splicing by altered splicesomal activity, mutations/SNP in the vicinity of splicing recognition sites or regulatory elements can give rise to a surprising number of human pathologies due to altered protein function of target genes or complete loss of function. These include cancers and neurodegenerative diseases (see Chapter 3).

Spliceosomes comprise of between 60 and 150 proteins and five small nuclear RNAs (snRNA; U_1, U_2, U_4, U_5, U_6). Whilst the snRNA, particularly U_6, is thought to be involved in the splicing reaction the exact role of the other snRNAs and proteins remain sketchy. What is known is that there are three core splicing sequences; two splice sites and a branch site. As Figure 8.13 shows, the $3'$ splice site and the $5'$ splice site flank an exon and contain conserved dinucleotides AG and GU respectively. These sites bind the snRNAs U_{2AF} and U_1 whereas the branch site binds U_2; although there is some debate as to whether U_6 binds to the branch site but is then displaced by U_2. Within the exons there are repressor elements where splicing silencer (ESS) complexes like heterogeneous nuclear ribonucleoproteins (hnRNP) can bind to prevent exon inclusion or splicing enhancers (ESE) domains where complexes such as serine/arginine-rich proteins (SR) can bind to promote exon inclusion. Introns also contain splicing enhancer (ISE) and silencing (ISS) domains for their selective inclusion or omission from the mature mRNA transcript. SNP at these splicing motifs can prevent enhancer/silencer from binding and therefore correct transcript processing (Ward and Cooper, 2010).

If the splicing site is not accurately targeted and occurs at a nucleotide either side of its intended site then the resultant mRNA will have its reading frame shifted to produce a transcript whose translation is prematurely terminated or gives rise to a 'nonsense' protein. Either way the resultant splicing error will result in a loss of function for that particular mRNA transcript. Cyclooxygenases (COX) mediate the inflammation response by triggering the formation of prostaglandins. Two isoforms of COX have been identified in mammals; COX1 and COX2. Since COX1 has an intron retained in theory the COX1 gene could express a splice variant, COX3, that has had this intron removed; although whether COX3 is actually expressed is debateable. Nevertheless if both COX1 and COX3 were translated the resultant proteins would have very different properties, due to a reading frame shift (Kis, Snipes and Busija, 2005).

In cystic fibrosis (see Chapter 6) the gene responsible has a mutation in exon 8 has a repetitive UG sequence and since the dinucleotide GU is characteristic of donor sites it leads to removal of exon 9. This deletion compromises the ability of this transporter to secrete mucous (Buratti et al., 2001). Repetitive sequences such as CUG can be found in the $3'$-untranslated region or the first intron of a gene that is associated with muscular dystrophy. This repeat cases exon skipping due to spliceosomal binding and mis-splicing (Wood, Gait and Yin, 2010).

Signalling pathways influence spliceosomal activity. For example the p38-MAPK pathway is involved in determining the cellular location of a member of the hnRNP family which is an ESS and responsible for exonic-exclusions. This affects the alternative splicing of target genes such as the fibroblast growth factor receptor 2 gene thereby altering the affinity of the receptor for its ligand. This in turn can cause abnormalities in cell growth as well as skin and bone development.

It has been proposed that over 90% of the genes in the human genome are alternatively spliced and that this essential process adds a further level of complexity to gene expression to give rise to specific tissue spatial and temporal effects. The ability of a single gene to produce a number of functionally different proteins affords cells with the capacity to tailor responses to specific stimuli and desired outcomes. However, this degree of control is not without a price as mis-splicing due to mutations in the regulatory elements (ISE, ISS, ESS, ESE) or acceptor or donor sites can give rise to a staggering number of pathologies. One of the causes of spinal muscular atrophy (SMA) has been found to be due to mutation in survival of motor neurons (SMN) protein. SMN is needed for spliceosome assembly and some variant forms of SMN lead to disrupted interaction with exon enhancers and silencers to promote exon skipping (Ward and Cooper, 2010).

Alternative splicing and pharmacogenomics

Genetic variation due to SNP within splicing sites, splicing enhancers/silencers of introns/exon or regulatory elements sequences can have profound effects on the properties and function of a particular protein as well as drug efficacy and metabolism. This probably explains why a particular drug when used within its therapeutic range for the majority can cause some patients to experience toxicity effects or lack of efficacy in others. By employing pharmacogenomics scientists can identify particular SNPs and/or transcripts to predict the optimal drug concentration for individual patients based on their genotype.

Cytochrome P_{450} (CYT) is one of the major family of metabolising enzymes in the liver and is responsible for drugs metabolism (see Chapter 7). Mutations in the splicing sequences of this enzyme, particularly the CYP2D6 isoform, results in expression of a truncated form which cannot break down its substrates. This leads to toxic levels of drugs and overdosing problems. Conversely some drugs are administered as inactive pro-drug that only become active in target tissue after metabolism and if their rate of breakdown is too slow then dosage and efficacy becomes a problem.

The dopamine 2 receptor (D2) has two main transcripts designated long and short. D2 is negatively coupled to adenylyl cyclase (AC) and the two isoforms have differing sensitivity to the antipsychotic drug, benzamide; with the shortened form exhibiting a greater inhibition of AC. Antipsychotic drugs that target D2 receptors have opposing effects depending upon whether the long or short variant of this gene is expressed. Targeting of drugs to the short form has been shown to reduce the side-effects of these antipsychotics. Another splice variant of the D2 receptor has been identified in the brains of psychotic patients (D2Longer) where the AG splice site has been mutated to TG so that part of intron five is retained. Since this transcript has not been isolated in control brains it is suggestive of a correlation between D2 mis-splicing and psychosis (Seeman et al., 2000); see Chapter 3.

8.8 RNA editing

As described earlier in this chapter, genes can be differently transcribed via transcriptional regulation involving transcription factors. Once produced, the stability and the distribution of mRNAs are determined by post-transcriptional modification. It is an important mechanism in eukaryotes and involves RNA binding proteins to select a specific form of a transcript according to the status of the cell. These mechanisms includes (a) capping – the 5' end of precursor mRNA is 'capped' usually with 7-methylguanosine by a 5'-5' triphosphate linkage to protect the mRNA from exonuclease activity; (b) alternative splicing – the removal of introns by spliceosomes and re-packaging exons together to make the mRNA ready for translation; (c) poly-adenylation – the addition of poly-A tail on the 3' end to increase the stability of mRNA during translation (Maas and Rich, 2000)(see figure 8.14); and (d) RNA editing.

The concept of RNA editing

Eukaryotic organisms can employ a variety of mechanisms to increase the number of functionally different proteins produced from a single gene. In 1981, Fox and Leaver postulated that different proteins could be derived from an identical transcript in mitochondrial genes. This could occur if there were minor chemical modifications in the structure of a particular nucleotide within the mRNA transcript. This was later confirmed by Covello and Gray (1989) and has been termed, RNA editing. Subsequent studies have revealed that RNA editing is widespread in many eukaryotic cells. It is now defined as *'post-transcriptional alterations of sequence information in the mRNA beyond what is encoded in the DNA genome'* (Homann, 2008). Therefore after RNA editing the nucleotide sequence of a transcript is changed such that the RNA sequence differs from the original DNA template. This type of re-coding of genomic information is carried out in a systematic and regulated manner to ensure the change of nucleotide identity at a specific position without affecting the total number of nucleotides within the sequence and hence codon shuffling. In some types of RNA editing, such as nucleotide insertion/deletion it is impossible to maintain the original codon sequences. To date, RNA editing has been seen in tRNA, rRNA, mRNA and micro-RNA molecules (Li et al., 2011).

Mechanisms of RNA editing

RNA editing is a highly diverse post-transcriptional process that differs from species to species as well as the type of RNA and the site of alteration. Editing usually occurs in either the nucleus, cytosol, mitochondria or in plastids (Homann, 2008). A plethora of RNA editing phenomena has been described in multi-cellular animals (Yang et al., 2008; Li et al., 2011). Most of them can be grouped into two basic classes namely (a) insertion/deletion editing (nucleotides are inserted into or deleted from the RNA molecule) and (b) substitution editing; also known as 'modification editing' where nucleosides cytosine (C) and adenosine (A) are converted to uracil (U) and Inosine (I) respectively.

Insertion/deletion

This type of RNA editing was first discovered in the mitochondrial RNA (mtRNA) of the protozoan, *Trypanosomes* (Benne et al., 1986) and involved the addition or removal of a U usually in a codon region. This type of editing can occur at several sites in the pre-mRNA transcript to create translation start and stop codons. In addition, it is an important process that allows the insertion of over half

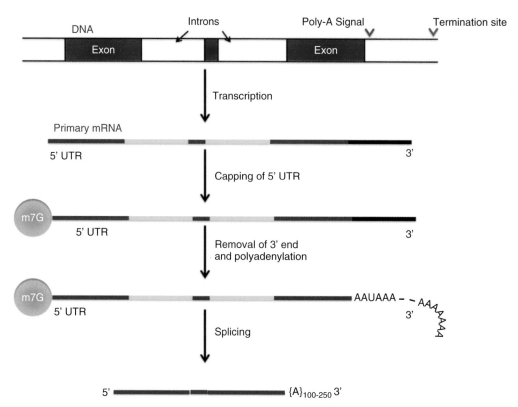

Figure 8.14 Schematic representation of common post-translational modifications. Transcription is usually followed by (1) the addition of 7-methylguanosine (m7G) as a cap on the 5′ end; (2) the addition of a poly-adenosine (A) tail at the 3′ end; and (3) splicing by which introns are removed and exons are joined by spliceosomes to produce a correct protein through translation. UTR = un-translated region.

the protein coding residues of certain mRNAs. Therefore these protozoans would not be viable without U insertion and deletion events.

Subsequent studies using other protozoans like, *Leishmania major*, found that the exact mechanisms involved in the enzymatic cleavage-ligation of U are species specific (Cruz-Reyes et al., 1998). This and other protozoa cause a variety of human diseases including sleeping sickness and Leishmaniasis. Therefore an understanding of the mechanisms involved in insertion or deletion of U residues are of pharmacological interest for the development of treatments against these parasites. The edited mRNAs encode for proteins involved in oxidative phosphorylation (components of the electron transport chain and F-ATPase) making them attractive cytotoxic targets. The pre-edited mRNAs are encoded in a larger mitochondrial DNA, termed the 'maxi-circles', whereas smaller mitochondrial DNAs or 'mini-circles' encode guide RNAs (gRNAs) that

specify the editing. Sequences within gRNA are complementary to the target mRNA (see Figure 8.15) and this gRNA determines the fate and number of U nucleotides to be inserted or deleted. Therefore it is also called RNA-mediated RNA modification (Simpson et al., 2003).

The gRNA first hybridises to pre-edited mRNA just downstream of the editing site (ES). This may be mediated by a RNA chaperone. Any base pairing mismatches will be removed by endonuclease activity. After that, in U insertion, RNA editing 3′-terminal uridyl transferase (TUTase) adds U's to 3′ end of the fragment guided by gRNA's A's and U's. The sites of U insertion and their number are specified within gRNA. On completion, the mRNA fragments are ligated back together by RNA Ligase. Finally, the activity of 3′-5′ exonuclease removes any bulged U's (urindine). On the other hand, in U deletion RNA editing, the unpaired U's from gRNA-mRNA complex are removed by 3′-5′ exonuclease activity. This is followed by RNA ligase activity similar to insertion

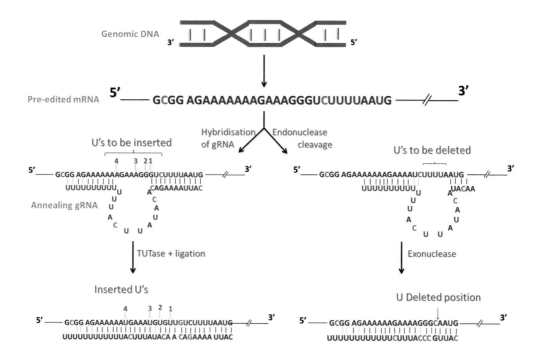

Figure 8.15 Schematic representation of mRNA editing by Uridine (U) insertion/deletion. Insertion and deletion pathways are given on the left and right sides respectively. Pre-edited mRNA can hybridise with guide RNA (gRNA) and either be processed by the 3′ terminal uridylyl transferase (TUTase)/ligation pathway for U nucleotides insertion or the exonuclease pathway for U nucleotide removal.

pathway. The sequence of events in RNA editing by insertion/deletion are summarised in Figure 8.15.

Substitution

Here the chemical conversion of one nucleotide to another alters the codon sequence and hence the amino acid that is inserted into the growing peptide during translation. The resultant protein may have slightly different properties to that of the parent gene. For example the calcium sensor, synaptotagmin-1 is involved in neurotransmitter release at the synapse and an A→I substitution has marked consequences on the potential speed of neurotransmission. In addition, new initiation/termination codons, or splicing sites can be created depending upon where the substitution occurs (Fox and Leaver, 1981).

Whilst in theory it is possible to interchange adenosine with inosine (or guanosine) or cytosine with uracil (or thymine) by removing or adding an amine group the most common known substitutions involve the chemical conversion of A→I and C→U. This involves the enzymes adenosine deaminase acting on RNA (ADAR) and

cytosine deaminase acting on RNA (CDAR) deamination (Figure 8.16) (Blanc and Davidson, 2003). These enzymes do not act serendipitously but are highly coordinated so that certain substitutions occur at the correct position and in the correct cells. When a nucleotide is selected for substitution the RNA molecule introduces specific secondary structures which allow the enzymes and their accessory proteins to interact. These can range from simple regions of double stranded RNA due to the lining up of antiparallel Alu elements as shown in Figure 8.18 or more complicated structures that make the RNA look like a 'knot'.

The first CDAR to be cloned was APOBEC-1, which is the catalytic subunit of the complex that edits Apo-B mRNA. The Apo-B protein plays an important role in lipid and cholesterol transport in the intestines and liver respectively. It achieves this dual role by RNA editing so that a truncated form of the protein is only expressed in the intestines because the substitution of a C for a U produces a stop codon (see Figure 8.17). Basically three adjacent elements within the RNA molecule allow the formation of a small loop. This is recognised by the APOBEC-1

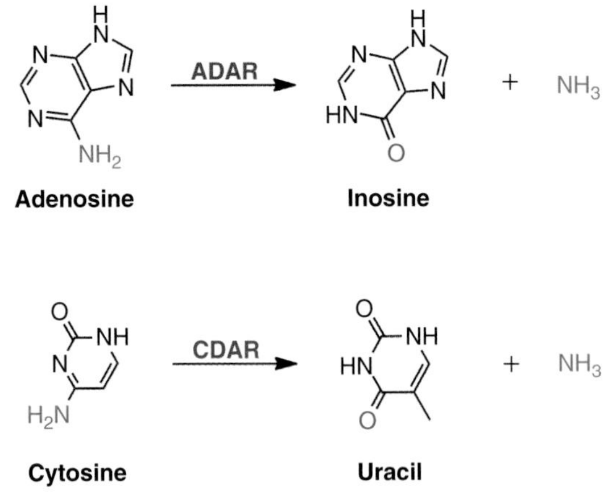

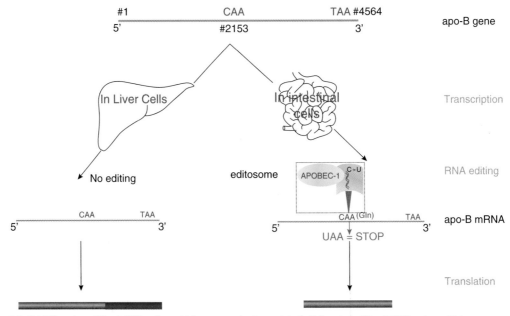

Adenosine → **Inosine** + NH₃ (via ADAR)

Cytosine → **Uracil** + NH₃ (via CDAR)

Figure 8.16 Deamination of adenosine and cytosine. The enzymes adenosine deaminase acting on RNA (ADAR) converts A→I and cytosine deaminase acting on RNA (CDAR) converts C→U.

dimer, which positions it so that the mRNA molecule is sandwiched between it and the target C nucleotide is adjacent to its active site. Accessory proteins such as ACF also interact with the APOBEC-1 complex. Recent studies have found that different ACFs are expressed in different tissue which gives rise to a further level of control.

There are four ADAR gene expressed in animals. Several splice variants with differing enzyme activity and editing-target sites can be expressed in an apparent tissue-specific manner. In fact, ADAR1 has been shown to contain three different promoters. ADAR1 and ADAR2 are expressed ubiquitously throughout the body with the highest expression in the brain. ADAR3 is primarily found in brain tissue whilst the final member of this gene family, TENR, is testis specific. It has been postulated that ADAR3 competes with ADAR1 or ADAR2 for target sequences and may be acting as an inhibitor to repress nucleotide substitution. Knocking out the genes for either ADAR1 or ADAR2 has proven to be lethal in mice illustrating the importance of this type of RNA editing.

Figure 8.17 Schematic representation showing C-to-U RNA editing of apolipoprotein. The apo-B gene in liver does not undergo RNA editing (left panel), therefore produces a polypeptide of 4563 amino acids. The right panel shows the apo-B mRNA in the intestine, which undergoes C→U RNA editing resulting in the change of codon CAA (for glutamine) to UAA (terminator codon). This editing is catalysed by a APOBEC-1 (apolipoprotein B mRNA-editing, enzyme-catalytic-1) deaminase, ACF (apobec-1 complementation factor) complex.

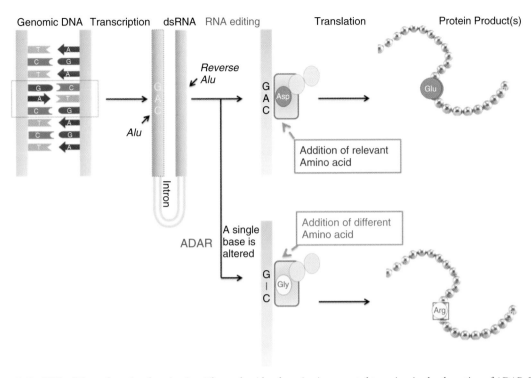

Figure 8.18 RNA editing: adenosine deamination. The nucleotide adenosine is converted to an inosine by the action of ADAR. The CAG codon encodes for a glutamine whereas the CIG codon encodes for an arginine. So in theory the same gene can encode for two different protein products. In practice, a short double-stranded RNA structure within the pre-mRNA is formed. This is because Alu sites within the pre-mRNA line up antiparallel. ADAR recognises this structure and causes the deamination of adenine into inosine.

Figure 8.18 illustrates how ADAR recognises a region of double stranded RNA that has been formed due to the interaction of two antiparallel Alu elements from two different exons. Exchanging an A for an I results in a codon that now encodes for an arginine rather than a glutamine. The effect of substituting this single amino acid can have profound effects upon the properties of a number of different proteins. For example it can alter the conductance of Ca^{2+} ions through the channel of glutamatergic AMPA receptors. This can give rise to brain region specific AMPA receptor expression that enables those neurones to perform a specific function or if they are expressed in other brain regions they can lead to neurodegeneration.

ADAR can also be promiscuous at perfectly double stranded RNA where it can play a role in gene silencing

(see Figure 8.27). It can also facilitate the proliferation and invasion of viruses such as HIV-1.

Another good example is the G-protein coupled receptor, 5-hydroxytryptamine subtype 2C (5-HT$_{2C}$). Several *in vitro* functional studies have shown that five RNA transcripts encoding 5-HT$_{2C}$ are expressed due to A being deaminated to I at five different sites (A, B, C, E, D) in the mRNA transcript (Niswender et al., 1999; Morabito et al., 2010). This results in proteins where an alternative amino acid has been inserted at three positions; 156, 158, and 160. In the unedited transcript these positions are filled by the amino acids, isoleucine (I), asparagine (N) and isoleucine (I). Therefore this transcript is referred to as 5-HT$_{2C}$-INI. If all the A nucleotides are deaminated to I then these amino acids become valine (V), glycine (G), and valine (V). Hence this transcript is known as

155	156	157	158	159	160	Codon
GCA	A B AUA Ile	CGU	C E AAU Asn	CCU	D AUU Ile	unedited
GCA	IUA Val	CGU	AAU Asn	CCU	IUU Val	partial edit
GCA	IUI Val	CGU	IAU Asp	CCU	IUU Val	partial edit
GCA	IUA Val	CGU	AIU Ser	CCU	IUU Val	partial edit
GCA	IUI Val	CGU	IIU Gly	CCU	IUU Val	full edit

Figure 8.19 Effect of nucleotide substitution on amino acid selection for the 5-HT$_{2C}$ gene. The 5HT$_{2C}$ gene has five possible sites for adenosine deamination at A, B, C, E and D. If the transcript is unedited then the protein sequence contains an isoleucine (Ile; I), asparagine (Asn; N) and isoleucine (Ile; I) at codons 156, 158 and 160 respectively. However, if all these adenosines are converted to inosine (full editing) then these codons now encode for valine (Val; V), glycine (Gly; G) and valine (Val; V). A number of partially edited transcripts are also expressed; only three are shown here for clarity. (Asp = aspartate, Ser = serine).

5-HT$_{2C}$-VGV. Up to 24 different partially edited transcripts can also be expressed (see Figure 8.19). These partially and fully edited transcripts have different affinities for the receptor's G-protein and hence activation of the secondary messenger paths that are couple to them (see Figure 8.20).

There is a causal relationship between 5-HT$_{2C}$R mRNA editing and depressive disorders (Thoda et al., 2006; Niswender et al., 2001). Gurevich et al. (2002) found an association with depression-related suicide and editing of the A at positions C and E in amino acid 158 (Herrick-Davis et al., 2001). Whereas, at position D it was more likely to be an A nucleotide that had not been deaminated. Interestingly, preliminary evidence suggests that the anti-depressive, fluoxetine, prevents editing of both A nucleotides at sites C and E whilst facilitating editing at position D (Gurevich et al., 2002).

As depicted in Figure 8.20, the non-edited form 5-HT$_{2C}$-INI can stimulate both the PLC and PLD (phospholipase C and D respectively) pathways. Whereas the fully edited form 5-HT$_{2C}$-VGV is only capable of activating the PLC pathway with reduced efficacy (Price et al., 2001). This could be due in part to 5-HT$_{2C}$-VGV having a five-fold decrease in its affinity for its ligand, 5-HT compared to 5-HT$_{2C}$-INI. The fully edited form has also

lost its constitutive activity (Parker et al., 2003). That is 5-HT$_{2C}$-VGV cannot stimulate inositol triphosphate (IP$_3$) formation in the absence of agonist.

The 5-HT$_{2C}$-VGV transcript is the most prevalent isoform expressed in the human brain and associated with a number of cognitive functions (Niswender et al., 1999). Although the exact functional importance of this type of editing is not clearly known, it has been suggested that it helps to reduce activity of the signalling pathway in certain parts of the brain. Therefore RNA editing of 5-HT$_{2C}$ receptor may play a beneficial role in cognitive disorders. For example, the efficacy of the hallucinogenic recreational drug LSD (lysergic acid diethylamide) is reduced in cells expressing the 5-HT$_{2C}$–VGV isoform (Herrick-Davis et al., 2000; Gresch et al., 2007). However these claims need to be substantiated by additional *in vitro* as well as clinical studies. It is also worth noting A→I editing may have other consequences too. Since I is recognised as guanosine by the splicing machinery A-I editing can also lead to modification of splice sites in introns, inducing premature termination, frame-shift, or new exon formation. In addition, it is also possible this type of RNA editing is widespread amongst the 5-HT receptor super family.

The importance of RNA editing

RNA editing has become an important mechanism of specific gene expression. It has been found to take place in tRNA, rRNA, mRNA and micro-RNA molecules. It is believed that editing has several unique roles (Gott and Emeson, 2000) in each of these types of RNAs; these are summarised in Table 8.6.

Apart from these class specific roles, RNA editing has important evolutionary functions. It not only determines the stable 'flow' of genetic information from DNA to protein but also produces an array of genetic variations with minimal energy expenditure. The introduction of an extra regulatory step helps to diversify protein expression (i.e. multiple proteins can be produced from one gene; Maas and Rich, 2000). It is also believed that by introducing considerable genetic diversity, RNA editing plays a vital part in protecting vertebrates against the infection of exogenous genetic elements such as virus and transposons expression (Hamilton et al., 2010). Above all it can speed up the evolutionary process by antagonising the deleterious effects of genomic mutations (Yang et al., 2008).

The discovery of several RNA editing enzymes such as ADAR, nucleases and ligases, which have the ability to produce functional changes at protein level has created

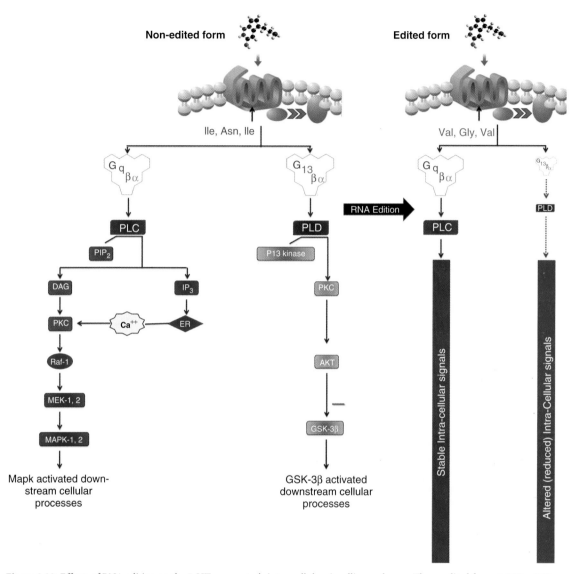

Figure 8.20 Effects of RNA editing on the 5-HT$_{2C}$ receptor's intra-cellular signalling pathways. The unedited form, 5-HT$_{2C}$-INI, can activate either the phospholipase C (PLC) or the phospholipase D (PLD) pathways. However, the fully edited 5-HT$_{2C}$-VGV version has a much lower affinity for the receptor's G-protein and hence severely reduced activation of these pathways. PIP$_2$, phosphatidyl-inostitol biphosphate; IP$_3$, inositol triphosphate; PKC, protein kinase C; P$_{13}$ kinase, phosphatidylinositol 3-kinases; PIP$_3$, Phosphatidylinositol (3,4,5)-triphosphate.

interest in exploring their potential to treat several CNS related and infectious disorders. These include alternations in several receptor mediated intracellular pathways via the 5HT$_{2C}$ receptor and apolipoprotein B (Hinsdale et al., 2002) and the development of therapeutic strategies for the treatment of their related disorders.

8.9 The importance of non-coding RNAs in gene expression

Non-coding RNAs, commonly defined as transcripts that are not translated into proteins, exist in simple as well

Table 8.6 Specific functions of RNA editing.

RNA Type	Type of RNA Editing	
	Base conversion	Base insertion
mRNA	1. Changes in encoded amino acids 2. Splice-site choice change 3. Removal of stop codon	1. Creation of new open reading frames
	1. Creation of START codon (involves conversion/insertion) 2. Creation of STOP codon (involves conversion/insertion)	
tRNA	1. Correcting stem mismatches 2. Creation of substitutes for base modification 3. Changes in tRNA identity	1. Creation of base paired stem 2. Addition of conserved sequence elements 3. Creation of substrates for 5′ and 3′ processing 4. Completion of overlapping tRNAs
rRNA	1. Creation of conserved structural elements 2. Potential modulation of translational efficiency	1. Insertion of nucleotides involved in translational fidelity and efficiency. 2. Creation of conserved structural elements

as in complex forms of life. But, until recently modern technology and traditional thinking failed to recognise their number, diversity, functional roles and importance in molecular diagnostics and drug discovery. Indeed, it now emerges that the complexity of organisms is not just dependant on the number of protein-coding genes but their non-coding RNAs, too (Ponting, 2008; Technau, 2008). These transcripts add an extra layer to the regulation of gene expression, by offering alternative, energetically favourable mechanisms. Hence, non-coding RNAs question the central dogma of biology and the definitions associated with it.

Non-coding RNAs are very diverse – as are their mechanisms of action and functions. The following section can only provide a concise overview of the current knowledge and recent findings in this quickly expanding area.

The discovery of large numbers of non-coding RNAs

The release of a draft sequence of the human genome, in 2001 (International Human Genome Sequencing Consortium, 2001; Venter et al., 2001), was eagerly anticipated by the scientific community, hoping that a genomic inventory would improve our understanding of the blueprint of life. However, the excitement and optimism were dampened by this initial analysis, which predicted a surprisingly low count of protein-coding genes, i.e. ~20,000 to 25,000 or just 1.5% of the entire sequence! In those days, the great majority of the human genome was believed to comprise

transcriptionally-silent nongenic regions, or 'junk' DNA that has no functional purpose, and rather represents genomic fossils of our evolutionary past. The low gene count was also perplexing, because it was little higher than the 19,000 genes of the nematode worm *Caenorhabditis elegans* (C. elegans Sequencing Consortium, 1998), an organism with a far less complex phenotype than the human body.

Over the last decade a very different, multifaceted picture has emerged of the structure of the human genome and how cells utilise this information. For example, RNA sequencing has revealed extensive alternative splicing, with more than 90% of human genes giving rise to different isoforms (Wang et al., 2008); alternative polyadenylation sites also contribute to this transcript diversity. The greatest surprise, however, is that the repertoire of protein-coding genes is complemented by an increasing number of RNA genes, which reside within protein-coding loci or the alleged non-genic regions. Indeed, a pilot project by the Encyclopedia of DNA Elements (ENCODE) consortium concluded that transcription of the human genome is pervasive, as primary transcripts were identified for 93% of bases in a selected region (ENCODE Project Consortium, 2007). Only a small fraction of these transcripts were mRNAs, which encoded proteins of considerable length. The remaining bulk of the transcriptome was rich in various types of non-coding RNA (ncRNA). Despite different sizes, all these untranslated transcripts are defined by a common feature – the lack of an extended open-reading frame, one of the main characteristics of protein-coding mRNAs.

The existence of a diverse range of ncRNAs is not new knowledge. Already in the pre-genomic era, several types of RNA had been intensively studied and classified, including ribosomal RNAs (rRNAs) and transfer RNAs (tRNAs), or spliceosomal small nuclear RNAs (snRNAs). This was followed by the discovery of other ncRNA species, such as natural antisense transcripts (NATs; Spencer et al., 1986) and micro RNAs (miRNAs; Lee et al., 1993). Although their purpose was poorly understood then, they appeared to be very common in prokaryotes and eukaryotes, as implied by the first sequenced microbial and invertebrate genomes (Eddy, 1999). Later, a first systematic search applied the BLAST algorithm and confirmed the existence of numerous human antisense transcripts (Lehner et al., 2002). However, until recently it was not necessarily the lack of available sequence data, but inadequate algorithms of the commonly applied gene prediction methods that failed to identify novel ncRNAs and to uncover the true extent of transcription.

Today, with a rapidly growing number of discovered non-coding RNAs, we are aware that a multitude of them is undoubtedly functional and not a consequence of leakage of transcription, as often argued in the past. They add previously unknown levels of complexity to the regulation of genes, that is, mechanisms which are versatile, quick and economical, as they do not act on the encoded proteins. Supporting evidence for this is drawn from different lines of research (reviewed by Lapidot and Pilpel, 2006; Wahlestedt, 2006; Ponting et al., 2009; Esteller, 2011), such as:

- comparative genomics – remarkably, the chromosomal position of many investigated ncRNA genes is conserved between species, and probably indicates their functional importance at that locus
- evolutionary studies – ncRNA genes appear to be under selective pressure, because they display reduced substitution rates in comparison to other neutrally-evolving sequences
- expression studies – some ncRNA genes are tightly regulated, with expression profiles specific to a tissue, subcellular location or developmental stage, or they are co-regulated with other genes; like mRNAs, various types of ncRNAs are even processed (e.g. spliced, polyadenylated)
- functional studies – dysfunction of ncRNAs through naturally-occurring or experimentally-evoked processes may result in states of diseases.

These examples demonstrate that the terms 'non-genic' and 'non-coding' are no longer synonymous to 'non-functional' or 'junk' DNA. Modern genetics now faces the challenge to revise the definition of 'gene' (see Box 8.1) – and the daunting tasks of annotating numerous RNA genes with yet unknown function, or perhaps no function. For pharmacologists, on the other hand, the study of ncRNAs is a fascinating area, since it is likely

---

Box 8.1 Genes and genomes – multiple layers of encoded information

Over the last 70 years, the definition of 'gene' and its coding potential has undergone several revisions. One early version was the 'one gene-one enzyme' hypothesis by Beadle and Tatum (1941), which was later generalised into the 'one gene-one polypeptide' theory (Ingram, 1957). Following the discoveries of introns in genes and post-transcriptional modifications, some genes were known to have the potential to encode multiple proteins (Berget et al., 1977; Chow et al., 1977). Since those bygone days, protein-coding genes are often (mis)understood as defined transcriptional units, containing exons and introns, untranslated regions, promoters, and perhaps enhancer and repressor elements – and the term 'coding' is associated with DNA sequences, which have an recognisable open-reading frame for the production of proteins. If genes are transcribed into non-translatable transcripts, they are commonly referred to as non-coding (RNA) genes.

These traditional views, however, are outdated as they do not consider the recent revelations from the RNA world (discussed by Brosius, 2009). Surprisingly, many loci in the genome are multigenic (Ponting et al., 2009), that is, RNA genes may reside within or are interleaved with protein-coding genes, and some promoters are bidirectionally transcribed. In nature's reality, the boundaries between transcriptional units are often blurred (see Figure 8.24). In addition, the coding capacity of a transcript is not just encrypted in the primary sequence, in the presence of a series of codons. For example, specific sequence elements influence the turnover of a transcript, while certain codons may slow down the elongation process during translation. Other codes, such as those for splicing or A-to-I editing, exist in secondary and tertiary structures, or combinations of them. In particular, the diversity among 'non-coding' RNAs and their interactions indicate that multiple layers of instructions are embedded in these transcripts – but how is largely unknown. This also applies to the post-transcriptional cleavage of a large number of RNAs, which give rise to smaller functionally-independent fragments (Tuck and Tollervey, 2011). In conclusion, the term 'non-coding RNA' is imprecise and should probably be replaced by 'non-protein-coding RNA', as suggested by several authors (Brosius, 2009).

to reveal a new spectrum of potential drug targets and means of applying a new generation of drugs.

Classes of non-coding RNA

The classification of non-coding RNAs is primarily based on functional aspects, and distinguishes two main groups: housekeeping RNAs and regulatory RNAs. Each group can be further divided into classes and subclasses according to structure, size and subcellular location of the non-coding transcripts (see Figure 8.21 and Table 8.7). This classification is a dynamic field, but the name of an annotated ncRNA is usually indicative of its class. Like for protein-coding genes in human, the nomenclature for ncRNA genes is standardised. Unique gene names and gene symbols (i.e. short-form abbreviations) are only assigned by the HUGO Gene Nomenclature Committee (HGNC; Seal et al., 2011). Similar nomenclature committees exist for several commonly used model organisms, such as the mouse or the nematode *C. elegans*.

The 'classical' group of housekeeping RNAs consists of constitutively expressed and well-characterised ncRNAs, such as those involved in protein biosynthesis (i.e. rRNAs, tRNAs), RNA maturation (e.g. snRNAs and small nucleolar RNAs [snoRNAs]) or RNAs with catalytic activity (i.e. ribozymes, such RNase P). Surprisingly, they are greatly outnumbered by the genes and transcripts of regulatory RNAs (Figure 8.21; Wright and Bruford,

2011), including long non-coding RNAs (lncRNAs), microRNAs (miRNAs), endogenous small-interfering RNAs (siRNAs), Piwi-interacting RNAs (piRNAs) and transcription initiation RNAs (tiRNAs). Although most of them have only been revealed recently, they now represent major classes of ncRNAs – and continue to grow in numbers due to advanced genomic and transcriptomic approaches. They are subject to intensive research in complex as well as primitive multicellular organisms, since they are involved in widespread and diverse forms of gene regulation (for details, see Table 8.7).

At present, the basic mechanisms of action of the major regulatory RNAs are understood, however the specific purposes of individual ncRNAs remain largely unknown. In addition to the major RNA classes, eukaryotic cells generate small ncRNAs, which only exist in a few different types and are expressed by a small number of genes. If they are functionally annotated, they may be grouped as 'miscellaneous' ncRNAs. Some databases also consider human pseudogene RNAs as a separate group, while others assign them to lncRNAs. This large group of ncRNAs (>7,400) arises from genomic loci that have lost their capacity to generate proteins, but may still play a role in gene regulation.

The following sections focus on three groups of regulatory RNAs, which have received significant interest from researchers in the field of drug discovery: siRNAs and miRNAs, and lncRNAs.

RNA interference through small interfering RNAs and microRNAs

In 1998, Fire and Mello published a scientific breakthrough that would earn them the Nobel Prize eight years later (Fire et al., 1998). By injecting single-stranded sense and antisense RNAs together into *C. elegans*, they were able to interfere with the expression of selected genes, in a very effective and specific manner. This observation of post-transcriptional gene silencing followed other earlier studies, such as those in plants by Jorgensen and coworkers (Napoli et al., 1990). However, the significance of Fire and Mello's work was the conclusion and the experimental proof that the interference was initiated by RNA duplexes, which had formed from the single-stranded RNAs used in their study.

Today, this phenomenon is known to occur naturally in plants and metazoan animals (Technau, 2008), and it is referred to as RNA interference (RNAi), or gene knockdown as it reduces the level of the corresponding transcript. RNAi involves

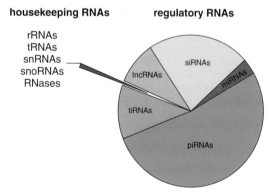

Figure 8.21 In humans, the number of the classical housekeeping RNAs account for only several hundred different types, while regulatory RNAs are believed to exist in tens of thousands of different types (see Table 8.7 for details). These data are based on a publication by Wright and Bruford (2011), Esteller (2011) and statistics on the HGNC website in 2011 (www.genenames.org).

Table 8.7 The major classes of human ncRNAs originating from the nuclear genome. The system here distinguishes characteristic functions and sizes in nucleotides (nt); pseudogene RNAs and other small miscellaneous RNAs are not presented as independent groups. It should be noted that there is no clear delineation between several classes of ncRNAs. The classification as well as the number of types in each category vary depending on the source of information, even among the most recent literature (Ghildiyal and Zamore, 2009; Wright and Bruford, 2010; Esteller, 2011). Some authors separate lncRNAs further into subclasses, and others do not mention siRNAs at all.

Name	Size (nt)	Number	Function
Classic ncRNAs			
rRNAs	120-5000	4	essential parts of ribosomes; site of protein translation
tRNAs	70-80	49	transport of amino acids; involved in protein translation
snRNAs	60-360	5	parts of spliceosomes; involved in splicing of primary transcripts
snoRNAs	60-300	>300	post-transcriptional modifications to rRNAs, tRNAs and snRNAs
RNases	260-320	2	processing of rRNA or tRNA precursors
Regulatory ncRNAs			
lncRNAs	>200	>4300?	gene regulation, post-transcriptional and epigenetic modifications
miRNA	19-24	>1,400?	post-transcriptional regulation
siRNA	~21	>10,000?	post-transcriptional regulation, transposon control, viral defence
piRNA	26-31	>23,400?	transposon defence during spermatogenesis
tiRNAs	17-18	>5,000?	regulation of transcription (?)

different intracellular pathways and small RNAs, including siRNAs, miRNAs and piRNAs, which act as gene-silencing effector molecules. The common feature of these RNAs is the interference with selected target transcripts, but they differ in their biogenesis from precursor molecules, the intracellular sorting and their molecular mode of action (reviewed by Ghildiyal and Zamore, 2009). However, our basic understanding of the RNAi mechanism has improved rapidly since its discovery. The fact that RNAi is a natural process with sequence-specific and potent mediators has fueled research in this field, and led to the development of RNAi technologies (reviewed by Davidson and McCray, 2011). Already in 2001, it was demonstrated that chemically-synthesised siRNAs can induce sequence-specific knockdown in mammalian cells (Elbashir et al., 2001).

The siRNA pathway

The early studies on RNAi and the siRNA pathway were predominantly carried out in invertebrates, such as *C. elegans* or *Drosophila*. Exogenous double-stranded RNAs (dsRNAs) served frequently as precursors, which were observed to be processed into siRNAs duplexes of ~21 bp and with two-nucleotide 3′ overhangs (Figure 8.23; Elbashir et al., 2001). This also led to the long-lasting view that the siRNA pathway mainly serves as a

defence mechanism against dsRNA, deriving from either invading viruses (exogenous source) or transposons (endogenous). However, other endogenous siRNAs (endo-siRNAs) and new genomic sources for their production have recently been identified in *Drosophila* and mice (e.g. Okamura et al., 2008; Tam et al., 2008). These findings suggest that another role of the siRNA pathway may be the regulation of genes. Apart from transposons, endo-siRNAs can originate from a) repeats of a pseudogene and its duplicated but inverted copy, b) duplex formation between transcripts from a parent gene and its pseudogene, or c) convergently and d) bidirectionally transcribed loci (Figures 8.22 and 8.23; Sasidharan and Gerstein, 2008).

The siRNA-mediated RNAi pathway is initiated in the cytoplasm (Ghildiyal and Zamore, 2009) by Dicer, a member of the RNase III family. It cleaves the dsRNA substrate molecules into 21 bp-siRNA duplexes and subsequently forms a loading complex that transfers the siRNA into the precursor RNA-induced silencing complex (pre-RISC). Here, the siRNA associates with an Argonaute (AGO) protein and is unwound into a guide strand, which is retained, and a passenger strand, which is degraded by AGO. This selection depends on the thermodynamic stabilities at the 5′ ends of the duplex, that is, a low GC content at the 5′ end of the guide strand facilitates the loading and unwinding of the duplex from

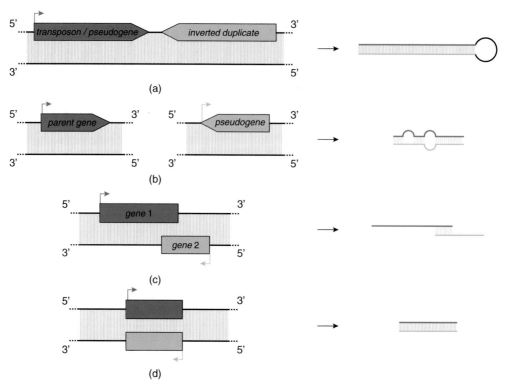

Figure 8.22 Precursors for endo-siRNAs can be intramolecular stem-loop structures, which are transcribed from a pseudogene/transposon and its duplicated but inverted copy (a). Other Dicer substrates are intermolecular dsRNAs, which formed after expression of a parent gene and its pseudogene (b), or convergently (c) and bidirectionally (d) transcribed loci.

one side (Kvorova et al., 2003; Schwarz et al., 2003). Following the release of the passenger strand, the guide strand directs the now-activated RISC to the target transcript, where it associates into an RNA duplex with fully matching sequences. In the final stage, the cleavage of the target mRNA, by AGO, leads to a reduced protein output.

Despite millions of years of species-specific evolution, the siRNA pathway is remarkably well-preserved across the animal kingdom. Differences exist mainly in the number of the involved key factors and auxiliary proteins; for example, only one Dicer exists in humans, but *Drosophila* has two isoforms with distinct functions, that is, Dicer-2 generates siRNAs, while Dicer-1 is involved in the miRNA pathway. Another exception is found in *C. elegans*, where the silencing effect can be amplified through secondary siRNAs (Sijen et al., 2001). These are synthesised by an RNA-dependent RNA polymerase (RdRP), after the formation of the duplex between the initial guide strand and its target mRNA; RdRP uses the mRNA as template.

The miRNA pathway

During the search for small antisense ncRNAs, the cloning of lin-4 from *C. elegans* marked the identification of the class of miRNAs (Lee et al., 1993). They are single-stranded RNAs of ~22 nucleotides, which exist in nearly all metazoan animals (Technau, 2008). In contrast to siRNAs, they bind with imperfect complementarity to the 3'UTR of target mRNAs and repress the translation.

The biogenesis of miRNAs typically starts in the nucleus with the synthesis of primary miRNAs (pri-miRNA; Figure 8.23; reviewed by Miller and Wahlestedt, 2010). These precursor molecules are often encoded by clusters of miRNA genes, or they originate from transcribed and spliced intronic sequences (mirtrons) of host genes (e.g. Okamura et al., 2007). Subsequently, the RNase III endonuclease Drosha in combination with an auxiliary protein trims the pri-miRNA into ~70-nucleotide pre-miRNAs, which have a characteristic stem-loop structure and a two-nucleotide 3' overhang. Exportin 5 now carries a pre-miRNAs through the nuclear pore into the

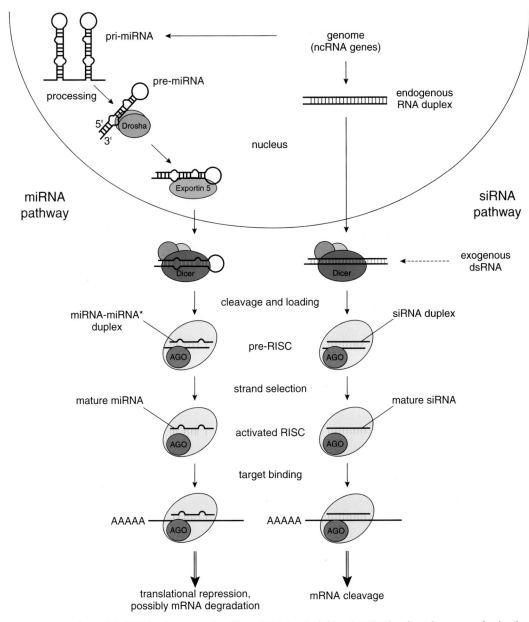

Figure 8.23 Comparison of the RNAi pathways mediated by miRNA (on the left) and siRNA (on the right; see text, for details on the biogenesis of the small interfering RNAs, the involved key molecules and the effects on the targeted transcripts) AGO, Argonaute.

cytoplasm, where a protein complex containing Dicer produces a miRNA-duplex of ~22 bp length. Comparable to the siRNA pathway, the duplex is loaded into the RISC complex and its thermodynamic signature determines, which of its arms produces the guide strand (miRNA) or the passenger strand (miRNA*). The latter is usually

degraded by AGO and rarely detectable in cell extracts, while the mature miRNA enables the target finding of the activated RISC complex. This recognition process only requires a limited degree of complementarity and is essentially mediated by the 'seed' sequence, a region spanning nucleotides 2–8 at the 5′ end of the miRNA

(Brennecke et al., 2005). Due to the partial binding, a single miRNA is able to target numerous transcripts; it causes translational repression, followed by mRNA degradation. Although the initial repression is reversible and may be a means of storing transcripts, miRNAs predominantly act to decrease mRNA levels (Guo et al., 2010). On the other hand, a perfect sequence match between the miRNA and its target, even though rare, results in the immediate mRNA destruction by AGO, as observed for siRNAs.

Overall, miRNAs are thought to be global regulators of gene activity during most processes including development, proliferation, differentiation and apoptosis. Their own expression is often regulated in a tissue and time-specific manner. Surprisingly, over half of the miRNAs discovered in mice were expressed in the brain (Landgraf et al., 2007), where miRNAs also contribute to synaptogenesis, dendrite morphogenesis and synaptic plasticity. Their functional significance can be illustrated by miR-134, a miRNA that derives from an activity-dependent cluster of pri-miRNAs. MiR-134 is located at postsynaptic sites, where it controls dendritic growth by down regulating the translational repressor Pumilio2, in response to neuronal activity (Fiore et al., 2009). In addition, miR-134 decreases the dendritic spine volume of mature neurons through the repression of the kinase Limk1, which otherwise polymerises actin (Schratt et al., 2006). Neuronal activation with BDNF, however, de-represses miR-134 function and consequently enlarges the spine size.

Long non-coding RNAs

Non-coding transcripts longer than 200 nucleotides are arbitrarily grouped into the class of long non-coding RNAs. Their characteristic length may distinguish them from smaller regulatory RNAs, such as siRNAs or miRNAs, but not necessarily from translatable mRNAs.

Indeed, despite their insignificant protein-coding capacity, many lncRNAs undergo processing. Like primary mRNA transcripts that are prepared for translation, they are spliced, capped and polyadenylated (Kapranov et al., 2007; Guttman et al., 2009). This phenomenon hampers a clear distinction in structure and function between lncRNAs and mRNAs – as evident by numerous incorrectly annotated protein-coding mRNAs, which now appear to be lncRNAs (Ponting, 2008). Functional characterisation is further complicated by the existence of bifunctional transcripts that can either encode a functional protein or serve as RNA with intrinsic function (see below, the RevErbAα RNA; Ulveling et al., 2011).

Genes of lncRNAs do not only reside within the previously alleged, non-genic regions, but also in loci that encode proteins. They can be arranged into five categories, which are based on their genomic positions in relation to the structure of protein-coding genes (see Figure 8.23; Ørom and Shiekhattar, 2011; Wright and Buford, 2011): i) The lncRNA gene is located on the opposite DNA strand and generates a complimentary transcript, ii) the lncRNA is entirely generated from an intron, iii) the transcriptional start site is found in the promoter or the 5′/3′ untranslated regions, iv) the lncRNA is transcribed from an exon of a protein-coding gene (and may also retain an intron), or v) it is located at an intergenic region, between two protein-coding units. The class of lncRNAs, however, is very heteromorphous, and some of their genes do not fit into a single category, as they are combinations of the scenarios above. These examples highlight that even the traditional view of distinct and non-overlapping transcriptional units is outdated (see Box 8.1).

Among these lncRNAs are *cis*-natural antisense transcripts (*cis*-NATs) that originate from the opposite DNA strand in close proximity to another transcriptional unit (see Figure 8.24 (a)). Due to their genomic position, they

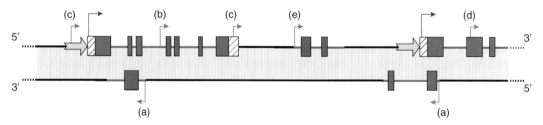

Figure 8.24 The transcriptional units of two protein-coding genes are schematised with their promoters (yellow arrows), transcriptional start sites (blue arrows), exons (blue boxes) and untranslated regions (UTRs; hatched boxes). This hypothetical genomic site also harbours several lncRNA genes (green), which may be transcribed (green arrows) from: the opposite (antisense) strand (a), introns of protein-coding genes (b), promoters or UTRs (c), exons of protein-coding genes (d), or more distal intergenic locations (e). In this greatly simplified diagram, promoter regions of lncRNA genes are not illustrated.

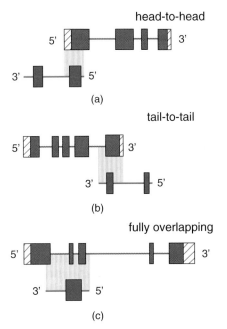

head-to-head

tail-to-tail

fully overlapping

Figure 8.25 Formation of sense-antisense pairs between primary transcripts. Depending on the degree of overlap, pairs of these primary transcripts are orientated in a head-to-head (5′ to 5′; divergent; a), tail-to-tail (3′ to 3′; convergent; b), or fully overlapping manner (c).

have some overlap and perfect sequence complementarity with the sense transcript, which facilitates the formation of sense-antisense pairs. Depending on the degree of overlap, these transcript pairs are orientated in a head-to-head (5′ to 5′) or divergent, tail-to-tail (3′ to 3′) or convergent, or fully overlapping manner (see Figure 8.25). Such configurations, of which the divergent arrangement is the predominant type, are also likely to occur between protein-coding mRNAs as well as non-coding transcripts (Katayama et al., 2005).

Cis-NATs are a well-studied and relatively common variety of lncRNAs; possibly around 20% of transcriptional units in humans harbour genes for *cis*-NATs (Chen et al., 2004). In addition, the transcriptome contains another fraction of antisense transcripts, termed *trans*-NATs, which are generated from intergenic regions. Sense-antisense pairs formed by these lncRNAs display imperfect sequence complementarity, as the genes of the *trans*-NATs and the target transcripts are positioned at separate chromosomal loci. However, this apparent lack in sequence specificity potentially enables *trans*-NATs to target several sense transcripts, as it is the case for

miRNAs. Overall, the functional roles of *trans*-NATs are poorly understood, and only a few have been functionally characterised (see below, other mechanisms of lncRNA function). Among other roles, it has been suggested that they act as precursors for small ncRNAs (Kapranov et al., 2007).

How many of the identified lncRNAs fulfil functional roles is currently unknown. However, data from expression profiling and genomic studies indicates that they are not random by-products of transcription. On the contrary, their genes appear to be subject to evolutionary constraints, with tightly-regulated expression patterns, reduced nucleotide substitutions compared to other non-genic DNA (e.g. transposable elements), and conserved genomic positions (Guttman et al., 2009; Ponting et al., 2009). For example, a comparison between human and chimpanzee lncRNA genes revealed expression profiles, which are tissue-specific and evolutionary conserved across both species (Khaitovich et al., 2006). Numerous other lncRNA genes are transcribed during a specific developmental stage, together with protein-coding genes in their genomic vicinity (Ponjavic et al., 2009). In addition, the regions within or near the 3′ termini of many protein-coding genes are rich in binding sites for transcription factors, which are correlated with the transcription of non-coding RNAs at that locus (Cawley et al., 2004).

Further support for a controlled expression of lncRNA genes and their regulatory roles derives from *cis*-NAT pairs. The regulation of sense and their antisense partners often follows either a concordant or a discordant expression pattern, and results in similar or inverse levels of transcript, respectively (Katayama et al., 2005). Other transcript pairs, however, do not show a clear correlation in their expression profiles. This possibly mirrors the complexities of interleaved transcriptional units within a chromosomal region – and the diverse mechanisms through which these non-coding RNAs act.

Function and mechanisms of action

Long non-coding RNAs are a heteromorphous group. They reside and act in different subcellular compartments of the nucleus or the cytoplasm, and influence the regulation of genes in close genomic proximity (*cis*-acting) or at distant sites (*trans*-acting). Frequently, their molecular mechanisms rely on the formation of Watson-Crick base pairs (bp) between natural antisense transcripts and their sense complements. However, functionality does not exclusively depend on the linear nucleotide sequence and perfect complementarity. Other lncRNAs interact with their molecular environment, including proteins, through secondary structures (structural complementarity), they may physically block cellular processes, or coat and thus epimodify chromosomal domains (see below). The *cis*-regulatory mechanisms fall into four groups (Lavorna et al., 2004; see Figures 8.26 to 8.28): i) transcriptional interference, the formation of RNA duplexes in ii) the nucleus or iii) the cytoplasm, and iv) chromatin remodelling (RNA-DNA interactions).

Transcriptional interference

According to the model of transcriptional interference, a sense gene is repressed by the simultaneous expression of an lncRNA gene from the opposite strand, rather than by the corresponding *cis*-NAT transcript itself. The hypothesis originally derived from studies in yeast (Peterson and Meyers, 1993; Prescott and Proudfoot, 2002), where reduced transcript levels were observed for opposing genes, if they overlapped. Similarly, an inverse correlation between the length of the overlapping regions and the level of expression of a *cis*-NAT pair was detected in human and mice, two more complex organisms (Osato et al., 2007). The levels of sense and antisense transcripts were comparably high, if the overlapping region was less than 200 bp, but they vanished if the overlap exceeded 2000 bp.

For genes on opposite strands, the interference is believed to occur during the elongation process of transcription, when the two RNA polymerase II complexes converge and eventually collide due to their sizes; the transcription either halts or continues on one strand only (see Figure 8.26). In addition, the expression of an lncRNA gene, which is located on the same DNA strand, can prevent or delay the initiation of transcription of an adjacent gene, while the RNA polymerase proceeds through the latter's promoter.

Formation of RNA duplexes

The formation of RNA duplexes in the nucleus and the cytoplasm is a common phenomenon, but the functional consequences of *cis*-NAT pairs are diverse. They depend on the spatiotemporal profiles of the sense and antisense transcripts as well as their subcellular locations. Post-transcriptional processes, which may be manipulated by double-stranded RNA, include alternative splicing and RNA editing (in the nucleus), and mRNA translation and stability (cytoplasm).

A well-characterised example for antisense-regulated splicing is the mammalian α-thyroid hormone receptor TRα (Hastings et al., 1997). The corresponding gene *erbAα* generates a pre-mRNA, which can give rise to two variants, α1 and α2, through alternative splicing of the 3′ end (see Figure 8.27a). Although both transcripts only differ in unique 3′ exons, they are translated into functionally-antagonistic proteins: The TRα1 isoform can bind α-thyroid hormone and trigger a genetic response, whereas TRα2 does not have this ability as it lacks the hormone-binding domain at the C terminus. However, TRα2 antagonises the activated TRα1 receptor by competing for the same DNA binding sites on target genes. Interestingly, the opposite strand of the *erbAα* locus harbours the *RevErbAα* gene, which is transcribed into a bifunctional RNA, holding the information either for a heme-binding receptor or an antisense transcript. In its capacity as antisense mRNA, the RevErbAα RNA is an important physiological regulator, because it overlaps in a tail-to-tail fashion with the erbAα pre-mRNA and masks splicing enhancers sites, which are involved in generating the α2 variant (Salato et al., 2010). Consequently, the splicing machinery favours the production of the hormone-responsive TRα1 receptor. This case illustrates how, in the nucleus, RNA masking through duplexes can restrict the splicing possibilities by blocking elements,

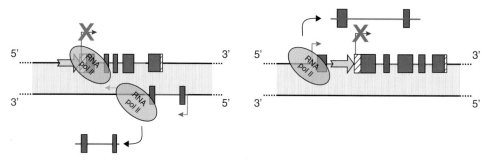

Figure 8.26 Transcriptional interference can result from the collision of two converging RNA polymerase II (RNA pol II) complexes (on the left), or when the expression of an ncRNA gene hinders the expression of a second gene located further downstream.

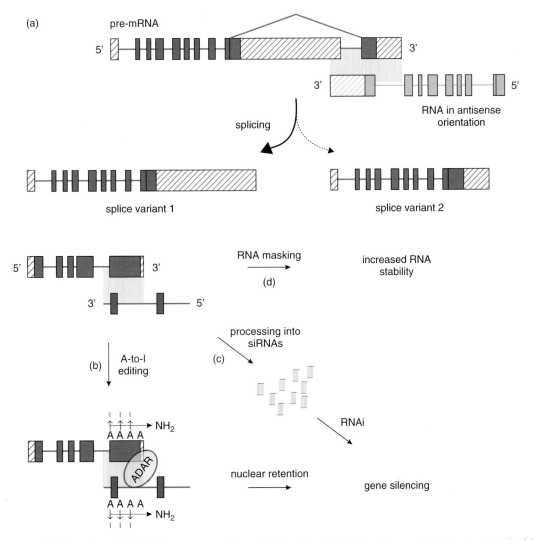

Figure 8.27 The formation of RNA duplexes may cause changes in the splicing (a), editing (b), processing (c) or stability (d) of the protein-coding transcripts (see text for details). ADAR, adenosine deaminase acting on RNA enzyme.

which are necessary for the interaction with *trans*-acting splicing factors. Similar scenarios may potentially obscure signals, on the pre-mRNA, for polyadenylation and termination, or translational repression by interfering RNAs (see below) A-to-I RNA editing is a post-transcriptional and dsRNA-dependent event, in which nuclear ADAR (adenosine deaminase acting on RNA) enzymes hydrolyse adenosine (A) to inosine (I), at selected nucleotide positions (Bass, 2002). Given that inosine is read as guanosine during the subsequent translation, the conversion potentially alters the amino acid sequence of the encoded protein and secondarily its physiological properties. The

molecular mechanisms for site-selective editing of the mRNA are not fully understood, but an essential step is probably the intramolecular formation of dsRNA, with imperfect complementarity. In contrast, long and perfect *cis*-NAT pairs (intermolecular duplexes) are randomly hyper-edited by ADAR (see Figure 8.27b), and can afterwards be retained in nuclear complexes by the RNA-binding protein p54[nrb] (Zhang and Carmichael, 2001). This process may contribute to the silencing of genes, as has been proposed for numerous human transcripts, which contain pairs of inverted and thus hyper-edited Alu elements in their 3′ UTRs (Chen et al., 2008). However, with respect to NATs, the current lack of experimental evidence argues against a significant role of this antisense-mediated mechanism, while other facts favour RNAi as the alternative pathway.

Indeed, some invertebrate and vertebrate RNA duplexes are believed to act as endogenous precursors for so-called endo-siRNAs, that is, interfering RNAs which do not originate from exogenous dsRNA (Okamura and Lai, 2008; Figure 8.27c). Support for this hypothesis comes from the pioneering work by Kapranov et al. (2007), who examined the genomic origins of different-sized RNAs in human cell lines. The genome-wide study strongly indicated that, based on sequence similarities, around 40% of short RNAs (<200 nucleotides) found in the cytosol may be processed from long polyadenylated RNAs in the nucleus. Whether these long precursors were sense-antisense duplexes, could not be resolved in this, but in a similar study on mouse oocytes a year later (Watanabe et al., 2008). For example, a cluster of over a hundred small RNAs (19–22 nucleotides in length) was linked to the *Pdzd/Kif4* locus, where two opposing genes are orientated in a divergent manner. Interestingly, the majority of these RNAs only derived from the overlapping region that the predicted *cis*-NAT pair is likely to form. Several other clusters of endo-siRNAs originated from *trans*-NAT duplexes, which were assemblies of an mRNA and its processed pseudogene transcript. One such pair, with ~90% sequence identity, comprised the RNAs from the *Ppp4r1* gene on chromosome 17 and its pseudogene that is located on chromosome 8, within an intron of another gene. They gave rise to siRNAs, which exclusively mapped either to the pseudogene locus or to exons of the *Ppp4r1* gene. Most other siRNAs in the growing mouse oocytes were generated from retrotransposons. In addition, mutant oocytes lacking Dicer showed significantly reduced levels of siRNAs, which derived from the investigated chromosomal loci, while the levels of the corresponding transcripts increased (Watanabe et al., 2008). Taken together, this demonstrates that naturally-formed dsRNAs can be substrates for endo-siRNAs, which down regulate protein-coding genes through a Dicer-dependent RNAi pathway.

RNA duplex formation in the cytoplasm may also affect the stability of a transcript (Faghihi et al., 2008), as hypothesised for the mRNA of the β-secretase 1 (*BACE1*). It overlaps by 104 nucleotides and in perfect complementarity with the antisense transcript *BACE1-AS* that is expressed from the opposite strand at the same locus.

Experimental knockdown of *BACE1-AS in vitro* did not only reduce the levels of *BACE1* and the β-secretase 1 protein, but also decreased the half-life of *BACE1*. It was concluded that both transcripts are regulated concordantly and that the duplex formation decelerates the degradation of mRNA through RNases (Figure 8.27d). Recently, the same authors identified RNA masking as a possible explanation, for *BACE1-AS* can occupy the binding site for the microRNA miR-485-5p, on *BACE1*, which otherwise would lead to translational repression and destabilisation of the *BACE1* mRNA (Faghihi et al., 2010).

Chromatin remodelling

RNA-DNA interactions can initiate epigenetic changes, that is, heritable alterations of the chromatin structure (chromatin remodelling), and lead to monoallelic expression of genes. The modifications frequently include alterations in the methylation status of histone proteins or DNA regions (not their sequence), but they can also involve changes in ubiquitylation and acetylation. Such epigenetic marks are stable and transmissible, and may be propagated clonally to daughter cells or from parents to their progeny, but they are not necessarily permanent. The two best studied examples of chromatin remodelling, which are induced by antisense transcripts, are X chromosome inactivation and genomic imprinting.

X chromosome inactivation (XCI) in mammals is a critical process that takes place during the early developmental stages of the female embryo (Pontier and Gribnau, 2011). It results in the inactivation of most genes on one X-chromosome (Xi), which afterwards appears morphologically as dense heterochromatic region, referred to as Barr body; the second X-chromosome (Xa) remains transcriptionally active. Whether the cell silences the female or male-inherited X-chromosome, is random. The purpose of XCI is to ensure equal expression of genes located on the X-chromosome in males (XY) and females (XX), as otherwise the differences in gene copy numbers are potentially harmful to the female gender.

This form of dosage compensation is a fascinating example of the complexities of RNA-mediated gene regulation, because it requires the interaction of several genes on the X-chromosome. Remarkably, many of them are transcribed into non-coding RNAs, and they are located within the X chromosome inactivation centre (Xic; Figure 8.28), from where the silencing process spreads out. Key to this cascade of events is the accumulation of Xist (X-inactivation specific transcript), a spliced and polyadenylated lncRNA of 19 kb (human;

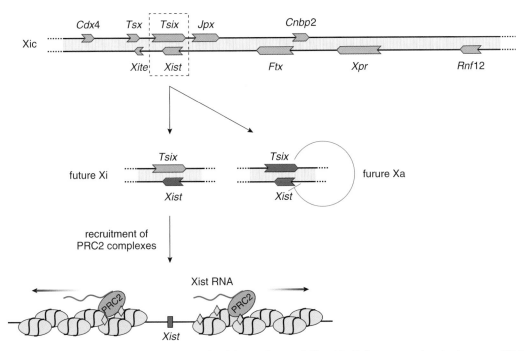

Figure 8.28 X chromosome inactivation as an example of chromatin remodelling. The X chromosome inactivation centre (Xic) comprises predominantly of ncRNA genes, including *Xist* and *Tsix*. Their expression as well as their transcripts orchestrate changes in the methylation signature, which leads to the inactivation of the X chromosome.

Brown et al., 1991) or 17 kb (mouse; Borsani et al., 1991). Once expressed Xist begins to coat the future Xi in *cis* and to recruit chromatin-modifying protein complexes, including the polycomb repressive complex 2 (PRC2), which leave their epigenetic marks. PRC2 methylates the *Xist* gene promoter and drastically enhances *Xist* expression, and eventually it trimethylates the lysine K 27 on histone H3 (H3K27me3) throughout Xi and inactivates its genes (Marks et al., 2009). Amongst other alterations are the gradual loss of the methylation on H3K4me3, the hypoacetylation of histone H4 and the ubiquitylation of a site on H2. Noteworthy, the silencing process excludes some genes on Xi, but it remains stable throughout mitosis and does not require the Xist RNA for maintenance.

On the active X-chromosome Xa, however, the Xist activity would be detrimental and needs to be suppressed. The cell achieves this through Tsix, another non-coding RNA that spans 40 kb in antisense orientation to Xist (Lee et al., 1999; Figure 8.28). It is believed to antagonise Xist via transcriptional interference, dsRNA-mediated RNAi or recruitment of chromatin remodelling complexes to the *Xist* promoter. Although the expression of the *Tsix* gene is initially observed on both X-chromosomes, it turns

monoallelic (i.e. from Xa) following the up-regulation of *Xist* on Xi, and it ceases once XCI is established. In addition, *Xist* expression is positively influenced by other non-coding RNAs originating within the inactivation centre (e.g. Ftx and Jpx), or inhibited by various autosomal-encoded transcription factors.

Genomic imprinting is also due to differential epigenetic marks on the homologous chromosomes, but the monoallelic expression occurs in a strictly parent-of-origin-specific manner, that is, either the maternally or the paternally-inherited allele is active. The second major difference to XCI is that the epimodifications are generally acquired during gametogenesis and then transmitted to the next generation, where they persist throughout life (Radford et al., 2011).

Currently, some 100 imprinted genes are known, which are predominantly located in clusters in the genome, such as the *Kcnq1* locus on chromosome 11 in human (Lee et al., 1999b; Smilinich et al., 1999). It contains at least eight, maternally-expressed protein-coding genes and the paternally-expressed lncRNA gene *Kcnq1ot1*, which lies in antisense direction within intron 10 of the *Kcnq1* gene (Kanduri, 2011). The expression of *Kcnq1ot1* depends on the DNA methylation status of its promoter, and it is thought to drive the bidirectional gene silencing on the paternal loci. While the introduced histone modifications (e.g. H3K27me3 and H3K9me3) repress the paternal alleles, others (e.g. H3K4me3) activate the genes on the maternal chromosome. Remarkably, the inactivation is initiated in *cis*, at a specific site, by an antisense transcript and finally covers a distance of 780 kb.

Other mechanisms of lncRNA function

Among the intergenic lncRNAs are two types that take an activating role in gene regulation, by acting at or as enhancers. These DNA elements are characterised by their location distally from the transcriptional start site, the ability to bind the co-activator protein p300, and the presence of the chromatin signatures H3K4me1 and H3K4me2 (Kim et al., 2010). In murine neurons, a recent study identified nearly 12,000 neuronal activity-regulated enhancers, 2000 of which were thought to recruit RNA polymerase II (RNAPII) and be bidirectionally transcribed. They generated so-called enhancer RNAs (eRNAs) of <2 kb length, in response to the membrane depolarisation (Kim et al., 2010). It was suggested that eRNAs take an active role, possibly by facilitating the transfer of RNAPII to downstream promoters, because the levels of eRNAs and transcripts of nearby genes correlated positively. The second type of stimulating lncRNA, termed activating ncRNAs (ncRNA-a), has been discovered in human cell lines (Ørom et al., 2010) and originates from sites >1 kb upstream of a protein-coding gene. Knockdown of individual ncRNA-a transcripts, using siRNAs, caused a concomitant decrease of the adjacent protein-coding gene and demonstrated that these ncRNAs have enhancer-like functions. The mechanism of action may be similar to the aforementioned, in that they first form larger complexes with specific proteins, which then interact with the promoter.

In addition, some lncRNAs are known to control the availability of essential proteins factors for cellular processes (e.g. splicing or transcription). One such example is MALAT-1 (metastasis-associated lung adenocarcinoma transcript-1; Ji et al., 2003), an lncRNA with an interesting biogenesis, subcellular location and function. In mammals, the mature MALAT-1 transcript has a length of ~6.7 kb and derives from a larger precursor RNA (>7 kb), following RNase P cleavage. This also produces a smaller RNA, which is further processed to mascRNA (MALAT-1-associated RNA), a 61-nt tRNA-like small RNA (Wilusz et al., 2008). While mascRNA is exported

to the cytoplasm, MALAT-1 is retained and enriched in nuclear 'speckles', that is, subnuclear bodies which play a role in the assembly of the pre-mRNA processing machinery. MALAT-1 is thought to modulate alternative splicing by sequestering inactive SR splicing factors into the speckles and altering their phosphorylation status (Tripathi et al., 2010). Experimentally-induced depletion of MALAT-1, which is normally present at high levels, leads to an increase in mislocalised and unphosphorylated SR proteins, and a higher rate of exon retention in mRNA transcripts. Likewise, trafficking of transcription factor NFAT (nuclear factor of activated T cells) in the cytoplasm can be controlled by NRON (ncRNA repressor of the NFAT; Willingham et al., 2005). Its interaction with the importin proteins in the nuclear envelope prevents NFAT from being transported into the nucleus and from activating genes. Increased NFAT activity, on the other hand, is observed if NRON is knockeddown. Both examples illustrate that important cellular processes can also be regulated indirectly by lncRNAs.

8.10 Summary

In this chapter we have seen that gene expression can be controlled at the level of transcription by transcription factors and their accessory proteins/complexes, noncoding RNAs and UTRs. The type of protein expressed is dependent upon splicing sites and the insertion/removal of specific exons. In addition, all of these factors are dependent upon SNP which can alter transcription factor and/or splicesome binding sites to prevent/enhance the expression of certain splice variants from a particular gene. All these elements can interact to produce cell-specific transcripts and hence responses to certain stimuli. This is an exciting area of research for the treatment of many types of disease.

The human genome project has revealed that there are fewer genes in our chromosomes, than originally thought. This actually means is that different cells are likely to have varying levels of selective expression of the same groups of genes (rather than completely different sets of genes). This is mainly achieved by three processes (i) transcriptional regulation; (ii) post-transcriptional modification such as RNA editing; and (iii) translation/post-translational modifications. However transcriptional regulation is the most important in that it can coordinate the expression of gene products that act antagonistically in physiological processes. The BTFs are essential to initiate the transcription, whereas MTFs help to select, regulate and/or modify the transcriptional events. Thereby cells minimise the energy expenditure.

The ability to control gene expression, along with knowledge obtained from studying the human genome and genomics in other organisms, has led to the theory that disease processes can be altered by manipulating the expression and functions of transcription factors.

References

Adcock IM, Ito K and Caramori G (2006). Transcription factors: Overview. Academic Press, Oxford 243–251.

Ali A, Christie PT, Grigorieva IV, Harding B, Van EH,Ahmed SF, Bitner-Glindzicz M, Blind E, Bloch C, Christin P, Clayton P, Gecz J, Gilbert-Dussardier B, Guillen-Navarro E, Hackett A, Halac I, Hendy GN, Lalloo F, Mache CJ, Mughal Z, Ong AC, Rinat C, Shaw N, Smithson SF, Tolmie J, Weill J, Nesbit MA and Thakker RV (2007). Functional characterization of GATA3 mutations causing the hypoparathyroidism-deafness-renal (HDR) dysplasia syndrome: insight into mechanisms of DNA binding by the GATA3 transcription factor. Human Molecular Genetics 16:265–275.

Al-Quobaili F and Montenarh M (2008). Pancreatic duodenal homeobox factor-1 and diabetes mellitus type 2 (review). International Journal of Molecular Medicine 21: 399–404.

Altarejos JY and Montminy M (2011). CREB and the CRTC co-activators: sensors for hormonal and metabolic signals. Nature Reviews Molecular Cell Biology 12:141–151.

Bass BL (2002). RNA editing by adenosine deaminases that act on RNA. Annual Review of Biochemistry 71:817–846.

Bartek J and Lukas J (2001). Pathways governing G1/S transition and their response to DNA damage. FEBS Letters 490: 117–122.

Beadle GW and Tatum EL (1941). Genetic control of biochemical reactions in Neurospora. Proceedings of the National Academy of Sciences USA 27: 499–506.

Benne R, Van den Burg J, Brakenhoff JP, Sloof P, Van Boom JH and Tromp MC (1986). Major transcript of the frameshifted coxII gene from trypanosome mitochondria contains four nucleotides that are not encoded in the DNA. Cell 46:819–826.

Berget SM, Moore C and Sharp PA (1977). Spliced segments at the 5′ terminus of adenovirus 2 late mRNA. Proceedings of the National Academy of Sciences USA 74: 3171–3175.

Biason-Lauber A. (2010). Control of sex development. Best Practical Research Endocrinology Metabolism 24:163–186.

Blanc V and Davidson NO (2003). C-to-U RNA Editing: Mechanisms Leading to Genetic Diversity. The Journal of Biological Chemistry. 278: 1395–1398.

Borsani G, Tonlorenzi R, Simmler MC, Dandolo L, Arnaud D, Capra V, Grompe M, Pizzuti A, Muzny D, Lawrence C, Willard HF, Avner P and Ballabio A (1991). Characterization of a murine gene expressed from the inactive X chromosome. Nature 351:325–329.

Bracco L and Kearsey J (2003). The relevance of alternative RNA splicing to pharmacogenomics. Trends Biotechnol 21:346–353.

Brennan J and Capel B (2004). One tissue two fates: molecular genetic events that underlie testis versus ovary development. Nature Reviews Genetics 5:509–521.

Brennecke J, Stark A, Russell RB and Cohen SM (2005). Principles of microRNA-target recognition. Public Library of Science Biology 3: e85.

Brosius J (2009). The fragmented gene. Annals of the New York Academy of Sciences 1178: 186–193.

Brown CJ, Ballabio A, Rupert JL, Lafreniere RG, Grompe M, Tonlorenzi R and Willard HF (1991). A gene from the region of the human X inactivation centre is expressed exclusively from the inactive X chromosome. Nature 349: 38–44.

Brown V, Elborn JS, Bradley J and Ennis M (2009). Dysregulated apoptosis and NFκB expression in COPD subjects. Respiratory Research 10:10–24.

Bulyk ML, Johnson PLF and Church GM (2002). Nucleotides of transcription factor binding sites exert interdependent effects on the binding affinities of transcription factors. Nucleic Acids Research 30:1255–1261.

Buratti E, Dork T, Zuccato E, Pagani F, Romano M and Baralle FE (2001). Nuclear factor TDP-43 and SR proteins promote in vitro and in vivo CFTR exon 9 skipping. EMBO J 20:1774–1784.

Carlezon J,William A., Duman RS and Nestler EJ (2005). The many faces of CREB. Trends in Neuroscience 28:436–445.

Carroll SB (2008). Evo-Devo and an Expanding Evolutionary Synthesis: A Genetic Theory of Morphological Evolution. Cell 134:25–36.

Cawley S, Bekiranov S, Ng HH, Kapranov P, Sekinger EA, Kampa D, Piccolboni A, Sementchenko V, Cheng J, Williams AJ, Wheeler R, Wong B, Drenkow J, Yamanaka M, Patel S, Brubaker S, Tammana H, Helt G, Struhl K and Gingeras TR (2004). Unbiased mapping of transcription factor binding sites along human chromosomes 21 and 22 points to widespread regulation of noncoding RNAs. Cell 116: 499–509.

C elegans Sequencing Consortium (1998). Genome sequence of the nematode C. elegans: a platform for investigating biology. Science 282: 2012–2018.

Chan L (1992). Apolipoprotein B, the major protein component of triglyceride rich and low density lipoproteins. The Journal of Biological Chemistry. 267:25621 25624.

Chen J, Sun M, Kent WJ, Huang X, Xie H, Wang W, Zhou G, Shi RZ and Rowley JD (2004). Over 20% of human transcripts might form sense-antisense pairs. Nucleic Acids Research 32: 4812–4820.

Chandra V, Huang P, Hamuro Y, Raghuram S, Wang Y, Burris TP and Rastinejad F (2008) Structure of the intact PPAR-gamma-RXR- nuclear receptor complex on DNA. Nature 456:350–356.

Chen LL, DeCerbo JN and Carmichael GG (2008). Alu element-mediated gene silencing. EMBO Journal 27:1694–1705.

Chow LT, Gelinas RE, Broker TR and Roberts RJ (1977). An amazing sequence arrangement at the 5′ ends of adenovirus 2 messenger RNA. Cell 12: 1–8.

Covello PS and Gray MW (1989). RNA editing in plant mitochondria. Nature 341:662–666.

Crick F (1970). Central dogma of molecular biology. Nature 227:561–563

Cruz-Reyes J, Rusché LN and Sollner-Webb B (1998). Trypanosoma brucei U insertion and U deletion activities co-purify with an enzymatic editing complex but are differentially optimized. Nucleic Acids Research 26(16): 3634–3639. Neuropsychopharmacology 24:478–491.

Davidson BL and McCray PB (2011). Current prospects for RNA interference-based therapies. Nature Reviews Genetics 12: 329–340.

Eddy SR (1999). Noncoding RNA genes. Current Opinion in Genetics and Development 9: 695–699.

Elbashir SM, Lendeckel W and Tuschl T (2001a). RNA interference is mediated by 21- and 22-nucleotide RNAs. Genes Development 15: 188–200.

Elbashir SM, Harborth J, Lendeckel W, Yalcin A, Weber K and Tuschl T (2001b). Duplexes of 21-nucleotide RNAs mediate RNA interference in cultured mammalian cells. Nature 411: 494–498.

ENCODE Project Consortium (2007). Identification and analysis of functional elements in 1% of the human genome by the ENCODE pilot project. Nature 447: 799–816.

Engelkamp D and van Heyningen V (1996). Transcription factors in disease. Current Opinion in Genetics & Development 6: 334–342.

Esteller M (2011). Non-coding RNAs in human disease. Nature Reviews Genetics 12: 861–874.

Faghihi MA, Modarresi F, Khalil AM, Wood DE, Sahagan BG, Morgan TE, Finch CE, St Laurent G 3rd,, Kenny PJ and Wahlestedt C (2008). Expression of a noncoding RNA is elevated in Alzheimer's disease and drives rapid feed-forward regulation of beta-secretase. Nature Medicine 14: 723–730.

Faghihi MA, Zhang M, Huang J, Modarresi F, Van der Brug MP, Nalls MA, Cookson MR, St-Laurent G 3rd, and Wahlestedt C (2010). Evidence for natural antisense transcript-mediated inhibition of microRNA function. Genome Biology 11: R56.

Fiore R, Khudayberdiev S, Christensen M, Siegel G, Flavell SW, Kim TK, Greenberg ME and Schratt G (2009). Mef2-mediated transcription of the miR379-410 cluster regulates activity-dependent dendritogenesis by fine-tuning Pumilio2 protein levels. EMBO Journal 28: 697–710.

Fire A, Xu S, Montgomery MK, Kostas SA, Driver SE and Mello CC (1998). Potent and specific genetic interference by double-stranded RNA in Caenorhabditis elegans. Nature 391: 806–811.

Fox TD and Leaver CJ (1981). The Zea mays mitochondrial gene coding cytochrome oxidase subunit II has an intervening sequence and does not contain TGA codons. Cell 26:315–323.

Germain P, Staels B, Dacquet C, Spedding M and Laudet V (2006). Overview of nomenclature of nuclear receptors. Pharmacological Reviews 58:685–704.

Ghildiyal M and Zamore PD (2009). Small silencing RNAs: an expanding universe. Nature Reviews Genetics 10: 94–108.

Gilbert SF and Singer S (2006). Developmental Biology, 8th Edition; Sinauaer Associates Ltd, Sunderland, USA.

Gill G (2001). Regulation of the initiation of eukaryotic transcription. Essays Biochemistry 37: 33–43

Glass MK and Rosenfeld MG (2000). The coregulator exchange in transcriptional functions of nuclear receptors. Genes & Development 14:121–141.

Gott JM and Emeson RB (2000). Functions and mechanisms of RNA editing. Annual Reviews in Genetics 34:499–531.

Gresch PJ, Barrett RJ, Sanders-Bush E and Smith RL (2007). 5-Hydroxytryptamine (serotonin) 2A receptors in rat anterior cingulate cortex mediate the discriminative stimulus properties of d-lysergic acid diethylamide. Journal of Pharmacological Experimental Therapeutics. 320:662–669.

Griffiths-Jones S, Bateman A, Marshall M, Khanna A and Eddy SR (2003). Rfam: an RNA family database. Nucleic Acids Research 31: 439–441.

Gualberto JM, Weil JH and Grienenberger JM (1990). Editing of the wheat coxIII transcript: Evidence for twelve C to U and one U to C conversions and for sequence similarities around editing sites. Nucleic Acids Research 18:3771–3776.

Guo H, Ingolia NT, Weissman JS and Bartel DP (2010). Mammalian microRNAs predominantly act to decrease target mRNA levels. Nature 466: 835–840.

Gurevich I, Tamir H, Arango V, Dwork AJ, Mann JJ and Schmauss C (2002). Altered editing of serotonin 2C receptor pre-mRNA in the prefrontal cortex of depressed suicide victims. Neuron 34:349–356.

Guttman M, Amit I, Garber M, French C, Lin MF, Feldser D, Huarte M, Zuk O, Carey BW, Cassady JP, Cabili MN, Jaenisch R, Mikkelsen TS, Jacks T, Hacohen N, Bernstein BE, Kellis M, Regev A, Rinn JL and Lander ES (2009). Chromatin signature reveals over a thousand highly conserved large non-coding RNAs in mammals. Nature 458: 223–227.

Halvorsen M, Martin JS, Broadaway S and Laederach A (2010). Disease-associated mutations that alter the RNA structural ensemble. Public Library of Science Genetics 6: e1001074.

Hamilton CE, Papavasiliou NF and Rosenberg BR (2010). Diverse functions for DNA and RNA editing in the immune system. RNA Biology 7:1–10

Harbour JW and Dean DC (2000). Rb function in cell-cycle regulation and apoptosis. Nature Cell Biology. 2: E65-E67.

Harjes P and Wanker EE (2003). The hunt for huntingtin function: interaction partners tell many different stories. Trends in Biochemical Sciences 28: 425–433.

Hastings ML, Milcarek C, Martincic K, Peterson ML and Munroe SH (1997). Expression of the thyroid hormone receptor gene, erbAalpha, in B lymphocytes: alternative mRNA processing is independent of differentiation but correlates with antisense RNA levels. Nucleic Acids Research 25: 4296–4300.

Herrick-Davis K, Grinde E and Teitler M (2000). Inverse agonist activity of atypical antipsychotic drugs at human 5-hydroxytryptamine2C receptors. Journal of Pharmacological. Experimental. Therapeutics. 295:226–232.

Hinsdale ME, Sullivan PM, Mezdour H and Maeda N (2002). ApoB-48 and apoB-100 differentially influence the expression of type-III hyperlipoproteinemia in APOE*2 mice. The Journal of Lipid Research 43:1520–1528.

Homann M (2008). Editing reactions from the prospective of RNA structure. In Nucleic acids and Molecular Biology – Hans Jochim Gross and Ulriech (eds). Springer 2–24.

Houmart B, Small C, Yang L, Naluai–Cecchinit, Cheng E, Hassold T and Griswold M. (2009). Global gene expression in human fetal testis or ovary. Biology Reproduction 81:438–443.

Ingram VM (1957). Gene mutations in human haemoglobin: the chemical difference between normal and sickle cell haemoglobin. Nature 180: 326–328.

International Human Genome Sequencing Consortium (2001). Initial sequencing and analysis of the human genome. Nature 409: 860–921.

Iwakuma T, Lozano G and Flores ER (2005). Li-Fraumeni syndrome: a p53 family affair. Cell Cycle 4: 865–867.

Ji P, Diederichs S, Wang W, Böing S, Metzger R, Schneider PM, Tidow N, Brandt B, Buerger H, Bulk E, Thomas M, Berdel WE, Serve H and Müller-Tidow C (2003). MALAT-1, a novel noncoding RNA, and thymosin beta4 predict metastasis and survival in early-stage non-small cell lung cancer. Oncogene 22: 8031–8041.

Kanduri C (2011). Kcnq1ot1: a chromatin regulatory RNA. Seminars in Cell and Developmental Biology 22:343–350.

Kapranov P, Cheng J, Dike S, Nix DA, Duttagupta R, Willingham AT, Stadler PF, Hertel J, Hackermüller J, Hofacker IL, Bell I, Cheung E, Drenkow J, Dumais E, Patel S, Helt G, Ganesh M, Ghosh S, Piccolboni A, Sementchenko V, Tammana H and Gingeras TR (2007). RNA maps reveal new RNA classes and a possible function for pervasive transcription. Science 316: 1484–1488.

Katayama S, Tomaru Y, Kasukawa T, Waki K, Nakanishi M, Nakamura M, Nishida H, Yap CC, Suzuki M, Kawai J, Suzuki H, Carninci P, Hayashizaki Y, Wells C, Frith M, Ravasi T, Pang KC, Hallinan J, Mattick J, Hume DA, Lipovich L, Batalov S, Engström PG, Mizuno Y, Faghihi MA, Sandelin A, Chalk AM, Mottagui-Tabar S, Liang Z, Lenhard B and Wahlestedt C; RIKEN Genome Exploration Research Group; Genome Science Group (Genome Network Project Core Group); FANTOM Consortium (2005). Antisense transcription in the mammalian transcriptome. Science 309: 1564–1566.

Kaufman B, Scharf O, Arbeit J, Ashcroft M, Brown JM, Bruick RK, Chapman JD, Evans SM, Giaccia AMJ, Harris AL, Huang E, Johnson R, Kaelin W, Koch CJ, Maxwell P, Mitchell J, Neckers L, Powis G, Rajendran J, Semenza GL, Simons J, Storkebaum E, Welch MJ, Whittelaw M, Melillo G and Ivy P (2004). Proceedings of the Oxygen Homeostasis/Hypoxia Meeting. Cancer Research (Meeting Report) 64:3350–3356.

Khaitovich P, Kelso J, Franz H, Visagie J, Giger T, Joerchel S, Petzold E, Green RE, Lachmann M and Pääbo S (2006). Functionality of intergenic transcription: an evolutionary comparison. Public Library of Science Genetics 2: 1590–1598.

Khvorova A, Reynolds A and Jayasena SD (2003). Functional siRNAs and miRNAs exhibit strand bias. Cell 115 : 209–216.

Kim TK, Hemberg M, Gray JM, Costa AM, Bear DM, Wu J, Harmin DA, Laptewicz M, Barbara-Haley K, Kuersten S, Markenscoff-Papadimitriou E, Kuhl D, Bito H, Worley PF, Kreiman G and Greenberg ME (2010). Widespread transcription at neuronal activity-regulated enhancers. Nature 465: 182–187.

Kis B, Snipes JA and Busija DW (2005). Acetaminophen and the cyclooxygenase-3 puzzle: sorting out facts, fictions, and uncertainties. Journal of Pharmacological Experimental Thererpeutics 315:1–7.

Kliewer SA, Umesono K, Noonan DJ, Heyman RA and Evans RM (1992). Convergence of 9-cis retinoic acid and peroxisome proliferator signalling pathways through heterodimer formation of their receptors. Nature 358:771–774.

Landgraf P, Rusu M, Sheridan R, Sewer A, Iovino N, Aravin A, Pfeffer S, Rice A, Kamphorst AO, Landthaler M, Lin C, Socci ND, Hermida L, Fulci V, Chiaretti S, Foà R, Schliwka J, Fuchs U, Novosel A, Müller RU, Schermer B, Bissels U, Inman J, Phan Q, Chien M, Weir DB, Choksi R, De Vita G, Frezzetti D, Trompeter HI, Hornung V, Teng G, Hartmann G, Palkovits M, Di Lauro R, Wernet P, Macino G, Rogler CE, Nagle JW, Ju J, Papavasiliou FN, Benzing T, Lichter P, Tam W, Brownstein MJ, Bosio A, Borkhardt A, Russo JJ, Sander C, Zavolan M and Tuschl T (2007). A mammalian microRNA expression atlas based on small RNA library sequencing. Cell 129: 1401–1414.

Landles C and Bates GP (2004). Huntingtin and the molecular pathogenesis of Huntington's disease EMBO reports 5:958–963.

Landschulz WH, Johnson PF and McKnight SL (1988). The leucine zipper: a hypothetical structure common to a new class of DNA-binding proteins. Science 240:1759–1764.

Lapidot M and Pilpel Y (2006). Genome-wide natural antisense transcription: coupling its regulation to its different regulatory mechanisms. EMBO Reports 7: 1216–1222.

Lavorgna G, Dahary D, Lehner B, Sorek R, Sanderson CM and Casari G (2004) In search of antisense. Trends in Biochemical Sciences 29: 88–94.

Lee JT, Davidow LS and Warhawsky D (1999a). Tsix, a gene antisense to Xist at the X-inactivation centre. Nature Genetics 21: 400–404.

Lee MP, DeBaun MR, Mitsuya K, Galonek HL, Brandenburg S, Oshimura M and Feinberg AP (1999b). Loss of imprinting of a paternally expressed transcript, with antisense orientation to KVLQT1, occurs frequently in Beckwith-Wiedemann syndrome and is independent of insulin-like growth factor II imprinting. Proceedings of the National Academy of Sciences USA 96: 5203–5208.

Lee RC, Feinbaum RL and Ambros V (1993). The C. elegans heterochronic gene lin-4 encodes small RNAs with antisense complementarity to lin-14. Cell 75: 843–854.

Lee, JA and Lupski J.R. (2006). Genomic rearrangements and gene copy-number alterations as a cause of nervous system disorders. Neuron 52:103–121.

Lennon PA, Cooper ML, Peiffer DA, Gunderson KL, Patel A, Peters S, Cheung SW and Bacino CA (2007). Deletion of 7q31.1 supports involvement of FOXP2 in language impairment: clinical report and review. American Journal of Medical Genetics A 143A:791–798.

Lehner B, Williams G, Campbell RD and Sanderson CM (2002). Antisense transcripts in the human genome. Trends in Genetics 18: 63–65.

Li M, Wang IS, Li Y, Bruzel A, Richards AL, Toung JM and Cheung VG (2011). Widespread RNA and DNA Sequence Differences in the Human Transcriptome. Science. 333:53–58.

Luconi M, Cantini G and Serio M (2010). Peroxisome proliferator-activated receptor gamma (PPARγ): Is the genomic activity the only answer? Steroids 75:585–594.

Lynch RA, Etchin J, Battle TE and Frank DA (2007). A small-molecule enhancer of signal transducer and activator of transcription 1 transcriptional activity accentuates the antiproliferative effects of IFN-gamma in human cancer cells. Cancer Res 67:1254–1261.

MacLaughlin DT and Donahoe PK. (2004). Sex determination and differentiation. New England Journal of Medicine 350:367–378.

Maestro MA, Cardalda C, Boj SF, Luco RF, Servitja JM and Ferrer J (2007). Distinct roles of HNF1beta, HNF1alpha, and HNF4alpha in regulating pancreas development, beta-cell function and growth. Endocrine Development 12:33–45.

Marks H, Chow JC, Denissov S, Françoijs KJ, Brockdorff N, Heard E and Stunnenberg HG (2009). High-resolution analysis of epigenetic changes associated with X inactivation. Genome Research 19: 1361–1373.

Maas S and Rich A (2000). Changing genetic information through RNA editing. BioEssays 22:790–802.

Markov GV and Laudet V (2011). Origin and evolution of the ligand-binding ability of nuclear receptors. Molecular Cellular Endocrinology. 334:21–30.

Matsuda M, Sakamoto N, and Fukunaki Y (1992). α-thalassemia caused by disruption of the site for an erythroid-specific transcription factor, GATA-1, in the gamma-globin gene promoter. Blood 80:1347–1351.

Metcalfe D (2007). Molecular Patterning of the Vertebrate Limb and Implications for Congenital Deformity. Journal of Young Investigators 22:130–135.

Miller BH and Wahlestedt C (2010). MicroRNA dysregulation in psychiatric disease. Brain Research 1338: 89–99.

Molenda-Figueira HA, Williams CA, Griffin AL, Rutledge EM, Blaustein JD and Tetel MJ (2006). Nuclear receptor coactivators function in estrogen receptor- and progestin receptor-dependent aspects of sexual behaviour in female rats. Hormonal Behaviour 50:383–392.

Morabito MV, Abbas AI, Hood JL, Kesterson RA and Jacobs MM (2010). Mice with altered serotonin 2C receptor RNA editing display characteristics of Prader–Willi syndrome. Neurobiological Disorders. 39:169–80.

Muchardt C and Yaniv M (2001). When the SWI/SNF complex remodels the cell cycle. Oncogene. 20:3067–3075.

Müller H and Helin K (2000). The E2F transcription factors: key regulators of cell proliferation. Biochimica et Biophysica Acta 1470:M1-12.

Mundlos S and Olsen M (1997). Heritable diseases of the skeleton. Part I: Molecular insights into skeletal development-transcription factors and signalling pathways. FASEB 11:125–132.

Nakayama KI, Hatakeyama S and Nakayama K (2001). Regulation of the cell cycle at the G1-S transition by proteolysis of cyclin E and p27Kip1. Biochemical & Biophysical Research Communications 282: 853–860.

Napoli C, Lemieux C and Jorgensen R (1990). Introduction of a chimeric chalcone synthase gene into petunia results in reversible co-suppression of homologous genes in trans. Plant Cell 2: 279–289.

Nelson EA, Walker SR, Kepich A, Gashin LB, Hideshima T, Ikeda H, Chauhan D, Anderson KC and Frank DA (2008). Nifuroxazide inhibits survival of multiple myeloma cells by directly inhibiting STAT3. Blood 112:5095–5102.

Niswender CM, Copelan SC, Herrick-Davis K, Emeson RB and Sanders-Bush E (1999) RNA editing of the human serotonin 5-hydroxytryptamine 2C receptor silences constitutive activity. Journal of Biological Chemistry 274:9472–9478.

Niswender CM, Herrick-Davis K, Dilley GE, Meltzer HY, Overholser JC, Stockmeier CA, Emeson RB and Sanders-Bush E (2001). RNA Editing of the Human Serotonin 5-HT2C Receptor: Alterations in Suicide and Implications for Serotonergic Pharmacotherapy Neuropsychopharmacology. 24:478–491.

Okamura K, Chung WJ, Ruby JG, Guo H, Bartel DP and Lai EC (2008). The Drosophila hairpin RNA pathway generates endogenous short interfering RNAs. Nature 453: 803–806.

Okamura K, Hagen JW, Duan H, Tyler DM and Lai EC (2007). The mirtron pathway generates microRNA-class regulatory RNAs in Drosophila. Cell 130: 89–100.

Okamura K and Lai EC (2008). Endogenous small interfering RNAs in animals. Nature Reviews Molecular Cell Biology 9:673–678.

Olsen BR, Reginato AM and Wang WF (2000). Bone development. Annual Review of Cell and Developmental Biology. 16:191–220.

Ørom UA, Derrien T, Beringer M, Gumireddy K, Gardini A, Bussotti G, Lai F, Zytnicki M, Notredame C, Huang Q, Guigo R and Shiekhattar R (2010). Long noncoding RNAs with enhancer-like function in human cells. Cell 143: 46–58.

Ørom UA and Shiekhattar R (2011). Long non-coding RNAs and enhancers. Current Opinion in Genetics & Development 21:194–198. Ponting CP (2008). The functional repertoires of metazoan genomes. Nature Reviews in Genetics 9: 689–698.

Osato N, Suzuki Y, Ikeo K and Gojobori T (2007). Transcriptional interferences in cis natural antisense transcripts of humans and mice. Genetics 176: 1299–1306.

Parker LL, Backstrom JR, Sanders-Bush E and Shieh B (2003). Agonist-induced phosphorylation of the serotonin 5-HT2C receptor regulates its interaction with multiple PDZ protein 1. Journal of Biological Chemistry 278:21576–21583.

Parma P, Radi O, Vidal V, Chaboissier MC, Dellambra E, Valentini S, Guerra L and Schedl A. (2006). R-spondin1 is essential in sex determination, skin differentiation and malignancy. Nature Genetics 38:1304–1309.

Pessler A, Daib L, Crona R and Schumacher HR (2006). NFAT transcription factors – new players in the pathogenesis of inflammatory arthropathies. Autoimmunity reviews 5: 106–110.

Peterson JA and Myers AM (1993). Functional analysis of mRNA 3' end formation signals in the convergent and overlapping transcription units of the S. cerevisiae genes RHO1 and MRP2. Nucleic Acids Research 21: 5500–5508.

Phu DT, Wallbach M, Depatie C, Fu A, Screaton RA and Oetjen E (2011). Regulation of the CREB coactivator TORC by the dual leucine zipper kinase at different levels. Cell Signal 23:344–353.

Ponjavic J, Oliver PL, Lunter G and Ponting CP (2009). Genomic and transcriptional co-localization of protein-coding and long non-coding RNA pairs in the developing brain. Public Library of Science Genetics 5: 1–14.

Ponting CP (2008). The functional repertoires of metazoan genomes. Nature Reviews Genetics 9:689–698.

Pontier DB and Gribnau J (2011). Xist regulation and function explored. Human Genetics 130: 223–236.

Ponting CP, Oliver PL and Reik W (2009). Evolution and functions of long noncoding RNAs. Cell 136: 629–641.

Prescott EM and Proudfoot NJ (2002). Transcriptional collision between convergent genes in budding yeast. Proceedings of the National Academy of Sciences USA 99: 8796–8801.

Price RD, Weiner DM, Chang MSS and Sanders-Bush E (2001). RNA Editing of the human serotonin 5-HT2C receptor alters receptor mediated activation of G13 protein. Journal of Biological Chemistry 276:44663–44668.

Radford EJ, Ferrón SR and Ferguson-Smith AC (2011). Genomic imprinting as an adaptive model of developmental plasticity. FEBS Letters 585:2059–2066.

Sadowski L, Pilecka I and Miaczynska M (2009). Signaling from endosomes: location makes a difference. Experimental Cell Research 315:1601–1609.

Sakabe NJ and Nobrega MA (2010). Genome-wide maps of transcription regulatory elements. Wiley Interdisciplinary Reviews Systems Biology and Medicine 2:422–437.

Salato VK, Rediske NW, Zhang C, Hastings ML and Munroe SH (2010). An exonic splicing enhancer within a bidirectional coding sequence regulates alternative splicing of an antisense mRNA. RNA Biology 7: 179–190.

Sanders-Bush E, Fentress H and Hazelwood L (2003). Serotonin 5-HT2 receptors: molecular and genomic diversity. Molecular Interventions 2: 319–330.

Sasidharan R and Gerstein M (2008). Genomics: protein fossils live on as RNA. Nature 453: 729–731.

Savinkova LK, Ponomarenko MP, Ponomarenko PM, Drachkova IA, Lysova MV, Arshinova TV and Kolchanov NA (2009). TATA box polymorphisms in human gene promoters and associated hereditary pathologies. Biochemistry (Moscow) 74:117–129.

Schratt GM, Tuebing F, Nigh EA, Kane CG, Sabatini ME, Kiebler M and Greenberg ME (2006). A brain-specific microRNA regulates dendritic spine development. Nature 439: 283–289.

Schwarz DS, Hutvágner G, Du T, Xu Z, Aronin N and Zamore PD (2003). Asymmetry in the assembly of the RNAi enzyme complex. Cell 115: 199–208.

Schwartz GA and Shah MA (2005). Targeting the Cell Cycle: A New Approach to Cancer. Therapy Journal of Clinical Oncology 23:9408–9421.

Seal RL, Gordon SM, Lush MJ, Wright MW and Bruford EA (2011). Genenames.org: the HGNC resources in 2011. Nucleic Acids Research 39(Database issue): D514-519.

Seeman P, Nam D, Ulpian C, Liu ISC and Tallerico T (2000). New dopamine receptor, D2Longer, with unique TG splice site, in human brain. Mol Brain Res 76:132–141.

Semenza GL (2007). Oxygen-dependent regulation of mitochondrial respiration by hypoxia-inducible factor 1. Biochemical Journal 405:1–9.

Shah N and Sukumar S (2010). The Hox genes and their roles in oncogenesis. Nature Reviews Cancer 10: 361–371.

Sijen T, Fleenor J, Simmer F, Thijssen KL, Parrish S, Timmons L, Plasterk RH and Fire A (2001). On the role of RNA amplification in dsRNA-triggered gene silencing. Cell 107: 465–476.

Simpson L, Sbicego S and Aphssizhev R (2003). Uridine insertion/ deletion RNA editing in trypanosome mitochondria: A complex business. RNA 9:265–276.

Smilinich NJ, Day CD, Fitzpatrick GV, Caldwell GM, Lossie AC, Cooper PR, Smallwood AC, Joyce JA, Schofield PN, Reik W, Nicholls RD, Weksberg R, Driscoll DJ, Maher ER, Shows TB and Higgins MJ (1999). A maternally methylated CpG island in KvLQT1 is associated with an antisense paternal transcript and loss of imprinting in Beckwith-Wiedemann syndrome. Proceedings of the National Academy of Sciences USA 96: 8064–8069.

Speijer D (2008). Evolutionary Aspects of RNA Editing - In RNA Biology Nucleic Acids and Molecular Biology Volume: 20, Issue: 2, Publisher: Springer Berlin Heidelberg:199–227.

Spencer CA, Gietz RD and Hodgetts RB (1986). Overlapping transcription units in the dopa decarboxylase region of Drosophila. Nature 322: 279–281.

Straus DS and Glass CK (2007). Anti-inflammatory actions of PPAR ligands: new insights on cellular and molecular mechanisms. Trends in Immunology 28:551–558.

Tam OH, Aravin AA, Stein P, Girard A, Murchison EP, Cheloufi S, Hodges E, Anger M, Sachidanandam R, Schultz RM and Hannon GJ (2008). Pseudogene-derived small interfering RNAs regulate gene expression in mouse oocytes. Nature 453: 534–538.

Technau U (2008). Evolutionary biology: Small regulatory RNAs pitch in. Nature 455: 1184–1185.

Tohda M, Nomura M and Nomura Y (2006). Molecular Pathopharmacology of 5-HT2C Receptors and the RNA. Journal of Pharmacological Sciences 100:427–432.

Tontonoz P and Spiegelman BM (2008). Fat and beyond: the diverse biology of PPARgamma. Annual Review of Biochemistry 77:289–312.

Tripathi V, Ellis JD, Shen Z, Song DY, Pan Q, Watt AT, Freier SM, Bennett CF, Sharma A, Bubulya PA, Blencowe BJ, Prasanth SG and Prasanth KV (2010). The nuclear-retained noncoding RNA MALAT1 regulates alternative splicing by modulating SR splicing factor phosphorylation. Molecular Cell 39: 925–938.

Tuck AC and Tollervey D (2011). RNA in pieces. Trends in Genetics 27: 422–432.

Tyagi S, Chabes AL, Wysocka J and Herr W (2007). E2F Activation of S Phase Promoters via Association with HCF-1 and the MLL Family of Histone H3K4 Methyltransferases. Molecular Cell 27:107–119.

Ulveling D, Francastel C and Hubé F (2011). When one is better than two: RNA with dual functions. Biochimie 93: 633–644.

Van der Vliet HJ and Nieuwenhuis EE (2007). IPEX as a Result of Mutations in FOXP3. Clinical & Developmental Immunology 89017.

Venter JC, Adams MD, Myers EW, Li PW, Mural RJ, Sutton GG, Smith HO, Yandell M, Evans CA, Holt RA et al. (2001). The sequence of the human genome. Science 291: 1304–1351.

Viswakarma N, Jia Y, Bai L, Vluggens A, Borensztajn J, Xu J and Reddy JK (2010). Coactivators in PPAR-Regulated Gene Expression. PPAR Res:250126.

Wahlestedt C (2006). Natural antisense and noncoding RNA transcripts as potential drug targets. Drug Discovery Today 11: 503–508.

Wang ET, Sandberg R, Luo S, Khrebtukova I, Zhang L, Mayr C, Kingsmore SF, Schroth GP and Burge CB (2008). Alternative isoform regulation in human tissue transcriptomes. Nature 456: 470–476.

Wang T, Furey TS, Connelly JJ, Ji S, Nelson S, Heber S, Gregory SG and Hauser ER (2009). A general integrative genomic feature transcription factor binding site prediction method applied to analysis of USF1 binding in cardiovascular disease. Human Genomics. 3:221–235.

Wang C, Tian L, Popov VM and Pestell RG (2011). Acetylation and nuclear receptor action. Journal of Steroid Biochemistry Molecular Biology 123:91–100.

Ward AJ and Cooper TA (2010). The pathobiology of splicing. Journal of Pathology 220:152–163.

Watanabe T, Totoki Y, Toyoda A, Kaneda M, Kuramochi-Miyagawa S, Obata Y, Chiba H, Kohara Y, Kono T, Nakano T, Surani MA, Sakaki Y and Sasaki H (2008). Endogenous siRNAs from naturally formed dsRNAs regulate transcripts in mouse oocytes. Nature 453: 539–543.

Werner F and Weinzierl ROJ (2005). Direct Modulation of RNA Polymerase Core Functions by Basal Transcription Factors. Molecular Cell Biology 25: 8344–8355.

Willingham AT, Orth AP, Batalov S, Peters EC, Wen BG, Aza-Blanc P, Hogenesch JB and Schultz PG (2005). A strategy for probing the function of noncoding RNAs finds a repressor of NFAT. Science 309:1570–1573.

Wilusz JE, Freier SM and Spector DL (2008). 3′ end processing of a long nuclear-retained noncoding RNA yields a tRNA-like cytoplasmic RNA. Cell 135: 919–932.

Wittwer J, Marti-Juan J and Hersberg M (2006). Functional polymorphism in ALOX15 results in increased allele specific transcription in macrophages through binding of the transcription factor SPI1. Human Mutations 27:78–87.

Wood MJ, Gait MJ and Yin H (2010). RNA-targeted splice-correction therapy for neuromuscular disease. Brain 133:957–972.

Wray GA, Hahn MW, Abouheif E, Balhoff JP, Pizer M, Rockman MV and Romano LA (2003). The evolution of transcriptional regulation in eukaryotes. Molecular Biology Evolution 20:1377–1419.

Wright MW and Bruford EA (2011). Naming 'junk': Human non-protein coding RNA (ncRNA) gene nomenclature. Human Genomics 5: 90–98.

Yang Y, Jianning L, Gui 1, Yin H, Wu X, Zhang Y and Jin Y (2008). A-to-I RNA editing alters less-conserved residues of highly conserved coding regions: Implications for dual functions in evolution. RNA 14:1516–1525.

Yessoufou A and Wahli W (2010). Multifaceted roles of peroxisome proliferator-activated receptors (PPARs) at the cellular and whole organism levels. Swiss Medicine Weekly 140:w13071.

Yu S and Reddy JK (2007). Transcription coactivators for peroxisome proliferator-activated receptors. Biochimica et Biophysica Acta (BBA) - Molecular and Cell Biology of Lipids 1771:936–951.

Zhang Z and Carmichael GG (2001). The fate of dsRNA in the nucleus: a p54(nrb)-containing complex mediates the nuclear retention of promiscuously A-to-I edited RNAs. Cell 106:465–475.

Zuccato C, Ciammola A, Rigamonti D, Leavitt BR, Goffredo D, Conti L, MacDonald ME, Friedlander RM, Silani V, Hayden MR, Timmusk T, Sipione S and Cattaneo E (2001). Loss of huntingtin-mediated BDNF gene transcription in Huntington's disease. Science 293:493–498.

Zuccato C, Tartari M, Crotti A, Goffredo D, Valenza M, Conti L, Cataudella T, Leavitt BR, Hayden MR, Timmusk T, Rigamonti D and Cattaneo E (2003). Huntingtin interacts with REST/NRSF to modulate the transcription of NRSE-controlled neuronal genes. Nature Genetics 35:76–83.

9 Cellular Calcium

9.1 Introduction

Over a century ago Sydney Ringer established the importance of calcium in the heart beat. Initially he mistakenly thought that calcium was of limited interest, since omitting it from the physiological saline appeared to have no effect on isolated hearts. However, it soon became clear that the 'distilled water' he used was instead ordinary tap water, and that distilled water actually caused the heart to stop. His subsequent experiments then demonstrated that calcium was critical for the heart beat (Miller, 2004). Since this pioneering work it has become clear that the most common intracellular messenger is a change in the intracellular free ionised calcium concentration, $[Ca^{2+}]_i$. Indeed, it is difficult to think of any physiological process that calcium does not affect at some point. Calcium is used as a signalling molecule in organisms as diverse as bacteria, fungi, plants, invertebrates and vertebrates. This widespread occurrence throughout the phyla is in contrast to other signalling molecules which have more restricted distribution. Calcium has a pervasive influence on cell physiology, participating in numerous processes such as muscle contraction, secretion, proliferation and differentiation of cells, in addition to many other roles. Such is calcium's importance that it is even intimately involved in the beginning and end of life. Calcium is required

for sperm capacitation (hyperactivation of sperm in the female reproductive tract), the acrosome reaction (to allow sperm to penetrate the zona pellucida), egg activation (cell division) and the zona reaction (to prevent further sperm penetrating the zona pellucida). Calcium also has a role in apoptosis (programmed cell death), which is critical to the continual renewal of organs.

Calcium as a signalling molecule

At first sight Ca^{2+} may not appear to have the appropriate properties of a signalling molecule. It is present in a high concentration outside cells, approximately 2.4 mM in human blood serum. In contrast to other signalling molecules such as cyclic adenosine 3′, 5′ monophosphate (cAMP), calcium can be neither made nor destroyed by cells. Calcium is also cytotoxic, a sustained high intracellular free ionised calcium concentration, $[Ca^{2+}]_i$, will lead to cell death. High $[Ca^{2+}]_i$ is actually a relative term as the normal $[Ca^{2+}]_i$ is around 100 nM (10^{-7}M) and can reach the low µM range (10^{-6} M) during stimulation with agonists. In contrast, the extracellular free ionised calcium concentration, $[Ca^{2+}]_o$, is around 1 mM (10^{-3} M) as much of the total serum calcium is bound to proteins such as albumin. There is in effect a 10,000 fold concentration gradient in free calcium across the cell membrane (10^{-3} M outside and 10^{-7} M inside). Hence

Molecular Pharmacology: From DNA to Drug Discovery, First Edition. John Dickenson, Fiona Freeman, Chris Lloyd Mills, Shiva Sivasubramaniam and Christian Thode.

Ca^{2+} will tend to enter cells down a diffusion gradient as the plasma membrane is not totally impermeable to calcium. In order to maintain a low $[Ca^{2+}]_i$ cells have developed mechanisms to actively export Ca^{2+} across the plasma membrane via plasma membrane Ca^{2+} ATPases, and sequester Ca^{2+} into intracellular stores such as the endoplasmic reticulum (ER). This uses another type of active Ca^{2+} pump, the sarco/endoplasmic reticulum Ca^{2+} ATPase (SERCA). There are also cellular macromolecules that can bind calcium, thereby limiting the rise in $[Ca^{2+}]_i$ and restricting Ca^{2+} diffusion.

It is thought that calcium signalling has evolved from mechanisms that were developed to protect cells from calcium. In a signalling system there is need of a message, a way to generate the message, and a way to remove the message. For calcium there is an abundant supply of this signalling molecule both outside the cell and within certain intracellular organelles such as the ER and SR (sarcoplasmic reticulum). Also there is a way of terminating the signal, actively removing the calcium via Ca^{2+} ATPases, across the plasma membrane into the extracellular environment, and/or into intracellular organelles. Thus a mechanism to facilitate the movement of Ca^{2+} ions across cell membranes was needed for a functioning Ca^{2+} signalling system to develop (Figure 9.1). Maynard Case et al. (2007) noted that Ca^{2+} selective channels were probably the earliest ion channels

in the phylogenetic tree of life and that they are even found in prokaryotes. Thus, the ability to alter $[Ca^{2+}]_i$ is an almost universal signalling system.

9.2 Measurement of calcium

Such is the importance of calcium to cell physiology that there are over 200,000 references in the PubMed database that include calcium and cell in the abstract or keyword list. In order to understand the role of calcium in cell signalling it is essential to be able to measure aspects of cell calcium. A brief overview of some of the approaches that could be used are considered below and summarised in Table 9.1.

Non-optical methods

Electron probe X-ray microanalysis uses the electron beam of an electron microscope to generate X-rays from the biological specimen. The X-ray emission spectrum contains energy peaks that are characteristic of certain elements such as sodium, potassium, calcium and so on (Fernandez-Segura and Warley, 2008). By quantifying the size of specific peaks the concentrations of elements of interest can be determined. Whilst this technique can be of low resolution, allowing measurement of clumps of cells, it is also capable of high resolution analysis, enabling

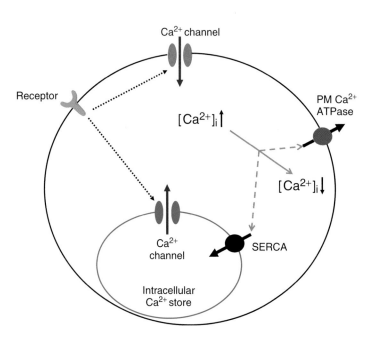

Figure 9.1 The basic cellular components required for calcium signalling. In non-excitable cells an extracellular hormone or neurotransmitter causes Ca^{2+} selective channels on the plasma membrane and/or intracellular organelles such as the endoplasmic reticulum to open. Calcium then enters the cytosol down a diffusion gradient causing a rise in $[Ca^{2+}]_i$, which then regulates cellular processes. The calcium signal is removed by the closing of the calcium selective channels and active pumping of Ca^{2+} out of the cytosol by Ca^{2+}-ATPases, either across the plasma membrane (plasma membrane Ca^{2+} ATPase, PMCA) and/or into intracellular stores (sarco/endoplasmic reticulum Ca^{2+} ATPase, SERCA). Whilst this is a highly simplified diagram, omitting intracellular signalling molecules, calcium induced calcium release, calcium binding proteins, and virtually all intracellular organelles, it does give a useful starting point for discussing calcium signalling that will be developed during this chapter.

Table 9.1 Methods for measuring aspects of cell calcium.

Method	Non invasive	Can Measure single cells	Can measure cell populations	Speed of response	Spatial information within cells	Additional comments
Radioisotopes	Yes	No	Needs a large number of cells	Seconds	No, but could be used for calcium fluxes in isolated organelles	Used for calcium influx and efflux measurements
Calcium selective microelectrodes	No, requires membrane puncture	Yes	No, each cell must be individually impaled with a microelectrode	Hundreds of milliseconds for microelectrodes, longer for minielectrodes (around 20–30 seconds for a large change in $[Ca^{2+}]_i$	Possible for large organelles such as the nucleus	
Calcium selective vibrating microelectrodes	Yes, but only measures calcium on the outside of cells	Yes	No, can only measure one small area at a time	3 seconds for calcium flux measurements	No	Can give some spatial information on calcium efflux
Calcium activated ion currents (patch clamp electrophysiology)	Generally requires membrane puncture (except cell attached)	Yes	No, but can be used in clusters of cells that are electrically coupled	Seconds	Cell attached mode can give information on the density and spatial distribution of plasma membrane ion channels, though it requires several experiments to achieve this	
NMR	Yes	Is possible with NMR microscopy	Yes	Seconds	Some spatial information possible, though less resolution than fluorescence microscopy	
Fluorimetry	Yes, if use AM ester loading	Yes	Yes	milliseconds for a full image or <1 msec for confocal line scan mode	Yes	The most commonly used technique to measure $[Ca^{2+}]_i$

(continued overleaf)

Table 9.1 (continued)

Method	Non invasive	Can measure single cells	Can measure cell populations	Speed of response	Spatial information within cells	Additional comments
Luminescence	Yes, if use genetically incorporated aequorin	Yes	Yes, but a single cell with a large $[Ca^{2+}]_i$ can severely bias the 'average' calcium signal of a population of cells. This arises as the relationship between calcium concentration and light output is a power function (i.e. an increase in calcium give a correspondingly greater rise in luminescence output)	Depends on the rate of photon emission, which in turn changes with calcium concentration. At a resting calcium concentration of around 100 nM there may only be a few photons/sec depending on the aequorin content. This count rate rapidly increases as the calcium concentration starts to rise, thereby allowing faster data capture.	Possible, though greatly dependant on the amount of light emitted. Will need an photon imaging detector	
Electron probe X-ray microanalysis	No, if intracellular measurement required	Yes	Yes	Dead cells only, so multiple samples needed for a time course	Yes, but not in areas where there is less than a few millimoles/Kg of calcium	Only measures total calcium (i.e. includes calcium bound to proteins)

No one technique on its own can cover all the desirable features of measuring calcium concentration and calcium fluxes, as well as being optimised for cell populations and high resolution spatial information. In most applications non-invasive measurements are required. However, in some experiments access to the cytosol is desirable. The choice of method will therefore depend on what aspect of cell calcium you wish to measure, equipment availability and your budget. Basic equipment for measuring cell populations in a fluorimeter is relatively cheap. However a top of the range multiphoton confocal system will cost over £500,000. Information in this table was based on Baudet et al., 1994; Benters et al., 1997; Chen et al., 1996; Cobbold and Lee, 1991; Fernandez-Segura and Warley, 2008; Matsuda et al., 1996; Metcalfe and Smith, 1991; Takahashi et al., 1999.

the determination of ion concentration in different intracellular compartments. Indeed, as this is based on an electron microscope, it can exceed the resolution of a confocal light microscope. However, there are significant disadvantages to this approach. The detection limit is in the order of a few millimoles/Kg and it cannot discriminate between free and bound elements, as both are measured. Further, it requires cryofixed freeze dried and sectioned cells. These features severely limit the use of this technique and it is not suitable for following $[Ca^{2+}]_i$. However, studies have shown that the calcium content of intracellular compartments does change upon agonist stimulation in the pancreas (Sasaki et al., 1996).

Nuclear magnetic resonance (NMR) involves applying electromagnetic radiation at characteristic resonance frequencies to ascertain structural information about substances. In order to measure $[Ca^{2+}]_i$, it is necessary to utilise a calcium chelator so that differences can be determined between the calcium bound and unbound state of the chelator. The fluorinated derivate of BAPTA, 1,2-bis(2-amino-5,6-diflurophenoxy)ethane-N,N,N′,N′-tetracacetic acid (5F-BAPTA) allows ^{19}F NMR to discriminate between unbound, calcium bound and heavy metal bound 5F-BAPTA. Although this technique is not commonly used, it does have some advantages. It has the ability to non-invasively determine $[Ca^{2+}]_i$ in isolated whole organs and can measure both cytosolic and SR calcium at the same time (Chen et al., 1996). In addition it is much less susceptible to measurement artefacts due to cellular proteins, and can even report on the intracellular free concentrations of heavy metals such as cadmium, lead and zinc (Matsuda et al., 1996; Benters et al., 1997). Both the presence of protein or heavy metals can seriously compromise measurement of $[Ca^{2+}]_i$ with fluorescent probes such as fura-2. Proteins can alter the apparent dissociation constant (K_d) of the probe for calcium, leading to a systematic error in estimation of $[Ca^{2+}]_i$. Also heavy metals often have an enhanced affinity for optical probes and/or affect their optical properties, again confounding attempts to estimate $[Ca^{2+}]_i$. However, there are some significant drawbacks to NMR. It has poor temporal resolution when compared to optical probes. This is compounded by the weak spatial resolution of NMR microscopy, which at present cannot achieve the resolution of normal fluorescence light microscopy. Thus NMR has only very limited application in studies of cell calcium.

Calcium selective microelectrodes contain a small amount of ion selective membrane solution at the tip that allows the passage of Ca^{2+} ions to the bulk filling solution of the electrode. This in turn is connected to a high impedance amplifier via an Ag-AgCl electrode. This system has the advantage of ease of calibration and has a much wider dynamic range than optical probes such as indo-1. The calcium selective microelectrode can cover the physiological calcium range (10 nM to 1 mM). This is in marked contrast to fluorescent optical probes such as indo-1 which are restricted to around two orders of magnitude (25 nM to 2.5 μM), rather than the five orders of magnitude achievable with calcium selective electrodes (Figure 9.2). However, calcium selective microelectrodes are infrequently used, as for most applications optical probes are the method of choice. Microelectrodes require puncture of the cell membrane, risking ingress of calcium into the cell. Of particular concern is their slow response time. Rapid changes in $[Ca^{2+}]_i$ detectable with optical probes will appear blunted with calcium selective microelectrodes, as the rise and fall measured will appear to be much slower than actually occurs. This restricted

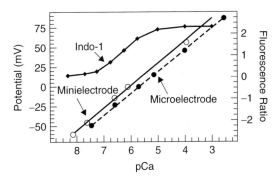

Figure 9.2 Comparison of the dynamic range of calcium sensitive mini and microelectrode with indo-1. Calcium sensitive microelectrodes have a larger dynamic range than fluorescent optical probes such as indo-1. The microelectrode response (mV) is linear when plotted on a log calcium concentration scale (pCa = $-\log_{10}$ of the molar calcium concentration). In contrast the sigmoid shape of the optical probe response (fluorescence ratio) limits the useful range of $[Ca^{2+}]_i$ measurement. Reprinted from Methods in Cell Biology volume 40, Baudet et al., 1994. How to make and use calcium-specific mini-and microelectrodes pp 94–113, Copyright (1994), with permission from Elsevier.

temporal resolution is compounded by a lack of spatial information as it records bulk cytosolic $[Ca^{2+}]_i$. Though some spatial information is possible if organelles such as the nucleus are targeted instead of the cytosol.

Whilst calcium sensitive microelectrodes are only infrequently used for intracellular measurement, minielectrodes are useful for extracellular calcium and can follow calcium fluxes. For example, the classic paper by Streb et al. (1983) used a calcium selective electrode to demonstrate for the first time that inositol 1,4,5,-trisphosphate (IP_3) caused calcium release from an intracellular store. They used permeabilised pancreatic acinar cells and measured the calcium concentration of the incubation medium. As the cell membrane was permeabilised, the medium calcium concentration was a surrogate for $[Ca^{2+}]_i$. The advantage of this approach is that the 'intracellular' environment can be easily manipulated, thereby allowing investigation of some of the factors influencing Ca^{2+} mobilisation from intracellular stores. However, it does risk loss of cytoplasmic factors that could influence $[Ca^{2+}]_i$.

Calcium sensitive vibrating microelectrodes

Although calcium selective electrodes can measure $[Ca^{2+}]_o$ (the extracellular free ionised calcium concentration), its spatial resolution has been improved by the introduction of so called 'self referencing' microelectrodes. As all calcium selective electrodes require an additional reference electrode, they are not strictly speaking self referencing. In this application the recording electrode is cycled between two positions 5 to $50\,\mu m$ apart, and is termed a vibrating electrode. As a measurement is made at both positions, approximately every 3 seconds, by the same electrode, it reduces the risk of electrical drift in comparison to the situation where two separate recording electrodes were used (Messerli and Smith, 2010). In essence if the recording electrode is positioned so that it travels back and forth in a perpendicular direction to the cell, it will give information on calcium efflux. By altering the electrode scanning position over the surface of the structure, this technique can localise calcium fluxes.

Measurement of the activity of calcium activated ion channels by **patch clamp electrophysiology** can give an indirect indication of $[Ca^{2+}]_i$. However, the sensitivity of the calcium activated channels to $[Ca^{2+}]_i$ will alter over time due to cellular events such as phosphorylation and so on. Hence this technique is best considered as an adjunct

to optical probes as it gives information on ion channel activity rather than $[Ca^{2+}]_i$ per se. It is sometimes used in combination with optical techniques as whole cell patch clamp gives access to the cytosol.

The **radioisotope** ^{45}Ca allows the non-invasive determination of calcium fluxes, but does not measure $[Ca^{2+}]_i$. Prior to the introduction of optical probes or the vibrating calcium selective microelectrode it was the only practical method available to measure calcium fluxes. However, it requires a large number of cells and has a low temporal resolution. Hence this technique is less common, though it is still used under certain conditions as it only requires relatively inexpensive equipment. For example, it has shown that some heavy metals can interfere with calcium uptake.

Optical probes

Optical probes are usually considered the method of choice for studies of cellular calcium. These are subdivided into two general areas, luminescent and fluorescent probes. Both of these methods use light to report on calcium concentration, but there are important differences between them (Table 9.2). Optical probes have revolutionised our understanding of cell physiology as they allow determination of $[Ca^{2+}]_i$ in real time (see Table 9.1 for a comparison with other techniques).

It is essential that optical probes have high specificity towards Ca^{2+} over other ions. In an ideal situation only calcium will bind to the optical probe. However, as long as the binding affinity for Ca^{2+} is several orders of magnitude greater than the other ions in the cell, it will be possible to use that optical probe to measure calcium. For example, the divalent cation Mg^{2+} is present at the mM level, whilst resting $[Ca^{2+}]_i$ is approximately 100 nM. The intracellular K^+ concentration is even higher, being approximately 140mM.

Fluorescence

Fluorescence requires a high intensity light source and a fluorescent molecule. The molecules absorb some of the light energy, which causes electrons to transiently jump from the ground state to a higher unstable energy state. The electrons rapidly return to the ground state and emit the energy as light for around 10 nano seconds. Since energy transfer is not 100% efficient some energy is lost and the emitted light is of a lower energy and hence longer wavelength. This is known as the Stokes shift, where the absorption spectrum is at a shorter wavelength than the emission wavelength.

Table 9.2 Comparison of optical techniques for measuring cell calcium.

Type of probe	Fluorescent probes	Fluorescent proteins	Aequorin
Underlying basis of probe	Fluorescence		Luminescence
Excitation light source	Essential		Absent
Background signals	Auto fluorescence can be a problem, particularly with cellular NADH and NADPH with near UV excitation, and FAD up to around 500 nm excitation		Ultra low background as no excitation light used
Calcium buffering	Can be a cause for concern		Unlikely to be a problem
Cytosolic lifetime	Limited to a few hours, though can be substantially shorter in some cell types	Long for cells expressing the protein based optical probe	
Compartmentalisation	Particularly a problem for AM loaded probes	GFP based probes are cytosolic proteins	Is a cytosolic protein
Targeting	Dextran coupled probes can help limit diffusion	Can be targeted to organelles	
Contrast	Significantly less than aequorin		High
Cost of equipment	More expensive than aequorin even if no spatial information required. At a minimum a systems requires an excitation light source, excitation wavelength selector, emission selector and detector.		Relatively low as it only needs a detector. If spatial information is required, suitable imaging cameras are expensive.
Photobleaching of probe during an experiment	Susceptible to photobleaching		Not a concern as no light source is used
Dynamic range	Limited to around 2 orders of magnitude		Can be up to 5 orders of magnitude

Information in this table was based on Thomas and Delaville, 1991; Cobbold and Lee, 1991; Miller et al., 1994; Webb et al., 2010 and Whitaker 2010a.

Types of fluorescent probe

The first generation calcium sensitive fluorescent probe quin-2 was based on the metal chelator ethylene glycol tetraacetic acid (EGTA). Whilst EGTA can bind several metals, it has around five orders of magnitude (10^5) higher affinity for calcium than magnesium at pH 7, though its buffering capacity is strongly influenced by pH. Quin-2 has an EGTA backbone with some fluorescent groups added. Although it was the first fluorescent probe to be used for measuring $[Ca^{2+}]_i$ it does suffer from a low quantum yield (number of photons absorbed per photon emitted). This means that relatively high intracellular concentrations of quin-2 are required to get a reasonable signal, risking excessive calcium binding. This can lead to the scenario whereby a hormone-induced intracellular calcium signal is effectively chelated, preventing calcium induced events, and potentially confounding the presumed role of calcium in that system. The second generation optical probe fura-2 was also based on EGTA, but with modified fluorescent groups. It has much better fluorescent properties than quin-2 and has been used extensively.

Fluorescent optical probes work on the principal that their fluorescent properties alter when calcium binds. Fluorescent probes fall into two general categories, single or dual wavelength probes. By looking at the excitation and emission spectra it is straightforward to determine the difference between them.

Single wavelength probes such as fluo-3 are excited at one wavelength and have only one peak in the emission spectrum (Figure 9.3a). It can be seen that for constant concentration of fluo-3 and fixed excitation intensity at 488 nm the emission spectrum peaks at around 525 nm. In particular, as the concentration of calcium increases the

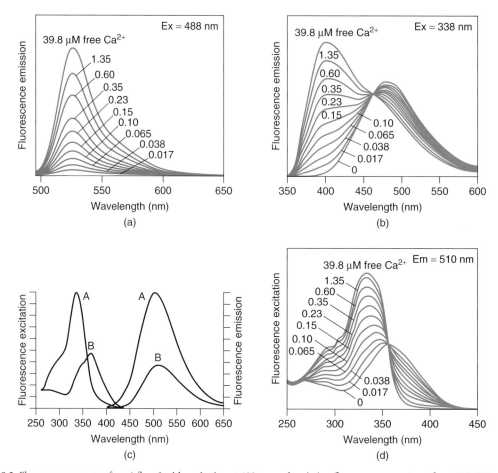

Figure 9.3 Fluorescence spectra for: a) fluo-3 with excitation at 488 nm and emission fluorescence spectrum from 500-650 nm, b) indo-1 emission spectrum from 350 to 600 nm with excitation at 388 nm, c) fura-2 excitation (left of panel) and emission spectra (right of panel) for calcium saturated (labelled A) and calcium free (labelled B) probe, d) fura-2 excitation scan (with emission at 510 nm) for a range of calcium concentrations. Figures from The molecular probes handbook, a guide to fluorescent probes and labelling technologies, 11th edition. Applied for permission, Invitrogen.com.

emission signal increases. Thus for fluo-3 the emission intensity is a function of cell calcium, assuming neither excitation intensity nor probe concentration varies throughout the experiment.

In contrast dual wavelength probes have two peaks either in their excitation spectra (e.g. fura-2) or emission spectrum (e.g. indo-1). For fura 2 (Figure 9.3c and d) the emission wavelength spectrum shows a single peak, which is similar to that of single wavelength probes. However the excitation spectrum is of much greater interest. If the emission wavelength is set at 510 nm and an excitation scan is run, it can be seen that the emission output is dependant on both the excitation wavelength and the calcium concentration. Where calcium saturates

fura-2 the peak excitation is around 340 nm. In contrast in calcium free media the peak excitation is shifted and is close to 380 nm. Notice that at one point the fluorescence spectra of calcium saturated and calcium free fura-2 cross at 360 nm. This is known as the isosbestic point and is where the fluorescence of fura-2 is independent of the calcium concentration. If a range of different calcium concentrations are shown (Figure 9.3d) it can be seen that an increase in calcium concentration causes the emission signal to increase when excited at 340 nm and decrease when excited at 380 nm, with no change when excited by 360 nm. In contrast, a fall in calcium concentration causes the emission to fall when excited by 340 nm and rise when excited by 380 nm, again with no

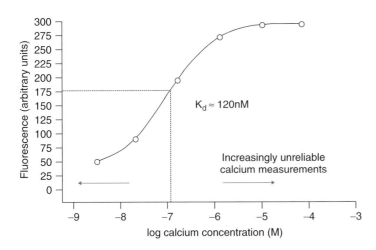

Figure 9.4 The importance of K_d for optical probes. As the K_d of this hypothetical probe is approximately 120 nm Ca^{2+}, this means that the probe should only be used to measure from around 12 nm to 1.2 µM calcium. Beyond these limits small errors in fluorescence measurement will result in large errors in estimation of the calcium concentration.

change when excited by 380 nm. This feature of differing calcium sensitive spectra with an isosbestic point is an indication that the probe can be used in dual wavelength mode (i.e. 340 and 380 nm excitation for fura-2) and is known as a ratiometric optical probe. This term means that rather than use the absolute fluorescence intensities, the ratio of the 340/380 signal is used instead.

Indo-1 is also a ratiometric probe (Figure 9.3b), but in this case it is the emission side that is ratiometric with excitation at a single wavelength of 335 nm and measurement of the emission signal at 400 and 480 nm.

These three probes cover the range of types of single fluorophore optical probes that are commonly encountered:
- single excitation and single emission, e.g. fluo-3
- dual excitation and single emission, e.g. fura-2
- single excitation and dual emission, e.g. indo-1

The change in fluorescent properties exhibited by fluorescent probes informing on the binding of calcium falls into one or more of the following categories (Thomas and Delaville, 1991):
1. alteration of quantum yield (i.e. the fluorescence emitted changes with calcium concentration). This occurs with all three optical probes considered above.
2. excitation spectrum shifts (e.g. fura-2).
3. emission spectrum shifts (e.g. indo-1).

Affinity of optical probes for calcium

There are over 40 calcium sensitive fluorescent optical probes commercially available. Thus it is necessary to consider some aspects that will affect the choice of probe. The relative merits of dual wavelength optical probes are considered elsewhere. Another important aspect is the calcium binding affinity, which is measured by K_d,

the calcium dissociation constant. This is determined by measuring the fluorescence emission of the probe in the absence of calcium and in a range of calcium concentrations up to that necessary to fully saturate the calcium binding sites of the probe. A graph of fluorescence emission plotted against calcium concentration will typically give a sigmoid curve (Figure 9.4). The calcium binding affinity is determined by interpolating the concentration of calcium that gives 50% of the maximum response, that is, (max–min response)/2. Notice that at the extremes of the range for both low and high calcium, large changes in calcium concentration only result in small changes in fluorescence emission. The central portion of the plot shows the largest change in fluorescence with a change in calcium. A rough rule of thumb is that you should not attempt to measure the calcium concentration less than 1/10th or more than 10 times the K_d of the probe.

Selection of single or dual wavelength optical probes

It all depends on your particular application. From a theoretical perspective dual wavelength probes are generally preferred if the equipment configuration allows this mode of operation. With this type of probe it is the ratio of the fluorescence at two wavelengths that is used to determine the calcium concentration. One wavelength represents the calcium bound and the other wavelength the calcium free forms of the optical probe. The use of ratios obviates the need to keep all other factors constant. Consider the situation where the fluorescence of a single wavelength optical probe changes. The assumption will be that this is due to an alteration in the calcium concentration.

However there are a variety of possible causes that don't involve calcium. These include:

i) anything that alters the amount of probe and therefore the fluorescence emission. This can be caused by photobleaching, whereby the high intensity light source actually degrades the optical probe. This is analogous to the loss of colour in brightly coloured plastic items left out in the sun. Also the cytosolic concentration of optical probes changes over time due to compartmentalisation (uptake into cellular organelles) and secretion from the cell. Differences in optical properties in various regions of the cell may also be a factor, particularly where the cell substantially varies in thickness (e.g. the nuclear region in an otherwise flattened cell).

ii) alteration of instrument parameters. Drift in equipment sensitivity and/or fluctuation in illumination intensity and so on is almost inevitable during experiments.

The net effect is that these effects will alter the fluorescence emission of optical probes, and could be taken to represent alteration in cellular calcium for single wavelength probes. In contrast dual wavelength ratiometric probes are much less susceptible to artifactual changes, provided the signal to noise ratio is sufficient. Consider the hypothetical situation for a dual wavelength probe. For wavelength one the initial signal is 100 and for wavelength two it is 200. If 50% of the probe is now removed the signal at wavelength one falls to 50 and that at wavelength two to 100. However, despite the 50% fall in actual fluorescence values, the ratio of fluorescence at wavelength one to fluorescence at wavelength two remains at 0.5 (fluorescence ratio moves from 100/200 to 50/100), and no change in $[Ca^{2+}]_i$ would be reported. This is in marked contrast to single wavelength optical probes. It is however important to recognise that this is only applicable for background corrected fluorescence signals. The effect of autofluorescence is considered later.

One of the drawbacks of dual wavelengths probes is that they are difficult to use on confocal microscopes. As fura-2 requires dual excitation, the maximum theoretical speed is half that of single wavelength probes. The dual emission probe indo-1 avoids the time penalty problem of dual excitation probes as it is only a single excitation probe. However, in order to use it on a confocal microscope it will require expensive UV lasers, which in turn will induce rapid photobleaching. Multiphoton confocal systems can reduce photobleaching, but are significantly more expensive.

Incorporation of optical probes into cells

Optical probes such as fura-2 are unable to cross cell membranes as the probes tend to be polyanions. Injection of optical probe is an invasive technique that risks damage to cells and ingress of Ca^{2+} through the injection site. In addition, if there is a need to measure several cells at once, each cell will need to be injected. The acetoxymethyl ester (AM) loading technique circumvents these problems. With calcium probes such as fura-2, fluo-3 and indo-1 four acetoxymethyl ester groups are attached to each molecule of the optical probe (though only one is shown in Figure 9.5). This has the effect of greatly increasing the hydrophobicity of the probe, thereby allowing it to readily penetrate cell membranes. However, as an AM form of an optical probe can now easily cross membranes, some of it will also enter various intracellular membrane compartments. In addition, the unmodified AM form of the optical probe can easily exit the cell. The reason why this is a very convenient loading technique is that there are intracellular esterases that hydrolyse the AM ester tag and remove it from the optical probe. This reveals the polyanionic form of the probe, which is now trapped within the cell as it is unable to cross membranes. Unfortunately, this process can also occur to AM labelled probe molecules inside intracellular membrane compartments, which then become trapped. This

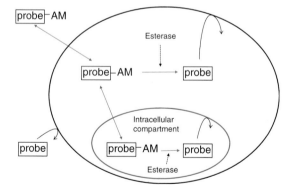

Figure 9.5 Acetoxymethyl ester loading technique. The optical probe is too hydrophilic to cross cellular membranes unaided (black arrows). The addition of an AM tag allows movement across membranes (blue arrows), but can also deliver the probe into intracellular compartments. Cellular esterases remove the AM tag, trapping the probe.

is known as compartmentalisation and can give rise to artifactual calcium signals, particularly if the intracellular membrane compartment has a high calcium concentration. For example, the calcium concentration of the ER is in the order of a few hundred micromolar, which will saturate incorrectly localised optical probes such as fura-2, as they are designed to measure cytosolic $[Ca^{2+}]_i$. The risk of compartmentalisation can be reduced by lowering the concentration of extracellular probe, reducing the loading time, and reducing the loading temperature. The optimum loading conditions aim to produce a good signal to noise ratio in the cytosol, but minimise compartmentalisation in intracellular membrane compartments. Thus, trials of a range of loading conditions are advised for a previously untried cell type.

Potential problems with fluorescent optical probes

Although fluorescent optical probes have revolutionised our understanding of cell physiology, it is important to recognise that they do have some significant potential problems. The risk of compartmentalisation, particularly a concern with AM ester loading of probes, has been mentionned previously. It is difficult to avoid, but optimal loading conditions can reduce the risk. Despite this, the longer an experiment is run, the higher the risk that at least some of the probe enters an intracellular membrane compartment. Related to this is where the AM ester loaded optical probe is incompletely de-esterified (Thomas and Delaville, 1991). As the AM form of the probe is fluorescent, but unable to bind calcium, its presence will impact on the estimation of $[Ca^{2+}]_i$. In addition, intracellular removal of the acetoxymethyl ester side groups results in the generation of toxic by products such as formaldehyde and H^+, which in turn can alter cell pH and ATP content. In practice both the problem of incomplete de-esterification and toxic by products can be ameliorated by an additional 30-minute incubation period after removal of extracellular probe. This incubation period allows complete de-esterification of the optical probe and recovery of the cell from the toxic by-products of de-esterification.

The excitation/emission spectrum produced by the manufacturers will have been obtained in a simple solution. The *in vivo* fluorescence properties may be altered by the cellular microenvironment. This could affect the peak excitation and/or emission wavelengths as well as the K_d. If the binding affinity to calcium is altered, then the reliability of the calibration from fluorescence to calcium concentration will be adversely affected. Other factors influencing the estimate of $[Ca^{2+}]_i$ include photobleaching of the probe, chelation of cellular calcium (both of which were previously discussed), autofluorescence (Table 9.2) and interference from other ions. The problem of metal interference arises as the optical probes tend not to be completely specific to calcium. They can also bind a variety of other cations. Usually Na^+, K^+ and Mg^{2+} are not a concern, even though the concentrations of these ions are several orders of magnitude greater than the calcium concentration. Rather, it is other metal ions, including both essential (e.g. copper, iron, manganese, zinc etc.) and non-essential metals (e.g. cadmium, mercury etc.) that can seriously impact on the fluorescent properties of optical probes such as fura-2. The actual effect on the emission spectrum will depend on the particular metal and its concentration. In some probes the metal will cause an increase in emission, whilst in others it will cause a decrease. Metal contamination is difficult to avoid, as even high purity salts will contain some low level contamination. Whilst membrane permeant heavy metal chelators such as TPEN (N,N,N',N'-tetrakis(2-pyridylmethyl)ethylenediamine) can remove the confounding influence of inappropriate metal binding, it does run the risk of removing metals from proteins to which they are normally bound, thereby altering their activity (Snitsarev and Kay, 2001). However, the metal induced change in fluorescence does offer the opportunity to estimate the free metal concentration in the cytosol. Indeed, the manganese quench technique even makes use of the quenching effect of Mn^{2+} on fura-2. As this is a dual excitation single emission ratiometric probe, a partial quench of the emission spectrum will not affect the measurement of calcium concentration, provided there is still a sufficiently high signal. Manganese will enter cells via calcium channels and bind to fura-2, which in turn reduces its fluorescence. This can be followed by monitoring the fluorescence at the isosbestic point (360 nm) of fura-2, which is the calcium independent fluorescence. Hence excitation at 340 and 380 nm will report on cellular calcium concentration, whilst excitation at 360 nm will give information on calcium influx, using manganese as a surrogate.

Protein-based optical probes

Protein-based optical probes include both luminescent and fluorescent types. The luminescent probe aequorin will be considered first, to allow subsequent comparison with fluorescent-based alternatives.

Bioluminescence is the ability of organisms to generate their own light. This is utilised for a variety of purposes including: communication (e.g. fireflies to attract mates); counter illumination, so that sea creatures blend in to the background when observed from below (a dark underside would otherwise clearly delineate their outline when viewed against the brighter light coming from above); warnings to predators that they contain toxic chemicals (e.g. firefly larvae); as a means of confusing predators (e.g. vampire squid); and in the lures of deep sea angler fish to attract prey and so on. Regardless of the function of the bioluminescence, the underlying mode of action is similar. There are a variety of calcium sensitive luminescent photoproteins, though aequorin is by far the most commonly used for determining $[Ca^{2+}]_i$, having been used for this purpose for over 40 years. Aequorin is found in the jellyfish *Aequorea victoria*, amongst other species. Hence natural aequorin is actually a mixture of various isoaequorins, due to the different species that are usually harvested together. Aequorin was first cloned in the 1980s and it is this form, rather than the natural aequorin, that is usually used to measure $[Ca^{2+}]_i$. Aequorin is a 21,000 Dalton protein that has three consensus EF hand sequences that represent calcium binding sites.

Aequorin is a photoprotein. This refers to the ability of the protein to emit light via luminescence under certain circumstances. It is important to consider the differences between luminescence and fluorescence as this has a major influence on how the optical probe can be used. In essence luminescence is where light can be emitted in the absence of an external light source. Bioluminescent reactions require a luciferin, which is the part that gives off the light, and a luciferase, which is an enzyme that oxidises the luciferin to generate light. The terms luciferin and luciferase are generic terms derived from the Latin lucifer that means 'light bearer'. In the case of aequorin the luciferin is coelentrazine and this is oxidised to coelentramide by the luciferase.

Natural aequorin actually has the prosthetic group coelentrazine bound to it. However, genetically engineered aequorin will lack coelentrazine as only the gene for aequorin is introduced into the cell, not the additional genes needed to allow the host cell to synthesise coelentrazine *de novo*. Upon calcium binding to aequorin, molecular oxygen oxidises the coelentrazine to coelentramide, which in turn causes the release of blue light (around 470 nm). Thus coelentrazine must be added extracellularly to cells expressing genetically engineered aequorin. Whilst coelentrazine can easily penetrate cell membranes, it can take up to 24 hours to fully reconstitute maximal activity as coelentrazine is unstable unless bound to aequorin (Campbell and Sala-Newby, 1993). When coelentrazine bound to aequorin is oxidised, the subsequent dissociation of calcium from aequorin results in the release of coelentramide from the photoprotein. The apoaequorin can then be reactivated by the binding of fresh coelentrazine. The use of recombinant aequorin has the advantage of restricting the aequorin to one type with known calcium binding properties, rather than a variable mixture that would otherwise occur with harvested natural aequorin.

As genetically engineered aequorin lacks coelentrazine, it is necessary to add it to the medium. This works well for transfected cells grown in culture, but is problematic for transgenic animals, where an injection into the blood stream will be required. Coelentrazine was first synthesised in the 1970s. Since then a variety of synthetic coelentrazines have been developed, including f-coelentrazine which produces greatly increased light emission, when the reconstituted aequorin binds to calcium (Webb et al., 2010).

The first fluorescent protein designed to measure calcium was developed from the naturally occurring green fluorescent protein (GFP). This is a small protein that is also a cytosolic protein found in the jellyfish *A. victoria*. Following the sequencing of GFP in 1992 a large variety of mutants have been produced. These have increased folding efficiency, shifted the excitation maximum and altered the emission characteristics. This has led to GFP being commonly used as a reporter gene and to follow proteins within cells. A rather beautiful example of labelling cells is brainbow, where individual nerve cells have been labelled with differing levels of expression of one of four fluorescent proteins to produce a colour palate of up to 100 different hues. This allows unambiguous determination of neuronal pathways (Livet et al., 2007). The technique of using fluorescent proteins has had a profound effect on our understanding of some aspects of proteins. Successful use of GFP to follow protein distribution and interaction with other proteins requires that the sequence for GFP is incorporated into the desired target protein, and that it does not unduly perturb the target protein. Thus the site of integration of GFP into the target protein must be carefully considered. The use of GFP to investigate G protein coupled receptors (GPCRs) is considered in Chapter 3. With regard to cell signalling, several GFP variants have been engineered to incorporate calcium binding domains, whilst others can sense pH, redox, cAMP (cyclic adenosine $3',5'$ monophosphate) and so on. The calcium sensing GFP-based probes include the chameleons, camgaroos and the pericams. Some are single wavelength, whilst others are dual wavelength ratiometric probes. Most are affected by changes in pH in the physiological range and emit less fluorescence than equivalent concentrations of non-protein-based optical probes. In addition they also suffer from some of the disadvantages of conventional fluorescent probes (Table 9.2). However, both aequorin and fluorescent proteins have some significant advantages over the conventional probes, namely cytosolic lifetime and targeting to the cytosol or organelles as desired (Table 9.2).

In order to direct proteins to selected organelles it is necessary to incorporate an organelle targeting sequence into the protein. Over the last few decades it has become apparent that certain sequences of amino acid help target proteins to particular organelles. These sequences might be cleaved of the protein on import into the organelle, or can be retained. In the case of the ER, there is a leader signal sequence that directs growing polypeptide chains in the cytosol to feed into the ER. This is then subsequently cleaved of from the polypeptide by a signal peptidase, thereby freeing the N terminal end of the polypeptide. However, there are also ER retention sequences, with the C terminal KDEL sequence being the most well known. KDEL refers to the single letter code for amino acids, namely lysine, aspartic acid, glutamic acid and leucine. The KDEL sequence does not actually prevent trafficking of proteins from the ER to the Golgi, but instead serves as a label that the protein is an ER resident protein. The retrieval (retrograde) transport pathway then returns any wayward KDEL labelled proteins back to the ER. Hence, if a recombinant calcium reporting protein is designed so that it also incorporates an organelle targeting or retention sequence (such as KDEL), it will be directed into the chosen organelle, thereby allowing investigation of organelle specific calcium handling. An alternative approach is to design a chimeric fusion protein whereby the calcium reporting protein incorporates another polypeptide that is normally resident in the desired organelle. Regardless of whether organelle localisation sequences are directly incorporated into the calcium reporting protein, or if the reporter is fused to a protein that itself localises to the organelle, it is essential that the calcium reporting ability of the construct is not subverted by the need to localise the probe to the desired organelle.

Fluorescent protein-based calcium sensors tend to have limited dynamic range, are susceptible to autofluorescence and photobleaching artefacts, and have lower contrast when compared to aequorin. However aequorin also has disadvantages. The need for a cofactor (coelentrazine) complicates the activation of aequorin, and the low light output compromises spatial information, generally requiring longer image capture times than with fluorescence-based alternative probes. The combination of aequorin and GFP into one calcium-sensing protein has resulted in improved performance. The aequorin component binds the calcium and the close proximity of the GFP component leads to non-radiative energy transfer to the GFP, which then emits light. This is known as bioluminescence resonance energy transfer (BRET). Its application in experiments to determine whether GPCRs dimerise is discussed in Chapter 3. BRET based calcium sensor proteins are an attempt to combine some of the advantages of luminescent (aequorin) and fluorescence (GFP) based approaches. Since the fusion construct is a protein it will have the advantages of protein-based probes. The GFP component will also allow non-invasive determination of which cells express the construct. Due to the aequorin, the fusion protein will have enhanced spatial discrimination over fluorescence-based probes as no excitation light is used. This almost eliminates autofluorescence, resulting in ultra low background signals, greatly improving contrast. BRET, due to energy transfer from aequorin to GFP, improves the light output over that which would be achievable with aequorin alone. The net result is a brighter image that will allow faster image capture, whilst still maintaining good spatial resolution. Future developments are likely to see light output increase even further.

In this book there is only sufficient space to give a brief overview of the techniques used to measure aspects of cell calcium. Readers interested in the area are advised to consult some of the many excellent reviews and books available such as McCormack and Cobbold (1991), Takahashi et al. (1999), Tepikin (2001) and Whitaker (2010b).

9.3 The exocrine pancreas

The exocrine pancreas is an important model system that has been extensively utilised to investigate calcium signalling in non-excitable cells, though it should be noted that there are significant differences with other cell types. For example, in contrast to most cell types the plasma membrane Na^+/Ca^{2+} exchanger plays little role in $[Ca^{2+}]_i$ homeostasis in exocrine pancreatic acinar cells (Hurley et al., 1992).

The typical human pancreas is a retroperitoneal elongated organ weighing about 100g that has both exocrine (secretes digestive enzymes) and endocrine (secretes hormones such as insulin and glucagon) components. It is located just below the stomach and its exocrine secretions empty into the duodenum. Although the pancreas has important endocrine functions, including, but not limited to, blood glucose regulation, the endocrine cells only account for around 2% of the volume of the pancreas.

In essence the structure of the exocrine pancreas can be thought of like a bunch of grapes. A single 'grape' represents a cluster of around 20–100 acinar cells, which is collectively known as an acinus. The stalk represents the pancreatic ducts that deliver the exocrine secretions to the duodenum. Whilst this is an oversimplification, it does allow an appreciation of the basic organisation.

The exocrine pancreas is divided into lobules that contain the acinar cells and each acinus has an intralobular duct. This intralobular duct then drains into interlobular ducts, which in turn feed into the main pancreatic duct. The bile duct from the liver joins with the main pancreatic duct just before exiting into the duodenum via the ampulla of Vater and the sphincter of Oddi. The juxtaposition of both these ducts draining into the duodenum via the same structure does give rise to the risk of developing acute pancreatitis, via blockage of the ampulla of Vater with gallstones. About one third of people have an additional accessory pancreatic duct that also drains into the duodenum via a different route. This feature reduces the risk of developing acute pancreatitis.

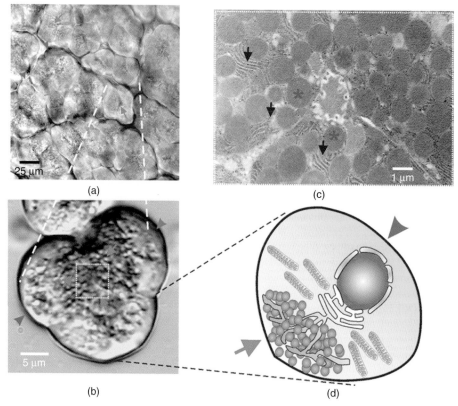

(a)

(c)

(b)

(d)

Figure 9.6 Pancreatic acinar cell morphology. (a) Transmitted light image of a mouse pancreatic lobule. (b) DIC image of three acinar cells separated by enzymatic digestion. (c) Transmitted electron microscopy image of the apical (secretory) pole region of three acinar cells with a central lumen. (d) Diagram of a single pancreatic acinar cell showing the characteristic organisation of organelles, with the nucleus positioned near the basal pole, zymogen (secretory) granules at the apical pole together with extensions of the ER, and mitochondria surrounding the secretory region. The red arrows indicate the apical pole whilst the blue arrows show the position of the basal pole. In panel (c) the blue asterisks denote zymogen granules whilst the black arrows indicate ER within the apical pole. Reprinted from The International Journal of Biochemistry and Cell Biology volume 42, Yule DI 2010. Pancreatic acinar cells: Molecular insights from signal-transduction using transgenic animals pp 1757–1761, Copyright (2010), with permission from Elsevier.

The acinar cells within an acinus are electrically coupled via gap junctions and form a functional unit. The gap junctions will allow the movement of small molecules to move between neighbouring cells. This may include signalling molecules and ions, contributing to the coordination of physiological responses in the acinar cluster. Acinar cells are highly polarised, with the apical pole facing the duct lumen, whilst the basal pole is on the outside of the cluster (Figure 9.6). The apical pole is readily recognisable as it contains the zymogen granules. The agonist receptors are however located on the basal pole of the cell, though some may also be present on the lateral membranes. Thus a central question is how does a hormone or neurotransmitter binding on the basal membrane lead to secretion at the apical membrane.

Although there is a continual low level of background constitutive secretion, a variety of hormones and neurotransmitters can greatly stimulate the regulated secretory pathway. The pancreas is innervated by both sympathetic and parasympathetic nerves, which release noradrenaline and acetylcholine (ACh) respectively. Noradrenaline tones down digestion, reduces pancreatic secretions, and diverts blood from the gastrointestinal (GI) tract to other areas such as the skeletal muscles. The parasympathetic nervous system stimulates digestive enzyme secretion and is mostly responsible for the low level basal secretion between meals, as the muscarinic antagonist atropine severely attenuates this. The actual rate of basal secretion varies between species, ranging from 10% in cats to up to 30% in rats, with humans around 20% of maximal rate. In contrast, bicarbonate secretion is much lower at around 2% (Solomon, 1994).

In essence the acinar cell secretes a mixture of digestive enzymes and some fluid that predominantly contains Na^+ and Cl^- ions. The pancreatic duct cells also secrete a bicarbonate rich fluid that helps wash pancreatic secretions down the ducts and into the duodenum. Whilst this occurs via Cl^-/HCO_3^- exchangers, the cystic fibrosis transmembrane conductance regulator (CFTR) Cl^- channel and the outwardly rectifying chloride channel are also involved in this process (see Chapter 6 for a discussion of this in relation to cystic fibrosis). Control of exocrine pancreatic secretions is complex and involves a variety of factors. The cephalic phase is where the smell, sight and taste of food can induce anticipatory secretions in the pancreas. This is mostly due to parasympathetic input via ACh. The gastric phase is where processing of food in the stomach causes hormones to be released that can impact on pancreatic secretions. Whilst this is partly due to the distension and movement of the

stomach, the composition of the meal will also have an influence as breakdown products of digestion can affect the hormonal environment. The intestinal phase occurs when substances exit the stomach. For example acid in the intestine will stimulate bicarbonate secretion, whilst breakdown products of protein and fat digestion will influence enzyme secretion from the pancreas. Cholecystokinin (CCK) is released from both enteroendocrine cells and neurons in the intestine. Other pancreatic secretagogues include bombesin, gastrin releasing peptide, neuropeptide Y, secretin, substance P and vasoactive intestinal peptide (VIP), whilst yet other hormones such as somatisation and pancreatic polypeptide inhibit pancreatic secretions.

Pancreatic secretagogues tend to fall into two basic categories, those that act via cAMP (e.g. secretin and VIP) and those that utilise Ca^{2+} (e.g. ACh and CCK). A full discussion of GPCRs and signal transduction pathways is given in Chapter 3 so is only briefly considered here. Secretin and VIP bind to their respective G protein coupled receptors (GPCRs). The occupation of the receptor by an agonist promotes binding of a heterotrimeric G-protein, in this case Gq. This leads to the dissociation of the Gsα subunit and activation of the enzyme adenylate cyclase which produces cAMP. The cAMP can either act on its own (e.g. cAMP activated ion channels), or more commonly binds to inactivated tetramers of protein kinase A (PKA), liberating the catalytic subunits to phosphorylate target proteins. As this chapter is focused on calcium signalling most attention will be given to ACh and CCK. Acetylcholine binds to muscarinic receptors that activate Gqα, which then stimulates the enzyme phospholipase C-β (PLCβ). This phospholipase cleaves the plasma membrane-attached phosphatidylinositol-4,5 bisphosphate (PIP_2) into diacylglycerol (DAG) and free inositol-1,4,5 trisphosphate (IP_3). DAG then activates protein kinase C (PKC), which in turn phosphorylates target proteins. IP_3 is water-soluble and rapidly diffuses through the cytoplasm to bind to IP_3 receptors (IP_3R) located in the endoplasmic reticulum (ER) membrane. These induce release of calcium into the cytosol. The calcium is then sequestered by calcium-binding proteins such as calmodulin, which in turn can activate a variety of proteins including kinases and phosphatases. These impact on the exocytotic pathway and stimulate secretion of digestive enzymes into the intralobular ducts.

Released calcium can either be removed from the cytosol by re-uptake into the ER calcium stores, and/or extruded to the outside of the cell by SERCA or plasma membrane Ca^{2+} ATPases respectively, in order to return the cell to resting calcium levels. There are two types of CCK receptor in pancreatic acinar cells. The CCK_A receptors are high affinity receptors preferentially stimulated by low concentrations of CCK (picomolar). This receptor has a much greater affinity for CCK than gastrin. The low affinity CCK_B receptors is roughly equally sensitive to CCK and gastrin. Although CCK can also act via the IP_3 pathway, the concentration that significantly increases $[Ca^{2+}]_i$ is around an order of magnitude less than that required to elevate the IP_3 concentration. Admittedly the IP_3 concentration actually refers to bulk IP_3, so it does not rule out a localised intracellular high IP_3 concentration. Whether IP_3 is actually the calcium mobilising second messenger for CCK in acinar cells is considered later.

Fluid secretion

In order to wash enzymes down the pancreatic duct it is also necessary to secrete fluid. Spatial organisation of ion channels, transporters and pumps allows the generation of an electrochemical Cl^- gradient that results in Cl^- secretion across the apical membrane into the intralobular duct (Figure 9.7).

9.4 Calcium signalling in pancreatic acinar cells

The exocrine pancreatic acinar cell was chosen to illustrate aspects of calcium signalling as it is a key model system of non-excitable cells and has been intensively studied. This section is not however intended as an extensive review of calcium signalling in the exocrine pancreas. Rather it aims to introduce some of the general themes of the multifactorial control of calcium signalling. This is a large and expanding area, as can be gauged by the observation that a PubMed search using the three terms calcium exocrine pancreas together gives over 500 hits.

With the advent of fluorescent optical probes much effort has focussed into understanding calcium signalling and how this relates to the physiological role of the acinar cell. Most of this work has used acutely isolated acinar cells which involves using enzymes such as collagenase and mechanical agitation to separate them. As the acinar cells now lack the support of their neighbours they take on a kidney bean-like shape, with the eye of the bean representing the secretory granule area (apical pole). Whilst these are much easier to investigate than intact tissue, they will have undergone damage during the isolation. Any damage to gap junctions, which is unavoidable, will disrupt communication between cell clusters. Park et al.

(2004) found that whilst polarised Ca^{2+} signals were relatively unaffected, gross disturbances to membrane potential and exocytosis were evident in single isolated cells. Despite this, acutely isolated pancreatic acinar cells are an important model system, though the development of multiphoton confocal microscopes will allow work on more physiologically relevant intact lobules.

Initial studies on isolated acinar cells revealed that both ACh and CCK can induce calcium oscillations. Yule et al. (1991) showed that 90 nM ACh induced oscillations in $[Ca^{2+}]_i$ that did not return to the baseline between oscillations (Figure 9.8). In contrast 60 pM CCK induced similar peak $[Ca^{2+}]_i$ of around 600 nM but in this case the Ca^{2+} oscillations did return to baseline between oscillations and were of a much lower frequency. In calcium free media the ACh Ca^{2+} response exhibited relatively rapid run down, whilst the CCK response persisted for several minutes (Figure 9.8). This shows that both ACh and CCK mobilise Ca^{2+} from both the intracellular and extracellular environment. Otherwise, removal of extracellular calcium would have resulted in an almost instantaneous block on calcium oscillations, if they were purely dependent on extracellular Ca^{2+}.

The spatial organisation of the acinar cell is such that neurotransmitters/hormones bind to receptors on the basal pole, leading to the production of calcium mobilising second messengers. The trigger for exocytosis is an increase in $[Ca^{2+}]_i$. As the secretory granules are at the opposite end of the cell to the GPCRs it would appear reasonable to expect the calcium signal to develop at the basal pole and spread to the apical pole to stimulate exocytosis. This is based on the realistic assumption that the highest concentration of second messengers is at the basal pole. However, experiments clearly demonstrate that the apical pole is the most sensitive region of the cell. The evidence for this derives from investigating different aspects of this initially unexpected observation. Low dose ACh and CCK can induce Ca^{2+} spikes (localised transient elevations of $[Ca^{2+}]_i$) that are confined to the apical region. In cases where the calcium signal spreads throughout the cell, the site of initiation tends to be the apical pole (Figure 9.9). This is followed by spreading of the calcium wave to the rest of the cell after a short time lag.

The data in Figure 9.9 were obtained with the calcium sensitive probe BTC. Similar experiments using fura-2 also show that the apical pole responds to 1 μM ACh before the basal pole. However, it generally fails to find much of a difference in peak $[Ca^{2+}]_i$ in these two regions (in contrast to the almost double $[Ca^{2+}]_i$ at the apical pole in Figure 9.9). This is due to the higher binding affinity of

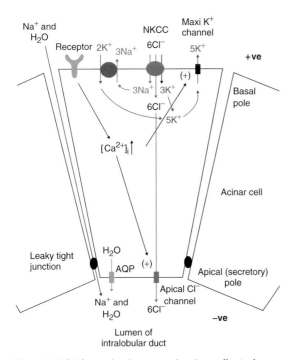

Figure 9.7 Fluid secretion in pancreatic acinar cells. At the basal membrane Na$^+$/K$^+$ ATPase maintains the transmembrane sodium gradient. This allows the basal Na/K/2Cl$^-$ transporter (NKCC) to deliver Na$^+$, K$^+$, and Cl$^-$ to the cytosol. The excess Na$^+$ is removed via Na$^+$/K$^+$ ATPase, whilst basolateral maxi K$^+$ channels allow the K$^+$ to exit. These ensure that cytosolic Na$^+$ and K$^+$ concentrations do not build up and impede the functioning of the NKCC transporter. The stoichiometry of the overall process is that 6Cl$^-$, 3K$^+$ and 3Na$^+$ ions enter via the NKCC transporter, whilst 3 Na$^+$ ions leave and 2 K$^+$ ions enter via Na$^+$/K$^+$ ATPase. The 5K$^+$ ions then leave the cell via the maxi K$^+$ channels, with the remaining 6Cl$^-$ ions exiting the cell via the apical Cl$^-$ channel. Thus these ion movements have the net effect of transport of Cl$^-$ ions from the interstitial fluid to the lumen. This creates a transepithelial electrical gradient, with the lumen negatively charged. Whilst there are tight junctions between cells, they are relatively leaky. This allows Na$^+$ to pass through them into the lumen. The movement of Na$^+$ and Cl$^-$ ions into the lumen causes water to follow, both via the leaky tight junctions and aquaporins (AQP) in the apical membrane. This results in fluid secretion which helps wash the digestive enzymes down the intralobular ducts. The [Ca^{2+}]$_i$ is instrumental in coordinating this as the maxi K$^+$ channel and the Cl$^-$ channel are Ca^{2+} activated, indicated by (+). Receptor activation leads to generation of an increase in [Ca^{2+}]$_i$ though the mechanisms by which this arises is omitted for clarity. Based on the model in Petersen (1988).

fura-2 for calcium (lower K$_d$). Thus, at peak [Ca^{2+}]$_i$ fura-2 is saturated, unlike the lower affinity probe BTC (Ito et al., 1997). Fura-2 therefore under reports peak [Ca^{2+}]$_i$ and thus emphasises the importance of K$_d$ when choosing optical probes (see section 9.2 for a fuller discussion of this).

The relative sensitivity of the different areas of the cell was also probed via addition of IP$_3$ or calcium into selected areas (Kasi et al., 1993). If a patch clamp microelectrode delivers 10 μM IP$_3$ to the cytosol at the basal pole a small local increase in [Ca^{2+}]$_i$ is observed in part of the basal pole. This is soon followed by a rise in [Ca^{2+}]$_i$ that starts in the apical pole and spreads throughout the apical pole, but does not progress to the basal pole. Thus there is a clear gap in calcium signal between the apical and basal poles. This is particularly informative as after initial breakthrough with the patch clamp pipette to adopt the whole cell configuration there will be an initial localised relatively high IP$_3$ concentration at the basal pole. This causes the initial small calcium response in the basal pole. However, as the IP$_3$ concentration reaches the same level throughout the cytosol, the apical pole responds in preference to the rest of the cell. These localised rises in [Ca^{2+}]$_i$ then diminish. If 50 μM IP$_3$ is delivered to the apical pole, via patch clamp pipette, a global Ca^{2+} signal initiates at the apical pole before spreading to the rest of the cell. Thus low and high dose IP$_3$ application have very similar effects to low and high dose ACh, where with low concentrations of ACh Ca^{2+} spiking is confined to the apical pole, but with a high dose of ACh the Ca^{2+} wave starts in the apical pole and spreads after a short delay (less than 1 sec) to the rest of the cell. Whether this is in part due to regional differences in IP$_3$R distribution is considered later.

Pancreatic acinar cells can also undergo calcium induced calcium release (CICR), where the act of raising [Ca^{2+}]$_i$ can itself induce a further increase in [Ca^{2+}]$_i$, as the intracellular calcium channels on the calcium stores are calcium sensitive (Figure 9.13). Similar to the results with IP$_3$, the site of addition of Ca^{2+} to the cytosol reflects regional differences in sensitivity. Basal injection of Ca^{2+} induces a slow gradual rise in [Ca^{2+}]$_i$ throughout the cell, from approximately 100 to 200 nM. In contrast, apical injection of calcium produced a rapid increase in [Ca^{2+}]$_i$ to around 700 nM in the apical pole within a second. The Ca^{2+} signal then spreads to the basal pole, though its amplitude was diminished (Kasi et al., 1993).

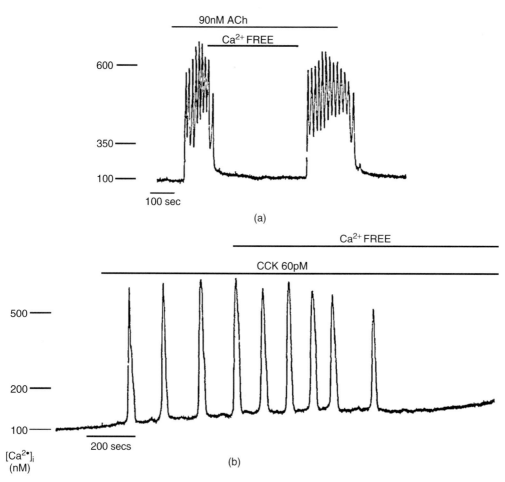

Figure 9.8 Effect of extracellular calcium removal on oscillations in (a) 90 nM ACh and (b) 60pM CCK treated pancreatic acinar cells. Reprinted from Cell Calcium volume 12, Yule et al., 1991. Acetylcholine and cholecystokinin induce different patterns of oscillating calcium signals in pancreatic acinar cells, pp. 145–151, Copyright (1991), with permission from Elsevier.

The relative contribution of Ca^{2+} extrusion and Ca^{2+} reuptake into stores as ways of removing Ca^{2+} from the cytosol

As calcium is toxic to cells it is essential that calcium signals are short lasting. Removal of Ca^{2+} from the cytosol to reduce $[Ca^{2+}]_i$ to resting levels is therefore of considerable importance. As mentioned previously the plasma membrane Ca^{2+} ATPase and SERCA can actively pump Ca^{2+} out of the cell and/or back into the intracellular calcium stores. By use of the calcium droplet technique (Figure 9.10) it is possible to demonstrate that following a rise in $[Ca^{2+}]_i$, a considerable amount of Ca^{2+} is extruded from the cell (Tepikin et al., 1992). In particular, extrusion

by calcium to the external environment after a Ca^{2+} spike starts to occur just as the peak $[Ca^{2+}]_i$ starts to decrease.

However, this technique gives no information on Ca^{2+} reuptake into stores. This can be investigated by measuring the rate at which Ca^{2+} is removed from the cytosol when it can be pumped both into stores and outside the cell, and comparing them to the situation where recovery to resting $[Ca^{2+}]_i$ can only occur via extrusion to outside of the cell (Figure 9.11). Exposing pancreatic acinar cells to 10 μM ACh (supramaximal dose) induces a large rise in $[Ca^{2+}]_i$. If the ACh is suddenly removed and a large excess of the muscarinic antagonist atropine is added (0.1mM), all ACh is displaced from GPCRs and further IP_3 production ceases. This leaves the cell with a high

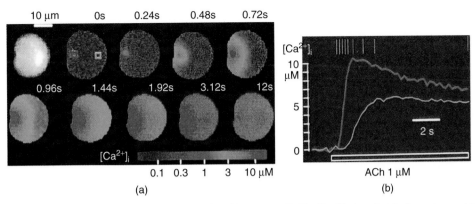

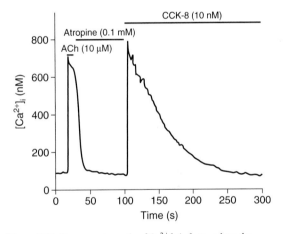

Figure 9.9 Regional differences in calcium mobilisation induced by 1 μM ACh. The first black and white image in panel (a) shows the fluorescent image, whereas the pseudocolour images represent the cellular calcium at the stated times after application of 1 μM ACh (indicated in panel (b) by the vertical lines above the graph). The red box in the first colour image indicates the area measured for the apical pole calcium dynamics, whilst the orange box shows the area measured for the basal pole. Panel (b) shows the $[Ca^{2+}]_i$ for the apical pole (red trace) and basal pole (orange trace). Adapted by permission from Macmillan Publishers Ltd [EMBO Journal] Ito et al. (1997). Micromolar and submicromolar Ca^{2+} spikes regulating distinct cellular functions in pancreatic acinar cells. EMBO Journal 16: 242–251. Copyright 1997.

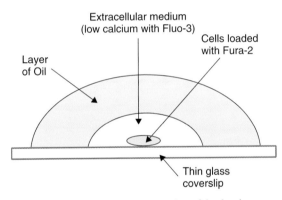

Figure 9.10 Diagrammatic representation of the droplet technique as devised by Tepikin et al. (1992). Pancreatic acinar cells were loaded with fura-2, isolated into a small cluster in a restricted volume of nominally Ca^{2+} free extracellular solution (approximately 50 times cell volume) containing fluo-3. A layer of oil is then applied to cover the extracellular solution, restricting evaporation. The calcium sensitive optical probes fluo-3 and fura-2 were chosen as they have different excitation wavelengths, allowing almost simultaneous measurement of both $[Ca^{2+}]_i$ and $[Ca^{2+}]_o$.

$[Ca^{2+}]_i$, and within a few seconds a low IP_3 concentration (IP_3 half life is approximately 1 second). Thus, the calcium can be removed from the cytosol by both calcium extrusion across the plasma membrane and reuptake into the calcium stores. This results in a rapid recovery to resting $[Ca^{2+}]_i$ (Camello et al., 1996). If this is followed

Figure 9.11 Recovery to resting $[Ca^{2+}]_i$ is faster when the agonist is removed. Camello et al. (1996). Calcium dependence of calcium extrusion and calcium uptake in mouse pancreatic acinar cells. Journal of Physiology 490: 585–593. With permission from John Wiley and Sons Ltd.

by a supramaximal dose of CCK (10 nM), a large rise in $[Ca^{2+}]_i$ will occur. It is necessary to use CCK, rather than a second application of ACh, as the muscarinic ACh receptor could have become desensitised due to the initial supramaximal dose of ACh (see Chapter 3 for a discussion of GPCR desensitisation). However, if the CCK remains in the extracellular solution, calcium mobilising second messenger production will still occur in the cytosol. Thus the calcium stores are functionally permeabilised as any Ca^{2+} pumped into the stores will leak out via the store calcium channels opened by the continued presence of second messengers. This means that a fall in $[Ca^{2+}]_i$ can only occur via extrusion across the plasma membrane, resulting in a much extended time for the $[Ca^{2+}]_i$ to fall to resting levels, approximately 200 seconds, compared to around 10 seconds (Camello et al., 1996).

The relationship between the relative Ca^{2+} pumping activity and the $[Ca^{2+}]_i$ can be revealed by plotting a graph of rate of change of $[Ca^{2+}]_i$, as given by $d[Ca^{2+}]_i/dt$, against $[Ca^{2+}]_i$ (Figure 9.12). In the situation with access to both stores and extrusion (ACh removal and Atropine addition), the relative removal of Ca^{2+} is much greater than that achieved by extrusion alone (Figure 9.12a), in the continued presence of CCK. The impression that reuptake into stores is the most important route is confirmed when the relative uptake into stores and extrusion across cells is directly compared (Figure 9.12b). Low rates of pumping into stores and out of the cell occur at resting $[Ca^{2+}]_i$. As the calcium concentration rises reuptake into stores occurs in preference to extrusion out of the cell (Camello et al., 1996).

As there is a spatial aspect to rises in $[Ca^{2+}]_i$, there may also be localised Ca^{2+} extrusion. The calcium jam technique (Belan et al., 1997) uses a high molecular weight dextran coupled to a fluorescent optical probe (calcium green 1-dextran) to assess the sites of calcium release. If pancreatic acinar cells are loaded with one optical probe (fura red via its AM ester form) and then added to a nominally Ca^{2+} free solution containing calcium green 1-dextran, it is possible to follow both $[Ca^{2+}]_i$ and extrusion of Ca^{2+} at the same time. The high molecular weight dextran limits the diffusion of calcium green 1, thereby revealing the sites of Ca^{2+} extrusion. Both localised ACh application (via iontophoresis), or flash photolysis of intracellular caged Ca^{2+}, generates a large rise in $[Ca^{2+}]_i$. This is accompanied by substantial Ca^{2+} extrusion that is greatest at the apical pole into the lumen (Belan et al., 1997). The caged form of Ca^{2+} uses a calcium buffer that releases Ca^{2+} on exposure of UV light. The source of the extruded Ca^{2+} into the lumen is apical plasma membrane Ca^{2+} ATPase. It should, however, be noted that zymogen granules contain substantial amounts of Ca^{2+}. When a sufficiently high $[Ca^{2+}]_i$ triggers exocytosis, some of the extruded Ca^{2+} will derive from zymogen granule fusion with the apical plasma membrane. Lee et al. (1997) found that plasma membrane Ca^{2+} ATPase was most concentrated in the luminal and lateral membranes, corresponding to the site of maximal Ca^{2+} extrusion. In addition, the SERCA 2a isoform was expressed in the

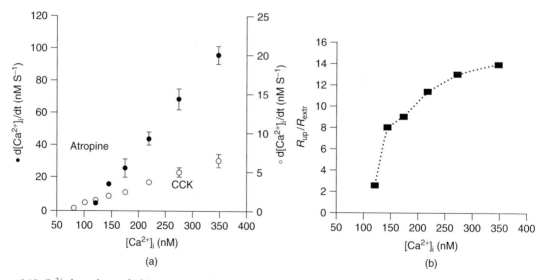

Figure 9.12 Ca^{2+} dependence of calcium recovery following supramaximal agonist stimulation. (a) Rate of uptake into stores and extrusion across the plasma membrane (Atropine) compared to extrusion across the plasma membrane alone (CCK). The difference between the two represents the rate of uptake into stores. (b) Ratio of relative rate of uptake into stores (R_{up}) to relative rate of extrusion across the plasma membrane (R_{extr}), Camello et al. (1996). Calcium dependence of calcium extrusion and calcium uptake in mouse pancreatic acinar cells. Journal of Physiology 490: 585–593. With permission from John Wiley and Sons Ltd.

apical region, whilst the SERCA 2b isoform was mostly in the basal area.

ER is mostly located in the basal area of the cell, though fine extensions of the ER network are present in the granular region at the apical pole. The ER does partly refill with Ca^{2+} between calcium signals via SERCA, though store operated calcium channels located on the basal pole are also involved. The store operated Ca^{2+} channels deliver Ca^{2+} to basal ER. However, as the lumen of the ER network is continuous, the ER effectively acts as a calcium tunnel, delivering Ca^{2+} to the apical pole. This was first demonstrated by Mogami et al. (1997). He maximally stimulated clusters of pancreatic acinar cells with $10\,\mu M$ ACh in calcium free media. After the first stimulation and recovery to resting $[Ca^{2+}]_i$ in the presence of ACh, no rise in $[Ca^{2+}]_i$ was detected after removing ACh and then reapplying it about 60 seconds later. This shows that the ER has been emptied of agonist releasable Ca^{2+}. One of the cells in the cluster was allowed access to Ca^{2+} via a cell attached patch pipette at the basal pole. However, by applying a charge across the pipette Ca^{2+} was only allowed to enter the cell during the brief 60 seconds between consecutive ACh applications. This cell, unlike the rest of the cluster, could now respond to the 2nd application of ACh with a rise in $[Ca^{2+}]_i$ that started at the apical pole, despite Ca^{2+} only being available at the basal pole. This elegant demonstration of Ca^{2+} tunnelling (movement of Ca^{2+} through the ER to distant locations within the cell, rather than via the cytosol) has been supported by Park et al. (2001). They found that localised photobleaching of an ER localised probe resulted in loss of probe throughout both regions of the cell regardless of whether the site of photobleaching was the basal or apical pole.

IP$_3$ receptors

IP$_3$R are composed of four subunits that oligomerise to form a functional Ca^{2+} channel. Whilst the IP$_3$R responds to the intracellular IP$_3$ concentration, it is also sensitive to the intracellular calcium concentration. At low $[Ca^{2+}]_i$ the IP$_3$R is relatively insensitive to Ca^{2+}. However, as the $[Ca^{2+}]_i$ increases, the sensitivity to Ca^{2+}, and hence CICR, rises to a maximum, and then falls on a further rise in $[Ca^{2+}]_i$. This gives a characteristic bell shaped curve (Figure 9.13).

There are three subtypes of IP$_3$R which vary in sensitivity to IP$_3$. Type I IP$_3$R has an EC$_{50}$ of approximately $4\,\mu M$, whilst for type II it is $0.3\,\mu M$ and for type III around $20\,\mu M$ IP$_3$. All three IP$_3$R subtypes occur in pancreatic acinar cells, though the type II is the most common at about 50% followed by type III at about 45%, with type

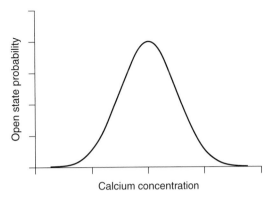

Figure 9.13 Diagrammatic representation of the calcium sensitivity of IP$_3$ receptors. As the calcium concentration increases the calcium starts to sensitise the IP$_3$ sensitive calcium channel, increasing the probability that the channel opens. However, once past a certain calcium concentration, negative feedback occurs. Further increase in calcium starts to desensitise the IP$_3$ sensitive calcium channel, reducing the probability that the channel will open.

I making up the rest (Wojcikiewicz, 1995). The most sensitive type II IP$_3$R is located to the area of the cell close to the luminal plasma membrane at the apical pole, whilst most type I and III IP$_3$ R are localised to the apical pole, though they are also found in the nucleus and basal pole (Yule et al., 1997). This helps to explain why even though IP$_3$ concentration is highest at the basal pole on agonist stimulation, the opposite side of the cell, the apical pole, responds first. Within the apical pole there are multiple hotspots of Ca^{2+} release sites where regenerative Ca^{2+} spikes occur (Thorn et al., 1996). Some of these hotspots release more Ca^{2+} than other sites (around a 300 fold difference between the smallest and largest events, Fogarty et al., 2000). The frequency distribution of calcium release events is not uniform, with most being small scale events, and only a few much larger events. Conceivably this could be due to differences in the density of local clusters of IP$_3$R and/or IP$_3$R subtypes. The larger the cluster and/or higher proportion of the most sensitive type II IP$_3$R, the larger the calcium event (Fogarty et al., 2000). IP$_3$R may also be mobile. IP$_3$R can permit the transit of cations, not just Ca^{2+}. Though, in relation to the high calcium concentration gradient across the ER membrane, Ca^{2+} is by far the most common cation moving through this channel into the cytosol. Thus, by following K^+ movement through the IP$_3$R channels in isolated patches it is possible to measure the activity of the channels without the confounding influence of Ca^{2+} sensitivity affecting the results (Taylor and Dale, 2012). It was found that in isolated nuclear membrane patches of DT40 cells (chicken lymphocyte B cell line) that the IP$_3$R were randomly distributed under resting conditions. However, increasing the IP$_3$ concentration led to clustering of IP$_3$Rs. Interestingly, the same elevated IP$_3$ concentration but with 1 μM Ca^{2+} in addition, negated the influence of IP$_3$ on IP$_3$R clustering (Taylor and Dale, 2012). This led them to develop a model (Figure 9.14) whereby as the IP$_3$ concentration increases, the IP$_3$Rs form clusters and calcium release events progress from localised calcium blips (release from a single IP$_3$R) to calcium puffs (release from a localised cluster of IP$_3$R), to calcium waves (progression from one cluster of IP$_3$Rs to the next). Whilst this hypothesis is attractive, calcium release sites do appear to occur from the same places within cells (Taylor and Dale, 2012). One possibility is that there are certain hotspots where IP$_3$R are fixed in position. A rise in IP$_3$ concentration might then lead to local recruitment of IP$_3$R so that calcium signals can progress outside the immediate vicinity of the hotspots, though this has yet to be demonstrated.

Ryanodine receptors

IP$_3$R are not the only intracellular Ca^{2+} channels opened by Ca^{2+} mobilising second messengers in pancreatic acinar cells. Ryanodine, which is a plant alkaloid, also mobilises Ca^{2+} release from intracellular Ca^{2+} channels on stores, though this occurs via the ryanodine receptor (RyR) rather than the IP$_3$R. Ryanodine actually has a biphasic effect, with nM concentrations opening the channel, but μM concentrations closing the channel. The structure of the ryanodine receptor is reminiscent of the IP$_3$R, being composed of four subunits, though they are substantially larger. There are three types of RyR, which are also calcium sensitive. Similar to IP$_3$R, they have a bell shaped curve of calcium sensitivity, where low to moderate calcium concentrations lead to CICR, but higher calcium concentrations inhibit the opening of the channel. Only the type II RyR has so far been found in pancreatic acinar cells. Whilst it is mostly present in the basolateral area, some is also found in the apical pole (Leite et al., 1999).

The physiological agonist of the RyR is actually cyclic adenosine diphosphoribose (cADPr). This has been shown to mobilise calcium from the secretory pole in pancreatic acinar cells (Thorn et al. 1994). However, both heparin (an IP$_3$R antagonist) and μM ryanodine (which blocks RyR) blocked the calcium spiking in acinar cells. This suggests that both IP$_3$R and RyR are involved in calcium spiking. The cADPr antagonist 8-NH$_2$ cADPr was found to block calcium spiking induced by intracellular cADPr applied via a patch clamp pipette, but did not affect the response to IP$_3$. In addition, it was found that the cADPr antagonist blocked the Ca^{2+} spikes induced by 5pM CCK. It was therefore concluded that low concentrations of CCK, which activate the high affinity CCK$_A$ receptor, leads to activation of RyR via cADPr (Cancella and Petersen, 1998).

NAADP

Nicotinic acid adenine dinucleotide phosphate (NAADP) was the last of the three currently known Ca^{2+} releasing intracellular messengers to be found in pancreatic acinar cells. NAADP is made by ADP-ribosyl cyclase which causes base exchange of nicotinamide from NADP$^+$ (nicotinamide adenine dinucleotide phosphate) with nicotinic acid (Cosker et al., 2010). The same enzyme can also make cADPr, though in this case NAD$^+$ (nicotinamide adenine dinucleotide) is used as the substrate instead of NADP$^+$. ADP ribosyl cyclase is found at various locations in the cell. A plasma membrane form, CD38, is found in pancreatic cells. However, the catalytic activity is on the extracellular side of the membrane. If NAADP was actually made extracellularly it would require transport into the cell in order to exert its effects. Using CD38 knockout mice Cosker et al. (2010) found

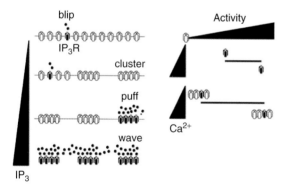

Figure 9.14 Elementary Ca^{2+} release events evoked by IP$_3$. At low IP$_3$ concentrations single IP$_3$Rs can only allow a small calcium blip to be released, though IP$_3$ also promotes IP$_3$R clustering. As the IP$_3$ concentration increases, the Ca^{2+} released by a single IP$_3$R in a cluster sensitises neighbouring IP$_3$Rs so that a calcium puff is emitted from the cluster. Further increased in IP$_3$ concentration allows calcium puffs to diffuse to other local clusters of IP$_3$Rs resulting in a developing calcium wave. Reprinted from Molecular and Cellular Endocrinology volume 353, Taylor and Dale 2012. Intracellular Ca^{2+} channels – a growing perspective pp 21–28, Copyright (2012), with permission from Elsevier.

that pancreatic acinar cells would no longer respond to 5pm CCK in Ca^{2+} free media, though in calcium containing media 5pm CCK still caused slow oscillations in $[Ca^{2+}]_i$. This was not due to reduced sensitivity of the calcium signalling machinery as NAADP, cADPr and IP_3 could still induce calcium spikes with the whole cell patch clamp technique. Subsequent investigation determined that the defect was due to a reduction in the ability to synthesise NAADP. Whilst CD38 is present on plasma membranes, subcellular localisation of CD38 in normal pancreatic acinar cells found that it co-localised with acidic compartments that were considered to be part of the endosomal system. This subcellular CD38 fraction was heavily concentrated at the apical pole. However, CD38 did not co-localise with either lysosomal or zymogen granule markers. Although some CD38 is already apically located, Cosker et al. (2010) suggested that endocytosis of plasma membrane CD38 induced by CCK could lead to enhanced intracellular generation of NAADP.

NAADP is an unusual calcium releasing messenger as at low concentrations (5-100 nM) it mobilises calcium, whereas at $1 \mu M$ and above it desensitises the NAADP receptor. This can be used to demonstrate the role of NAADP in calcium signalling. One hundred μM NAADP abolished the Ca^{2+} spikes elicited by 2pm CCK, but did not influence the response to IP_3 or cADPr (Cancella et al., 1999). The cADPr antagonist 8-NH_2-cADPr inhibited calcium spiking caused by 2pm CCK, cADPr and NAADP, but not IP_3, whilst heparin inhibited calcium spiking in IP_3, cADPr, NAADP and 2pM CCK treated pancreatic acinar cells (Cancella et al., 1999). This suggests that all three calcium mobilising second messengers are intimately involved in the control of calcium signalling in these cells.

The physiological receptor for NAADP is thought to be the two pore channel (TPC). The TPCs are found in acidic stores of the endo-lysosomal system within cells. Recent evidence has shown that these acidic compartments are functional Ca^{2+} stores. During the formation of endocytic vesicles, the plasma membrane invaginates and therefore 'samples' the extracellular fluid. This contains around 1 mM free Ca^{2+}. Indeed, the lysosomal calcium concentration of pancreatic acinar cells has been estimated to be around $40 \mu M$ (Sherwood et al., 2007). The cell permeant peptide glycyl-L-phenylalanine-2-napthylamide (GPN) enters subcellular compartments and is cleaved by the enzyme cathepsin C, which is resident in lysosomes. This causes osmotic swelling due to the liberation of free amino acids from the peptide. The resultant lysis of lysosomes leads to loss of Ca^{2+} from this pool. This in turn prevents

2pm CCK induced calcium oscillations, but did not affect 50 nM ACh induced calcium oscillations (Yamasaki et al., 2004). Thus, the lysosomal Ca^{2+} pool is likely to be significant in acinar cell calcium signalling. A convincing demonstration that TPCs are NAADP gated calcium channels was provided by Brailoiu et al. (2010). They mutated a lysosomal targeting sequence in the TPC so that it was redirected towards the plasma membrane. This channel was now accessible to patch clamp studies. They showed that excised patches of plasma membrane had NAADP gated Ca^{2+} channels. Mutating the conserved leucine residue at position 265 within the proposed pore region of the TPC to proline abolished the NAADP sensitive Ca^{2+} channel (Brailoiu et al., 2010). However, this does not rule out the possibility that other Ca^{2+} release channels are affected by NAADP. Indeed, the type II RyR, which is present in the apical pole of pancreatic acinar cells, has been shown to be activated by NAADP where Ca^{2+} is also present (Mojzisova et al., 2001).

NAADP on its own only produces small localised Ca^{2+} signals, and unlike the IP_3R and RyR, does not exhibit CICR. If NAADP is applied in the presence of IP_3 and/or cADPr the resultant Ca^{2+} signal is amplified, allowing a global calcium signal to develop. IP_3 also potentiated the response to CCK, whereas NAADP and cADPr did not (Cancella et al., 2002). Yamasaki et al. (2005) investigated NAADP and cADPr production in pancreatic acinar cells. They found that up to $1 \mu M$ ACh had no effect on NAADP production, but that for 10pM CCK there was a four fold transient increase in NAADP concentration. This peaked within 5 seconds and returned to basal levels within a minute. In contrast, both 50 nM ACh and 10pM CCK caused a three and four fold elevation in cADPr concentration respectively. This takes 1 to 2 minutes to fully develop, but remains elevated for several minutes. Thus the initial response to CCK is an increase in NAADP that rapidly declines just as the cADPr production increases.

The vacuolar H^+ ATPase inhibitor (V type ATPase) bafilomycin A1 destroys proton gradients in acidic compartments. This has the effect of abolishing the response to NAADP, 2pM CCK, but does not affect the response to 50 nM ACh. The SERCA inhibitor thapsigargin however inhibits both 2pM CCK and ACh induced Ca^{2+} signalling (Yamasaki et al., 2004).

The results described above (and others) have led to the development of a conceptual model of Ca^{2+} signalling in pancreatic acinar cells (Figure 9.16). This cell has densely packed zymogen granules, together with thin extension of the ER and lysosome like acidic compartments in the apical pole. The exact location of the three types of second messenger activated intracellular Ca^{2+} channels is the subject of some debate. It is generally accepted that IP_3R and RyR are located on the ER; it is the identity of the Ca^{2+} channels on the acidic stores that are disputed. The evidence clearly demonstrates that NAADP sensitive TPCs are present, but whether IP_3R and/or RyR are also located there is less certain. Regardless of this, low physiological doses of CCK (e.g. 5pM) leads to occupation of the high affinity CCK_A receptor and the transient production of NAADP. The NAADP then releases calcium via TPCs on the acid store, producing spatially restricted local calcium release events. This increase in $[Ca^{2+}]_i$ then sensitises RyR (and IP_3R) in the immediate vicinity. When cADPr production increases after a short delay, the sensitised RyR then releases additional Ca^{2+} which sets in train CICR, which, combined with the increase in cADPr results in a global Ca^{2+} wave. Part of the controversy may be related to the ability of NAADP to cause release from RyR directly, rather than require cADPr. Thus if an experiment shows that μM ryanodine or thapsigargin can inhibit NAADP evoked calcium release, it could actually be due to inhibition of the RyR receptors on the ER Ca^{2+} pool, rather than TPCs on the ER or RyR receptors on the acidic Ca^{2+} pool.

ACh induced Ca^{2+} signalling does not involve NAADP, but rather IP_3 and cADPr. The initial rise in Ca^{2+} will again sensitise IP_3R and RyR so that the initially localised Ca^{2+} release can result in a global Ca^{2+} wave.

The actual Ca^{2+} signalling dynamics will depend on the concentrations of NAADP, IP_3, cADPr and $[Ca^{2+}]_i$. As IP_3R and RyR are calcium sensitive, whilst an initial rise in $[Ca^{2+}]_i$ can give rise to CICR, a large rise in $[Ca^{2+}]_i$ will actually desensitise the IP_3R and RyR, thus imposing negative feedback.

Mitochondria

Mitochondria are often thought of as the powerhouse of the cell as they are responsible for the generation of most of the ATP used within the cell. However, they are also involved in a variety of other processes, including cell signalling. As the inside of mitochondria are negatively charged, cations such as Ca^{2+} will tend to enter via any channels that allow them passage (Figure 9.15). The voltage dependent anion channel (VDAC) in the outer membrane of mitochondria is only weakly selective and is permeable to metabolites and Ca^{2+}. VDAC is therefore the main route of Ca^{2+} uptake across the outer mitochondria membrane. In order to cross the inner mitochondrial membrane Ca^{2+} can move via the mitochondrial Ca^{2+} uniporter (MCU). Whilst it is highly selective for Ca^{2+},

other divalent (and trivalent) cations can enter. Although the MCU has a very large transport capacity, there is another route, known as rapid mode uptake (RaM). This, as its name implies, is a much faster mode of Ca^{2+} influx than that which occurs via MCU. Where the cytosolic Ca^{2+} concentration is less than 200 nM, Ca^{2+} uptake into the mitochondria is predominantly via RaM. However, as the cytosolic Ca^{2+} concentration exceeds 200 nM the RaM rapidly inactivates (Pan et al., 2011). Mitochondrial RyR have recently been identified in the inner mitochondrial membrane of heart cells and appear to be involved in allowing Ca^{2+} to move into the matrix. Other possible candidates involved in Ca^{2+} transport across the inner mitochondrial membrane into the matrix include the Letm1 Ca^{2+}/H^+ antiporter and the voltage dependent mCa1 and mCa2 calcium channels, though the evidence for these is limited (Pan et al., 2011).

Calcium efflux pathways from the matrix across the inner mitochondria membrane involve the mitochondrial Na^+/Ca^{2+} antiporter which probably transports 3 Na^+ ions for every Ca^{2+} ion (and is thus electrogenic) and the mitochondrial H^+/Ca^{2+} antiporter that probably transports 2 H^+ for every Ca^{2+} ion and is therefore electroneutral. There may also be an additional diacylglycerol activated Ca^{2+} channel on the inner nuclear membrane that allows Ca^{2+} to leave the matrix (Ryu et al., 2010). Under certain pathological conditions the RyR may run in reverse mode, allowing Ca^{2+} transit from the matrix to the inter membrane space. Calcium in the inter membrane space between the inner and outer mitochondrial membranes can then exit the mitochondrion via VDAC.

An alternative exit route for Ca^{2+} is the mitochondrial permeability transition pore (mPTP). Irreversible opening of the mPTP leads to cell death. However transient opening of the mPTP, known as flickering, may permit the exit of some Ca^{2+}, thereby contributing to cell homeostasis (Rasola and Bernardi, 2011). Calcium in mitochondria stimulates oxidative phosphorylation and thus ATP generation. However a by-product of this is reactive oxygen species (ROS). Thus, as the free calcium concentration of the mitochondria increases, the production of ROS also rises, risking damage to mitochondria. As ROS stimulates RyR and IP_3R, but inhibits SERCA and plasma membrane Ca^{2+} ATPase, ROS could actually contribute to calcium signalling within cells (Rasola and Bernardi, 2011). Indeed, ROS sensitises the mPTP, making it more likely to open. The molecular identity of the mPTP is currently uncertain. It is a non-selective channel that allows movement of substances up to about 1500 Daltons. It does contain cyclophilin-D, and the adenine

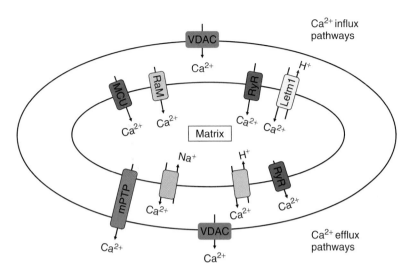

Figure 9.15 Routes of calcium movement within mitochondria. Mitochondrial Ca^{2+} uptake occurs via the voltage dependant anion channel (VDAC) on the outer mitochondrial membrane. The mitochondrial Ca^{2+} uniporter (MCU), rapid mode of uptake (RaM), mitochondrial ryanodine receptor (RyR) and Letm1 H$^+$/Ca^{2+} exchanger transport the Ca^{2+} into the matrix. Calcium efflux occurs via the Na$^+$/Ca^{2+} calcium exchanger, H$^+$/Ca^{2+} exchanger, and may involve transient flickering of the mitochondrial permeability transition pore (mPTP). The mitochondrial RyR may also run in reverse mode, allowing Ca^{2+} to leave the matrix. The mCa1 and mCa2 calcium influx channels and the DAG activated calcium efflux channel on the inner mitochondrial membrane are not shown as evidence for these is equivocal at present. Model based on Giacomello et al. (2007), Ryu et al. (2010), Pan et al. (2011) and Rasola and Bernardi (2011).

nucleotide translocase is thought to have a regulatory function, but may not actually be part of the channel. There is also some evidence for other components such as the mitochondrial phosphate carrier. Whether the mPTP actually spans both mitochondrial membranes is also unclear (Baines, 2009).

The pancreatic acinar cell has mitochondria localised to three general regions of the cell, namely: (i) at the boundary of the apical and basal zones (perigranular), (ii) close to the plasma membrane in the basolateral area, and (iii) around the nucleus (Park et al., 2001). Mitochondria can act as localised cellular calcium buffers, shaping the spread of calcium signals through the cell. The matrix functions as a calcium store as calcium phosphate precipitate starts to form when the calcium concentration increases above certain levels. This is a dynamic process and the calcium can be remobilised as the mitochondrial calcium concentration falls. The positioning of the perigranular mitochondria is ideally placed to affect the spread of Ca^{2+} signals throughout the acinar cell. Small calcium spikes can be converted into global calcium waves by the uncoupling agent carbonyl cyanide *m*-chlorophenylhydrazone (CCCP) that acts as an ionophore, or antimycin which is an electron transport inhibitor. As this work was done

in conjunction with patch clamp electrophysiology with 2 mM ATP in the whole cell configuration, this is not due to cellular ATP depletion (Tinel et al., 1999). Thus, the perigranular mitochondria act as a barrier to propagation of calcium waves that originate in the apical pole. This has been termed the mitochondrial firewall. The mitochondria around the nucleus may also have a similar function in helping to isolate the nucleus from changes in cytosolic calcium concentration (Park et al., 2001). However, the calcium buffering capacity of mitochondria can be exceeded, allowing larger calcium signals in the apical pole to develop into global calcium waves.

Other organelles are also likely to be involved in Ca^{2+} signalling. For example Pinton et al. (1998) found that the Golgi have IP$_3$ sensitive Ca^{2+} stores. Since Golgi are located between the apical region and the mitochondrial calcium firewall in pancreatic acinar cells, they may also contribute to shaping Ca^{2+} signals.

Crosstalk

Crosstalk is a common feature of intracellular signalling pathways. This is where activity in one pathway can influence another. Since the main secretagogues in the exocrine pancreas tend to act via calcium or cAMP, these pathways have been investigated for possible crosstalk. It was found that cAMP can impact on the calcium signalling pathway on several levels (Bruce et al., 2003). This can occur via:

i) Generation of IP_3. This can occur via PKA induced phosphorylation of either the GPCR directly, G proteins, or even $PLC\beta$ itself. Also the activity of some of the enzymes that metabolise IP_3 can be altered by phosphorylation. Indeed, cAMP can even directly activate $PLC\varepsilon$.

ii) IP_3 receptors. Phosphorylation of IP_3R can either potentiate or inhibit Ca^{2+} release depending on the receptor subtype and the cell. In the pancreatic acinar cell cAMP causes a reduction in the response to IP_3, mainly via PKA induced phosphorylation of type III IP_3R. This is partly reflected in the different basic types of oscillation in $[Ca^{2+}]_i$ observed with low doses of ACh or CCK. For ACh the oscillations are faster and tend to occur around an elevated baseline. In contrast, CCK induced calcium oscillations tend to be slower and return to the normal resting $[Ca^{2+}]_i$ between oscillations. As CCK can phosphorylate the type III IP_3R, the difference in spatiotemporal calcium oscillations may be partly attributable to this, though RyR and NAADPR also play a role.

iii) Ca^{2+}-ATPases. These act to remove calcium from the cytosol, either into stores (SERCA) or into the extracellular environment (PMCA). Due to the presence of several different isoforms of PMCA and SERCA, the effect of their phosphorylation is tissue specific. In some tissues PKA induced phosphorylation increases PMCA activity. The exact nature of this interaction is the subject of some debate. With SERCA it has been suggested that the phosphorylation of a SERCA associated protein causes it to dissociate from SERCA, thereby reducing its calcium pumping activity. However, with PMCA it has been proposed that the Ca^{2+} binds to calmodulin (CaM) forming a Ca-CaM complex that in turn binds to PMCA and activates it. The binding of Ca-CaM induces a conformational change that may expose an otherwise inaccessible PKA phosphorylation site. If PKA phosphorylation did indeed further activate PMCA, it would impact on calcium signalling (Bruce et al., 2003).

Whilst cAMP impacts on calcium signalling pathways, the converse is also possible. Calcium, via Ca-CaM can activate isoforms of adenylate cyclase, increasing the concentration of cAMP. Also calcium can inhibit and Ca-CaM stimulate various classes of phosphodiesterases which are responsible for metabolising cAMP and/or cGMP. Thus calcium and cAMP can exhibit crosstalk between their respective pathways. It is also important to recognise that interactions between calcium, cAMP and PKC can affect exocytosis.

Store operated calcium channel

Thapsigargin is a sesquiterpene lactone that was first isolated form the plant *Thapsia garganica*. It has been extensively used in calcium signalling as a selective inhibitor of SERCA pumps. If the ER Ca^{2+} ATPase is inhibited, the ER will no longer be able to maintain its high calcium concentration. The ER sequestered calcium thus enters the cytosol and causes an increase in $[Ca^{2+}]_i$. In calcium free media thapsigargin causes a transient rise in $[Ca^{2+}]_i$ as excess calcium is removed from the cytosol by plasma membrane Ca^{2+} ATPase. However, in Ca^{2+} containing medium thapsigargin causes a prolonged rise in $[Ca^{2+}]_i$. This importantly occurs without activating PLC. The interpretation was that a fall in store (ER) calcium content led to the opening of a calcium channel on the plasma membrane, which was termed the store operated calcium channel (SOC).

In the normal situation a fall in ER calcium concentration would lead to the opening of SOC, allowing Ca^{2+} to enter the cell and replenish the ER calcium content. This process does not require $[Ca^{2+}]_i$ to actively rise if the rate of entry of calcium into the cytosol, via SOC, is matched by uptake into the store. Indeed, Mogami et al. (1998) calcium clamped the cytosol to 90 nM, but failed to prevent the ER refilling after hyperstimulation with $10\,\mu M$ ACh.

The identification of a calcium release activated Ca^{2+} channel (I_{crac}) lent support to the idea of SOC. I_{crac} appeared to be an unusual Ca^{2+} channel in several respects. It had very low conductance (20-30fS), was inhibited by intracellular Ca^{2+} and stimulated by extracellular Ca^{2+} (Putney, 2007). However, the question arises as to how a reduction in ER calcium concentration can lead to opening of SOC. The main contenders were that a fall in ER luminal calcium concentration triggered:

i) release of a soluble diffusible messenger termed the calcium influx factor (CIF).

ii) conformational coupling between the SOC and component(s) of the ER.

At present, whilst there is a body of evidence to support the existence of CIF, the identity of this factor remains to be established. By the use of various chromatography techniques CIF has been shown to be a small non-protein molecule around 600Da in size. Based on its susceptibility to attack by proteases and other treatments, it has been suggested that CIF may be a phosphorylated sugar nucleotide (Bolitina and Csutora, 2005). The link between CIF and SOC is thought to involve the β isoform of Ca^{2+}

independent phospholipase A_2 (i$PLA_2\beta$). This enzyme produces arachidonic acid and lysophospholipids. Whilst arachidonic acid is involved with calcium signalling, via arachidonic acid regulated Ca^{2+} channels (ARC channels) that are independent of store depletion, lysophospholipids can activate SOC. This led to the suggestion that CIF displaces inhibitory calmodulin on i$PLA_2\beta$, which in turn produces lysophospholipids that activate SOC. Thus CIF may have an indirect effect on SOC. However, over the last few years considerable progress has been made in the alternative hypothesis, so studies on CIF have tended to be neglected.

Conformational coupling originally started out as a proposed interaction between IP_3R and the SOC that required close contact between them. It is now known that it is not IP_3R that communicate with SOC, but another protein known as stromal interaction molecule (STIM). STIM was identified via RNAi gene silencing screens of thapsigargin treated cells. Two STIM proteins have been identified. Both STIM1 and STIM2 are found in the ER and have EF hand calcium binding sites. When ER calcium stores are depleted STIM relocates to areas of the ER which are close to the plasma membrane to form punctuate structures. This is accompanied by activation of SOC. Under normal luminal ER calcium concentration both STIM1 and STIM2 will have calcium bound and be inactive. STIM2 has a lower calcium binding affinity than STIM1. Hence STIM2 will preferentially activate before STIM1 as the luminal ER calcium concentration declines. The initial fall in luminal calcium concentration will require a smaller calcium influx in order to replenish stores. This is consistent with the finding that in STIM2 deficient cells the basal $[Ca^{2+}]_i$ is significantly less than in normal cells. This led to the suggestion that STIM2 may influence basal calcium fluxes to maintain basal $[Ca^{2+}]_i$ (Várnai et al., 2009). Upon removal of Ca^{2+} from the EF hand binding sites the STIM proteins form oligomers.

Most attention has focused on STIM1 as this appears to have the largest influence on SOC. However, there may be several mechanisms that activate SOC. An interesting recent development is a link between CIF and STIM1. If STIM1 is down regulated the thapsigargin induced production of CIF is impaired. In contrast, if STIM1 is overexpressed CIF production is stimulated. This was shown to be specific to STIM1 as loss of a few amino acids at glycosylation site(s) in the intraluminal sterile α motif (SAM) of STIM1 abolished its ability to rescue CIF production (Csutora et al., 2008). These authors consider that STIM1 is not actually a CIF synthase, but rather the ER luminally located SAM domain of STIM1 might interact with the currently unknown CIF synthase. CIF production has a faster time course than migration of STIM to puncta formation. Conceivably a fall in ER luminal calcium concentration will lead to a conformational change in STIM1 that activates CIF synthase (Csutora et al., 2008). Thus both CIF and STIM1 are probably involved in SOC.

Although STIM1 and 2 act as ER calcium sensors, they do not form the SOC channel. Orai proteins were discovered via genetic analysis of a form of severe combined immunodeficiency that had defective I_{crac}, and a whole genome screen of a *Drosophila* cell line. It has subsequently been demonstrated that Orai proteins form the SOC calcium pore. Three Orai proteins are known, with Orai1 giving the greatest Ca^{2+} fluxes in reconstituted channels. As four Orai proteins are required for pore formation, heterotetramers with different subunit composition may exist with differing channel characteristics. Regardless of the exact molecular configuration(s) of the channel, STIM1 is intimately involved in SOC activation. Coexpression of STIM1 and Orai1 in cell lines resulted in a large rise in I_{crac}. Mutation studies with single amino acid substitutions demonstrated that Orai proteins form the central calcium pore. Prior to agonist stimulation Orai proteins are distributed throughout the plasma membrane. As the calcium concentration of the ER falls STIM proteins form oligomers. The STIM proteins interact with microtubules via the plus end tracking protein EB1 which brings about their concentration in punctuate regions that underlie the plasma membrane. The STIM oligomers then interact with Orai proteins in the plasma membrane resulting in their concentration to regions of the plasma membrane that overlie the punctuate regions. It is not yet known whether there are additional proteins needed for activation of SOC. The observation that SERCA also co-localises with STIM1 and Orai1 would allow the generation of small micro domains of high $[Ca^{2+}]_i$ in the vicinity of the STIM1-Orai1 complex (Figure 9.16). SERCA would then refill the ER calcium store without leading to elevation of bulk cytosolic calcium (Alonso et al. 2012).

9.5 Nuclear calcium signalling

It has previously been shown that alteration in calcium concentration can influence nuclear processes. This includes fertilisation, prevention of polyspermy and therefore polyploidy (more than two copies of each chromosome), nuclear envelope breakdown, metaphase to

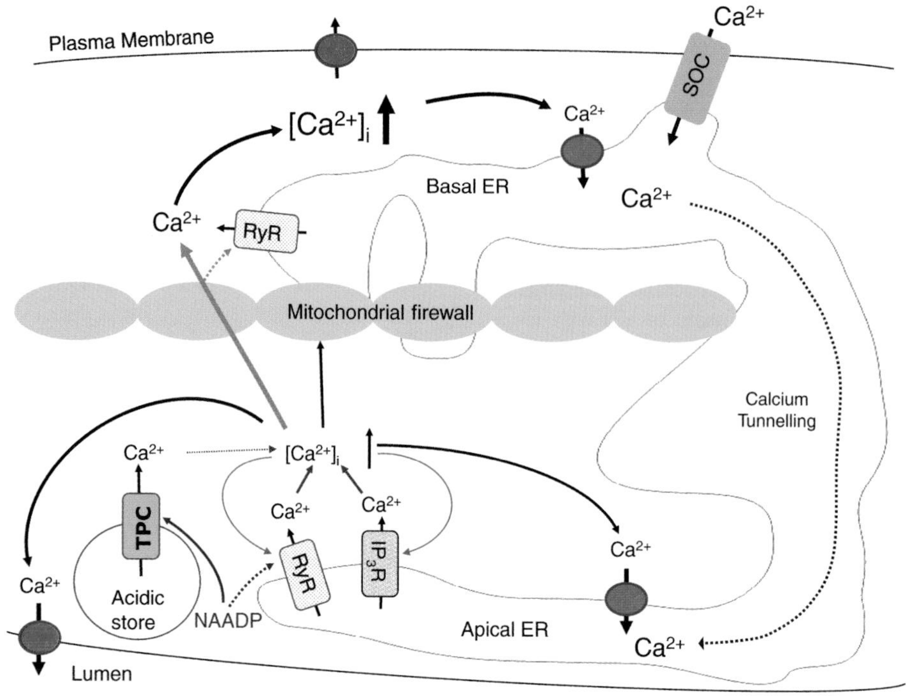

Figure 9.16 Simplified model of Ca^{2+} signalling in the pancreatic acinar cell. Low dose CCK causes an initial release of Ca^{2+} via a transient increase in NAADP acting on TPCs on the acidic stores in the apical pole (NAADP might also stimulate RyR). The local increase in Ca^{2+} concentration sensitises the RyR on the ER, which together with cADPr causes more Ca^{2+} release. The mitochondrial firewall prevents the local Ca^{2+} signals developing into a global response. Higher doses of CCK cause more NAADP and cADPr production, leading to a larger Ca^{2+} signal that can now breach the mitochondrial firewall (grey arrow) and spread to the basal pole (aided by RyR on the ER in the basolateral areas). Low dose ACh causes generation of IP$_3$ and cADPr, resulting in localised release of calcium from IP$_3$R and RyR on the ER, but does not spread to the basal pole. Higher doses of ACh cause more IP$_3$ and cADPr to be produced, resulting in a sufficiently large amount of Ca^{2+} being released by the IP$_3$R and RyR to breach the mitochondrial firewall. As most IP$_3$R are in the apical pole, the spread to the basolateral areas mostly involves RyR. IP$_3$R are also sensitised by Ca^{2+}. Return to resting [Ca^{2+}]$_i$ involves SERCA (blue circles) and PMCA (red circles) that pump Ca^{2+} back into the ER and out of the cell respectively. Most Ca^{2+} extruded from the cell exits via the apical plasma membrane into the lumen. The SOC helps maintain ER calcium levels, and the lumen of the ER delivers Ca^{2+} to the apical pole via calcium tunnelling. ACh, CCK, GPCRs, G proteins, second messenger generating enzymes, IP$_3$ and cADPr are omitted for clarity.

anaphase transition and cytokinesis, which is division of a eukaryotic cell into two daughter cells (Matchaca, 2011). Calcium has also been shown to regulate gene expression. There is therefore considerable interest in nuclear calcium signalling. Unfortunately these studies on nuclear calcium have been complicated by uncertainties as to whether the properties of optical probes are affected by the nuclear environment. Indeed, many optical probes actually appear brighter in the nucleoplasm (Alonso and Sanchez, 2011). This might arise via concentration of the probe in the nucleus and/or a change in the calcium binding affinity of the optical probe due to differences in the nuclear

and cytoplasmic environment. Whilst ratiometric optical probes will be less influenced by changes in probe concentration, both ratiometric and single wavelength probes will be affected by changes in calcium binding affinity.

The ER network joins onto the outer nuclear membrane and the lumen of the ER is continuous with the nuclear endoplasmic space (NES). Since the ER has a high calcium concentration, this raises the possibility that the NES could function as a nuclear calcium store. In many cell types invagination of the nuclear envelope, known as nucleoplasmic reticulum (NR), have been observed (Figure 9.17). These may function as calcium release sites within the nucleus. This could be due to Ca^{2+} release channels on the NR. In addition, as there is a cytosolic 'lumen' in the NR, cytosolic second messengers could gain access to deeper areas of the nucleus via the nuclear pore complex (NPC) on the NR (Bootman et al., 2009).

IP$_3$, cADPR and NAADP have all been shown to be able to induce Ca^{2+} release from isolated pancreatic acinar cell nuclei (Gerasimenko et al., 2003). IP$_3$R are located on both the inner and outer nuclear membrane. This was demonstrated by both biochemical and functional assays. By injecting IP$_3$ into the nucleus, IP$_3$R located on the inner nuclear membrane release calcium from the NES into the nucleoplasm. Conceivably nuclear IP$_3$ could leave the nucleus via the NPC, act on IP$_3$R located on the outer nuclear membrane, with the released calcium then being able to enter the nucleus via the NPC to elevate the nuclear free ionised calcium concentration, $[Ca^{2+}]_n$. This long winded route may occur, but it can be demonstrated that there are functional IP$_3$R inside the nucleus by the use of the IP$_3$R blocker heparin. In permeabilised GH$_3$ cells (pituitary cell line) high molecular weight heparin abolishes the cytoplasmic response to IP$_3$, but hardly reduces the peak response in the nucleus (Chamero et al., 2008). It is important to note that heparin actually has a variety of effects apart from blocking the IP$_3$R. Whilst other more specific IP$_3$R antagonists are available such as 2-aminoethoxydiphenyl borate (2-APB) and xestospongin C, high molecular weight heparin has the advantage that its large size restricts entry into the nucleus. Similarly, Luo et al. (2008) found that IP$_3$ increased the rate of cytosolic and nuclear calcium sparks in permeabilised neonatal rat cardiomyocytes, with nuclear calcium sparks 1.5 times as frequent as cytosolic sparks. This was attributed to the higher density of IP$_3$R in the nucleus. In addition, nuclear calcium waves were observed that were confined to the nucleus. However, other authors have found that nuclear calcium signals require initiation in the cytosol, before spreading to the nucleus. Allbritton et al. (1994) found that cytosolic calcium signals preceded nuclear calcium signals and that cytoplasmic injection of a heparin-dextran severely attenuated the ability of cytosolic IP$_3$ to mobilise nuclear calcium.

Nuclear calcium signals do not simply reflect passive diffusion of calcium from the cytosol via the nuclear pore complex. Indeed, in many instances calcium spiking in the cytosol does not travel to the nucleus. Free calcium ions in the cytosol have only a very short diffusion distance (around $1\,\mu m$) before they are sequestered (Allbritton et al., 1992). This contrasts with the nucleus, where a lower calcium buffering capacity will allow Ca^{2+}

to travel further. Hence, if localised cytosolic calcium release occurs close to the nucleus, the calcium signal may propagate into the nucleus, whilst the cytosolic calcium is rapidly buffered.

It has been suggested that there may also be small IP$_3$ sensitive calcium stores in the nucleus associated with chromogranins, though little is currently known about them (Bootman et al., 2009). Since IP$_3$, cADPr and NAADP can all cause Ca^{2+} release from the inner nuclear membrane, receptors for all three second messengers are also thought to be present on the inner nuclear membrane, though only IP$_3$R and RyR have so far been found. However, this would represent a departure from the current model of NAADP receptors confined to acidic stores, though NAADP may actually be acting on RyR. As the nucleus has second messenger generating mechanisms (PLC and ADP ribosyl cyclase) it would be expected that IP$_3$, cADPr and NAADP receptors are nuclear located.

The role of calcium on the regulation of gene expression

It is generally accepted that the nuclear pore complex (NPC) is permeable to Ca^{2+}, though NPCs might be able to slow down, though not eliminate, movement of Ca^{2+} through them. Nuclear calcium and/or $[Ca^{2+}]_i$ may affect NPC opening and hence movement of proteins through the NPC. Some groups have found that depletion of nuclear Ca^{2+} reduces the movement of proteins into the nucleus, whilst others have found that $[Ca^{2+}]_i$ appears to control this.

Since changes in nuclear free calcium concentration $[Ca^{2+}]_n$ do occur, consideration must be given to the likely physiological consequences. As has been previously mentioned calcium is implicated in many nuclear processes. This section will be confined to aspects of its role in regulating the expression of some genes.

Calcium can influence gene expression in a variety of ways:

1. Changes in cytosolic $[Ca^{2+}]_i$ allow cytosolic transcription factors to migrate to the nucleus and affect gene expression (e.g. NFAT and NFκB).
2. Changes in the nuclear free calcium concentration $[Ca^{2+}]_n$ can affect the activation of transcription factors (e.g. transcription enhancer factor domains, TEF/TEAD).
3. Changes in $[Ca^{2+}]_n$ can influence the activity of transcriptional repressors (e.g. DREAM).

Since there is a variety of transcription factors that are sensitive to calcium, it is reasonable to expect that the spatiotemporal dynamics of calcium signalling determines which transcription factors are affected. As calcium is

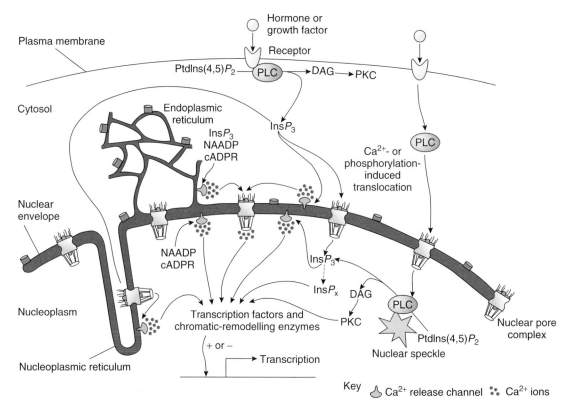

Figure 9.17 Potential nuclear calcium signalling pathways. Second messengers produced in the cytosol can enter the nucleus via the nuclear pore complex and bind to receptors on nuclear calcium stores. Similarly, perinuclear calcium release into the cytosol may result in calcium entering the nucleus. Nucleoplasmic reticulum can deliver signals deep into the nucleus. Whilst some PLC may be resident in the nucleus, additional PLC can migrate to the nucleus. Production of IP_3 within nuclei is thought to occur at nuclear speckles. As ADP ribosyl cyclase is also present in the nucleus, cADPr and NAADP may also be synthesised here. Ca^{2+} ATPases (small blue cylinders) found on the outer nuclear membrane (cytoplasmic face) and the ER remove Ca^{2+} from the cytosol and deliver it to the lumen of both these organelles. Alteration in nuclear calcium will influence gene expression. Adapted with permission from the Journal of Cell Science, Bootman et al. (2009).

toxic to cells calcium signals tend to be oscillatory rather than sustained elevations. Thus oscillations in calcium concentration can carry a message in two general ways (Figure 9.18):

- Amplitude coding, where the amplitude of the calcium oscillation varies, but the frequency remains the same.
- Frequency coding, where the amplitude of the calcium oscillation remains the same, but the frequency varies.

Amplitude coding and frequency coding are the two extremes and are not mutually exclusive. Indeed, it is likely that cells use a combination of these to drive differential expression of calcium sensitive genes. In order to study the calcium coding it will be necessary to induce reproducible calcium oscillations and then measure the resultant induced gene expression. Unfortunately it is not practical to achieve reproducible calcium oscillations in a cell population for a sustained period by the use of agonists acting on GPCRs. This is because the prolonged stimulus necessary will induce receptor desensitisation and down regulation. Thus a method is needed to bypass GPCRs to generate reproducible calcium oscillations. Two independent groups using different techniques to achieve this reported their findings in the very same issue of Nature. Li et al. (1998) used caged IP_3, whilst Dolmetsch et al. (1998) manipulated the store operated calcium channel (SOC) to generate calcium signals that circumvent GPCRs.

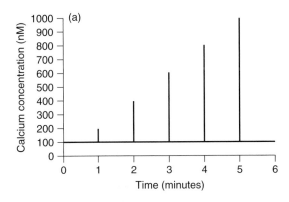

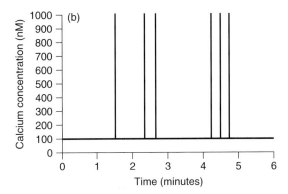

Figure 9.18 Panel (a) represents amplitude coding, where one calcium oscillation occurs each minute, though its amplitude varies from 200 to 1000 nM (100 to 900 nM above the resting calcium concentration). In contrast panel (b) represents frequency coding, where the amplitude of the calcium oscillation is from a resting level of 100 nM to 1000 nM, which occurs either 0, 1, 2 or 3 times a minute.

Caged IP_3 is a form of IP_3 that does not activate the IP_3 receptors. Using the AM form it is possible to load up cells with hundreds of micromolar of caged IP_3. Pulses of UV light at 365 nm were used to hydrolyse the caged IP_3 to convert it to a form that is recognised by the IP_3 receptor, giving rise to a release of calcium and a rise in $[Ca^{2+}]_i$ via IP_3 sensitive calcium channels. A stable reporter gene construct consisting of an NFAT (nuclear factor of activated T cells) response element upstream of a reporter gene was used in RBL-2H3 cells (rat basophilic leukaemia cell line). A range of different photolysis protocols were then used to generate different frequencies and amplitudes of calcium oscillations. Then the effect on reporter gene activity was measured.

Each of the protocols for a–f was designed to cause approximately 30% of the caged IP_3 to be hydrolysed.

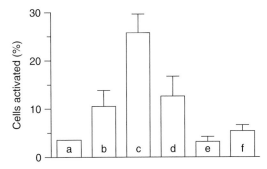

Figure 9.19 Calcium induced gene expression due to photolysis of caged IP_3. The panels depict the effect of NFAT driven reporter gene expression induced by: a) a single 10 second pulse of UV light. (b-e) a cycle of 12 pulses of UV light, four lasting 0.3 seconds, four at 0.8 seconds and then four at 1.5 seconds, spaced over 30 seconds (b), 1 minute (c), 2 minutes (d) and 8 minutes (e). (f) low intensity illumination for 21 minutes. Adapted by permission from Macmillan Publishers Ltd [Nature] Li et al. (1998). Cell-permeant caged $InsP_3$ ester shows that Ca^{2+} spike frequency can optimize gene expression. Nature 392: 936–941. Copyright 1998.

From the results it can be seen that either a single high intensity stimulation, or a long very low intensity stimulation induces little gene expression (Figure 9.19). However, b–e demonstrate that the frequency of stimulation has a large influence on gene expression, with the 12 UV pulses delivered over one minute being the most effective protocol (Li et al., 1998).

An alternative approach was used by Dolmetsch et al. (1998) to generate reproducible calcium oscillations. They poisoned Jurkat T cells (T lymphocyte cell line) with thapsigargin, a specific inhibitor of ER Ca^{2+} ATPase. This causes the ER calcium store to empty, which leads to activation of the store operated calcium channels (SOC) on the plasma membrane. Hence cells bathed in 1.5 mM Ca^{2+} containing solution will rapidly take up Ca^{2+} via SOC and cause a rise in $[Ca^{2+}]_i$. By rapidly switching between two solutions 0 and 1.5 mM Ca^{2+} bathing the cells, the rate of calcium influx into the cell, and therefore the resultant $[Ca^{2+}]_i$ can be carefully controlled. The plasma membrane Ca^{2+} ATPase will pump Ca^{2+} out of cells to return the $[Ca^{2+}]_i$ to pre stimulus levels. For example, exposing thapsigargin treated cells to 1.5 mM Ca^{2+} for 10 seconds every 100 seconds produced reproducible calcium oscillations that peak around 400 nM, whereas exposure to 1.5 mM Ca^{2+} for 30 seconds every 100 seconds produced peak calcium oscillations of over 1000 nM. Dolmetsch et al. (1998) generated reproducible calcium oscillations for three hours and then measured gene expression in cells transfected with a reporter gene construct. Three alternative transcription binding sites were incorporated into different constructs.

At normal resting $[Ca^{2+}]_i$ there is little calcium sensitive gene expression. However, as the steady state $[Ca^{2+}]_i$ increases from 10 to 400 nM there is a large increase in gene expression, with a half maximal activity at 270 nM calcium (Figure 9.20). It is unlikely that cells are sensitised to steady state $[Ca^{2+}]_i$ as all three transcription factors respond equally. If this reflected the true *in vivo* situation there would be no need for all three calcium sensitive transcription factors. Hence it is likely that coding is in the form of calcium oscillations. By varying the frequency of $[Ca^{2+}]_i$ oscillations it was found that with a strong stimulation (i.e. low oscillation period) of 100 seconds that gene expression was approximately 90% with NFκB (nuclear factor kappa of activated B cells), 75% with Oct/OAP (octomer/octomer associated proteins) and 50% with NFAT driven reporter gene expression. However a reduction in stimulation, via an increase in the period between $[Ca^{2+}]_i$ oscillations, caused a fall in gene expression. NFκB was least affected by this. A lower calcium signal will still switch on the suite of genes activated by NFκB, whilst a higher stimulation of an oscillation more than once every 400 seconds will cause an increase in gene expression activated by NFAT, Oct/OAP and NFκB (Figure 9.20). This difference in behaviour of transcription factors is linked to their residence time in the nucleus. Following the return of $[Ca^{2+}]_i$ to resting levels after a large Ca^{2+} signal NFκB can remain in the nucleus for more than 16 minutes, whilst NFAT is rapidly dephosphorylated and returns to the cytosol (Dolmetsch et al., 1998). In essence the transcription factors are 'tuned' to different cytosolic calcium signals (Li et al., 1998).

How a change in Ca^{2+} activates NFAT and NFκB

In the unstimulated state most of the cellular NFAT is present in the cytosol as associations of phosphorylated NFAT. A rise in the $[Ca^{2+}]_i$ activates calmodulin, forming a calcium calmodulin complex, which in turn activates calcineurin. This is a calcium calmodulin dependant phosphatase that dephosphorylates NFAT in the cytosol. This causes the NFAT aggregates to disaggregate and exposes a nuclear localisation sequence. NFAT then enters the nucleus where it binds to the NFAT binding sequence in the promoter region of some genes, thus inducing gene expression. Nuclear export of NFAT into the cytosol is driven by kinases that phosphorylate NFAT

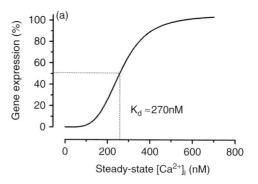

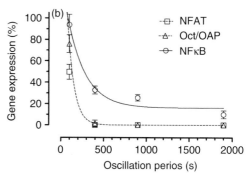

Figure 9.20 The effect of calcium on gene expression driven by NFAT, Oct/OAP and NFκB: (a) at steady state $[Ca^{2+}]_i$ and (b) with 1 μM calcium oscillations (100 to 1000 nM) with varying frequency. Separate data points are not shown for panel (a) as the trend line represents the response for all three transcription factors. Adapted by permission from Macmillan Publishers Ltd [Nature] Dolmetsch et al. (1998). Calcium oscillations increase the efficiency and specificity of gene expression. Nature 392: 933–936. Copyright 1998.

and expose a nuclear export sequence. Hence the balance between kinase and phosphorylase activity regulates the location of NFAT and therefore NFAT driven gene expression. As calcium (via calcium calmodulin) regulates the activity of the phosphatase calcineurin, NFAT is a calcium sensitive transcription factor. Indeed, calcineurin translocates into the nucleus, possibly as a complex with NFAT. As long as $[Ca^{2+}]_i$ remains high the phosphatase activity of calcineurin will outcompete the nuclear located kinases, thereby maintaining NFAT in the nucleus (Bootman et al., 2009).

NFκB is a transcription factor that is located in the cytosol under resting calcium concentrations via its interaction with IκB, which is an inhibitor of NFκB. A rise in $[Ca^{2+}]_i$ activates calmodulin, forming a Ca^{2+} calmodulin complex that activates CaM kinase. This kinase then phosphorylates IκB kinase (IKK2). An alternative route is the increase in $[Ca^{2+}]_i$ activates PKC, which can also phosphorylate IκB kinase. The IκB kinase then phosphorylates IκB, reducing its interaction with NFκB and thereby uncovering a nuclear localisation sequence on NFκB. This transcription factor then moves into the nucleus via the nuclear pore complex.

Calcium regulated transcriptional repression

Prodynorphin is an opiate polypeptide that can be converted into dynorphins and neoendorphins. It is involved in pain pathways and also has a role in learning and memory. Prodynorphin expression is controlled by the downstream regulatory element (DRE). DRE is so named because when it was first discovered it functioned as a regulatory element that was positioned downstream of the TATA box (a sequence that is found within many promoter regions which is a binding site for transcription factors and histones). Introduction of a mutation into DRE enhanced basal prodynorphin expression. This led to the suggestion that DRE actually functions as a gene silencer that tones down the level of gene expression to below that which would otherwise occur. Another protein can further reduce gene expression by binding to DRE. This is termed the DRE antagonist modulator (DREAM). Southwestern blotting (which identifies DNA binding proteins) of nuclear extracts of DREAM transfected HEK293 cells found a 110 kDa band. This represents four DREAM protein units bound to DRE (Carrión et al., 1999).

The link with calcium is that DREAM codes for four putative EF hand Ca^{2+} binding sites. By comparing predicted amino acid sequences to other related calcium binding proteins, such as recoverin and hippocalcin, it was found that the 1st site is less well conserved than the 2nd to 4th EF hand calcium binding sites. The 1st site is now thought to not bind Ca^{2+}. EF hand binding sites do not only bind Ca^{2+}, they can also interact with Mg^{2+}. Cellular magnesium concentrations are typically in the low millimolar range. Thus it is likely that magnesium is extensively bound to EF hand binding sites at resting calcium concentration (Grabarek, 2011). Whilst EF hand binding sites are generally conserved, differences can occur between them. The four EF hand binding sites on DREAM are around 50% identical to recoverin (Osawa et al., 2005). In the case of the 2nd EF hand site of DREAM, a notable difference is the presence of aspartate at the position of the 12th amino acid, rather than the more common glutamate. It is known that in other proteins having this substitution it reduces the ability of Ca^{2+} to

bind in preference over Mg^{2+} (Lucin et al., 2008). Indeed, an NMR study on DREAM found that Mg^{2+} binds at the 2nd EF hand, whilst Ca^{2+} binds at the 3rd and 4th, which maintain the normal glutamate in the 12th position (Lucin et al., 2008).

At resting calcium concentration Mg^{2+} is bound to the high affinity magnesium binding site in the 2nd EF hand and at two low affinity sites in the 3rd and 4th EF hand binding sites respectively. The three magnesium atoms bound to DREAM stabilise it and allow it to bind to DNA. When the calcium concentration rises, Ca^{2+} displaces the single Mg^{2+} bound at each of the 3rd and 4th EF hands. This causes the DREAM to detach and to dimerise, thereby permitting DRE regulated gene expression to occur (Osawa et al., 2005). Mutating two amino acids in one or more of the 2nd to 4th EF hand binding sites of DREAM resulted in EF hand mutants that severely impacted on the ability of mutated DREAM to bind calcium (Carrión et al., 1999).

Figure 9.21 demonstrates that the calcium binding ability of DREAM has a functional consequence. HEK293 cells were transfected with DREAM or an EF hand mutant DREAM (4EFmut DREAM). Southwestern blotting revealed that both wild type and EF hand mutant DREAM form a 110 kDa complex. This shows that mutating the EF hand binding sites does not affect the ability to bind to DRE. However, by raising the calcium concentration to 10 μM, the effect of the EF hand mutant becomes evident. It is clear that in the case of the wild type DREAM, the increase in calcium causes much of the wild type DREAM to no longer bind. In marked contrast, the rise in calcium concentration has no effect on the ability of the EF hand mutant to bind to DNA.

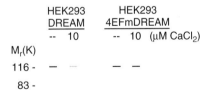

Figure 9.21   DREAM is a calcium binding protein. Southwestern blotting of HEK293 cells expressing DREAM or a 4th EF hand mutant DREAM (4EFmDREAM) show a 110 kDa DNA binding protein. Ten micromolar CaCl$_2$ was added prior to southwestern blotting where indicated. Reprinted by permission from Macmillan Publishers Ltd [Nature] Carrión et al. (1999). DREAM is a Ca^{2+} -regulated transcriptional repressor. Nature 398: 80–84. Copyright 1999.

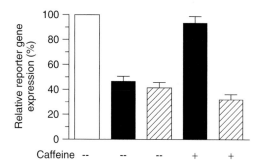

Figure 9.22 DREAM is a Ca^{2+} dependant transcriptional repressor. The open bar represents reporter gene expression in the absence of DREAM, the black bars expression in the presence of DREAM and the hatched bars expression in the presence of 4EFmDREAM (means ± sd). Ten millimolar caffeine was added where indicated by +. Adapted by permission from Macmillan Publishers Ltd [Nature] Carrión et al. (1999). DREAM is a Ca^{2+} -regulated transcriptional repressor. Nature 398: 80–84. Copyright 1999.

Co-transfection of a DRE reporter construct with either wild type or an EF hand mutant DREAM (4EFmDREAM) allowed investigation of the role of calcium on DRE dependant transcription. In Figure 9.22 the control gene expression, in the absence of DREAM, is set to 100% and is given by the open bar. The other conditions either have DREAM (black bars), or an EF hand mutant (hatched bars). In the absence of stimulation both the wild type and EF hand mutant DREAMs bind to DRE and restrict reporter gene expression to around 40% of control values. However, treatment with 10 mM caffeine has the effect of raising intracellular calcium. The wild type DREAM binds calcium, reduces its affinity for DRE, dissociates from DRE and enhances gene expression. This causes a rise in reporter gene expression to nearly that of the control, which has no DREAM present. In contrast, the EF hand mutant DREAM does not bind calcium, so the mutant DREAM remains bound to DRE, thereby inhibiting reporter gene expression.

Caffeine actually has a variety of effects in cells. It is a methyl xanthine and can act as a non-selective phosphodiesterase (PDE) inhibitor (raising the concentration of cAMP and cGMP by reducing their breakdown by PDEs), and is a non-selective antagonist of adenosine receptors. Caffeine sensitises ryanodine receptors to calcium, thereby increasing the probability of calcium-induced calcium release, and it can also inhibit IP$_3$ sensitive calcium channels. In this experiment

it is simply used to mobilise intracellular calcium (via its effect on ryanodine receptors).

DREAM can be found in both the nucleus and cytosol. In order to modify gene expression DREAM will need to be present in the nucleus. However, DREAM does not have classical nuclear localisation sequences. Instead, there are at least two small ubiquitin like modifier (SUMO) sites. A single amino acid substitution at both sites reduced nuclear localisation and failed to suppress DRE regulated gene expression in transfected cells. As both sumoylated and non sumoylated DREAM coexist in cells, it has been suggested that sumoylation increases nuclear import, whilst desumoylation will result in nuclear export (Palczewska et al., 2011).

DREAM is also known as calsenilin 3 or KChIP3 (K^+ channel interacting protein 3). These were independently named due to their effects in various systems. Calsenilin for interactions with calcium fluxes induced by presenilin and its possible role in Alzheimer's disease, KChIP3 for its role in expression and trafficking of K^+ channels, and DREAM for its role in DRE induced gene expression (Rivas et al., 2011). Since the initial studies on prodynorphin, DREAM has been shown to be involved in the regulation of a number of genes including calcitonin, Na^+/Ca^{2+} exchanger 3 and a range of intermediate early transcription factors such as c-fos. In addition, DREAM can interact with various other transcription factors.

9.6 Conclusions

The intention of this chapter was to introduce some themes pertinent to an appreciation that the control of calcium signalling is multifactorial, using the exocrine pancreas as an example. Spatial organisation of Ca^{2+} release sites results in hot spots of calcium release events. Whether these proceed from localised to global Ca^{2+} signals depends on a myriad of potential interactions, which include local second messenger concentration, receptor clustering, CICR, cross talk and shaping by mitochondria and so on. Physiological concentrations of agonists produce calcium spikes and waves rather than sustained high $[Ca^{2+}]_i$. SOC on the basal plasma membrane maintain ER calcium pools in conjunction with SERCA. Extrusion of Ca^{2+} mostly across the luminal plasma membrane also helps to ensure $[Ca^{2+}]_i$ does not remain elevated for long periods, thereby alleviating the risk of pathological events that can lead to cell death, such as acute pancreatitis. Nuclear calcium signals turn on suites of calcium responsive genes, whether via Ca^{2+} sensitive transcription factors or by Ca^{2+} sensitive transcriptional repressors. Whilst the pancreatic acinar cell has told us much about calcium signalling in non-excitable cells, much still remains to be said as there are still many more questions to answer.

References

Allbritton NL, Meyer T and Stryer L (1992). Range of messenger action of calcium ions and inositol 1,4,5-trisphosphate. Science 258: 1812–1815.

Allbritton NL, Oancea E, Kuhn MA and Meyer T (1994). Source of nuclear calcium signals. Proceedings of the National Academy of Sciences USA 91: 12458–12462.

Alonso MT, Manjarrés IM and García-Sancho J (2012). Privileged coupling between Ca^{2+} through the plasma membrane store-operated Ca^{2+} channels and the endoplasmic reticulum Ca^{2+} pump. Molecular and Cellular Endocrinology 353: 37–44.

Alonso MT and Sanchez JG (2011). Nuclear Ca^{2+} signalling. Cell Calcium 49: 280–289.

Baines CP (2009). The composition of the mitochondrial permeability transition pore. Journal of Molecular and Cellular Cardiology 46: 850–857.

Baudet S, Hove-Madsen L and Bers DM (1994). How to make and use calcium-specific mini- and microelectrodes. Chapter 4. In: Methods in cell biology volume 40. (R Nuccitelli ed.) pp 94–113. Academic Press, San Diego.

Belan P, Gerasimenko O, Petersen OH and Tepikin AV (1997). Distribution of Ca^{2+} extrusion sites on the mouse pancreatic acinar cell surface. Cell Calcium 22: 5–10.

Benters J, Flögel U, Schäfer T, Leibfritz D, Hechtenberg S and Beyersmann D (1997). Study of the interactions of cadmium and zinc with cellular calcium homeostasis using ^{19}F-NMR spectroscopy. Biochemical Journal 322: 793–799.

Bolitina VM and Csutora P (2005). CIF and other mysteries of the store-operated Ca^{2+} entry pathway. Trends in Biochemical Sciences 30: 378–387.

Bootman MD, Fearnley C, Smyrnias I, MacDonald F and Roderick HL (2009). An update on nuclear calcium signalling. Journal of Cell Science 122: 2337–2350.

Brailoiu E, Rahman T, Churamani D, Prole DL, Brailoiu CG, Hooper R, Taylor CW and Patel S (2010). An NAADP-gated two pore channel targeted to the plasma membrane uncouples triggering from amplifying Ca^{2+} signals. Journal of Biological Chemistry 286: 38511–38516.

Bruce JIE, Straub SV and Yule DI (2003). Crosstalk between cAMP and Ca^{2+} signalling in non-excitable cells. Cell Calcium 34: 431–444.

Campbell AK and Sala-Newby G (1993). Bioluminescent and chemiluminescent indicators for molecular signalling and function in living cells. Chapter 5. In: Fluorescent and luminescent probes for biological activity. A practical guide to technology for quantitative real-time analysis. (WT Mason ed.) pp 58–82. Academic press. London.

Camello P, Gardner J, Petersen OH and Tepikin AV (1996). Calcium dependence of calcium extrusion and calcium uptake in mouse pancreatic acinar cells. Journal of Physiology 490: 585–593.

Cancela JM, Churchill GC and Galione A (1999). Coordination of agonist induced Ca^{2+} -signalling patterns by NAADP in pancreatic acinar cells. Nature 285: 74–76.

Cancela JM and Petersen OH (1998). The cyclic ADP ribose antagonist 8NH$_2$ cADP-ribose blocks cholecystokinin evoked cytosolic Ca^{2+} spiking in pancreatic acinar cells. Pflugers Archiv 435: 746–748.

Cancela JM, Van Coppenolle F, Galione A, Tepikin AV and Petersen OH (2002). Transformation of local Ca^{2+} spikes to global Ca^{2+} transients: the combinatorial roles of multiple Ca^{2+} releasing messengers. EMBO journal 21: 909–919.

Carrión AM, Link WA, Ledo F, Mellström B and Naranjo JR (1999). DREAM is a Ca^{2+} -regulated transcriptional repressor. Nature 398: 80–84.

Chamero P, Manjarres IM, García-Verdugo JM, Villalobos C, Alonso MT and García-Sancho (2008). Nuclear calcium signalling by inositol trisphosphate in GH$_3$ pituitary cells. Cell Calcium 43: 205–214.

Chen W, Steenbergen C, Levy LA, Vance J, London RE and Murphy E (1996). Measurement of free Ca^{2+} in sarcoplasmic reticulum in perfused rabbit heart loaded with 1,2-bis(2-amino-5,6-diflurophenoxy)ethane-N,N,N′,N′-tetracacetic acid by ^{19}F NMR. Journal of Biological Chemistry 271: 7398–7403.

Cobbold PH and Lee JAC (1991). Aequorin measurements of cytoplasmic free calcium. Chapter 2. In: Cellular calcium a practical approach. (JG McCormack and PH Cobbold eds.) pp 55–81. Oxford University Press, Oxford.

Cosker F, Cehevion N, Yamasaki M, Menteyne A, Lund FE, Moutin M-J, Galione A and Cancela J-M (2010). The ecto-enzyme CD38 is a nicotinic acid adenine dinucleotide phosphate (NAADP) synthase that couples receptor activation to Ca^{2+} mobilization from lysosomes in pancreatic acinar cells. Journal of Biological Chemistry 285: 38251–38259.

Csutora P, Peter K, Kilic H, Park KM, Zarayskiy V, Gwozdz T and Bolotina VM (2008). Novel role for STIM1 as a trigger for calcium influx factor production. Journal of Biological Chemistry 283: 14524–14531.

Dolmetsch RE, Xu K and Lewis RS (1998) Calcium oscillations increase the efficiency and specificity of gene expression. Nature 392: 933–936.

Fernandez-Segura E and Warley A (2008). Electron probe X-ray microanalysis for the study of cell physiology. In: Introduction to electron microscopy for biologists. Methods in cell biology volume 88. (TD Allen ed.) pp 19–43. Elsevier, Amsterdam.

Fogarty KE, Kidd JF, Tuft RA and Thorn P (2000). A bimodal pattern of InsP$_3$-evoked elementary Ca^{2+} signals in pancreatic acinar cells. Biophysical Journal 78: 2296–2306.

Gerasimenko JV, Maruyama Y, Yano K, Dolman NJ, Tepikin AV, Petersen OH and Gerasimenko OV (2003). NAADP mobilizes Ca^{2+} from thapsigargin-sensitive store in the nuclear envelope by activating ryanodine receptors. Journal of Cell Biology 163: 271–282.

Giacomello M, Drago I, Pizzo P, and Pozzan T (2007). Mitochondrial Ca^{2+} as a key regulator of cell life and death. Cell Death and Differentiation 14: 1267–1274.

Grabarek Z (2011). Insights into modulation of calcium signalling by magnesium in calmodulin, troponin C and related EF-hand proteins. Biochimica et Biophysica Acta 1813: 913–921.

Hurley TW, Dale WE and Rovetto MJ (1992). Differing significance of Na^+–Ca^{2+} exchange in the regulation of cytosolic Ca^{2+} in rat exocrine gland acini and cardiac myocytes. Canadian Journal of Physiology and Pharmacology 70: 461–465.

Ito K, Miyashita Y and Kasai H (1997). Micromolar and submicromolar Ca^{2+} spikes regulating distinct cellular functions in pancreatic acinar cells. The EMBO Journal 16: 242–251.

Kasi H, Li YX and Miyashita Y (1993). Subcellular distribution of Ca^{2+} release channels underlying Ca^{2+} waves and oscillations in exocrine pancreas. Cell 74: 669–677.

Lee MG, Xu X, Zeng W, Diaz J, Kuo TH, Wuytack F, Racymaekers L and Mullem S (1997). Polarized expression of Ca^{2+} pumps in pancreatic and salivary gland cells. Role in initiation and propagation of $[Ca^{2+}]_i$ waves. Journal of Biological Chemistry 272: 15771–15776.

Leite MF, Dranoff JA, Gao L and Nathanson MH (1999). Expression and subcellular localization of the ryanodine receptor in rat pancreatic acinar cells. Biochemical Journal 337: 305–309.

Li WH, Llopis J, Whitney M, Zlokarnik G and Tsien RY (1998) Cell-permeant caged $InsP_3$ ester shows that Ca^{2+} spike frequency can optimize gene expression. Nature 392: 936–941.

Livet J, Weissman TA, Kang H, Draft RW, Lu J, Bennis RA, Sanes JR and Lichtman JW (2007). Transgenic strategies for combinatorial expression of fluorescent proteins in the nervous system. Nature 450: 56–62.

Lucin JD, Vanarotti M, Li C, Valiveti A and Ames JB (2008). NMR structure of DREAM: Implications for Ca^{2+}-dependant DNA binding and protein dimerization. Biochemistry 47: 2252–2264.

Luo D, Yang D, Lan X, li K, Li X, Chen J, Zhang Y, Xiao R-P, Han Q and Cheng H (2008). Nuclear Ca^{2+} sparks and waves mediated by inositol 1,4,5-trisphosphate receptors in neonatal rat cardiomyocytes. Cell Calcium 43: 165–174.

Matchaca K (2011). Ca^{2+} signalling, genes and the cell cycle. Cell Calcium 49: 323–330.

Matsuda S, Kusuoka H, Hashimoto K, Tsujimura E and Nishimura T (1996). The effects of proteins on $[Ca^{2+}]$ measurement: different effects on fluorescent and NMR methods. Cell Calcium 20: 425–430.

Maynard Case R, Eisner D, Gurney A, Jones O, Muallem S and Verkhratsky A (2007). Evolution of calcium homeostasis: from birth of the first cell to an omnipresent signalling system. Cell Calcium 42: 345–350.

McCormack JG and Cobbold PH (1991) *eds*. Cellular calcium a practical approach. Oxford University Press. Oxford.

Messerli MA and Smith PJS (2010). Construction, theory and practical considerations for using self-referencing of Ca^{2+}-selective microelectrodes for monitoring extracellular Ca^{2+} gradients. *In*: Methods in cell biology volume 99. (M Whitaker ed.) pp 91–111. Elsevier, Amsterdam.

Metcalfe JC and Smith GA (1991). NMR measurement of cytosolic free calcium concentration by fluorine labelled indicators. *In*: Cellular calcium a practical approach. (JG McCormack and PH Cobbold eds.) pp 123–132. Oxford University Press, Oxford.

Miller AL, Karplus E and Jaffe LF (1994). Imaging $[Ca^{2+}]_i$ with aequorin using a photon imaging detector. *In*: Methods in cell biology volume 40. (R. Nuccitelli ed.) pp 305–338. Academic Press Inc, San Diego.

Miller DJ (2004). Sydney Ringer; physiological saline, calcium and the contraction of the heart. Journal of Physiology 555: 585–587.

Mogami H, Nakano K, Tepikin AV and Petersen OH (1997). Ca^{2+} flow via tunnels in polarized cells: recharging of apical Ca^{2+} stores by focal Ca^{2+} entry through basal membrane patch. Cell 88: 49–55.

Mogami H, Tepikin AV and Petersen OH (1998). Termination of cytosolic Ca^{2+} signals: Ca^{2+} reuptake into intracellular stores is regulated by the free Ca^{2+} concentration in the store lumen. EMBO Journal 17: 435–442.

Mojzisova A, Krizanova O, Zacikova L, Kominkova V and Ondrias K (2001). Effect of nicotinic acid adenine dinucleotide phosphate on ryanodine calcium release channel in heart. Pflugers Archiv 441: 674–677.

Osawa M, Dace A, Tong KI, Valivetti A, Ikura M and Ames JB (2005). Mg^{2+} and Ca^{2+} differentially regulate DNA binding and dimerization of DREAM. Journal of Biological Chemistry 280: 18008–18014.

Palczewska M, Casafont I, Ghimire K, Rojas AM, Valencia A, Lafarga M, Mellström B and Naranjo JR (2011). Sumoylation regulates nuclear localization of repressor DREAM. Biochimica et Biophysica Acta 1813: 1050–1058.

Pan S, Ryu S-Y and Sheu S-S (2011). Distinctive characteristics and functions of multiple mitochondrial Ca^{2+} influx mechanisms. Science China Life Sciences 54: 763–769.

Park MK, Ashby MC, Erdemil G, Petersen OH and Tepikin AV (2001). Perinuclear, perigranular and sub-plasmalemmal mitochondria have distinct functions in the regulation of cellular calcium transport. EMBO Journal 20: 1863–1874.

Park MK, Lee M and Petersen OH (2004). Morphological and functional changes of dissociated single pancreatic acinar cells: testing the suitability of the single cell as a model for exocytosis and calcium signalling. Cell Calcium 35: 367–379.

Park MK, Petersen OH and Tepikin AV (2000). The endoplasmic reticulum as one continuous Ca^{2+} pool: visualization of rapid Ca^{2+} movements and equilibration. The EMBO Journal 19: 5729–5739.

Petersen OH (1988). The control of ion channels and pumps in exocrine acinar cells. Comparative Biochemistry and Physiology 90A: 717–720.

Pinton P, Pozzan T and Rizzuto R (1998). The Golgi apparatus is an inositol 1,4,5-trisphosphate-sensitive Ca^{2+} store, with functional properties distinct from those of the endoplasmic reticulum. The EMBO Journal 17: 5298–5308.

Putney JW (2007). Recent breakthroughs in the molecular mechanism of capacitative calcium entry (with thoughts on how we got here). Cell Calcium 42: 103–110.

Rasola A and Bernardi P (2011). Mitochondrial permeability transition in Ca^{2+}-dependent apoptosis and necrosis. Cell Calcium 50: 222–233.

Rivas M, Villar D, González P, Dopazo XM, Mellström B and Naranjo JR (2011). Building the DREAM interactome. Science China Life Sciences 54: 786–792.

Ryu S-Y, Beutner G, Dirksen R, Kinnally KW and Sheu S-S (2010). Mitochondrial ryanodine receptors and other mitochondrial Ca^{2+} permeable channels. FEBS Letters 584: 1948–1955.

Sasaki S, Nakagaki I, Kondo H and Hori S (1996). Changes in element concentrations induced by agonist in pig pancreatic acinar cells. Pflugers Arch. 432: 538–545.

Sherwood MW, Prior IA, Voronina SG, Barrow SL. Woodsmith JD, Gerasimenko OV, Petersen OH and Tepikin AV (2007). Activation of trypsinogen in large endocytic vacuoles of pancreatic acinar cells. Proceeding National Academy of Science 104: 5674–5679.

Solomon TE (1994). Control of exocrine pancreatic secretions. *In*: Physiology of the gastrointestinal tract (LR Johnson ed.) 3rd edition, Raven Press, New York pp 1499–1529.

Snitsarev V and Kay AR (2001). Detecting and minimizing errors in calcium-probe measurements arising from transition metals and zinc. *In*: Calcium signalling a practical approach (AV Tepikin ed.). 2nd edition, Oxford University Press, Oxford pp 45–57.

Streb H, Irvine RF, Berridge MJ and Schultz I (1983). Release of Ca^{2+} from a non-mitochondrial intracellular store in pancreatic acinar cells by inositol-1,4,5,-trisphosphate. Nature 306: 67–69.

Takahashi A, Camacho P, Lechleiter JD and Herman B (1999). Measurement of intracellular calcium. Physiological Reviews 79: 1089–1125.

Taylor CW and Dale P (2012). Intracellular Ca^{2+} channels – a growing perspective. Molecular and Cellular Endocrinology 353: 21–28.

Tepikin AV editor (2001). Calcium signalling a practical approach. 2nd edition Oxford University Press, Oxford

Tepikin AV, Voronia SG, Gallacher DV and Petersen OH (1992). Pulsatile Ca^{2+} extrusion from single pancreatic acinar cells during receptor-activated cytosolic Ca^{2+} spiking. Journal of Biological Chemistry 267: 14073–14076.

Thomas AP and Delaville F (1991) The use of fluorescent indicators for measurements of cytosolic-free calcium concentrations in cell populations and single cells. *In*: Cellular calcium A Practical Approach. (JG McCormack and PH Cobbold eds.), pages 1–54. Oxford University Press, Oxford.

Thorn P, Gerasimenko O and Petersen OH (1994). Cyclic-ADP-ribose regulation of ryanodine receptors involved in agonist evoked cytosolic Ca^{2+} oscillations in pancreatic acinar cells. The EMBO Journal 13: 2038–2043.

Thorn P, Moreton R and Berridge M (1996). Multiple coordinated Ca^{2+}-release events underlie the inositol trisphosphate-induced local Ca^{2+} spikes in mouse pancreatic acinar cells. The EMBO Journal 15: 999–1003.

Tinel H, Cancela JM, Mogami H, Gerasimenko JV, Gerasimenko OV, Tepikin AV and Petersen OH (1999). Active mitochondria surrounding the pancreatic acinar granule region prevent spreading of inositol trisphosphate-evoked local cytosolic Ca^{2+} signals. The EMBO Journal 18: 4999–5008.

Várnai P, Hunyady L and Balla T (2009). STIM and Orai: the long-awaited constituents of store-operated calcium entry. Trends in Pharmacological Sciences 30: 118–128.

Webb SE, Rogers KL, Karplus E and Miller AL (2010). The use of aequorins to record and visualise Ca^{2+} dynamics: from subcellular microdomains to whole organisms. *In*: Methods in cell biology volume 99. (M Whitaker ed.) pp 263–300. Elsevier, Amsterdam.

Whitaker M (2010a). Genetically encoded probes for the measurement of intracellular calcium. *In*: Methods in Cell Biology volume 99 (M Whitaker ed.). Elsevier, San Diego, pp 153–182.

Whitaker M (2010b) Calcium in living cells. Methods in cell biology volume 99. Elsevier, San Diego pp 316.

Wojcikiewicz RJH (1995). Type I, II and III inositol 1,4,5-trisphosphate receptors are unequally susceptible to down-regulation and are expressed in markedly different proportions in different cell types. Journal of Biological Chemistry 270: 11678–11683.

Yamasaki M, Masgrau R, Morgan AJ, Churchill GC, Patel S, Ashcroft SJH and Galione A (2004). Organelle selection determines agonist-specific Ca^{2+} signals in pancreatic acinar and β cells. Journal of Biological Chemistry 279: 7234–7240.

Yamasaki M, Thomas JM, Churchill GC, Garnham C, Lewis AM, Cancela JM, Patel S and Galione A (2005). Role of NAADP and cADPr in the induction and maintenance of agonist-evoked Ca^{2+} spiking in mouse pancreatic acinar cells. Current Biology 15: 874–878.

Yule DI (2010). Pancreatic acinar cells: molecular insights from signal-transduction using transgenic animals. The International Journal of Biochemistry and Cell Biology 42: 1757–1761.

Yule DI, Ernst SA, Ohnishi H, and Wojcikiewicz RJH (1997). Evidence that zymogen granules are not a physiologically relevant calcium pool. Defining the distribution of inositol 1,4,5-trisphosphate receptors in pancreatic acinar cells. Journal of Biological Chemistry 272: 9093–9098.

Yule DI, Lawrie AM and Gallacher DV (1991), Acetylcholine and cholecystokinin induce different patterns of oscillating calcium signals in pancreatic acinar cells. Cell Calcium 12: 145–151.

10 Genetic Engineering of Mice

10.1 Introduction to genetic engineering

Genetic engineering techniques enable us to introduce defined and stable modifications into the genomes of animal models. It is a widely-applied process, which facilitates the functional characterisation of genes, the dissection of complex physiological processes, the identification of drug targets or the development of animal models for human diseases. The insertion of new genes or point mutations, and the elimination of endogenous genes can tailor the host genome to fit almost any scientific question. In the post-genomic era, the genetic modification has become an important approach that complements the analysis and utilisation of increasing quantities of sequence data.

This chapter is a concise overview of the two main techniques that are used for the genetic manipulation of the mouse, the favourite model for human genetics. The focus of the chapter is on the technical aspects and introduces the reader to a selection of essential molecular tools.

10.2 Genomics and the accumulation of sequence data

The development of DNA cloning and sequencing techniques in the 1970s marked the beginning of an era that enabled scientists to generate an enormous amount of genetic data – the era of genomics (Jackson et al., 1972; Cohen et al., 1973; Sanger et al., 1977; see Box 10.1). Initially this culminated in the completion of the Human Genome Project (HGP), after it had taken over a decade to sequence the human genome (International Human Genome Sequencing Consortium, 2001; Venter et al., 2001). Back then, it was the first and with nearly 3 billion base pairs the largest vertebrate genome that had been sequenced. But around the same time, similar projects successfully deciphered the genomes of the mouse (2002) and the rat (2004), two commonly used model organisms. In subsequent years genome sequences of a number of very diverse organisms were generated – at ever increasing speed and lower costs due to advances in sequencing technologies and strategies,

Molecular Pharmacology: From DNA to Drug Discovery, First Edition. John Dickenson, Fiona Freeman, Chris Lloyd Mills, Shiva Sivasubramaniam and Christian Thode.
© 2013 John Wiley & Sons, Ltd. Published 2013 by John Wiley & Sons, Ltd.

Box 10.1 Scientific milestones in genetics

Since their establishment in the 1980s, the protocols for pronuclear injection and gene targeting have given insights into complex biological processes and improved our understanding of them. They also led to the development of other DNA technologies. Scientific milestones, such as these, have revolutionised biotechnology and the study of genetics that began some 150 years ago, in plants, with Gregor Johann Mendel.

In the 1850s, the Austrian monk Mendel began a series of experiments on the mechanisms of heredity in garden peas. He observed that certain characteristics are transmitted in distinct entities to the next generation, and he deduced from this the laws of inheritance (Mendel, 1866). His work marks the beginning of classic genetics or forward genetics, which seeks to identify the gene(s) for a given phenotype or a particular trait. This traditional approach was initially based on creating hybrids by crossing species with distinct characteristics, and the study of naturally-occurring mutants (Morgan, 1911). In later years, it was complemented by the use of mutagenic chemicals or ionising radiation to generate random mutations (Muller, 1925). However, it was not until a century after Mendel's pioneering work that finally the structure and function of DNA – and with this the molecular nature of genes – had been determined (Avery et al., 1944; Franklin and Gosling, 1953; Watson and Crick, 1953; Wilkins et al., 1953; Söll et al., 1965; Nirenberg et al., 1966). With the help of several newly-discovered molecular tools (e.g. ligases, restriction enzymes, reverse transcriptase; Lehman et al., 1958; Linn and Arber, 1968; Baltimore, 1970; Smith and Wilcox, 1970; Temin and Mizutani, 1970; Danna and Nathans, 1971), it was then possible to manipulate the genetic material in a controlled manner and to study the effects on the resultant phenotype. This new era of molecular genetics or reverse genetics is characterised by techniques such as DNA recombination and gene cloning (Cohen et al., 1972; Jackson et al., 1972; Cohen et al., 1973), DNA sequencing (Maxam and Gilbert, 1977; Sanger et al., 1977), transgenesis (Gordon and Ruddle, 1981), gene targeting (Evans and Kaufman, 1981; Doetschman et al., 1987; Thomas and Capecchi, 1987), polymerase chain reaction (PCR; Mullis and Faloona, 1987) and animal cloning (Campbell et al., 1996), all of which have been introduced to research in relative quick succession. It illustrates how progress in the acquisition of scientific knowledge is paralleled by advances in the experimental technology and vice versa.

1854–	Gregor Mendel starts experiments on heredity in garden peas and observes that certain 'factors' determine 'characters', which are transmitted to the next generation; he formulates the laws of inheritance.
1869–	Friedrich Miescher isolates the molecule 'nuclein' (i.e. nucleic acid) from white blood cells; however he believes that proteins hold the hereditary information.
1910–	Thomas Hunt Morgan concludes from his studies of naturally-occurring fruit fly mutants that genes being the inheritable traits are located on chromosomes. The term 'gene' was already introduced by the botanist Wilhelm Johannsen in 1909.
1925–	Hermann Muller, Morgan's former students, publishes his discovery in fruit flies that X-ray irradiation produces gene mutations and structural changes in chromosomes.
1944–	Oswald Avery, Colin MacLeod and Maclyn McCarty publish their experiments about bacterial transformation proving that genetic information is stored in the form of DNA and not protein as assumed by many at the time.
1953–	James Watson and Francis Crick determine the double-helix structure of DNA.
1956–	Arthur Kornberg and colleagues isolate the first DNA polymerase from *E. coli* bacteria.
1966–	Har Gobind Khorana's and Marshall Nirenberg's groups complete to decipher the genetic code.
1967–	Martin Gellert identifies DNA ligase in *E. coli* extracts.
1968–	Several research groups describe the first restriction endonucleases and apply the isolated enzymes to cleave DNA sequences.
1970–	David Baltimore, Howard Temin and Satoshi Mizutani discover reverse transcriptases in preparations of retroviruses.
1970s–	Paul Berg, Herb Boyer and Stanley Cohen generate the first recombinant DNA; subsequently this leads to the first cloning of an animal gene.
1977–	Alan Maxam and Walter Gilbert, and Frederick Sanger publish two methods for DNA sequencing.
1980–	Jon Gordon and Frank Ruddle create the first transgenic mouse using the method of pronuclear injection of DNA.
1983–	Kary Mullis develops the polymerase chain reaction (PCR).
1987–	Mario Capecchi, Martin Evans and Oliver Smithies establish the gene targeting technique to create knockin and knockout mice.
1996–	Keith Campbell and Ian Wilmut clone the first adult mammal by nuclear transfer.
2003–	The sequencing of the human genome has been completed.

and computational power (Collins, 2010; Metzker, 2010; Venter, 2010). Towards the end of 2010, the number of sequenced human genomes alone approached 3000.

The scientific community has benefited from this development, because publicly funded genome projects provide them with these reference genomes via rapidly expanding international databases. Such data can be utilised to address a wide range of questions, from elementary to complex ones. For example, the HGP has revealed the structure of the human genome and led to the unexpected discovery that it only contains ~20,000 to 25,000 protein-coding genes – or 1.5% of the whole genome. Alternatively, comparative analysis may use genomes of a variety of organisms to investigate their phylogenetic relationship or to shed light onto the molecular evolution of multi-gene families. And yet other disciplines, such as molecular medicine and pharmacogenomics, respectively, can screen human genomes for genetic predispositions to diseases, or to identify variations in genetic backgrounds, which may be considered in the development of improved or personalised medicine.

Following on from the publications of the first vertebrate genome sequences, the annotations of the raw data have provided important answers, while other optimistic expectations for biomedical research (e.g. gene therapy; see Chapter 6) have not been met yet (Collins, 2010). Interestingly, these projects have also uncovered previously unknown complexities within genomes and raised a multitude of new questions. These cannot be investigated through sequence analysis alone, as illustrated by the different aspects of drug target discovery (see section below).

New genes – new drug targets?

Genome sequencing projects are of particular interest to the pharmaceutical industry, as it is hoped that these data accelerate the discovery of novel drug targets and the development of pharmaceutically-active compounds. Indeed, target innovation is a key concern in drug discovery: The number of therapeutic drugs is in excess of 21,000 but it has been proposed that they only modulate 266 molecular targets in humans, the majority of which are distributed among ten protein families (Overington et al., 2006; see Chapter 1). The number of unique drug targets is small considering the total estimate of protein-coding genes in humans, and it has triggered a genome-wide search for new and 'druggable' gene loci, that is, gene products which can be modulated by small molecules (Hopkins and Groom, 2002). Even though this search has been successful, functionally-unclassified gene products can only be considered as potential drug targets if they fulfil two general requirements. Firstly, drug targets are expected to possess protein folds or domains, which facilitate a strong interaction with therapeutic compounds (Hopkins and Groom, 2002). And,

secondly, the biological target should play a key role in physiological processes, if a significant therapeutic effect is to be achieved.

To address the first aspect, several groups have taken the *in silico* approach, that is, the use of computer programs to predict genes, amino acid sequences and protein folds from raw genomic data. Their early studies have suggested that the human genome contains ~3,000 druggable gene loci (Hopkins and Groom, 2002, Russ and Lampel, 2005). Although the outcome of such analysis is dependent on the accuracy of the available sequence data and the precision of the programs, it facilitates the process of drug target identification. It may even give insights into the physiological functions of predicted gene products, as putative protein domains are unveiled. Furthermore, 3D models of pharmacologically-interesting proteins can be generated and used to screen existing chemical libraries *in silico* for compounds with potential binding affinities. However, serious limitations of computational analysis are the inability to determine how individual cells use the underlying genetic instructions in a biological context, and what the function of the encoded products are: Cellular processes in eukaryotes, for example alternative splicing of precursor mRNAs, RNA editing or post-translational modifications, can create an astonishing diversity of structurally - and functionally - distinct proteins from a single gene (Nilsen and Graveley, 2010).

The general challenge in the post-genomic phase is to translate *in silico* into functional data (for review, see Bogue, 2003). Both, *in vitro* and *in vivo* studies are indispensible to elucidate the physiological roles of the encoded proteins. With respect to drug target discovery, novel molecular targets also need to be tested pharmacologically for their response to drugs. Initially, this may be achieved through *in vitro* assays, but the final target validation requires pre-clinical research in appropriate model organisms.

The need for the functional characterisation of gene products

Prior to the advent of recombinant DNA technology, classic genetics (forward genetics) commonly relied on naturally-occurring or induced mutations in species. This allowed the identification of genes involved in the phenotype and gave insights into their functions. In molecular or reverse genetics, this process is reversed – usually the genes of interest have been mapped to chromosomal locations and sequenced, but the roles of the encoded proteins are unknown.

Today, sophisticated *in vitro* techniques can be applied to characterise the molecular structure of a gene product and its function on a cellular level (e.g. metabolism, cell cycle). Mutagenesis may facilitate this line of research further. *In vitro* studies, however, are inadequate to determine the role of a molecule in complex physiological systems, for example the endocrine, nervous, immune, urinary or cardiovascular system. In multicellular organisms, such as mammalian species, these systems are integrated; together they enable survival, growth, reproduction and other forms of behaviour. In an integrated system the influence of a key molecule frequently reaches far beyond its immediate cellular environment, and may simultaneously affect different tissues and organs. Likewise, long-ranging effects may be observed in a pathophysiological context, where this molecule only exists in a mutated form or is entirely absent. For instance, deletions in the growth hormone gene in humans can result in hormonal deficiencies (Phillips et al., 1981), which cause primarily reduced somatic growth, but they have also a negative effect on the cardiovascular system, the metabolism or the mental abilities.

For most gene products, the functional characterisation needs to be carried out *in vivo* in that species or, if required due to ethical or practical reasons, in suitable animal models and with the help of genetic manipulation.

10.3 The mouse as a model organism

Traditionally the house mouse has been and still is the favourite animal model, when insights into human genetics need to be gained. Mice are easy to keep and, with a relatively short life cycle and gestation period (18–22 days), easy to breed in large numbers, that is, female mice reach sexual maturity after 6 weeks, males after 8 weeks. After mice have been widely used in research for decades, their genetics is well understood and their genome can be manipulated with relative ease.

Why the mouse?

Besides practical and economic reasons, the close similarities to the human genetics, physiology and anatomy are of greater importance, as they offer advantages for research. In total, 99% of the genes in mouse and human are homologous, and even 80% of the murine genes have a direct human counterpart or orthologue (Mouse Genome Sequencing Consortium, 2002; Guénet, 2010). Extensive conservation is also observed for entire chromosomal regions and the relative positions of genes. Both species share nearly 400 conserved syntenic segments (Bourque et al., 2004), despite chromosome rearrangements during the mammalian evolution and, hence, differences in chromosome numbers (40 in mice vs. 46 in human).

In addition, mice naturally develop neurological disorders, obesity, hypertension, atherosclerosis, cancer and other pathologic conditions, which mimic those in humans. Hundreds of mice strains, where these conditions are triggered by spontaneous mutations, are phenotypically characterised and available for research (see the Mouse Phenome Database from The Jackson Laboratory; Grubb et al., 2009). Epileptic seizures in the *stargazer* mouse, for example, are the consequence of a natural mutation in the subunit gene of an ion channel (Letts et al., 1998; Hunter et al., 2000).

Genetic manipulation of the mouse

Natural mutant strains offer invaluable insights into the function of genes as well as into the pathogenesis and progression of mammalian diseases. However, spontaneous mutations are rare, random and affect a relative small proportion of the total number of genes. To generate new gene mutations, two different types of mutagenesis can be employed.

In the first and classic approach (forward genetics), mutations are induced in mice through radiation or chemicals, followed by a series of physiological and behavioural tests, in which the animals are screened for genetic alterations (Hunter et al., 2000; Godinho and Nolan, 2006). *N*-ethyl-*N*-nitrosourea (ENU) is one such chemical mutagen. Today ENU is used in research centres around the globe, because it induces point mutations at high frequency and often at multiple loci within the same allele. Depending on the affected site, the mutant phenotypes can vary from the complete loss of gene function to partial loss-of-function or even gain-of-function. In other cases the mutation is silent with no apparent effect on either the encoded amino acid sequence or a non-coding region. The fact that ENU-induced mutations occur in a random fashion, is often considered to be of advantage, as this situation is more likely to resemble that in humans, where inherited disorders are frequently caused by spontaneously occurring single nucleotide changes.

In contrast to randomly-induced mutations, the second type of mutagenesis is genotype-driven (reverse genetics), and may result in the addition of new DNA to the host genome or in the predetermined modification of an endogenous site. In this approach it is DNA itself that, by being introduced into the animal host, acts as the mutagen. The advantage of this procedure is that many manipulations can be implemented in a more controlled manner, as the introduced exogenous DNA carries desired the genetic information. Together with the recent access to sequence information from the murine and human genomes, it has opened and improved the technical possibilities to create a wide range of genetically-modified organisms, such as mice carrying point mutations (Löw et al, 2000), animal models for human diseases with an aberrant gene expression (Harper, 2010) or humanised mice (Thomsen et al, 2005). The two main methods which are applied in genotype-driven mutagenesis will be covered in the following section.

10.4 Techniques for genetic engineering

The existing molecular tools and protocols for genetic engineering are as diverse as the types of mutant mice that are generated with them. The majority of methods, however, are variations of two techniques which have been widely used since their origin in the 1980s: Pronuclear injection and gene targeting. They differ in their experimental protocols and in the technical possibilities/limitations associated with them, but they share the same principles (Figures 10.2 and 10.5):

- The ultimate aim of both techniques is to manipulate the genome of every nucleated cell in the animal, in such a way that the modification is stable and transmittable to the next generation, via the germ cell lineage.
- This is achieved if the procedure is carried out during the first stages of embryogenesis, when the developing organism consists of only one or a few cells. The genetic manipulation itself results from introducing a fragment of exogenous DNA, often referred to as transgene or DNA construct, into the genome of early embryo.
- The exact nature of the integrated DNA and the applied technique predetermine the mode of modification. A fundamental difference between the two techniques is that pronuclear injection only allows the addition of genetic material (gain-of-function), while gene targeting can add a new gene function (knockin) or abolish an existing one (null mutant or knockout), or even introduce subtle alterations to the genome.
- Any process of genetic engineering can be divided into phases of *in vitro* and *in vivo* work. Indeed, prior to the actual *in vivo* manipulation, a considerable amount of time is spent on planning the experiment and preparing the exogenous DNA. The preparatory work is a decisive factor in determining success, since the following *in vivo*

phase relies on naturally occurring processes within the cell and is less controllable (Figure 10.1).

- Irrespectively of the desired outcome, the initial integration of the exogenous DNA is mandatory, even if a selected region of DNA is to be 'removed' from the genome (Figure 10.7a).
- The resultant mutant offspring can give rise to a generation of founder animals. They form the basis for a programme of interbreeding, which is necessary to obtain a generation of mice that is homozygous for the engineered locus.

An important aspect in genetic engineering of mice is the choice of the strain. Genetic manipulations are usually introduced to inbred strains, such as C57BL/6, BALB/c, FVB/N and NMRI (Nagy et al., 2003). These mice have well-defined genetic backgrounds and show reduced genetic variability between individual animals. The use of one or even several inbred strains in a project (Figure 10.5) facilitates the identification of phenotypic changes, which arise from the manipulation. Certain strains are also chosen for their physiological features. For example, C57Bl/6 mice breed well, and are characterised by longevity and low susceptibility to tumours, but they show severe hearing loss with age (for more details, see the Mouse Mutant Resource Web Site from The Jackson Laboratory; http://mousemutant.jax.org).

Pronuclear injection

Today pronuclear injection is the dominating technique in genetic engineering. It enables the artificial addition of genetic information to the host genome, often with the purpose of heterologous gene expression. Other applications range from the overexpression of endogenous genes or mutant genes, to promoter analysis, labelling of subpopulations of cells with molecular markers and the inhibition of gene expression. The protocol for this technique was established by two groups of scientists in 1980s. It was based on their discoveries that injection of mRNA and DNA into mouse embryos resulted in the translation and expression of these foreign nucleic acids, respectively (Brinster et al., 1980, 1981). This led to the creation of the first transgenic mice (Gordon et al., 1980), which artificially expressed the thymidine kinase gene of the herpes simplex virus (HSV).

Although the term 'transgenic' originally referred to mice, which had been genetically modified with this particular method (i.e. the transmission of a gene into the embryo; Gordon and Ruddle, 1981), it is also frequently

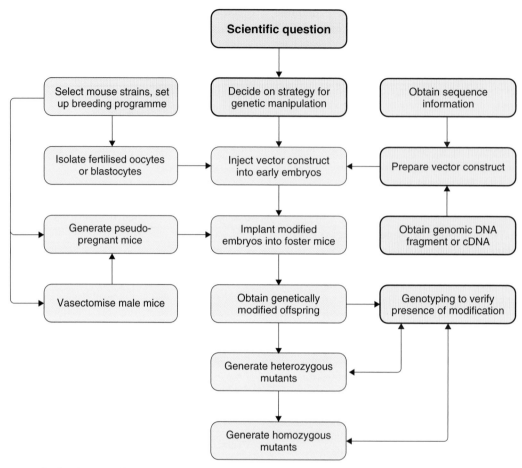

Figure 10.1 The flowchart provides a generic overview of the various steps involved in genetic engineering of mice. The hypothesis or scientific question (highlighted in green) determines the strategy and the subsequent practical work, which is carried out either *in vitro* (yellow) or *in vivo* (blue).

used in the context of other types of gene transfer. Likewise, the term 'transgene' is imprecise if the exogenous DNA has not the structural characteristics of a typical gene (e.g. introns). In some cases the transgene consists of complementary DNA (cDNA) only, in others it comprises of several fragments of coding sequence.

The procedure

The approach is straightforward and consists of three main steps, which are carried out subsequently: collection of fertilised eggs (oocytes) from mated mice, *in vitro* manipulation of the eggs (pronuclear injection) and reimplantation into mice (Gordon et al., 1980). The technical intricacies of this protocol, however, are complex (Figure 10.1) and require careful planning. For

the researcher, the necessary commitment of time and the costs involved are significant factors in the project (Ittner and Götz, 2007).

To obtain sufficient numbers of fertilised eggs, female mice are first treated with hormones to induce multiple ovulations (superovulation), and are then mated with males. For a short period after the fertilisation, when the one-cell embryo is in the oviduct, it still has the two haploid nuclei (pronuclei) from the female egg and the male sperm (Figure 10.2). It is at this stage that the fertilised oocytes are collected and prepared for the *in vitro* manipulation.

For the DNA-injection, a harvested oocyte is immobilised through suction of a blunt-ended holding pipette,

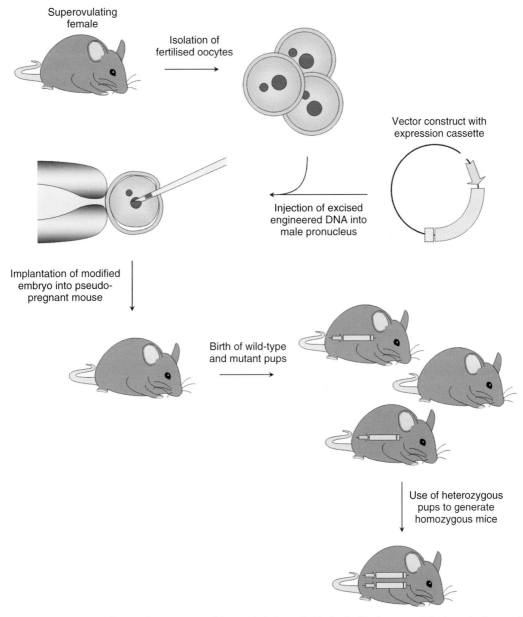

Figure 10.2 For the process of pronuclear injection, a blunt-ended pipette holds the fertilised oocyte, while the excised expression cassette is microinjected into the male pronucleus. The modified embryo is then re-implanted into a foster mouse, which can give birth to heterozygous offspring, if the transgene has successfully integrated into the genome of the one-cell embryo. Due to the random incorporation of the transgene, the heterozygous mutants are not genetically identical, and further breeding is required to generate a homozygous mutant line.

while a finer capillary penetrates the membranes of the cell and the larger paternal pronucleus and injects a solution containing the transgenic construct (Figure 10.2). After a few hours, the oocytes that survived the procedure (~40-90%; Rülicke and Hübscher, 2000) develop into zygotes with a single diploid nucleus, following the fusion of the two pronuclei. This natural process triggers the cleavage of the zygotes into a multicellular embryo.

The transgenic zygotes can be kept in culture medium until they reach the morula stage. Finally, multiple modified embryos are re-implanted into the oviducts of pseudo-pregnant surrogate mothers, that is, female mice which have been mated with vasectomised males. If these embryos are heterozygous for the transgene and develop into live-born offspring, they form a generation of founder animals (F0). Male F0 mutants can be crossed with wild-type females to obtain 50% of genetically-identical heterozygous mice (F1 generation), following the Mendelian laws of inheritance. Mating of two heterozygous siblings gives rise to a line of homozygous mutants.

However, obtaining live founders depends on the cumulative success of numerous factors, including the pronuclear injection, the re-implantation and the embryonic development, as well as the integration of the exogenous DNA. Only 2-3% of the microinjected oocytes are estimated to develop into transgenic founders (Brinster et al., 1985; Rülicke and Hübscher, 2000). It is worth noting that the overall efficiency is also influenced by the genetic background of the chosen inbred mouse strain (Auerbach, 2004).

Alternative protocols have been developed in an attempt to increase the efficiency of gene transfer in transgenesis. In intracytoplasmic sperm injection, the mouse sperm heads are coated with the DNA construct and then injected into the oocytes (Perry et al., 1999). In another approach the transgene is transferred into the undifferentiated spermatogonia of male mice, through *in vivo* electroporation of the testis (Dhup and Majumdar, 2008). Transgenic offspring can be obtained after natural mating, as the sperm from the male donor already carry the transgene. Despite these and other technical innovations, the traditional pronuclear injection remains the most widely applied method.

Integration of the transgene

The integration of the injected DNA into the host genome can be verified at different molecular levels. Initially, Southern blot analysis and PCR genotyping may confirm the presence of the transgene and to identify founder animals. These screens are done on genomic DNA from either ear punches or tail biopsies from young mice, and they are repeated for successive generations during the establishment of the transgenic lines (Figure 10.1). Larger tissue samples can be subjected to Western blot analysis or PCR to detect the corresponding gene products and, thus, demonstrate the expression in the mutant offspring. The inclusion of protein tags or reporter genes into the DNA construct may provide further support for the detection of transgene expression in the host. However, as discovered in early studies (Gordon et al., 1980, Brinster et al., 1981), the level of transgene expression is highly variable, due to the mechanism of integration.

The transgenic construct integrates into the genome in a random, non-reproducible fashion, predominantly as multiple copies (10-100s) in a head-to-tail array, called concatemer. Double-strand breaks in chromosomes probably contribute to the incorporation of the exogenous DNA (Brinster et al., 1985); the exact mechanisms are yet unknown. The integration occurs mainly (~80%) at one chromosomal site, but double-integration events on the same or two different chromosomes are possible, too, as detectable with fluorescence *in situ* hybridisation (FISH; Nakanishi et al., 2002).

A major disadvantage of this randomness is that the same DNA construct can produce genetically very different founder animals. Variable levels of expression may be observed for the recombinant gene – frequently in inverse correlation to the number of incorporated copies. The expression is also affected by positional effects, specifically by the chromosomal regions that flank the integration site (Rülicke and Hübscher, 2000). Among the possible consequences are transgene silencing in transcriptionally-inactive regions, for example in heterochromatin, or the stimulation through regulatory elements in the host genome. Otherwise, the incorporated construct itself can cause chromosomal rearrangements, such as translocations or deletions (Nakanishi et al., 2002). In ~10% of cases, this results in the disruption of endogenous genes and can further lead to pathological phenotypes.

The inconsistencies in the phenotype generally hamper the comparison of different transgenic lines and their selection for subsequent studies. Usually, several independent transgenic founders are investigated in the same project. It is also not uncommon that the studies are carried out on heterozygous mutants instead, to minimise a possible accumulation of negative effects as observed in homozygous mice.

Another complicating factor in establishing a homozygous mouse mutant is the time point of transgene integration. Frequently, this event occurs after the early divisions of the zygote and results in genetic mosaicism. The resultant mice contain transgenic and non-transgenic cells, and are not suitable as founders if none of the germ cells carries the transgene.

The nature of the DNA construct (transgene)

The DNA construct that was used to generate the first transgenic mouse contained the cloned gene of the herpes simplex virus thymidine kinase (HSV-tk) fused to the simian virus 40 (SV40) promoter (Gordon et al., 1980). It integrated successfully and led to robust and ubiquitous expression, as evident from assays for thymidine kinase activity.

This example illustrates that transgene expression also depends on the presence of essential regulatory elements, the majority of which are found in the promoter region. In the case of HSV-tk, an intronless viral gene, a small promoter may be sufficient to achieve the desired effect. However, transcription of eukaryotic genes is a more complex process, as reflected by the diversity of regulatory elements and sequence motifs in their promoters as well as within the genes. The core promoter initiates the transcription and, together with binding sites for enhancers or suppressors, determines the temporal, spatial and level of expression. Some of these elements can be located within introns of genes (see Chapter 8), while other sequences in the genes' exons signal the transcriptional stop (Figure 10.3). In addition, the use of alternative promoters and the splicing process may produce different mRNA transcripts in a tissue-dependent manner. With respect to the transgene, it is the quantity and quality of sequence information in the DNA construct that largely predetermines the characteristics of the expression pattern.

The choice of the vector

The first constructs used in transgenesis were based on plasmid vectors, which can be easily manipulated *in vitro* and multiplied in bacterial hosts. Prior to pronuclear injection, the exogenous DNA is usually excised with restriction endonucleases, and unnecessary prokaryotic vector sequences are removed. However, a disadvantage of plasmids is their low cloning capacity, because it limits the size of the expression cassette to about 10kb (reviewed by Auerbach, 2004) and makes the cloning of entire genes often impractical. In particular eukaryotic genes are prone to exceed the upper cloning limit due to large intronic regions. Thus, many plasmids only carry the protein coding sequence of a eukaryotic gene in the form of the full-length cDNA; though the inclusion of intronic sequences seems to enhance transgene expression (Figure 10.3).

A considerable weakness related to the small insert size of recombinant plasmid vectors is that the transgene expression is likely to be influenced by the site of integration. This problem can be overcome with chromosome-based vectors, namely the bacterial artificial chromosome (BAC), the bacteriophage P1 artificial chromosome (PAC) and the yeast artificial chromosome (YAC). BACs and PACs can take up large DNA fragments of 100kb to 300kb, YACs even up to 1Mb. Their higher cloning capacities permit the cloning of large genomic loci, including entire genes and their promoters. Due to their size and the integrity of sequence information, the transgenes in such constructs are less affected by regulatory elements flanking the integration site, and they may be expressed in their native pattern. Multiple integrations (up to ~10 copies) are possible but, contrary to the insertional cassettes of plasmid-based vectors, the level of expression is positively correlated with the copy number.

The choice of the promoter

The choice of the promoter in the expression cassette is an important one that needs to be a well-considered, because the promoter has a major impact on the qualitative and quantitative expression pattern of the transgene.

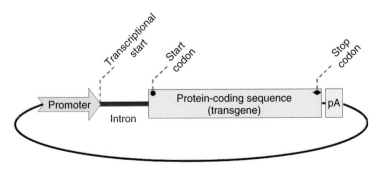

Figure 10.3 A typical vector construct for pronuclear injection contains the expression cassette with a minimum of elements, which are required for expression: a promoter with regulatory elements, such as the transcriptional start site; the protein-coding sequence or cDNA of the transgene, including the start (●) and stop (◆) codons; and a polyadenylation (pA) sequence. The level of transgene expression can be further increased by including at least one intronic sequence.

Regulatory elements in the construct may derive from the gene's own or a heterologous promoter. Various minimal promoters, such as those from SV40, the human cytomegalovirus (CMV) or the mammalian β-actin gene, lead to a constitutive, wide-spread and high transcription. Others are specific to a tissue or cell type, a developmental stage and the level of expression. Control over the onset of expression can be achieved with inducible promoters, which respond to either exogenously administered small molecules (e.g. drugs) or physiological factors (e.g. hypoxia, hypothermia; for details, see Guo et al., 2008). The promoter of the metallothionein-1 gene, for example, can be induced with the heavy metal cadmium (Brinster et al., 1982).

A tightly-regulated or conditional expression is possible with binary systems. For one category, the control mechanisms are based on the interaction of a ligand-induced transactivator and the promoter of the gene of interest (Figure 10.4). The most widely applied system utilises elements of the tetracycline resistance operon

from *Escherichia coli* (Gossen and Bujard, 1992), and the antibiotic doxycycline (a stable tetracycline analogue) as ligand. In the *Tet-off* version of this system, the administered antibiotic binds to the transactivator, which thus is unable to induce expression of the target transgene. Here, transcriptional activation is obtained in the absence of the ligand. The opposite is the case for the *Tet-on* version, that is, the ligand's presence is obligatory to induce expression of the gene of interest. Similar systems are based on the use of steroid hormones or synthetic derivatives as inducers. Since the control over expression is mediated through the presence or absence of a ligand, the respective effects on the gene of interest are reversible.

A second category of binary systems utilises DNA recombinases, instead of transactivators, to control expression (Lakso et al., 1992). Once the synthesis of these enzymes has been induced, they carry out site-specific DNA recombination in the host genome at sites that had been modified previously; this process is irreversible. Two possible applications in transgenesis

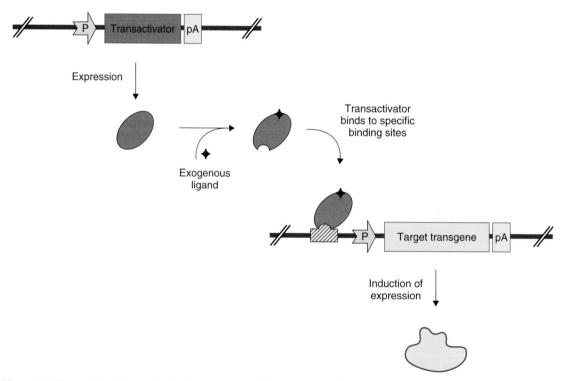

Figure 10.4 Transcriptional transactivation is one category of binary systems, where control over gene expression is achieved with an effector molecule (pink). In the example above, an exogenously administered ligand (◆) binds to the transactivator and causes a conformational change. This enables the effector to attach to a specific binding site (shaded) upstream of the target transgene (blue) and to induce its transcription. P, promoter; pA, polyadenylation signal.

are the inactivation of the transgene by removing it, or its activation by excising an intervening stop sequence. The exact mechanisms are discussed below.

Binary systems provide scientists with a range of molecular tools for a tight and yet flexible regulation of transcription. For example, the inducible transactivator of the tetracycline system can be placed under the control of a tissue-specific promoter and would limit the regulation of the target transgene to the corresponding tissue. However, as the name indicates, binary systems require the establishment of a bi-transgenic mouse line in a labour and time-intensive process.

The use of protein tags and reporter genes

A major concern in transgenesis is the verification of transgene expression in the tissue. Two groups of markers are available that facilitate the detection and quantification of the transgenic product; these are short non-functional protein tags or reporter genes.

Protein or epitope tags are short peptide sequences and functional protein domains, which were originally developed to purify recombinant proteins through immunoaffinity, chromatography or specific substrates (Brizzard, 2008). In transgenesis, a sequence encoding the epitope tag is fused to the gene of interest, either at the 5' or the 3' end, followed later by the detection of the fusion product with a tag-specific antibody. Commonly used tags are 6xHis, a synthetic peptide consisting of six histidine residues (single-letter code: HHHHHH), and peptides derived from the influenza hemagglutinin protein (YPYDVPDYA) or the human c-myc protein (EQKLISEEDL).

In contrast to this, the majority of reporter genes code for bacterial or invertebrate enzymes, and are activated by their own promoter and set of regulatory elements. Their presence in the cells is visualised on the basis of substrate-dependent reactions. For example, the activity of the bacterial β-galactosidase (*lacZ* gene) or the firefly luciferase can be identified and measured through the conversion of substrates into colorimetric products or light, respectively. In contrast, another popular marker, that is, the jellyfish green fluorescent protein (GFP) and its numerous engineered variants, is autofluorescent (Shimomura et al., 1962; Shaner et al., 2008). It can be easily localised in living cells or even whole animals, since its detection does not require any substrate.

Like small epitope tags, a reporter gene can be employed to create a fusion protein, consisting of the products from the transgene and the reporter gene. However, as this larger tag may interfere with the physiological function of the transgenic protein, the expression of reporter genes is frequently mediated through bicistronic expression cassettes. Such constructs generate single transcripts comprising the mRNAs from the transgene and the marker, which are then simultaneously translated into two separate proteins of equal amounts. Alternatively, the reporter gene can be placed under the control of a cell-specific promoter to selectively mark a group of cells, or an uncharacterised promoter to identify the corresponding expression pattern.

Generating loss-of-function mutants

Technical improvements and new molecular tools have expanded the range of potential applications for the traditional pronuclear injection method. The unpredictable nature of DNA integration, however, remains a limiting factor: It only allows new genetic material to be added to the host genome. Gain-of-function mutants can be generated with relative ease, but it appears to be technically unfeasible to disrupt selected endogenous genes, in order to create loss-of-function mutants.

It is possible to address the problem on a transcriptional rather than on a genomic level. A traditional approach is to inject DNA constructs into the pronucleus, which express the antisense strand of the gene of interest. This antisense transcript is likely to hybridise to the corresponding sense mRNA and contributes to the formation of a double-stranded molecule. Eventually this results in reduced levels of both transcript and translated protein. A similar outcome is achieved with transgenes that express small interfering RNAs, double-stranded RNAs or catalytically active ribozymes (Nagy et al., 2003). The process is commonly referred to as gene silencing or gene knockdown; though the gene is still active the levels of the corresponding products are down-regulated. Gene silencing is a naturally-occurring mechanism that is mediated through several classes of small interfering and sequence-specific RNAs. In recent years, it gained significant attention as potential and effective therapeutic application (Scherer and Rossi, 2003; Ghildiyal and Zamore, 2009; see Chapter 8).

An alternative approach is the overexpression of truncated or otherwise mutated versions of endogenous proteins, which interfere with the normal regulation of cellular processes. This is frequently used to generate mouse models for Alzheimer's disease.

The gene targeting technique, however, proves to be a true alternative. With respect to engineering loss-of-function mutants, it has superseded the pronuclear injection protocol, because it can be utilised to target and directly abolish the function of a selected gene. Gene targeting will be covered in the next section.

Gene targeting

In 2007, Capecchi, Evans and Smithies were awarded the Nobel Prize in Physiology or Medicine for their pioneering work in developing a technology, which has revolutionised many aspects of scientific research: Gene targeting. Unlike pronuclear injection, where the transgene incorporation is random, it is a precise and more versatile strategy for the manipulation of the mammalian genome. New genetic traits can be added to create knockin mutants, but endogenous genes can also be rendered non-functional to produce knockout mice. The genetic alterations may affect large regions of the host genome, or they are subtle in the form of point mutations.

The protocol for gene targeting was established in the late 1980s, following a series of groundbreaking studies. Back then, Smithies demonstrated that he could repair a mutant version of the hypoxanthine phosphoribosyl transferase (HPRT) gene *in vitro* (Doetschman et al., 1987). Cells with a functional copy of this gene were now able to survive in a selection medium. In contrast, Capecchi used a very similar approach to disrupt the HPRT gene in those cells, by inserting the neomycin resistance gene (Thomas and Capecchi, 1987). Albeit the different outcomes, the success of both studies was based on the scientists' earlier discovery that exogenous DNA can be incorporated into a cell's genome through homologous recombination. A second key discovery was that of embryonic stem cells by Evans (Evans and Kaufman, 1981), because these cells allowed the transition of the targeted change from an *in vitro* system to *in vivo*, in order to achieve inheritance.

Embryonic stem cells

The early stages of mammalian embryogenesis are characterised by rapid divisions of the embryo from the single-cell stage (zygote) to a multicellular organism. When the blastocyst stage is reached, it resembles a hollow sphere consisting of a fluid-filled cavity (blastocoel), a surrounding outer layer of cells (trophoblast) and an inner cell mass (embryoblast). Later the trophoblast contributes to the placenta, while the embryoblast grows into the foetus.

The inner mass cells were identified by Evans as embryonic stem (ES) cells, that is, undifferentiated or pluripotent cells, which have the ability to develop into any cell type of the foetus (Evans and Kaufman, 1981). Another finding was that isolated ES cells proliferate in cell culture and maintain their pluripotency, if they are grown on a layer of fibroblasts serving as feeder cells; removal of the fibroblasts induces differentiation. Evans and colleagues took advantage of these properties of ES cells to genetically modify them *in vitro*, through infection with a retroviral vector. After reintroducing the recombinant ES cells first into blastocysts and then foster mice, they obtained chimeric offspring (Robertson et al., 1986). Although only some of the pups' tissues carried the retroviral DNA, this was a breakthrough, because it showed the prospect of introducing exogenous DNA into the mouse germ line.

The procedure

Like pronuclear injection, the gene targeting protocol requires a vector construct or targeting vector that is introduced during the organism's early embryogenesis. However, in gene targeting, the use of ES cells with their unique biological characteristics offers an alternative and advantageous route for the DNA insertion.

After being harvested from mouse blastocysts, ES cells are initially cultured and then transfected with the linearised targeting vector through electroporation. Cells surviving this treatment are maintained in culture medium, where they may proliferate to increase the pool of genetically-modified cells. Here is an important opportunity for selecting those recombinant cells, which have integrated the construct at the desired chromosomal site, through homologous recombination. The success of the recombination and the selection of clones much depends on the sequence information in the targeting vector.

Following selection, the recombinant ES cells are microinjected into the cavities of fresh blastocysts, which are later re-implanted into the uterus of a pseudopregnant foster female. Offspring arising from the modified embryos are chimeras, as the implanted blastocysts contained recombinant as well as wild-type ES cells. Hence, at least two rounds of breeding are required to generate homozygous mutants (Figure 10.5).

To facilitate the identification of chimeras/mutants in this lengthy process, mouse strains with different fur colours are used in gene targeting studies. For example, a common strategy is to inject recombinant ES cells that derive from the brown-coloured strain 129 into blastocysts from C57BL/6 mice, a black strain. Since the coat colour brown is dominant, chimeric pups are easily recognisable by their brown and black fur, whereby the percentage of coat colour indicates how much of the animal's tissue derive from the 129 ES cells. In the first round of breeding, these chimeras need to be backcrossed with wild-type C57BL/6 mice to obtain a progeny with a

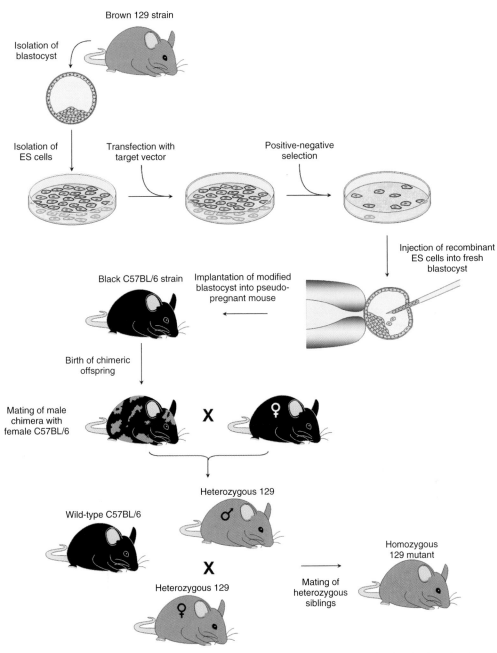

Figure 10.5 In gene targeting, the genetic modification of the host genome is introduced via isolated and cultured embryonic stem (ES) cells. Following the transfection of the cells with the target vector, the positive–negative selection enriches the recipient ES cells, which have incorporated the DNA through homologous recombination. The selected cells are injected into a blastocyst that is then re-implanted into a foster mouse. The born offspring are chimeric and recognisable as such, because the modified blastocyst contained recombinant and wild-type ES cells, which originate from the brown-coated 129 and the black C57BL/6 mouse strain, respectively. Homozygous mutants are eventually obtained after backcrossing the chimeras with the wild-type, to generate true heterozygotes, and mating the heterozygous siblings with each other.

pure brown coat. Such animals arise if the recombinant ES cells have contributed to the germ cells of the chimeras; they represent the heterozygote founder generation. In the final round of breeding, the heterozygote siblings are mated with each other to create mice with a genetic background, which is homozygous for the engineered site. Typically, along the visual selection, Southern blot analysis is carried out for each generation to confirm the stable transfer of the modified allele(s) via the germ line.

Homologous recombination and the targeting vector

Homologous recombination forms the basis for the success of the gene targeting technology. The term refers to a naturally occurring process in living cells, where genetic material is exchanged between DNA molecules with homologous sequences. It is a relatively frequent event during the production of gametes (meiosis), but rare in somatic cells. Yet, it was early recognised as a possible route to integrate exogenous DNA into specific genes of somatic cells *in vitro* (Folger et al., 1982; Smithies et al., 1985). When ES cells were microinjected with a vector construct, one out of 1000 modified cells incorporated the insert at the desired site (homologous recombination), while the others integrated of the vector randomly (non-homologous recombination; Thomas and Capecchi, 1987).

In gene targeting, the double-reciprocal DNA exchange is probable, if the targeting vector contains fragments, which have a high degree of sequence homology to the selected endogenous site in the host. Usually, the engineered DNA in the vector is flanked by chromosomal fragments of identical (isogenic) sequence. They need to be of sufficient length (>4–5 kb) to enable the genetic exchange through cross-over (Figure 10.6A). The required genomic fragments for the construction of the targeting vector often derive from commercially available BAC libraries, which contain 130–180 kb long clones of genomic DNA. Other, supplementary sequence information of cloned and characterised genes or entire genomes may be gathered from public databases (see 10.2); it is often crucial for the design and assembly of the targeting vector.

Two other key components in the target vector are selectable markers. They significantly increase the efficiency of the gene targeting procedure, because they enable the enrichment of ES cells containing the engineered change. The two classic genes for this positive–negative selection are those for the neomycin resistance (i.e. neomycin phosphotransferase; neoR) as positive marker and the HSV-tk as the negative marker (Mansour

et al., 1988). In the targeting construct, the positive selectable gene is located within the recombining region, while its negative counterpart is positioned outside the isogenic sequences on one vector arm (Figure 10.6). In the case of homologous recombination only the positive marker neoR is transferred to the ES cells and permits them to grow in the presence of the antibiotic Geneticin (G418). The addition of the nucleoside analogue and HSV-tk substrate ganciclovir, to the culture medium, has no effect. Non-homologous recombination, on the other hand, may result in the integration of the entire targeting vector including the positive and the negative selectable gene. It renders the recipient ES cells resistant to G418, but the treatment with ganciclovir causes cell death, since the drug is phosphorylated by HSV-tk and then inhibits the DNA polymerase in dividing cells. ES cells with no recombination event are already elimdinated by G418. Some alternatives for positive markers (i.e. antibiotic resistance) are the puromycin-*N*-acetyltransferase or the hygromycin B phosphotransferase. The diphtheria toxin A fragment is another negative marker, which provides selection without the need of a drug.

Knockin and knockout mice

The efficiency and the precision of the gene targeting technique become evident when DNA is inserted to create a knockin mouse. As the exogenous DNA is flanked by isogenic sequences (Figure 10.6), it is incorporated as a single copy at a predetermined and possibly non-critical site. In contrast to pronuclear injection, the reproducibility of this approach results in a more consistent level of transgene expression, and it can minimise the disruption of endogenous genes. It is also common to remove the positive selectable gene later from the targeted recombinants (Figure 10.7b), since high levels of the marker may have adverse effects in the embryo or the fully-grown animal.

A widely used system in this context is the Cre-*loxP* recombination system from the bacteriophage P1 (Lakso et al., 1992). It requires that the selectable gene is flanked ('floxed') by 34bp-long *loxP* sites (locus of cross-over (x) in P1), the recognition motifs for the Cre recombinase. Following the selection process, the recombinant ES cells are transiently transfected with a vector expressing the Cre recombinase, which subsequently excises the floxed DNA in a highly site-specific manner. A second popular system is the Flp-*FRT* recombination system from the yeast *Saccharomyces cerevisiae*; here, the target site needs to be 'flrted', that is, contain the enzyme-specific FRT sites of 48bp length. In addition to the excision, both systems allow other highly efficient recombination

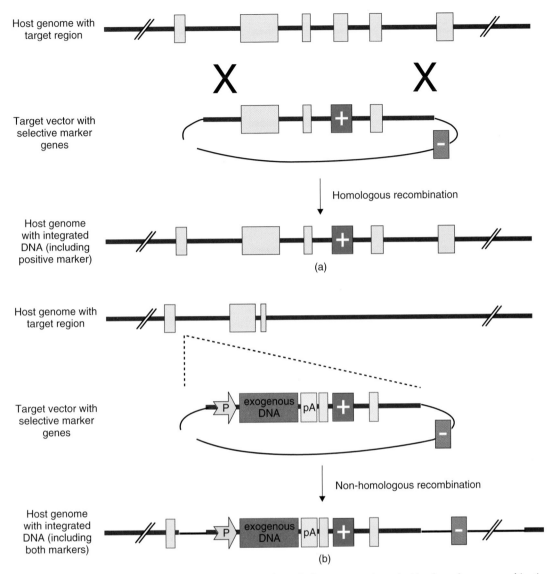

Figure 10.6 The targeting fragment in the vector can be inserted into the host genome through either homologous recombination (a) at the selected region or non-homologous recombination (b) at a random site. (a) Homologous sequences (dark blue line) in the vector lead to a cross-over (**X**) with the genomic site and a genetic exchange. Only the desired DNA, including a positive marker gene (green), is inserted, but not the negative marker gene (red) outside the recombining region. (b) The entire vector construct, including the expression cassette (pink) and both marker genes, is detectable in the host genome, as recombination between homologous sequences did not occur. The following positive–negative selection eliminates all cells without a homologous recombination event. P, promoter; pA, polyadenylation signal.

reactions, namely inversion, insertion, duplication and translocation of genetic material, depending on the orientation of the enzymes' target sites (van der Weyden et al., 2002). Recombinases are also an important tool in conditional gene targeting.

The knockin method is commonly utilised to add genes coding for reporters, inducible transactivators and recombinases. In the host genome, these genes are either placed under the control of an endogenous promoter or inserted with their own expression cassette. Another

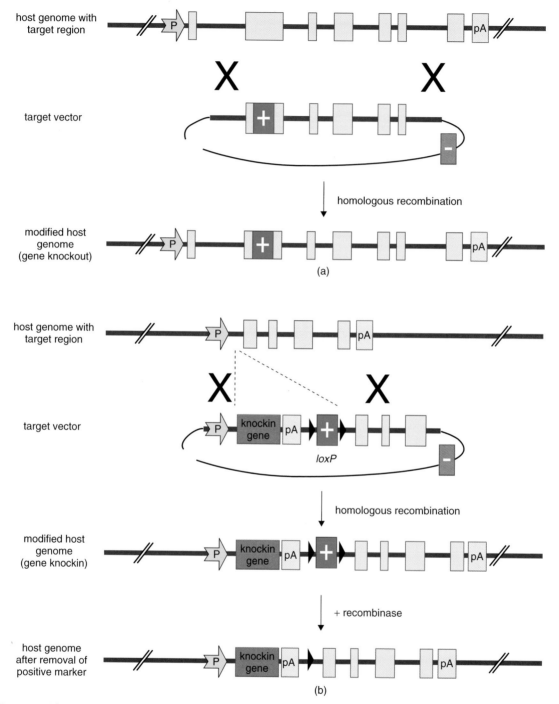

host genome with target region

target vector

homologous recombination

modified host genome (gene knockout)

(a)

host genome with target region

target vector

homologous recombination

modified host genome (gene knockin)

+ recombinase

host genome after removal of positive marker

(b)

Figure 10.7 The outcome of the gene targeting technique depends on the targeting vector. Provided that the exogenous DNA in the vector is flanked by isogenic sequences (dark blue line), it can site-specifically disrupt an endogenous gene or sequence to create a knockout animal (a), or insert a new gene to produce a knockin (b). (a) The positive marker (green) partly replaces the second exon (light blue) of an endogenous gene, and renders it non-functional. (b) Homologous recombination adds a gene (pink) in front of an endogenous promoter (P) sequence. The positive marker gene (green), which is flanked by *loxP* sites, is excised by a recombinase after the selection process. P, polyadenylation signal.

attractive knockin application is the introduction of point mutations (e.g. substitutions, insertion, deletions). The substitution of a few nucleotides, for example, may reveal a link between a gene locus and a disease, or identify an amino acid that serves as the binding site on a drug target. Otherwise, point mutations can be an invaluable means to create animal models, which mimic human genetic diseases.

The introduction of subtle modifications is technically more challenging, as it requires a two-step strategy, such as the 'in-out' or 'hit-and-run' procedure (Valancius and Smithies, 1991). This strategy uses an insertion-type vector, which has been linearised in such a way that homologous recombination inserts the whole construct, including the mutant form of the target gene and the selectable genes. The second step relies on the single-reciprocal or intrachromosomal recombination between the wild-type gene and its modified portion. This spontaneous event eliminates all superfluous sequences, with the exception of the modified version of the gene.

Gene knockouts or null alleles are predominantly created with replacement vectors, where the isogenic sequence in the vector is partially substituted or interrupted by the positive selectable marker (Figure 10.7a). The successful integration in the host genome then replaces an essential part of the endogenous gene (e.g. an exon) and/or leads to a shift in the reading frame, which is likely to cause the premature end of translation of the corresponding gene transcript. An alternative approach for producing a knockout mouse uses point mutations, either to create a premature stop codon in the targeted gene or to delete essential elements in the regulatory sequence upstream of the gene. It has to be noted that the outcome of a knockout experiment not only depends on the mode of disruption but also the animal strain and its genetic background. Disabling a functionally-important gene may lead to lethal defects in one strain, while a second strain survives the same modification and has no obvious phenotype, in comparison to the wild-type (Pearson, 2002). This possibly reflects the natural variations in the genotypes, whereby in the surviving mutant other genes functionally compensate for the eliminated locus. It is often true for members of multi-gene families, where the encoded proteins differ slightly in their sequence, but not significantly in their physiological function.

Conditional gene targeting

Despite its technical advances over pronuclear injection, conventional gene targeting, as described above, has the major disadvantage, that the targeted changes – and their consequences – become effective immediately after the homologous recombination event in the ES cells. This leaves the researcher without any control over the onset of either the expression of a knockin gene or the loss of gene function in a knockout mutant. In particular during embryogenesis, the untimely and perhaps ubiquitous expression of a knockin gene may lead to physiological abnormalities, while the early deletion of an indispensable gene may cause death of the embryo *in utero* or the neonate. Such undesirable effects are not necessarily apparent in the heterozygous mutant, but likely to become more prominent in the homozygous mutant. In this instance, the study is frequently carried out in the heterozygous offspring only. Another limiting factor is that the conventional approach makes it impractical to investigate the role of a selected gene within a specific developmental window.

Conditional gene targeting techniques can overcome the problems associated with the temporal expression or elimination of a gene by utilising binary systems. These molecular tools depend on the interaction of an effector protein, such as an inducible transactivator or a recombinase, on the engineered target region. In combination with cell or tissue-specific promoters, they can be applied to control the implementation of the desired manipulation simultaneously in a temporal and spatial manner. Unfortunately, a considerable drawback of binary systems is the necessity to generate double-mutant animals, which carry the gene encoding the effector molecule and the responding modified target site. This process is labour and time-intensive because it first, entails the creation of two independent mouse lines, that is, one each for the effector and the responder construct. Subsequently, both lines of homozygous mutants are crossed to produce the double mutant. The two types of binary systems for conditional gene targeting, which can be established in this way, are transcriptional transactivation and site-specific DNA recombination.

Conditional knockin experiments generally use binary systems for transcriptional transactivation, such as the tetracycline-dependant regulatory systems (Gossen and Bujard, 1992), which have been covered earlier. Here, the transcription of the responding gene can be controlled in a reversible way, that is, an exogenous inducer is either added or removed to (de)activate the effector molecule (as detailed in Figure 10.4). In contrast, site-specific DNA recombination is not reversible and is mainly applied to produce conditional knockout mice. The double-mutant mouse, in this case, needs to be a carrier of a recombinase gene (e.g. Cre or Flp recombinase) and a modified target locus, where an exon or any other essential part is flanked by the recombination-specific DNA motifs (e.g. *loxP* or *FRT*; see Figure 10.7A). Following the expression of the recombinase, the flanked fragment is excised and the gene rendered non-functional (Gu et al., 1993). The onset of the gene inactivation can be directed, if the recombinase gene has been placed under the control of an inducible promoter. This was achieved, for the first time, by Rajewsky and colleagues (Kühn et al., 1995), who used the interferon-responsive Mx1 promoter. Recently, the possible range of conditional knockout experiments has been increased with systems, which can be induced through administering tetracycline or hormones (e.g. ecdysone), and tissue-specific promoters. Variation of these can also be used to generate inducible knockin mice. For example, a knockin gene could finally be activated, after inducing a recombinase that excises an intervening stop sequence.

10.5 Examples of genetically-engineered mice

Point mutations to identify and characterise drug targets

In the vertebrate central nervous system, $GABA_A$ receptors are the major neurotransmitter receptors for fast synaptic inhibition. They are the target for numerous therapeutic drugs with anxiolytic, sedative, hypnotic and/or anticonvulsive actions, such as benzodiazepines (BZs), barbiturates and general anaesthetics. However, mammalian $GABA_A$ receptors exist in a variety of subtypes, since they are pentameric combinations from up to 16 different subunits ($\alpha1$–$\alpha6$, $\beta1$-$\beta3$, $\gamma1$-$\gamma3$, δ, ϵ, π and θ). Even though many of the aforementioned drugs potentiate the action of the natural ligand GABA, their pharmacologic spectra seem to be largely dependent on the subunit combination in the receptor subtype (Rudolph et al., 2001).

Over the last two decades, gene targeting has been employed to assess the physiological relevance of the BZ-binding site and to identify which receptor subtypes with a high affinity for the BZ agonist diazepam (Valium®) are responsible for the anxiolytic and sedative actions of this compound. Early attempts, which used a target vector with a neomycin resistance cassette to knockout selected subunit genes, caused the expected loss of BZ-binding sites, but these changes were often accompanied by reduced growth and a lethal phenotype in the homozygous mutants (e.g. Günther et al., 1995). Unexpectedly, other non-targeted subunit genes in the genomic vicinity

were down regulated, too. These studies revealed the significance of the ablated target genes, for survival, but also negative side effects arising from the presence of the positive marker (i.e. neoR) in the host.

Follow-up studies approached the subject with knockin point mutations that substituted a conserved amino acid believed to be essential for BZ binding, that is, the histidine residue at position 101 (encoded by CAC). The change of this wild-type histidine residue in the $\alpha1$ and $\alpha2$ subunits to an arginine residue (CGG) was subtle, but had profound effects on the animals' behavioural responses to diazepam. In $\alpha1$(H101R) mutant mice, the sedative and amnesic activities of diazepam were absent, while its anxiolytic and myorelaxant properties were entirely unaffected (Rudolph et al., 1999). However, the $\alpha2$(H101R) strain failed to show the drug's anxiolytic action in a light–dark choice test (Löw et al., 2000). Like untreated wild-type mice, the treated $\alpha2$(H101R) mice demonstrated the fear behaviour that such brightly-lit environment normally elicits. On the contrary, the anxiety was not evident in either wild-type or $\alpha1$(H101R) mutant animals, if those were treated with diazepam.

In conclusion, this indicates that $\alpha2$ subunit-containing $GABA_A$ receptors mediate the anxiolytic actions of diazepam. Moreover, it illustrates that, unlike gene knockouts, small mutations do not necessarily compromise the animal's development and life span. Concerning the development of highly selective therapeutics, they are a helpful tool in identifying the drug's molecular target(s) and binding sites as well as their unwanted off target effects.

Creating an animal model for Alzheimer's disease

Alzheimer's disease (AD) is the most prevalent form of progressive neurodegeneration and dementia among the elderly, accounting for about 65% of all cases of mental decline. AD is mainly diagnosed after the age of 65 (late-onset dementia), although in about 5% of sufferers the disease becomes apparent prior to this age, probably due to genetic predispositions (early-onset familial dementia). The initial symptoms are an impairment of memory and other cognitive functions, however rapid mood swings, and changes in personality and social behaviour develop as the disease progresses. These clinical features are the consequence of extensive neurodegeneration in the brain, which disturbs the integrity of intra- and extracortical circuits and leads to imbalances of neurotransmitter systems. On a microscopic level, the two pathological hallmarks of AD are extracellular aggregates of amyloid β (Aβ) peptide (amyloid plaques) and intracellular neurofibrillary tangles (NFT) of hyperphosphorylated tau proteins. The amyloid cascade hypothesis suggests that the formation of amyloid plaques precedes the presence of NFTs and initiates the pathogenic processes in AD (Harper, 2010).

Unlike many epidemics and forms of cancer, there is no cure for Alzheimer's disease, as the currently available drugs can only treat the associated symptoms and reduce its progression. However, since the mid 1990s, genetic engineering has facilitated the design of numerous mouse models for AD, which endeavour to resemble the disease phenotype. They assist in the investigation of the pathogenesis a molecular, cellular and behavioural level, and the development of treatments. The early mouse models were generated through pronuclear injection, and they overexpressed mutant versions of the human amyloid precursor protein (APP). This strategy was based on the discovery of mutations in the APP gene linked to a few cases of early-onset familial dementia and the fact that Aβ peptides originate from APP isoforms, which are cleaved by secretases into smaller fragments.

The PDAPP mouse was the first transgenic model that successfully developed an AD-like phenotype including the neuronal Aβ deposits (Games et al., 1995). The expression cassette consisted of the platelet derived growth factor promoter and a cDNA for the human APP carrying the Indiana mutation, where the valine at residue 717 was substituted by phenylalanine, that is, APP(V717F). In addition to the deposits, the brain showed the characteristic loss of cholinergic neurons, and animals displayed abnormalities in their learning and general behaviour, but no NFTs were detected. A year later, a publication reported the study of the Tg2576 transgenic mouse (Hsiao et al., 1996). Here, the hamster prion protein drove overexpression of another human APP isoform, bearing the Swedish double mutation APP(K670N/M671L). As observed previously, the mutant mouse had the Aβ aggregates and behaviour abnormalities resembling an AD-like phenotype, but the brain was devoid of authentic NFTs. Also the APP23 mouse, where the expression of APP(K670N/M671L) was controlled by the neuron-specific Thy-1 promoter, showed the incomplete disease phenotype (Stürchler-Pierrat et al., 1997). In all these studies, the complete absence of the second pathological hallmark, that is, the tangles, was a particular problem, since it did not support the amyloid cascade hypothesis.

Progress in the development of improved AD models followed, after the identification of pathogenic mutations, in different genes, which could also be linked to this and related disorders. Mutations were discovered in human

tau itself, and the corresponding transgenic mice, such as the Tau(P301L) mutant, successfully developed NFTs in the nervous tissue (Ballatore et al., 2007). Other mutations were found in the presenilin (PS) genes *PSEN1* and *PSEN2*, which code for the catalytic subunits of the γ secretase, one of the enzymes responsible for the proteolytic processing of APP. This led to the generation of the PS1(M146V) knockin and the PS1 knockout mice.

Newer AD models are no longer single transgenic mice, since one mutation cannot fully mimic the human neuropathology. Instead, they carry mutant versions of several genes believed to be involved in AD. The triple transgenic 3xTg-AD (Oddo et al., 2003), for example, combined the three mutant genes APP(K670N/M671L), Tau(P301L) and PS1(M146V). In this model, the formation of amyloid plaques prior to the occurrence of neurofibrillary tangles did support the amyloid cascade hypothesis. The aggregation of Aβ peptides was further accelerated in mutant mouse with five familial Alzheimer's disease mutations (Oakley et al., 2006).

In summary, animal models can provide invaluable insights into the aetiology, pathophysiology and symptoms of a human disorder, and they aid the development of suitable pharmacotherapies. However, the majority of model systems are frequently only partial models. They cannot fully recapitulate the human disease phenotype, since not all key elements are yet known and incorporated into the model system. Sometimes the human body's very own responses to environmental factors and administered drugs hamper the development of a valid animal model for research.

Humanised mice

Mice are the favourite animal model for genetic engineering due to their close homologies in genetics and physiology to humans. However, the immune systems of both species are clearly distinct. Hence, research on the human immunology and drug development requires mouse models, which show human-specific immune responses. This issue has been addressed by creating so-called humanised mice, which possess some components of the human immune system. A key characteristic of the majority of such strains is their immunodeficiency, which is the consequence of spontaneous mutations or gene targeting (i.e. knockout). In addition, they are often transgenic for human genes or they are reconstituted with human haematopoietic stem cells (HSCs; Thomsen et al., 2005).

Early efforts to generate humanised mice used the CB17 inbred strain with severe combined immunodeficiency (SCID; Bosma et al., 1983) that manifests itself by a complete lack of mature T and B cells, and a susceptibility to numerous infections. The reconstitution of the immune system with its human counterpart, via HSC grafts, was unsuccessful although the HSCs engrafted. It was hampered by the residual activities of the innate immunity and natural killer cells in the recipient mice. The successive development of the non-obese diabetic (NOD) mouse, with autoimmune diabetes (Makino et al., 1980), and the NOD-SCID strain decreased those residual activities further, but still limited the success of engraftment. The necessary progress came, when Rajewsky's team eliminated the gene of the interleukin-2 receptor γ (IL-2Rγ) chain, an essential component of the family of cytokine receptors (DiSanto et al., 1995). Their target vector inserted the neoR marker gene into the IL-2Rγ gene, and *loxP* sites flanking several exons and the marker gene. The following Cre-*loxP*-mediated recombination rendered the target locus non-functional. In the knockout mouse, it led to the complete disappearance of the natural killer cells, and a large reduction in the number of mature T and B cells. It significantly improved the engraftment of HSCs and other human cells into mice. Further progress in the development of a functional human immune system was achieved after abolishing the IL-2Rγ gene in the NOD-SCID and other immunodeficient mouse strains.

Humanised mice have enhanced our understanding of the fundamental aspects of our immune system, including autoimmunity, allergy, infectious diseases, cancer and transplantation biology. This research field began with the discovery of immunodeficient strains, but adequate model systems were only created with the available techniques for genetic engineering, in later years.

10.6 Summary

Pronuclear injection and gene targeting are the two major techniques for the genetic engineering of the mouse. In contrast to spontaneous or chemically-induced mutations, these techniques are forms of genotype-driven mutagenesis – the genetic changes are introduced in a controlled manner, with the help of sequence information about a gene of interest or a particular chromosomal locus, and a vector construct carrying engineered DNA. The manipulation of the host genome takes place during early embryogenesis, so that it is later present in every cell of the adult organism and can be stably transmitted to the next generation. In pronuclear injection, the desired alteration is introduced into the male pronucleus of fertilised

oocytes, while genetic targeting involves the transfection of embryonic stem cells with a targeting vector. Despite some technical limitations, pronuclear injection is the dominating approach in genetic engineering, since it is less labour and time intensive than gene targeting.

Today, the range of applications of both techniques is continuously expanding, due to technical refinements and the discovery of new molecular tools. These developments enable science to meet the demand for improved model systems, which are required to address scientific questions in greater detail.

References

Auerbach AB (2004). Production of functional transgenic mice by DNA pronuclear injection. Acta Biochimica Polonica 51: 9–31.

Avery OT, Macleod CM and McCarty M (1944). Studies on the chemical nature of the substance inducing transformation of pneumococcal types: induction of transformation by a desoxyribonucleic acid fraction isolated from pneumococcus type III. The Journal of Experimental Medicine 79: 137–158.

Ballatore C, Lee VM and Trojanowski JQ (2007). Tau-mediated neurodegeneration in Alzheimer's disease and related disorders. Nature Reviews Neuroscience 8: 663–672.

Baltimore D (1970). RNA-dependent DNA polymerase in virions of RNA tumour viruses. Nature 226: 1209–1211.

Bogue CW (2003). Genetic models in applied physiology functional genomics in the mouse: powerful techniques for unraveling the basis of human development and disease. Journal of Applied Physiology 94: 2502–2509.

Bosma GC, Custer RP and Bosma MJ (1983). A severe combined immunodeficiency mutation in the mouse. Nature 301: 527–530.

Bourque G, Pevzner PA and Tesler G (2004). Reconstructing the genomic architecture of ancestral mammals: lessons from human, mouse, and rat genomes. Genome Research 14: 507–516.

Brinster RL, Chen HY, Trumbauer ME and Avarbock, MR (1980). Translation of globin messenger RNA by the mouse ovum Nature 283: 499–501.

Brinster RL, Chen HY, Trumbauer ME, Senear AW, Warren R and Palmiter RD (1981). Somatic expression of herpes thymidine kinase in mice following injection of a fusion gene into eggs. Cell 27: 223–231.

Brinster RL, Chen HY, Warren R, Sarthy A and Palmiter RD (1982). Regulation of metallothionein-thymidine kinase fusion plasmids injected into mouse eggs. Nature 296: 39–42.

Brinster RL, Chen HY, Trumbauer ME, Yagle MK and Palmiter RD (1985). Factors affecting the efficiency of introducing foreign DNA into mice by microinjecting eggs. Proceedings of the National Academy of Sciences USA 82: 4438–4442.

Brizzard B (2008). Epitope tagging. Biotechniques 44: 693–695.

Campbell KH, McWhir J, Ritchie WA and Wilmut I (1996). Sheep cloned by nuclear transfer from a cultured cell line. Nature 380: 64–66.

Cohen SN, Chang ACY and Hsu L (1972). Nonchromosomal antibiotic resistance in bacteria: genetic transformation of *E. coli* by R-factor DNA. Proceedings of the National Academy of Sciences USA 69: 2110–2114.

Cohen SN, Chang ACY, Boyer HW and Helling RB (1973). Construction of biologically functional bacterial plasmids *in vitro*. Proceedings of the National Academy of Sciences USA 70: 3240–3244.

Collins F (2010). Has the revolution arrived? Nature 464: 674–675.

Danna K and Nathans D (1971). Specific cleavage of simian virus 40 DNA by restriction endonuclease of *Hemophilus influenza*. Proceedings of the National Academy of Sciences USA 68: 2913–2917.

Dhup S and Majumdar SS (2008). Transgenesis via permanent integration of genes in repopulating spermatogonial cells *in vivo*. Nature Methods 5: 601–603.

DiSanto JP, Müller W, Guy-Grand D, Fischer A and Rajewsky K (1995). Lymphoid development in mice with a targeted deletion of the interleukin 2 receptor gamma chain. Proceedings of the National Academy of Sciences USA 92: 377–381.

Doetschman T, Gregg RG, Maeda N, Hooper ML, Melton DW, Thompson S and Smithies O (1987). Targeted correction of a mutant HPRT gene in mouse embryonic stem cells. Nature 330: 576–578.

Evans MJ and Kaufman MH (1981). Establishment in culture of pluripotential cells from mouse embryos. Nature 292: 154–156.

Folger KR, Wong EA, Wahl G and Capecchi MR (1982). Patterns of integration of DNA microinjected into cultured mammalian cells: evidence for homologous recombination between injected plasmid DNA molecules. Molecular and Cellular Biology 2: 1372–1387.

Franklin RE and Gosling RG (1953). Molecular configuration in sodium thymonucleate. Nature 171: 740–741.

Games D, Adams D, Alessandrini R, Barbour R, Berthelette P, Blackwell C, Carr T, Clemens J, Donaldson T, Gillespie F, Guido T, Hagopian S, Johnson-Wood K, Khan K, Lee M, Leibowitz P, Lieberburg I, Little S, Masliah E, McConlogue L, Montoya-Zavala M, Mucke L, Paganini L, Penniman E, Power M, Schenk D, Seubert P, Snyder B, Soriano F, Tan H, Vitale J, Wadsworth S, Wolozin B, and Zhao J (1995). Alzheimer-type neuropathology in transgenic mice overexpressing V717F beta-amyloid precursor protein. Nature 373: 523–527.

Gellert M (1967). Formation of covalent circles of lambda DNA by *E. coli* extracts. Proceedings of the National Academy of Sciences USA 57: 148–155

Ghildiyal M and Zamore PD (2009). Small silencing RNAs: an expanding universe. Nature Reviews Genetics 10: 94–108.

Godinho SI and Nolan PM (2006). The role of mutagenesis in defining genes in behaviour. European Journal of Human Genetics 14: 651–659.

Gordon JW, Scangos GA, Plotkin DJ, Barbosa JA and Ruddle FH (1980). Genetic transformation of mouse embryos by injection of purified DNA. Proceedings of the National Academy of Sciences 77: 7380–7384.

Gordon JW and Ruddle FH (1981). Integration and stable germ line transformation of genes injected into mouse pronuclei. Science 214: 1244–1246.

Gossen M and Bujard H (1992). Tight control of gene expression in mammalian cells by tetracycline-responsive promoters. Proceedings of the National Academy of Sciences USA 89: 5547–5551.

Grubb SC, Maddatu TP, Bult CJ and Bogue MA (2009). Mouse phenome database. Nucleic Acids Research 37 (Database issue): D720-730.

Guénet JL (2010). The mouse genome. Genome Research 15: 1729–1740.

Gu H, Zou YR and Rajewsky K (1993). Independent control of immunoglobulin switch recombination at individual switch regions evidenced through Cre-loxP-mediated gene targeting. Cell 73: 1155–1164.

Günther U, Benson J, Benke D, Fritschy JM, Reyes G, Knoflach F, Crestani F, Aguzzi A, Arigoni M, Lang Y, Bluethmann H, Möhler H and Lüscher B (1995). Benzodiazepine-insensitive mice generated by targeted disruption of the gamma 2 subunit gene of gamma-aminobutyric acid type A receptors. Proceedings of the National Academy of Sciences USA 92: 7749–7753.

Guo ZS, Li Q, Bartlett DL, Yang JY and Fang B (2008). Gene transfer: the challenge of regulated gene expression. Trends in Molecular Medicine 14: 410–418.

Harper A (2010). Mouse models of neurological disorders – a comparison of heritable and acquired traits. Biochimica et Biophysica Acta 1802: 785–795.

Hopkins AL and Groom CR (2002). The druggable genome. Nature Reviews Drug Discovery 1: 727–730.

Hsiao K, Chapman P, Nilsen S, Eckman C, Harigaya Y, Younkin S, Yang F and Cole G (1996). Correlative memory deficits, Abeta elevation, and amyloid plaques in transgenic mice. Science 274: 99–102.

Hunter AJ, Nolan PM and Brown SD (2000). Towards new models of disease and physiology in the neurosciences: the role of induced and naturally occurring mutations. Human Molecular Genetics 9: 893–900.

International Human Genome Sequencing Consortium (2001). Initial sequencing and analysis of the human genome. Nature 409: 860–921.

Ittner LM and Götz J (2007). Pronuclear injection for the production of transgenic mice. Nature Protocols 2: 1206–1215.

Jackson DA, Symons RH and Berg P (1972). Biochemical method for inserting new genetic information into DNA of simian virus 40. Proceedings of the National Academy of Sciences USA 69: 2904–2909.

Kühn R, Schwenk F, Aguet M and Rajewsky K (1995). Inducible gene targeting in mice. Science 269: 1427–1429.

Lakso M, Sauer B, Mosinger B Jr,, Lee EJ, Manning RW, Yu SH, Mulder KL and Westphal H (1992). Targeted oncogene activation by site-specific recombination in transgenic mice. Proceedings of the National Academy of Sciences USA 89: 6232–6236.

Lehman IR, Bessman MJ, Simms ES and Kornberg A (1958). Enzymatic synthesis of deoxyribonucleic acid. I. Preparation of substrates and partial purification of an enzyme from *Escherichia coli*. Journal of Biological Chemistry 233: 163–170.

Letts VA, Felix R, Biddlecome GH, Arikkath J, Mahaffey CL, Valenzuela A, Bartlett FS 2nd,, Mori Y, Campbell KP and Frankel WN (1998). The mouse stargazer gene encodes a neuronal Ca^{2+}-channel gamma subunit. Nature Genetics 19: 340–347.

Linn S and Arber W (1968). Host specificity of DNA produced by *Escherichia coli*, X. *In vitro* restriction of phage fd replicative form. Proceedings of the National Academy of Sciences USA 59: 1300–1306.

Löw K, Crestani F, Keist R, Benke D, Brünig I, Benson JA, Fritschy JM, Rülicke T, Bluethmann H, Möhler H and Rudolph U (2000). Molecular and neuronal substrate for the selective attenuation of anxiety. Science 290: 131–134.

Makino S, Kunimoto K, Muraoka Y, Mizushima Y, Katagiri K and Tochino Y (1980). Breeding of a non-obese, diabetic strain of mice. Jikken Dobutsu 29: 1–13.

Mansour SL, Thomas KR and Capecchi MR (1988). Disruption of the proto-oncogene int-2 in mouse embryo-derived stem cells: a general strategy for targeting mutations to non-selectable genes. Nature 336: 348–352.

Maxam AM and Gilbert W (1977). A new method for sequencing DNA. Proceedings of the National Academy of Sciences USA 74: 560–564.

Metzker ML (2010). Sequencing technologies - the next generation. Nature Reviews Genetics 11: 31–46.

Mendel G (1866). Versuche über Pflanzen-Hybriden. Verhandlungen des naturforschenden Vereines in Brünn 4, 3–47.

Miescher F (1871). Über die chemische Zusammensetzung der Eiterzellen. Medizinisch-chemische Untersuchungen 4: 441–460.

Morgan TH (1911). The origin of five mutations in eye color in *Drosophila* and their modes of inheritance. Science 33: 534–537.

Mouse Genome Sequencing Consortium (2002). Initial sequencing and comparative analysis of the mouse genome. Nature 420: 520–562.

Müller HJ (1925). The Regionally Differential Effect of X Rays on Crossing over in Autosomes of *Drosophila*. Genetics 10: 470–507.

Mullis KB and Faloona FA (1987). Specific synthesis of DNA *in vitro* via a polymerase-catalyzed chain reaction. Methods in Enzymology 155: 335–350.

Nakanishi T, Kuroiwa A, Yamada S, Isotani A, Yamashita A, Tairaka A, Hayashi T, Takagi T, Ikawa M, Matsuda Y and Okabe M (2002). FISH analysis of 142 EGFP transgene integration sites into the mouse genome. Genomics 80: 564–574.

Nagy A, Gertsenstein M, Vinterstein K and Behringer R (2003). Manipulating the Mouse Embryo – A Laboratory Manual (3rd edn). Cold Spring Harbor Press, Cold Spring Harbor, New York.

Nilsen TW and Graveley BR (2010). Expansion of the eukaryotic proteome by alternative splicing. Nature 463: 457–463.

Nirenberg M, Caskey T, Marshall R, Brimacombe R, Kellogg D, Doctor B, Hatfield D, Levin J, Rottman F, Pestka S, Wilcox M and Anderson F (1966). The RNA code and protein synthesis. Cold Spring Harbor Symposia on Quantitative Biology 31: 11–24.

Oakley H, Cole SL, Logan S, Maus E, Shao P, Craft J, Guillozet-Bongaarts A, Ohno M, Disterhoft J, Van Eldik L, Berry R and Vassar R (2006). Intraneuronal beta-amyloid aggregates, neurodegeneration, and neuron loss in transgenic mice with five familial Alzheimer's disease mutations: potential factors in amyloid plaque formation. Journal Neuroscience 26: 10129–10140.

Oddo S, Caccamo A, Shepherd JD, Murphy MP, Golde TE, Kayed R, Metherate R, Mattson MP, Akbari Y and LaFerla FM (2003). Triple-transgenic model of Alzheimer's disease with plaques and tangles: intracellular Abeta and synaptic dysfunction. Neuron 39: 409–421.

Overington JP, Al-Lazikani B and Hopkins AL (2006). How many drug targets are there? Nature Reviews Drug Discovery 5: 993–996.

Pearson H (2002). Surviving a knockout blow. Nature 415: 8–9 .

Perry AC, Wakayama T, Kishikawa H, Kasai T, Okabe M, Toyoda Y and Yanagimachi R (1999). Mammalian transgenesis by intracytoplasmic sperm injection. Science 284: 1180–1183.

Phillips JA 3rd,, Hjelle BL, Seeburg PH and Zachmann M (1981). Molecular basis for familial isolated growth hormone deficiency. Proceedings of the National Academy of Sciences USA 78: 6372–6375.

Robertson E, Bradley A, Kuehn M and Evans M (1986). Germ-line transmission of genes introduced into cultured pluripotential cells by retroviral vector. Nature 323: 445–448.

Rudolph U, Crestani F, Benke D, Brünig I, Benson JA, Fritschy JM, Martin JR, Bluethmann H and Möhler H (1999). Benzodiazepine actions mediated by specific gamma-aminobutyric acid(A) receptor subtypes. Nature 401: 796–800.

Rudolph U, Crestani F and Möhler H (2001). GABA(A) receptor subtypes: dissecting their pharmacological functions. Trends in Pharmacological Sciences 22: 188–194.

Russ AP and Lampel S (2005). The druggable genome: an update. Drug Discovery Today 10: 1607–1610.

Sanger F, Nicklen S and Coulson AR (1977). DNA sequencing with chain-terminating inhibitors. Proceedings of the National Academy of Sciences USA 74: 5463–5467.

Scherer LJ and Rossi JJ (2003). Approaches for the sequence-specific knockdown of mRNA. Nature Biotechnology 21: 1457–1465.

Shaner NC, Lin MZ, McKeown MR, Steinbach PA, Hazelwood KL, Davidson MW and Tsien RY (2008). Improving the photostability of bright monomeric orange and red fluorescent proteins. Nature Methods 5: 545–551.

Shimomura O, Johnson FH and Saiga Y (1962). Extraction, purification and properties of aequorin, a bioluminescent protein from the luminous hydromedusan, *Aequorea*. Journal of Cellular and Comparative Physiology 59: 223–239.

Smith HO and Wilcox KW (1970). A restriction enzyme from *Hemophilus influenza*. I. Purification and general properties. Journal of Molecular Biology 51: 379–391.

Smithies O, Gregg RG, Boggs SS, Koralewski MA and Kucherlapati RS (1985). Insertion of DNA sequences into the human chromosomal beta-globin locus by homologous recombination. Nature 317: 230–234.

Söll D, Ohtsuka E, Jones DS, Lohrmann R, Hayatsu H, Nishimura S and Khorana HG (1965). Studies on polynucleotides, XLIX. Stimulation of the binding of aminoacyl-sRNA's to ribosomes by ribotrinucleotides and a survey of codon assignments for 20 amino acids. Proceedings of the National Academy of Sciences USA 54: 1378–1385.

Stürchler-Pierrat C, Abramowski D, Duke M, Wiederhold KH, Mistl C, Rothacher S, Ledermann B, Bürki K, Frey P, Paganetti PA, Waridel C, Calhoun ME, Jucker M, Probst A, Staufenbiel M and Sommer B (1997). Two amyloid precursor protein transgenic mouse models with Alzheimer disease-like pathology. Proceedings of the National Academy of Sciences USA 94: 13287–13292.

Temin HM and Mizutani S (1970). RNA dependent DNA polymerase in virions of Rous sarcoma virus. Nature 226: 1211–1213.

Thomas KR and Capecchi MR (1987). Site-directed mutagenesis by gene targeting in mouse embryo-derived stem cells. Cell 51: 503–512.

Thomsen M, Yacoub-Youssef H and Marcheix B (2005). Reconstitution of a human immune system in immunodeficient mice: models of human alloreaction *in vivo*. Tissue Antigens 66: 73–82.

Valancius V and Smithies O (1991). Testing an "in-out" targeting procedure for making subtle genomic modifications in mouse embryonic stem cells. Molecular and Cellular Biology 11: 1402–1408.

van der Weyden L, Adams DJ and Bradley A (2002). Tools for targeted manipulation of the mouse genome. Physiological Genomics 11: 133–164.

Venter JC (2010). Multiple personal genomes await. Nature 464: 676–677.

Venter JC, Adams MD, Myers EW, Li PW, Mural RJ, Sutton GG, Smith HO, Yandell M, Evans CA, Holt RA, et al. (2001). The sequence of the human genome. Science 291: 1304–1351.

Watson JD and Crick FHC (1953). Molecular structure of nucleic acids: a structure for deoxyribose nucleic acid. Nature 171: 737–738.

Wilkins MH, Stokes AR and Wilson HR (1953). Molecular structure of deoxypentose nucleic acids. Nature 171: 738–740.

11 Signalling Complexes: Protein-protein Interactions and Lipid Rafts

11.1 Introduction to cell signalling complexes

It is well established that many signal transduction pathways are organised into large multi-protein complexes which enable spatial and temporal control of cell signalling cascades. The formation of these macromolecular complexes involves protein-protein interactions and from a drug discovery perspective there is considerable interest in developing novel therapeutics that target the boundary or interface of such interactions. This chapter will describe some important examples of cell signalling complexes with a particular emphasis on G-protein coupled receptors (covered in Chapter 3). In certain cases the initiation of intracellular signalling cascades involves the endocytosis of activated receptors from the plasma membrane in a process known as endosome-based signalling. Our understanding and knowledge of cell signalling complexes comes from the various genetic and biochemical-based techniques that have been developed to study protein-protein interactions, some of which are described in this chapter. Finally, whilst the formation of cell signalling complexes involves protein-protein interactions is also becoming increasingly apparent that micro-domains within the plasma membrane also play a role in the organisation and regulation of cell signalling cascades. Understanding how these specialised micro-domains in the plasma membrane called 'lipid rafts' regulate the clustering of receptors and associated

Molecular Pharmacology: From DNA to Drug Discovery, First Edition. John Dickenson, Fiona Freeman, Chris Lloyd Mills, Shiva Sivasubramaniam and Christian Thode.
© 2013 John Wiley & Sons, Ltd. Published 2013 by John Wiley & Sons, Ltd.

signalling proteins is a hot topic in cell physiology. Overall, these exciting developments in our understanding of the complexity of cell signalling cascades will fuel future drug discovery research.

11.2 Introduction to GPCR interacting proteins

During the last decade it has become apparent that GPCRs interact not only with heterotrimeric G-proteins, arrestins and GRKs (see Chapter 3) but also with a host of other proteins known collectively as GPCR interacting proteins. These accessory proteins are involved in the modulation of GPCR signalling and pharmacology, the targeting of GPCRs to particular sub-cellular compartments, the regulation of GPCR trafficking to the plasma membrane, receptor desensitisation/resensitisation, and the formation of GPCR signalling complexes (reviewed by Magalhaes et al., 2012; Bockaert et al., 2010; Ritter and Hall, 2009; Bockaert et al., 2004). In this section we will review some prominent examples of GPCR interacting proteins illustrating how they modulate GPCR function.

Some of the GPCR interacting proteins identified to date are transmembrane proteins and include other GPCRs (dimerisation), ion channels, ligand-gated ion channels (ionotropic receptors) and single transmembrane proteins (e.g. RAMPs). However, the vast majority of GPCR interacting proteins are soluble cytoplasmic proteins that predominantly interact with the C-terminal tail of the receptor. Proteins containing a PDZ domain are the most common class of GPCR interacting protein which interact with a short consensus amino acid sequence usually found at the extreme end of the receptor's C-terminus.

11.3 Methods used to identify GPCR interacting proteins

The identification and characterisation of novel protein-protein interactions is an intense area of research in the quest to fully understand the complexity of cell signalling pathways and protein networks in living systems. A wide variety of genetic and biochemical-based approaches have been adopted and developed in order to identify novel GPCR interacting proteins. The long-term goal of such research is the potential identification of novel drug targets that can be used to modulate GPCR function independently of the classical pharmaceutical approach of targeting GPCRs using agonists and antagonists. However there are many pitfalls and problems that need to be addressed when studying protein complexes involving membrane proteins including solubilisation. Approaches to study GPCR interacting proteins fall into two main categories: those that use the entire receptor as 'bait' and those that use a specific GPCR domain such as the C-terminal tail as 'bait'. Although the use of specific receptor domains overcomes the problems of receptor solubilisation it cannot be used for interactions involving transmembrane domains. It is beyond the scope of this

Table 11.1 Examples of GPCR interacting proteins.

Interacting Protein	GPCR	Site of interaction	Functional role
Arrestin2	Ubiquitous	CT	Desensitization
GRKs	Ubiquitous	CT	Desensitization
AKAP5	β_2AR	CT	Localises PKA to the receptor
Calmodulin	D2-R	i3	Ca^{2+}-dependent attenuation of G-protein signalling
GASP1	D2-R	CT	Targets receptor to lysosomes for degradation
Homer	mGlu$_1$	CT	Regulates receptor Ca^{2+} signalling
Jak2	AT$_1$	CT	Triggers Jak/STAT signalling
NHERF-1	β_2AR	CT	Promotes activation of Na^+/H^+ exchanger
NHERF-2	mGlu$_5$	CT	Prolongs receptor-mediated Ca^{2+} signalling
RAMP1	CLR	NT, TM	Forms functional adrenomedullin receptors

Abbreviations: AT$_1$, angiotensin type 1 receptor; β_2AR, β_2-adrenoceptor; CLR, calcitonin-like receptor; CT, C-terminus; D2-R, dopamine D2 receptor; i3, third intracellular loop; mGlu, metabotropic glutamate receptor; NT, N-terminus; TM, transmembrane domain.

section to describe all the approaches used to identify GPCR interacting proteins but they are reviewed by Daulat et al. (2008). When investigating GPCR interacting proteins it is important to remember the dynamic and temporal nature of protein-protein interactions and the possible influence post-translational modifications may have on such events since many GPCRs are phosphorylated and/or ubiquitinated following receptor activation.

Molecular biology-based approaches
Yeast two-hybrid assay

The yeast two-hybrid system is a genetic-based approach used to identify novel protein-protein and protein-DNA interactions. The technique was developed by Fields and Song (1989) and is based upon the activation of a reporter gene (typically the LacZ gene which encodes for β-galactosidase) by the Gal4 transcription factor in yeast. Gal4 triggers gene transcription by binding to the upstream activating sequence (UAS), a *cis*-acting regulatory DNA sequence. An essential feature of the yeast two-hybrid assay is the splitting of the Gal4 transcription factor into two key protein fragments; the DNA-binding domain (Gal4-BD) and activating domain (Gal4-AD), which are responsible for UAS binding and activation of transcription, respectively (Figure 11.1). Although Gal4 is split it can still trigger gene transcription if the two protein fragments are brought together in close proximity. This is analogous to fluorescent protein-fragment complementation assays involving fragments of fluorescent protein which recombine to form a functional protein when brought into close proximity following GPCR dimerisation (see Chapter 3). Initially yeast two-hybrid screening

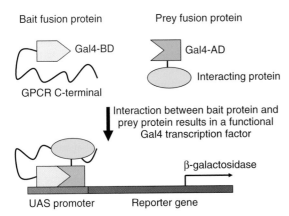

Figure 11.1 The yeast two-hybrid assay for detecting protein-protein interactions.

involves generating DNA plasmids containing Gal4-BD and Gal4-AD fusion proteins. Generally, the protein fused onto Gal-BD is referred to as the 'bait' and could for example be the C-terminal tail of a GPCR, whereas the protein fused onto Gal4-AD is referred to as the 'prey' and this could be a single known protein or a library of known or unknown proteins. A library in molecular biology terms is a collection of DNA fragments (usually cDNA derived) each inserted into an appropriate cloning vector. When the 'bait' and 'prey' plasmids are transfected into yeast cells reporter gene expression will only occur if the protein products interact to generate a functional Gal4 protein. The plasmids encoding the Gal4-BD and Gal4-AD fusion proteins also contain selection genes which typically encode for enzymes involved in the synthesis of specific amino acids essential for cell growth. When grown on minimal media only yeast cells containing both plasmids will survive. Furthermore, yeast cells that survive and display functional Gal4 activity will express β-galactosidase and stain blue when exposed to a suitable colorimetric substrate. Yeast cells expressing both plasmids but without functional Gal4 activity will survive but not stain blue. When using an expression cDNA library of unknown proteins the identity of the interacting protein is achieved via DNA sequencing of the positive 'prey' plasmids. Thus, in theory, the yeast two-hybrid system is a simply and efficient method for investigating protein-protein interactions which are not dependent upon post-translational modifications.

Split-ubiquitin yeast two-hybrid assay

The yeast two-hybrid assay is only suitable for binary detecting interactions between soluble proteins. To overcome this limitation the split-ubiquitin yeast two-hybrid assay was developed which allows screening for protein-protein interactions involving soluble and membrane proteins. The assay is also based upon fragment complementation and involves the 76 amino acid regulatory protein ubiquitin split into C-terminal (Cub; residues 35–76) and N-terminal halves (Nub; residues 1–34). The 'bait' protein, for example the full-length GPCR sequence, is fused to Cub, whereas the 'prey' proteins are fused to Nub. How do interacting Cub and Nub fragments trigger reporter gene expression? The Cub fragment is also fused to a transcription factor that is cleaved off by ubiquitin-specific proteases. Hence, when the 'bait' protein interacts with a 'prey' protein the Cub and Nub fragments re-assemble allowing the split-ubiquitin protein to be recognised by ubiquitin-specific proteases. The transcription factor which is cleaved from the Cub

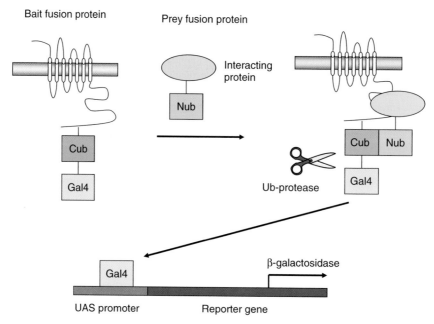

Figure 11.2 The split-ubiquitin yeast two-hybrid assay for detecting protein-protein interactions.

fragment translocates to the nucleus, leading to the activation of a reporter gene (Figure 11.2).

Although two-hybrid screens are widely used in many laboratories they can result in a large number of false positive and false negative interactions. The reasons for false positives are varied may include the following; (i) the over-expression of proteins that may result in non-specific interactions; (ii) the use of fusion proteins that may influence protein interactions; and (iii) lack of post-translational modifications to mammalian proteins as a consequence of using yeast cells.

Biochemical-based approaches
Immunoprecipitation assays
Immunopreciptation is a well-established biochemical method that allows the isolation of protein complexes from mammalian cell and/or tissue lysates. When studying GPCRs this can be achieved either by using epitope-tagged receptors in combination with an anti-epitope antibody or if available specific GPCR antibodies (Figure 11.3). In both cases it allows for detection of proteins interacting with the full-length of the receptor. The use of specific GPCR antibodies also has the distinct advantage of allowing GPCR interacting proteins to be studied in native tissue and cells expressing endogenous

receptors. However, from a practical viewpoint it is important to remember that solubilisation of hydrophobic membrane proteins may destabilise protein interactions and/or generate artificial aggregations.

GST pull-down assays
Glutathione-S-transferase (GST) is a protein of 220 amino acids that has a high affinity for glutathione and is frequently used to facilitate the purification of protein-protein complexes. The first stage in a typical GST-pull down experiment is the expression in bacteria of a GST fusion protein which is comprised of GST attached to a suitable 'bait' protein (e.g. C-terminus of a GPCR). The GST fusion protein is subsequently purified by affinity chromatography using glutathione-agarose beads. To identify or 'fish-out' proteins interacting with the GPCR C-terminus, the purified GST fusion protein is simply incubated with an appropriate cell lysate in the presence of glutathione-agarose beads. The beads are washed to remove any contaminating bacterial proteins and complexes analysed using either one-dimensional (1D) or two-dimensional (2D) gel electrophoresis to separate proteins and aid identification of interacting proteins by mass spectrometry analysis (Figure 11.4).

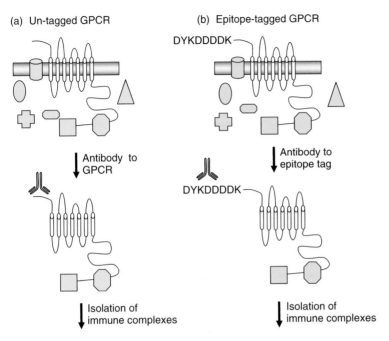

(a) Un-tagged GPCR

(b) Epitope-tagged GPCR

DYKDDDDK

Antibody to GPCR

Antibody to epitope tag

DYKDDDDK

Isolation of immune complexes

Isolation of immune complexes

Figure 11.3 Identifying protein-protein interactions using immunoprecipitation-based assays. GPCRs and their associated proteins can quickly be isolated using either (a) GPCR-specific antibodies or (b) anti-epitope antibodies if using epitope-tagged receptors. In this case the GPCR has the FLAG epitope (DYKDDDDK; single letter amino acid code) located at the end of its N-terminus.

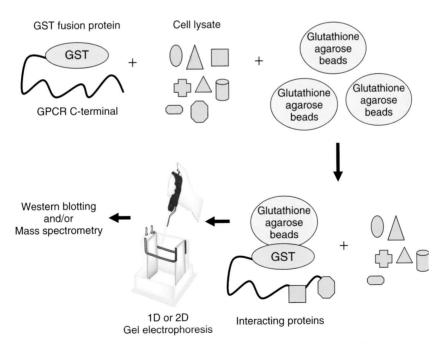

GST fusion protein

GST

GPCR C-terminal

Cell lysate

Glutathione agarose beads

Glutathione agarose beads

Glutathione agarose beads

Western blotting and/or Mass spectrometry

Glutathione agarose beads

GST

Interacting proteins

1D or 2D Gel electrophoresis

Figure 11.4 Identification of protein-protein interactions using GST fusion proteins.

Peptide affinity chromatography

Although the techniques for identifying GPCR interacting proteins covered so far are valid they do have a number of limitations including the generation of many false positives (yeast two-hybrid screens), detection of only binary interactions (yeast two-hybrid), and contamination with bacterial proteins (GST pull-down assays). Some of these problems have been overcome by the use of peptide affinity chromatography using chemically synthesised peptides containing an affinity tag of six consecutive histidine residues (His_6) coupled to the C-terminus of the GPCR under investigation (Pascal et al., 2008). The polyhistidine tag enables the rapid purification of recombinant proteins due to its high-affinity for nickel or cobalt-based affinity resins which have the metal chelating group nitrotriacetic (NTA) covalently attached. To 'fish-out' interacting proteins cell lysates are simply incubated with the His_6-tagged peptide, applied to the Ni-NTA agarose resin and then extensively washed to remove non-interacting proteins (Figure 11.5). Peptides are eluted from the resin and proteins interacting with the His_6-tagged peptide identified using 1D or 2D gel electrophoresis followed by mass spectrometry analysis. With this approach it is also possible to use very small 'bait' sequences such as PDZ domain binding motifs.

Protein micro-array analysis

Several recent investigations have employed protein micro-array methodology to identity novel GPCR interactions with PDZ domains. Protein micro-arrays are produced by spotting a range of different purified proteins or in this case specific PDZ protein domains onto nylon membranes (typically 96-spot formats). The protein array is first probed with an appropriate GPCR domain fusion protein (e.g. GPCR C-terminus tagged with GST) and then extensively washed to remove non-bound GST fusion protein. Specific binding of the GPCR fusion protein to any of the spotted proteins in the array is detected by incubating the membrane with an anti-GST antibody coupled to horseradish peroxidise (HRP). Antibody binding is visualised either via HRP-catalysed generation of a coloured product or if using a chemiluminescent substrate by detecting the light emitted (Figure 11.6). Although protein micro-arrays provide an alternative approach for detecting novel GPCR interacting proteins they are initially very time consuming due to the need for purified proteins and are limited to binary interactions.

The techniques described above are not only applicable for the identification of GPCR interacting proteins but also for exploring protein complexes associated

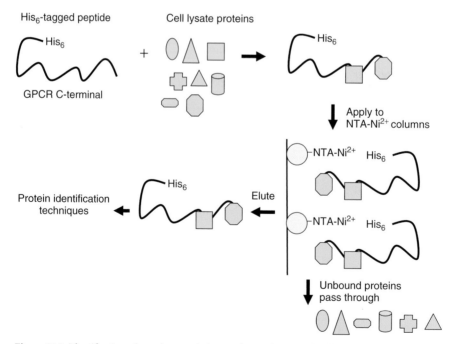

Figure 11.5 Identification of protein-protein interactions using peptide-affinity chromatography.

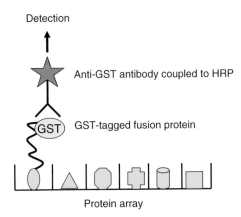

Figure 11.6 Identification of GPCR interacting proteins using protein micro-array analysis.

with many other important drug targets including ion channels, tyrosine kinase-linked receptors, transcription factors and transporters. Finally, it is important to determine whether proteins shown to interact using the above techniques are co-expressed in the same tissue and/or cells. This can be achieved through *in-situ* hybridisation assays to confirm mRNA co-expression and/or if suitable antibodies are available through protein co-expression in tissue (immunohistochemistry) or cells (immunocytochemistry).

11.4 Functional roles of GPCR interacting proteins

This section will discuss three prominent examples of GPCR interacting proteins illustrating how such proteins can influence receptor signalling, pharmacology and trafficking.

GPCR signalling independent of heterotrimeric G-proteins

It is now well known that some GPCRs can modulate cell signalling pathways independently of heterotrimeric G-proteins. For example, following agonist activation the angiotensin type 1 receptor (AT_1) associates with a non-receptor tyrosine kinase called Jak2. The recruitment of Jak2 to the C-terminal tail of the AT_1 receptor leads to the activation of Jak2-dependent signalling pathways including phosphorylation of the transcription factor STAT. Once phosphorylated, STAT proteins dimerise and translocate to the nucleus where they trigger gene transcription (Figure 11.7a).

The Na^+/H^+ exchange regulatory factor 1 (NHERF1) is a PDZ domain containing protein which associates with the β_2AR following agonist activation of the receptor (Figure 11.7b). Interestingly this association prevents NHERF1 from inhibiting the Na^+/H^+ exchanger 3 (NHE3) and in doing so enables the β_2AR to activate Na^+/H^+ exchange in the kidney via a G-protein independent pathway. NHE3 is a membrane transporter found in the nephron which is partly responsible for regulating sodium balance.

The above examples illustrate how agonist-activated GPCRs can stimulate cell signalling pathways independently of G-proteins. There are also some interesting cases where agonist-activation of a GPCR reduces the interaction between receptor and associated protein(s). For example, association of the sst_2 receptor with the p85 subunit of phosphoinositide 3-kinase (PI-3K) is reduced following agonist stimulation (Figure 11.7c). This results in reduced activation of PI-3K (an enzyme involved in promoting cell survival pathways) and hence increased sensitivity to apoptotic stimuli.

Modulation of GPCR pharmacology

So far we have discussed cytoplasmic GPCR associated proteins that interact with the C-terminal tails of such receptors. What about interactions with transmembrane proteins? Although there are several interesting examples of single transmembrane domain proteins that interact and modulate GPCR function it was the discovery of receptor-activity modifying proteins (RAMPs) that significantly changed the understanding of GPCR pharmacology. Indeed, the discovery of RAMPs is an interesting story which partly illustrates some of the problems that can be encountered during expression cloning of GPCRs. RAMPs were reported in 1998 by McLatchie et al. whilst trying to identify the receptor for the neuropeptide calcitonin gene-related peptide (CGRP). Previous studies had shown that an orphan GPCR named the calcitonin-like receptor (CLR; now classified as a class B GPCR) responded to CGRP when expressed in the HEK293 cells. These cells generated in the 1970s from human embryonic kidney cells are widely used by molecular pharmacologists as a heterologous expression system. However, these results were in stark contrast to a prior study performed using transfected COS-7 cells (another widely used model cell line), which had not responded to CGRP. At the time it was suggested that a 'factor' expressed by HEK293 cells (but not COS-7 cells) was required for the detection of CGRP binding in cells expressing the calcitonin-like receptor. This proved to be the case when McLatchie

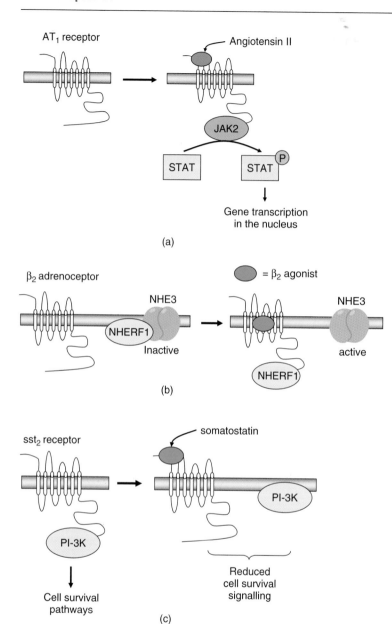

(a)

(b)

(c)

Figure 11.7 GPCR signalling independent of heterotrimeric G-proteins. The concept that GPCRs can regulate cell signalling pathways independently of classical heterotrimeric G-protein coupling is illustrated by (a) AT_1 receptor-mediated activation of JAK/STAT signalling, (b) β_2-adrenoceptor-mediated activation of the NHE exchanger and (c) sst_2 receptor-mediated attenuation of PI-3K signalling.

and colleagues reported that RAMP1 was essential for the trafficking or 'chaperoning' of the calcitonin-like receptor from the endoplasmic reticulum/Golgi apparatus to the cell membrane. Thus in the absence of RAMP1, the calcitonin-like receptor is not glycosylated within its N-terminus and remains 'trapped' in the endoplasmic reticulum. The reason for the absence of CGRP binding to transfected COS-7 cells is due to the fact that these cells do not endogenously express RAMP1.

McLatchie and co-workers also reported the existence of two additional members of the RAMP family; namely RAMP2 and RAMP3. The most intriguing observation was that interactions between RAMP2 and the calcitonin-like receptor generated a high-affinity receptor for a related peptide called adrenomedullin. Therefore the pharmacology of the calcitonin-like receptor is dependent upon its association with RAMP1 (generating the CGRP receptor) or RAMP2 (generating the adrenomedullin receptor; AM_1). The calcitonin-like receptor also interacts

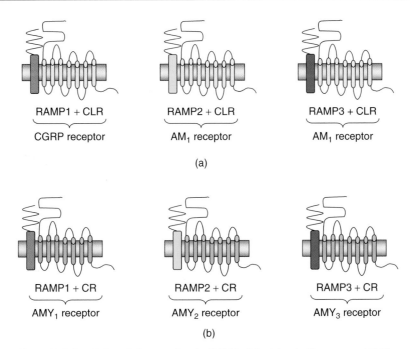

Figure 11.8 Regulation of pharmacology by RAMPs. (a) calcitonin-like receptor (CLR) and (b) calcitonin receptor (CR).

with RAMP3 producing a pharmacologically distinct adrenomedullin receptor (AM_2). These interactions are summarised in Figure 11.8a.

RAMP proteins also interact with the calcitonin receptor and in doing so generate three subtypes of amylin (AMY) receptor, named AMY_{1-3} (Figure 11.8b). There is also evidence for RAMP interactions with other class B GPCR family members including the $VPAC_1$ receptor (all RAMPs), glucagon receptor (RAMP2), and parathyroid hormone receptors (PTH_1 with RAMP2 and PTH_2 with RAMP3). The exact significance of these RAMP/GPCR interactions remains to be fully established. Finally, recent investigations have shown that RAMP interactions with GPCRs are not restricted to class B GPCRs. The calcium-sensing receptor which belongs to class C requires RAMP1 or RAMP3 for translocation to the cell membrane (Bouschet et al., 2008). Hence RAMPs may have a widespread role in regulating GPCR function.

Since RAMPs modulate GPCR function they potentially represent exciting drug targets. In order to design and develop novel therapeutics based on RAMP/GPCR binding it is important to understand the regions involved in such interactions. For example, in the case of the calcitonin receptor it appears that the long N-terminus sequence of the RAMP is important for determining receptor pharmacology, whereas RAMP transmembrane domains are involved in binding to the GPCR. Another important question relating to RAMPs concerns the mechanism of precisely how they modulate GPCR pharmacology. It is likely that the GPCR ligands bind directly to a novel binding site involving protein domain(s) associated with the RAMP and GPCR interface. Alternatively, RAMPs may influence GPCR pharmacology indirectly in an allosteric manner by altering GPCR conformation. Identifying which of these two mechanisms operates is experimentally difficult and it is likely that both contribute to the dramatic influence of RAMPs on GPCR pharmacology. In summary, RAMPs interact with GPCRs to modulate pharmacology and promote cell surface expression by functioning as a chaperone molecule. The PDZ domain present in RAMP3 also enables interaction with a host of other proteins which influence GPCR trafficking. For further in-depth reading on the varied functions of RAMPs see Sexton et al. (2009), Hay et al. (2006) and Parameswaran and Spielman (2006).

Regulation of GPCR trafficking

As previously explained in Chapter 3 (section 3.4) most GPCRs are removed from the plasma membrane and internalised into endosomes following agonist activation. A number of GPCR interacting proteins are involved in the post-endocytic trafficking of receptors either back to the plasma membrane or for degradation via lysosomes or the 26S proteasome. GPCRs also need to be chaperoned from their site of biosynthesis to the cell membrane and this also involves a host of GPCR interacting proteins. Examples of GPCR interacting proteins involved in GPCR trafficking and endocytosis are briefly described below.

An increasing number of proteins are associated with the biosynthetic trafficking of GPCRs following translation including, as we have already covered, other GPCRs (the process of heterodimerisation) and RAMPs. Additional proteins found to regulate GPCR trafficking to the cell membrane are GEC1 (κ-opioid receptor), RACK1 (thromboxane receptor), and DRIP78 (Dopamine D1 receptor). Understanding the molecular mechanisms associated with GPCR biosynthetic trafficking is of clinical importance since a number of congenital diseases are linked to GPCR mutations that cause retention of the misfolded protein in the endoplasmic reticulum (Bernier et al., 2004). Examples include mutations in the V_2 vasopressin receptor which are responsible for nephrogenic diabetes insipidus. Indeed a relatively new concept in the treatment of such conditions is the use of small molecule pharmacological chaperones which stabilise the misfolded protein and promote export from the endoplasmic reticulum. There are also GPCR interacting proteins which target receptors to specific regions of the plasma membrane. A prominent example being the Homer proteins which promote the clustering of $mGlu_1$ and $mGlu_5$ receptors to post-dendritic spines: a small membranous region of a dendrite that receives excitatory input from axons. This enables the $mGlu_{1/5}$ receptors to respond rapidly to glutamate released into the synaptic cleft. The $5\text{-}HT_{2A}$ receptor is also localised to post-dendritic spines via its interaction with post-synaptic density protein 95 (PSD-95). Other interesting examples include clustering of the $mGlu_7$ receptor to pre-synaptic sites via interaction with the PDZ scaffold protein PICK1 and targeting of the somatostatin sst_3 receptor to tight junctions in epithelial cells through Mupp1.

Many proteins initiate the endocytosis of GPCRs from the plasma membrane including GRKs and arrestins. A host of other proteins also control the post-endocytic trafficking of GPCRs including GPCR-associated sorting proteins (GASPs) which promote receptor sorting to lysosomes. In contrast, interaction of certain GPCRs with proteins such as NHERF-1 facilitates rapid recycling back to the plasma membrane. Hence, the sorting fate of some GPCRs is dependent upon the type of interacting protein associated with its C-terminus (Figure 11.9).

11.5 GPCR signalling complexes

It is known that many GPCRs and ion channels exist in large multi-protein complexes. In the case of GPCRs the term 'receptosome' is frequently used to describe the interaction of receptors with a specific group of proteins. Receptosome complexes regulate many aspects of GPCR life including anchoring and positioning of GPCRs at specific sites within the cell membrane, modulation of cell signalling events, as well as receptor internalisation and recycling. For molecular pharmacologists understanding the complex and dynamic interactions of specific receptosome proteins with a receptor will be critical for assessing whether such interactions are potential future drug targets.

GPCR-arrestin receptosome and arrestin-selective biased agonists

An increasing number of examples illustrate the concept of GPCR receptosomes. One of the first families of proteins shown to directly interact with GPCRs was the arrestins which are traditionally associated with the process of receptor desensitisation and internalisation (see Chapter 3). The visual arrestins (arrestin1 and 4) are solely expressed in visual sensory tissue where they bind to light-activated phosphorylated rhodopsin. The non-visual arrestins, arrestin2 (also known as β-arrestin1) and arrestin3 (β-arrestin2) are ubiquitously expressed and bind to many GPCRs. Once bound to GPCRs, arrestins recruit a host of proteins involved in the process of receptor endocytosis and trafficking including clathrin, AP-2 (adaptor protein 2) and N-ethylmaleimide-sensitive factor (NSF; see Figure 11.10). Interestingly, an obligatory step in β_2-adrenergic receptor internalisation is the ubiquitination of arrestin which is mediated by the recruitment of E3 ubiquitin ligase by arrestin itself.

Whilst the above consequences of arrestin binding are associated with terminating receptor responses, the role of arrestins extends beyond this and involves the recruitment and activation of cell signalling pathways (so called arrestin-dependent) once the receptor has internalised. Protein kinases including Src tyrosine kinase, ERK1/2 and c-Jun N-terminal kinase 3 (JNK3) bind to arrestins and are recruited to agonist-occupied

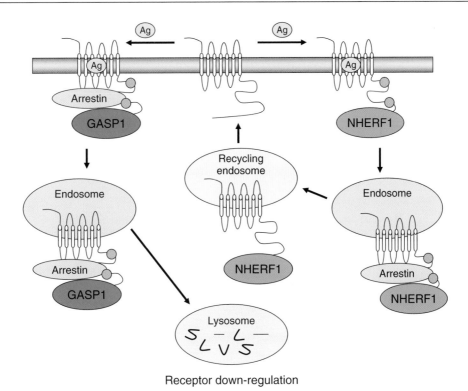

Receptor down-regulation

Figure 11.9 GPCR interacting proteins regulate post-endocytic trafficking of GPCRs. Following receptor activation GPCRs are rapidly removed from the plasma membrane and internalised into endocytic compartments. The fate of the internalised GPCR is determined by specific GPCR interacting proteins that interact with the C-terminus of the receptor. Interaction with NHERF-1 promotes recycling of receptors back to the plasma membrane (resensitisation), whereas interaction with GASP1 targets receptors for degradation (down-regulation).

receptors (Figure 11.10). The topic of arrestin-dependent signalling is extensively covered in two recent review articles (Luttrell and Gesty-Palmer, 2010; Shenoy and Lefkowitz, 2011). Indeed, arrestin-dependent signalling is partly responsible for the phenomenon of agonist-directed signalling covered in Chapter 3. Investigations using molecular-biology based approaches including arrestin knockouts and transgenic expression of G protein-uncoupled receptor mutants (useful for studying G-protein independent aspects of GPCR function) have revealed some of the physiological functions of arrestin-dependent signalling. Such roles include regulating cardiomyocyte hypertrophy and cell survival, promoting tumour growth, and embryonic development. The development of arrestin-selective biased agonists is an exciting prospect involving ligands that promote arrestin-dependent signalling in the absence of G-protein activation (Figure 11.11).

That is they behave as neutral antagonists or inverse agonists of G-protein signalling whilst functioning as agonists for arrestin-recruitment to the receptor and hence promote arrestin-dependent signalling. The non-selective β_2-adrenergic receptor ligands propranolol and carvedilol (both widely used beta-blockers), which are partial inverse agonists for G_s-protein signalling, function as agonists for arrestin-dependent activation of ERK1/2 by recruiting arrestins. In the future it may be useful to incorporate screening for arrestin-dependent signalling during drug discovery programmes.

Biased agonists in clinical trials

In this section we will briefly cover some very recent developments in biased agonists that target the angiotensin type 1 receptor (AT_1R). The AT_1R mediates the physiological effects of the peptide hormone angiotensin II;

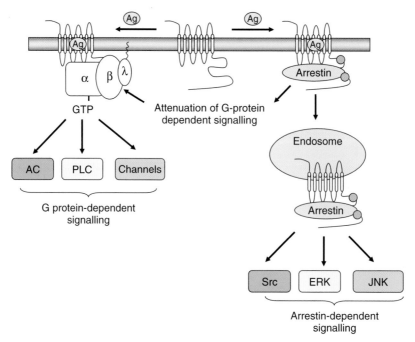

Figure 11.10 Arrestin-dependent endocytosis and cell signalling. Classical GPCR signalling dependent upon coupling to heterotrimeric G-proteins is rapidly attenuated by arrestins which are recruited to the agonist-occupied receptor in response to GRK-mediated receptor phosphorylation (red circles). Paradoxically the internalised GPCR/arrestin complex also functions as a scaffold for the recruitment and activation of several protein kinase cascades. Abbreviations: AC, adenylyl cyclase; Ag, agonist; ERK, extracellular signal-regulated kinase; PLC, phospholipase C; Src, Src tyrosine kinase; JNK, C-Jun N-terminal kinase.

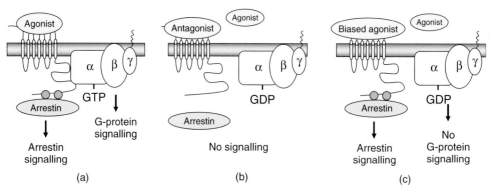

Figure 11.11 Classical agonist versus biased-agonist GPCR signalling. (a) Classical GPCRs agonist promote both G-protein-dependent and arrestin-mediated signalling. (b) Classical GPCR antagonists block agonist binding to the receptor preventing both G-protein and arrestin-mediated signalling. (c) Biased agonists stimulate arrestin-mediated signalling and block G-protein-dependent signalling.

a classical vasopressor whose levels are often elevated in patients with hypertension and heart failure. As such angiotensin-converting enzyme inhibitors and AT_1R antagonists are heavily used in the treatment of hypertension and other cardiovascular diseases.

The AT_1R activates numerous signalling pathways that are either G-protein dependent or arrestin-dependent (Figure 11.12). From a physiological perspective G-protein-dependent signalling is associated with classical AT_1R-induced vasoconstriction, whereas

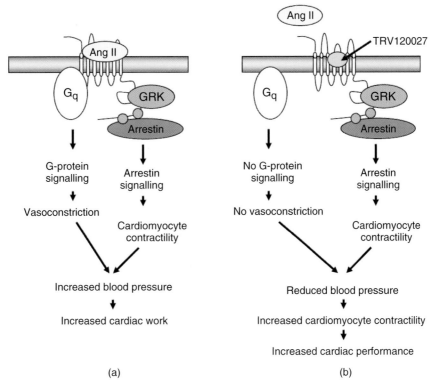

Figure 11.12 Targeting the AT_1R with biased agonists to treat acute heart failure. (a) When activated by angiotensin II the AT_1R triggers G_q-protein dependent and arrestin-dependent signalling pathways that promote vasoconstriction and cardiomyocyte contraction, respectively. (b) The biased agonist TRV120027 only promotes activation of arrestin-dependent signalling thus triggering cardiomyocyte contractility. This novel pharmacology may be explained by TRV120027 inducing a conformation in the AT_1R which promotes GRK-mediated phosphorylation of the receptor (red circles) and subsequent arrestin binding that is independent of classical agonist-induced G-protein activation. Figure modified from DeWire and Violin (2011) Circulation Research 109: 205–216.

arrestin-dependent signalling promotes AT_1R-mediated cell survival (anti-apoptotic) and cardiac contractility. Whilst traditional AT_1R antagonists, which block all AT_1R-mediated functions, are used widely to treat high blood pressure they may not be suitable for acute heart failure patients who would benefit from reduced hypertension but increased cardiac performance. Recently an AT_1R biased agonist (TRV120027) has been developed which competes with angiotensin II for the AT_1R (Violin et al., 2010). TRV120027 reduces angiotensin II-induced hypertension in animal models whilst promoting cardiac contractility suggesting it blocks classical G-protein dependent signalling whilst engaging arrestin-dependent signalling (Figure 11.12). TRV120027 is currently undergoing phase 2 clinical trials for acute heart failure and as such is the first biased ligand to do so. It is likely that research into biased agonist-based therapeutics will intensify as our

knowledge of GPCR signalling complexity increases thus allowing for the development of drugs that selectively activate or block specific signalling pathways mediated by a particular GPCR. For a comprehensive review discussing the concept of AT_1R biased ligands see DeWire and Violin (2011).

β_2-AR signalling complexes

β_1AR and β_2ARs play prominent roles in the regulation cardiac excitation-contraction coupling via the phosphorylation of key regulatory proteins. However, although both receptors are G_s-coupled and stimulate cAMP/PKA signalling, activation of the β_2AR results in the phosphorylation of a restricted range of proteins as a consequence of localised PKA activation within the cell. For example, whilst both receptors increase Ca^{2+} influx into cardiac myocytes through the activation of plasma membrane-bound voltage-dependent Ca^{2+} channels, the β_1AR but not the β_2AR, also phosphorylates phospholamban in the sarcoplasmic reticulum membrane, troponin I and C proteins in myofilaments, and glycogen phosphorylase kinase in the cytoplasm. These differences in target protein phosphorylation result in some marked physiological differences between β_1AR and β_2AR function in cardiac myocytes. Whilst both receptor subtypes exert a positive inotropic effect (increased force of muscle contraction) only the β_1AR accelerates muscle relaxation (shortens duration of contraction) and promotes glycogen breakdown via PKA-mediated phosphorylation of phospholamban and glycogen phosphorylase kinase, respectively. How is the spatial localisation or compartmentalisation of β_1AR and β_2AR signalling achieved?

The spatial localisation of β_2AR signalling involves the receptor interacting with scaffold proteins called A-kinase anchoring proteins (AKAPs). Scaffold proteins help localise and organise cell signalling proteins to specific areas of the cell (Figure 11.13).

The β_2AR interacts via its C-terminus with two members of the AKAP family called AKAP5 (also known as AKAP79/150) and AKAP12 (also known as gravin and AKAP250). Association of the β_2AR with AKAP12 is agonist-dependent and is enhanced by PKA-mediated phosphorylation of the receptor, whereas AKAP5 is constitutively associated with the receptor. Association with AKAP12 is involved in the internalisation and resensitisation of the β_2AR after agonist stimulation. However, it is the association with AKAP5 that is responsible for localised β_2AR signalling in cardiac myocytes. The β_2AR signalling complex contains the L-type voltage-dependent Ca^{2+} channel subunit $Ca_v1.2$, G_s-protein, adenylyl cyclase, and PKA all anchored together via AKAP5 (Figure 11.14). This complex partly explains the differences between β_2AR signalling, which is restricted to the cell membrane, and β_1AR signalling which occurs throughout the cell. However, there are some additional mechanisms responsible for the restriction of β_2AR-induced cyclic AMP formation. Firstly, the β_2AR can temporally limit cyclic AMP formation by switching from G_s-protein to G_i-protein coupling (see Chapter 3). This switching in G-protein coupling is achieved via PKA-mediated phosphorylation of the receptor and results in β_2AR-mediated inhibition of adenylyl cyclase thus restricting cyclic AMP generation. Secondly, the activity of adenylyl cyclase isoforms V and VI, which are known to associate with AKAP5, is inhibited when phosphorylated by PKA. Although it is not known if this precise mechanism occurs in cardiac myocytes it would provide an effective negative feedback mechanism for restricting cyclic AMP formation. Finally, the lifetime of cyclic AMP may be limited by the recruitment of phosphodiesterases (cyclic AMP degrading enzymes) to the active β_2AR signalling complex. This may involve arrestins and/or AKAP12 but as yet it is not known whether these proteins are associated with the β_2AR-$Ca_v1.2$ signalling complex (Figure 11.14). The above example illustrates how the spatial and temporal aspects of GPCR signalling can be

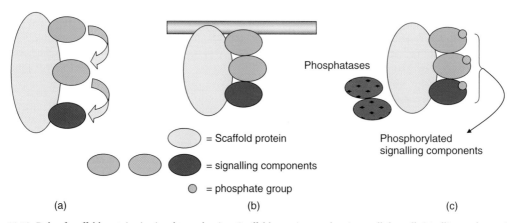

Phosphatases

Phosphorylated signalling components

= Scaffold protein

= signalling components

= phosphate group

(a)   (b)   (c)

Figure 11.13 Role of scaffold proteins in signal transduction. Scaffold proteins regulate intracellular cell signalling pathways in a number of ways including the tethering of several signalling proteins together (a). A good example is the linking of a protein kinase with its substrate protein to ensure specificity. Other roles include localisation of signalling molecules to a specific area of the cell (b) and in the case of protein kinases cascades protecton from inactivation by phosphatases (c).

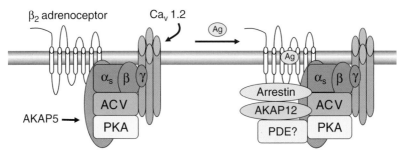

Figure 11.14 Compartmentalisation of β_2-adrenoceptor-mediated cell signalling. The β_2 adrenoceptor constitutively associates with the scaffold protein AKAP5 enabling the co-localization of G_s/AC/PKA signalling for voltage-sensitive Ca^{2+} channel activation ($Ca_v1.2$). Following agonist stimulation both arrestin and AKAP12 are recruited to the phosphorylated receptor prompting internalisation and arrestin-dependent signalling. Phosphodiesterases (PDEs) may also be recruited to spatially restrict cAMP formation.

'fine-tuned' and regulated by the assembly of large multi-protein complexes. Understanding the complex nature of β_1AR and β_2AR signalling may lead to the development of novel therapeutics to treat heart disease as a condition which involves significant changes in βAR signalling.

GPCR signalling complexes in the central nervous system

Receptors for several prominent neurotransmitters including glutamate, 5-HT, and dopamine engage with a host of GPCR interacting proteins. These multi-protein complexes play an important role in modulating CNS physiology and in certain cases disruption of such interactions promotes several neurological and psychological disorders (see Bockaert et al., 2010 for a comprehensive review on this topic). This section will briefly describe three examples of GPCR signalling complexes in the CNS.

Post-synaptic mGlu$_1$ and mGlu$_5$ receptor complexes

Metabotropic glutamate receptors (mGlu$_{1-8}$) are predominantly expressed in the CNS where they modulate synaptic plasticity events associated with learning and memory. There is considerable interest in the development of selective mGlu receptor ligands for the treatment of several CNS disorders including anxiety, depression, schizophrenia and epilepsy. The post-synaptic mGlu$_1$ and mGlu$_5$ receptors, which exists as constitutive homodimers (see Chapter 3), also interact with a scaffold protein known as Homer. Homer proteins interact with various Ca^{2+} channels including inositol triphosphate (IP$_3$) and ryanodine receptors, store-operated transient receptor channels (TRP), and the $Ca_v2.1$ subunit of P/Q type

voltage sensitive Ca^{2+} channels (Figure 11.15) creating a multi-protein complex that regulates mGlu$_1$ and mGlu$_5$ receptor Ca^{2+} signalling. Finally, a post-synaptic density protein called Shank links mGlu$_1$ and mGlu$_5$ receptors to the ionotropic NMDA glutamate receptor enabling further 'fine-tuning' of glutamatergic transmission. Dissecting out the functional consequences of disrupting such complex interactions is a difficult task that is gradually being explored. For example disrupting the mGlu$_5$-homer interaction prevents metabotropic receptor-induced long-term depression (LTD) of synaptic plasticity. In the future it may be possible to modulate mGlu$_5$-homer interactions to exploit the therapeutic potential of the mGlu$_5$ receptor as a target for the treatment of anxiety disorders.

Pre-synaptic mGlu$_7$ receptor complexes

The mGlu$_7$ receptor is located pre-synaptically on glutamatergic and GABAergic axon terminals where it attenuates neurotransmitter release by inhibiting P/Q type voltage sensitive Ca^{2+} channels. PICK1 (protein interacting with C kinase 1), a protein that interacts with protein kinase Cα, associates with the C-terminal of the mGlu$_7$ receptor and facilitates phosphorylation of the P/Q type voltage sensitive Ca^{2+} channel (Figure 11.16). The *in vivo* function of the mGlu$_7$-PICK1 interaction has been explored in rats and mice injected with a cell permeable peptide that blocks the association between mGlu$_7$ and PICK1. This uncoupling of the mGlu$_7$ and PICK1 caused absence-like seizures in the rodent models, a phenotype associated with a particular type of epilepsy known as absence epilepsy. Similar conclusions were obtained using knockin mice which expressed a mutant mGlu$_7$ receptor not able to bind PICK1. These observations highlight the

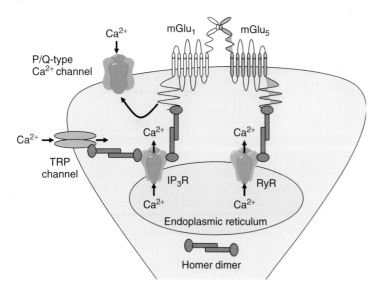

Figure 11.15 Post-synaptic metabotropic glutamate receptor signalling complexes. Homer proteins bind to proline-rich domains within the C-terminus of metabotropic glutamate 1 and 5 receptors facilitating interactions between these receptors and Ca^{2+} release channels located on the endoplasmic reticulum. IP_3 receptors (IP_3R) are opened by the second messenger inositol 1,4,5-trisphophate (generated via G_q/PLC), whereas ryanodine receptors (RyR) are opened by Ca^{2+} itself (known as Ca^{2+}-induced Ca^{2+} release). Homer can also associate with TRP channels which are involved in Ca^{2+} influx into the cell following depletion of endoplasmic reticulum Ca^{2+} stores.

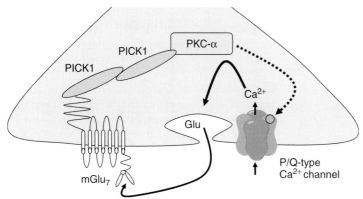

Figure 11.16 Pre-synaptic metabotropic glutamate receptor signalling complexes. The metabotropic glutamate 7 receptor negatively regulates the release of glutamate from pre-synaptic nerve terminals by inhibiting P/Q type voltage-sensitive Ca^{2+} channels. This is achieved by protein kinase C-α (PKCα) mediated phosphorylation of the Ca^{2+} channel and requires interaction of the mGlu$_7$ receptor with PICK1.

importance of GPCR signalling that is independent of heterotrimeric G-protein coupling.

5-HT$_{2C}$ receptor complexes

The 5-HT$_{2C}$ receptor is widely distributed CNS where it regulates many functions including mood, anxiety, feeding, sleep and reproductive behaviour. It is also associated with mediating the actions of many psychoactive drugs (e.g. LSD) and is the target of several antidepressants. The antidepressant action of 5-HT$_{2C}$ receptor antagonists relates to the disinhibition of the mesolimbic dopamine system, a pathway that is involved in modulating behavioural responses associated with feelings of motivation. Similarly, the mechanism of action of selective 5-HT uptake inhibitors (alternatively known as selective serotonin reuptake inhibitors; SSRI) may partly

involve the long-term down-regulation of 5-HT$_{2C}$ receptors which would also enhance the mesolimbic dopamine pathway. The C-terminal of the 5-HT$_{2C}$ receptor associates with many interesting GPCR interacting proteins including the PDZ-domain containing proteins MPP3 and PSD-95 which differentially control receptor desensitisation and internalisation (Gavarini et al., 2006). For example, when anchored to MPP3 the rate of 5-HT$_{2C}$ receptor internalisation decreases, whereas association with PSD-95 increases both receptor desensitisation and internalisation (Figure 11.17). Bockaert et al. (2010) have proposed targeting 5-HT$_{2C}$ receptor-PDZ protein interactions to increase receptor desensitisation as a novel approach to improve the therapeutic efficacy of current antidepressants.

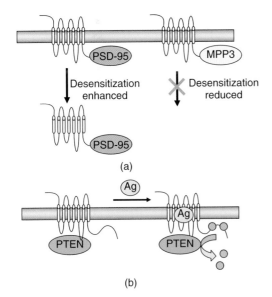

Figure 11.17 5-HT$_{2C}$ receptor interacting proteins.
(a) Differential regulation of 5-HT$_{2C}$ receptor desensitisation
by PSD-95 and MPP3. (b) The phosphatase PTEN associates
with the C-terminus of the 5-HT$_{2C}$ receptor and suppresses
agonist-induced phosphorylation (red circles) of the receptor.

The third intracellular loop of the 5-HT$_{2C}$ receptor
interacts with the tumour suppressor PTEN (protein
phosphatase and tensin homolog) which is a lipid and
protein phosphatase (Ji et al., 2006). This interaction
restricts agonist-induced phosphorylation of the 5-HT$_{2C}$
receptor (Figure 11.17). Interestingly this interaction was
observed in dopaminergic neurons located in the ventral
tegmental area (VTA), an area of the brain in which
most drugs of abuse exert rewarding effects by activating
dopaminergic neurons. The firing rate of VTA dopaminergic neurons in the VTA is reduced by 5-HT$_{2C}$ receptor
agonists and enhanced by 5-HT$_{2C}$ receptor antagonists
indicating that VTA dopaminergic neurons are tonically
inhibited by constitutive 5-HT$_{2C}$ receptor activity. Ji et al.
(2006) postulated that disrupting the interaction between
PTEN and the 5-HT$_{2C}$ receptor (which would increase
levels of receptor phosphorylation) would mimic the
inhibitory effects achieved by 5-HT$_{2C}$ receptor activation.
On reflection this seems at odds with the expected reduction of 5-HT$_{2C}$ receptor signalling if agonist-induced
phosphorylation of the receptor is increased. Remember
agonist-induced phosphorylation of GPCRs is important
in desensitisation and internalisation. However, it is also
believed that receptor phosphorylation is important in the

process of resensitisation and hence preventing agonist-
induced phosphorylation may in some cases reduce
receptor signalling. Therefore, disrupting the interaction between PTEN and the 5-HT$_{2C}$ receptor would
increase receptor phosphorylation and hence promote
resensitisation and receptor signalling. To investigate
this hypothesis the *in vivo* consequences of disrupting the interaction of PTEN with the 5-HT$_{2C}$ receptor
were explored using a synthetic peptide that mimics the
PTEN-binding sequence of the receptor. When given
intravenously to rats the peptide decreased the electrophysiological activity of VTA dopaminergic neurons
and suppressed behavioural responses induced by THC
(tetrahydrocannabinol; the psychoactive component of
marijuana) and nicotine. These effects are comparable
to those observed using 5-HT$_{2C}$ agonists but without
the associated side-effects such as anxiety, penile erec-
tion, hypophagia, and suppression of locomotor activity.
The authors of this work suggested that disrupting the
interaction of the 5-HT$_{2C}$ receptor with PTEN may represent a novel strategy for treating drug addiction (Ji
et al., 2006).

11.6 GPCR and ion channel complexes

In neurones GPCRs also interact with ion channels to
form signalling complexes that modulate synaptic activity. This was first reported by Liu et al. (2000) when the
dopamine D5 receptor was found to directly interact with
the inhibitory ligand-gated GABA$_A$ ion channel, both of
which are located in dendritic shafts (Figure 11.18). In
this case activation of the dopamine D5 receptor attenuates the functioning of the GABA$_A$ receptor (and *vice
versa*) possibly via co-internalisation of the ionotropic
receptor following D5 receptor activation. This allows
for the regulation of synaptic function by GPCRs to
occur independently of second-messenger dependent signalling pathways, which was the accepted paradigm prior
to these findings. Similarly, the dopamine D1 receptor
has been shown to directly interact with the excitatory ionotropic NMDA glutamate receptor subunits NR1
and NR2A with different functional consequences. The
attenuation of NMDA receptor currents following D1
receptor activation is dependent upon interaction with
NR2A, whereas the interaction with NR1 is associated
with suppressing neuronal cell death signalling events
that are also stimulated following NMDA receptor activation. These interesting examples highlight complex
signalling interactions between two major families of

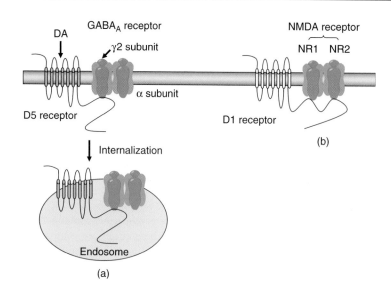

Figure 11.18 Interactions between GPCRs and ion channels. (a) Dopamine D5 receptor and GABA$_A$ receptor interactions. Activation of the D5 receptor with dopamine (DA) promotes internalisation of the GABA$_A$ receptor. (b) Dopamine D1 receptor and NMDA receptor interactions.

transmembrane proteins (GPCRs and ligand-gated ion channels) that may be exploited therapeutically in the future. The interaction between dopamine receptors and ion channels is expanded upon in a short review by Salter (2003).

11.7 Ion channel signalling complexes

We have already covered in this section the concept that multi-protein complexes involving GPCRs and GPCR/ion-channel interactions are prevalent in neuronal cells especially at the synapse where they regulate electrical activity. A number of signalling complexes involving ion channels have also been identified using proteomic-based approaches. For example, the ionotropic NMDA receptor exists in a multi-protein complex containing an incredible 77 proteins! These include various glutamate receptors (see above), scaffold and adaptor proteins, protein kinases, protein phosphatases, monomeric G-proteins, cell-adhesion and cytoskeletal proteins (Husi et al., 2000). The task for the future is to understand how this supramolecular signalling complex regulates synaptic plasticity and learning and whether alterations in the complex are associated with neuropsychiatric disorders. Other examples of ion channel signalling complexes include the ATP-gated P2X7 receptor (Kim et al., 2001) and the inward rectifier potassium channel (Leonoudakis et al., 2004).

11.8 Development of pharmaceuticals that target GPCR interacting proteins

Looking ahead it should be feasible to develop therapeutics that either modulate or disrupt the binding of a GPCR interacting protein to a specific GPCR. This has already been achieved in experimental models using cell permeable synthetic peptides to disrupt 5-HT$_{2C}$ receptor/PTEN and mGlu$_7$ receptor/PICK1 interactions. However, the Holy Grail of drug discovery would be the development of small molecule drugs that either disrupt or allosterically modulate GPCR protein-protein interactions. Some progress is being made since several small molecule drugs that target protein-protein interactions are currently under clinical trial (Wells and McClendon, 2007). Finally, since GPCR interacting proteins are often expressed in specific tissues/cell types targeting such proteins may provide a method to selectively modulate GPCR function in a particular tissue without altering receptor function in other tissues.

11.9 Development of pharmaceuticals that target protein-protein interactions

As indicated above the development of small molecule drugs that disrupt protein-protein interactions would be a major advance in the search for novel therapeutic approaches. In this section the potential to disrupt protein-protein interactions using small molecule drugs is highlighted with two examples from recently published work.

Bcl-2 protein interactions

The process of apoptotic cell death is tightly regulated by members of the Bcl-2 family of proteins. For example, the anti-apoptotic Bcl-2 protein, which is over-expressed in many forms of cancer, prevents cell death by forming heterodimers with pro-apoptotic proteins such as BAD and Bax (Figure 11.19). Hence it may be possible to develop novel anti-cancer drugs that disrupt the interaction between Bcl-2 and BAD/Bax and in doing so initiate the apoptosis of cancer cells. Abbott Laboratories have developed several small molecule drugs which bind to a key helical domain within Bcl-2, disrupting its interaction with BAD and/or Bax, thus triggering apoptosis (Tse et al., 2008). One of these ABT-263 is currently undergoing Phase II clinical trials.

p53 interaction with HDM2

About 50% of all human cancers have mutations in the gene encoding the tumour-suppressor protein p53 that result in its inactivation. In a normal cell p53 protein is inactive but in response to DNA damage the p53 protein is activated triggering cell cycle arrest and/or initiation of apoptosis. Furthermore, the level of p53 protein in the cell is tightly regulated by ubiquitin-dependent degradation involving an E3 ubiquitin ligase called MDM2 that constitutively interacts with p53. Under conditions of stress and DNA damage the interaction between p53 and MDM2 is disrupted and the levels of activated p53

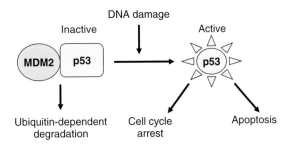

Figure 11.20 p53-mediated cell cycle arrest and apoptosis. The tumour suppressor protein p53 is inactive in normal cells due to its interaction with MDM2. Following stress or DNA damage the levels of activated p53 increase due to its dissociation from MDM2 promoting either cell cycle arrest or apoptosis. Cell cycle arrest allows the cell time to repair damaged DNA, whereas cells beyond repair are removed via apoptosis.

increase (Figure 11.20). Structural studies have shown that MDM2 binds to a hydrophobic 15 amino acid α-helical region of p53. Recently small molecule inhibitors of the p53-MDM2 interaction have been developed by Hoffman La Roche as novel anti-cancer drugs (Vassilev et al., 2004). These so-called 'nutlins' which do not interfere with normal p53 activity are likely to undergo clinical trials in cancer patients in the near future.

11.10 Lipid rafts

Lipid rafts are specialised membrane domains that are involved in the compartmentalisation of cellular processes. They are stable but dynamic lateral assemblies of heterogeneous protein together with sphingolipid- and cholesterol-enriched membrane, which can facilitate protein-protein interactions. Typically they are between 10 and 100 nm in size. Sometimes they can be derived from the coalescence of several micro-domains through protein-protein or protein-lipid interactions (for recent reviews see Pike, 2006; Simons and Gerl, 2010).

Caveolae are a type of lipid raft that appear as small flask-shaped, non-coated plasma membrane invaginations in electron micrographs (Yamada, 1955). They are specialised membrane domains rich in cholesterol, sphingolipids, saturated fatty acids, signalling proteins and a family of structural proteins called caveolins (types 1, 2 and 3). Flotillins are integral membrane proteins that are also associated with lipid rafts and they are thought to behave as caveolin homologs by contributing to lipid raft architecture and organisation (Babuke and Tikkanen,

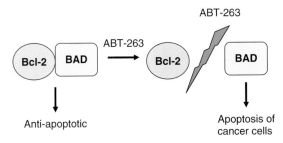

Figure 11.19 Interaction of Bcl-2 with BAD regulates cell apoptosis. The pro-apoptotic functions of BAD are prevented when it forms heterodimers with Bcl-2. Disrupting the Bcl-2-BAD interaction with the small molecule drug ABT-263 enables the BAD protein to initiate apoptosis.

2007). By clustering proteins such as receptors and/or signalling complexes within membrane domains, lipid rafts are thought to play pivotal roles in a myriad of cellular functions which include cholesterol transport, endocytosis, exocytosis, and signal transduction. Lipid rafts have also been associated with a number of pathologies like cancer, viral infections and neurodegenerative diseases. Drugs that target lipid rafts are currently being developed.

Evidence for the existence of lipid rafts is controversial mainly due to them being too small to observe using conventional microscopic techniques; the light microscope can only resolve membrane structures that are greater than 200 nm. However, this is less of an issue as time goes on due to the development of increasingly sophisticated microscopes with ever greater resolving powers that are used to visualise biological membranes. Currently most of our knowledge regarding lipid rafts are inferred using techniques such as fluorescence resonance energy transfer (FRET), homo-FRET, fluorescence correlation spectroscopy (FCS), atomic-force microscopy (AFM), electron microscopy (EM), deuterium-based nuclear magnetic resonance (^{2}H-NMR) and differential calorimetry (for a description of these techniques see Sharma et al., 2006). The study of lipid rafts can also be hampered by the fact that some lipid rafts can form and disassociate relatively quickly (within nano seconds). There is also the added problem of the techniques used to isolate lipid rafts for subsequent biochemical analysis: for example cholesterol-rich membranes or detergent resistant membrane fractions may not represent functional lipid raft compartments (Hancock, 2006). Despite all these drawbacks, data from different techniques offer compelling evidence for the existence of these specialised membrane units.

Membrane structure

Cellular membranes have a lipid bilayer containing proteins that is mainly composed of: i) glycerophospholipids with the main examples being phosphatidylcholine which is found in the exoplasmic leaflet and phosphatidylethanolamine and phosphatidylserine which are located in the inner-leaflet; ii) sphingolipids, glycosphingolipids and sphingomyelin (which is also a phospholipid) which are predominantly found in the exoplasmic leaflet and; iii) sterols which are found on both sides of the membrane with cholesterol being the only sterol found in mammalian membranes. The exact lipid composition of membranes can vary depending upon their cellular or organelle location. For example sphingolipids are particularly abundant in the myelin sheath that surrounds many types of neurones, whereas glycerophospholipids are plentiful in the endoplasmic reticulum and Golgi complex.

Phospholipids have a single hydrophilic polar head that faces outside and two non-polar hydrophobic fatty acid (acyl) tails which form the core of the membrane. Glycolipids, like phospholipids, have two acyl tails that vary in length (usually C_{16}, C_{18} and C_{20}) and as such will affect membrane depth. Their sugar groups project into the extracellular space and function to insulate, for example, neurones during action potential propagation, protect the cell from potential toxins (e.g. cholera and tetanus) or act as anchoring sites for receptors to bind. The acyl tails can be either straight (saturated) or have a 'bend' due to the presence of a double carbon bond (unsaturated). Saturated fatty acids can line up closely to each other whereas unsaturated chains need more space (Figure 11.21). This affects lipid packing and lateral movement which in turn alters membrane fluidity. Reduced fluidity results in a

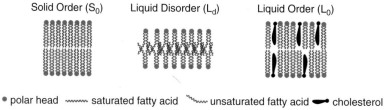

Figure 11.21 Artificial membranes can exist in three phases. Solid Order (S_o) phase membranes are composed of phospholipids with saturated acyl groups that allow uniform packing of the non-polar fatty acid tails. In the liquid disorder (L_d) phase the acyl chains contains a double bond, causing the fatty acid tail to bend so that the phospholipids are not tightly packed. Also the depth of the membrane is considerably shorter. The liquid order (L_o) phase contains sterols like cholesterol which allows uniform packing of saturated acyl tails. The inclusion of cholesterol is thought to concentrate the saturated acyl into a functional domain so that the membrane depth is large enough to accommodate proteins with long trans-membrane spanning domains.

more impermeable membrane whereas increased fluidity increases the likelihood of spontaneous rotation of lipids from one face of a membrane to the other; a flip:flop model of membrane activity. Membrane fluidity is an important factor in protein insertion and removal from specific membrane compartments. For example at the synapse, receptors are exocytosed at extra synaptic sites where they are then move by lateral diffusion to their synaptic membrane compartment and conversely receptors targeted for removal laterally diffuse to extracellular sites where they are endocytosed.

Cholesterol is a lipid that is found in many types of membranes and is thought to add stability as well as increase water permeability. Like phospholipids, cholesterol has a polar head and a non-polar tail which lines up in the lipid bilayer. Studies using artificial membranes have shown that they exist as three basic lipid-bilayer phases: solid order (S_o), liquid disorder (L_d) and liquid order (L_o) (see Figure 11.21). In the S_o phase the lateral mobility of lipids is restricted due to tighter packing of the fatty acid tails, whereas in the L_d phase there is less packing and greater membrane fluidity. The L_o phase is similar to the S_o phase except the inclusion of molecules like cholesterol (or any other sterols) functions as a scaffold to maintain membrane fluidity as well as tight fatty acid tail packing. Interestingly, the introduction of unsaturated fatty acid tails in the L_d domains can also reduce membrane thickness compared to areas with L_o domains, so that

proteins with relatively small trans-membrane spanning domains can only exist in membrane regions that are in the L_d phase. Within artificial membranes, lipid rafts are considered to consist of L_o domains whereas L_d domains represent non-raft areas. These phases are considered to be important in the formation, maintenance and dissolution of lipid rafts. However, this simplistic delineation between membrane phases may not be appropriate in more heterogeneous situations like biological membranes (see Lingwood and Simons, 2010). Nevertheless, this simple model has helped our understanding into how and when lipid rafts are formed as well as predicting their life span and which proteins (based on transmembrane size) can concentrate in them.

Lipid raft markers

A number of components of the membrane have been found to be associated with or concentrated in lipid rafts (Figure 11.22). These include cholesterol, the sphingolipids, ganglioside 1 and 2 (GM1 and GM2) and sphingomyelin, as well as scaffolding proteins that interact with the carboxyl terminal of many proteins and are thought to be involved in the stabilisation and assembly of lipid rafts such as the glycosylphosphatidylinositol (GPI)-anchored proteins family or flotillins. Removal from the membrane of any one of these examples has been shown to prevent clustering of proteins as well as activation of any associated downstream signal transduction cascades.

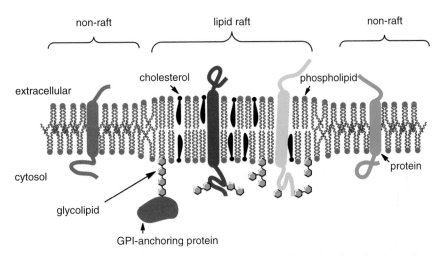

Figure 11.22 Diagram illustrating lipid rafts. Note how the non-raft region is shallower than the raft region and any protein that has a short transmembrane spanning domain cannot become part of a lipid raft. Glycosylation sites on glycolipids or proteins embedded in the membrane provide another possible site of anchorage with scaffolding proteins such as GPI-anchoring protein or lectins, as well as potential sites of interaction with signalling cascade molecules.

This makes them useful markers for lipid rafts as well as aid in their isolation for further analysis.

Biological functions of lipid rafts

Lipid rafts play important roles in signal transduction, endocytosis, exocytosis and cholesterol transport. Furthermore, a number of bacterial, parasitic and viral pathogens are associated with lipid rafts which exploit them as either a method of entry, replication, amplification or dispersal. They are also associated with the pathogenesis of a number of neurodegenerative diseases where they play a role in the conversion of proteins such as β-amyloid and prion from non-pathogenic to pathogenic forms.

Lipid rafts are found at immunological synapses and hence are involved in immunological surveillance. This specialist synapse is formed when the T cell antigen receptor (TCR) on the cell surface of T-lymphocytes interacts with an antigen (peptide) attached to the class I major histocompatibility complex (MHC) located on the surface of an antigen presenting cell (APC). Binding of antigen to the TCR triggers its interaction with another membrane bound protein, CD3, to form a TCR-CD3 complex. This complex mediates T cell activation by recruiting a number of signalling molecules; including src-family kinase, lymphocyte cell specific protein tyrosine kinase (Lck) and the tyrosine kinase 70 kDa ζ-associated protein (ZAP-70). T cell activation causes the clustering of TCR-CD3 complexes at the centre of an immune synapse to form a central supra-molecular activation complex (cSMAC) which is surrounded by peripheral SMAC formed by the integrin LFA1 (Saito et al., 2010; Simons and Gerl, 2010). If antibodies are employed to cross link GPI-anchored proteins this promotes T cell signalling whereas removal of cholesterol from the membrane inhibits signalling.

Viruses such as HIV can exploit T cell activation to facilitate its spread. HIV gain entry into cells by coating themselves with portions of the host cells membrane. These 'membrane-enveloped' viruses can then fuse with the membrane of another host cell so that they are endocytosed into the cell. Lipid rafts play a role in the formation of this lipid envelope and its sequential budding. Phosphoinositides (PI) which are abundant within the inner leaflet of the viral membrane envelope are thought to play a role in the oligomerisation of HIV particles. Since one of the acyl tails of PI is polyunsaturated, its inclusion in a lipid raft would appear to contradict the theory that unsaturated fatty acids cannot be a part of a lipid raft. However, when the Gag region of the HIV particle interacts with the polar head of PI it causes the polyunsaturated tail to flip so that it now interacts with the matrix domain of the Gag region. Hence, only the saturated acyl chain of PI is now inserted into the plasma membrane which allows a number of HIV particles to cluster within the membrane to form a lipid raft. This lipid raft has also been shown to be rich in cholesterol and sphingolipids as well as another viral protein, Env, which is incorporated into its outer leaflet. The raft can then bud-off so that viral particles are contained within the core of the 'micelle' and Env is exposed to the outside environment. The Env protein recognises receptors that are clustered into rafts on the surface of T cells as well as facilitating fusion of both viral and cellular membranes thus allowing 'naked' HIV particles to enter and infect a new T cell (Waheed and Freed, 2009).

Bacterial toxins such as shiga and ricin use lipid rafts to gain access into cells. Shiga toxins are produced by some classes of bacteria and cause dysentery by inhibiting proteins within infected cells. These toxins enter the host cell by interacting with a glycosphingolipid receptor (globotriaosylceramide; Gb3). Binding of toxin to these receptors causes them to coalesce into lipid rafts that form invaginations within the membrane leading to their endocytosis.

Lipid rafts are also thought to play roles in protein trafficking at various stages through the secretory pathway, from the endoplasmic reticulum through the Golgi complex into secretory vesicles and membrane insertion. It has been proposed that lipid rafts help maintain suitable levels of certain cytosol protein pools by altering their membrane properties. For example, the transmembrane depth of some proteins is too small for entry into lipid rafts so they are retained within the trans-Golgi membrane until an overriding signal is received.

Drugs that interact with lipid rafts

A number of drugs are known to deplete cholesterol from membranes. These include β-cyclodextrins, 3-hydroxy-3-methylglutaryl (HMG)-coenzyme A reductase inhibitors (statins e.g. mevastatin), cytochalasin (fumonisim B) and ceramide. Ceramide is a signalling molecule that is implicated in apoptosis, cellular differentiation, proliferation and cell migration. The sphingolipid, sphingomyelin, can also be hydrolysed to ceramide by sphingomyelinase (Smase). So a number of drugs that act as various members of the Smase family have been developed in an attempt to treat a number of pathologies including Alzheimer's disease (He et al., 2010). Since no direct inhibitors of Smase exist, pharmaceutical companies are screening naturally-occurring endogenous candidates. Organic bases like desipramine, which cause the detachment of Smase from the inner membrane and subsequent inactivation, have been used to study the role of Smase's in disease states. However, these compounds are too weak to be used as functional inhibitors. In addition, work on animal models has failed to find a therapeutic effect for a variety of functional Smase inhibitors.

Dietary factors can alter raft composition and hence cellular activities. These include omega-3 polyunsaturated fatty acids (Ω3-PUFA) which have been used to reduce the risk of a whole host of pathologies ranging from heart disease to malaria. Ω3-PUFA can alter lipid raft composition and hence the activation of downstream signalling molecules. Plant derived fats such as phytosterols, which are structurally related to cholesterol but have different biological effects in animals, have also been used to alter lipid raft composition. In fact, studies show that phytosterols, such as triterpenes, can be incorporated into mammalian membranes causing lipid raft destabilisation by depleting their cholesterol content and interfering with downstream signalling cascades (Verma, 2009).

11.11 Receptor-mediated endocytosis

A number of cell membrane receptors (e.g. GPCRs; see Chapter 3) are internalised into endosomes in a process known as receptor-mediated endocytosis. The extracellular domain of the receptor and any bound ligand is found within the lumen of the endosome and the cytosolic receptor domain remains in the cytoplasm. Since the receptor's activated tail is still exposed to the cytosolic compartment, it maintains the ability to interact with other proteins and take part in signalling cascades. Once endocytosed, ligand can either be removed from the receptor in either early or late endosomes or directed to the lysosomal compartment for destruction. Endosomal feedback can influence protein processing by the Golgi complex and/or the endoplasmic reticulum and hence protein trafficking and their plasma membrane insertion (Figure 11.23).

Signalling endosomes

Not all receptors found within endosomes are destined for recycling, degradation or providing feedback for regulation of receptor trafficking. In these cases they are

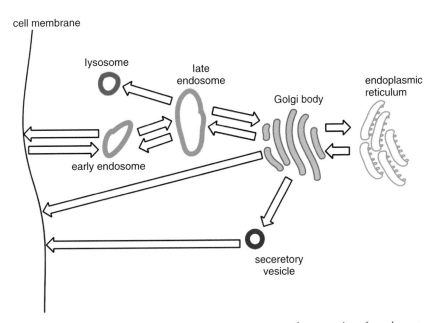

Figure 11.23 Cross talk between endosomal compartments. To prevent over- or under-expression of membrane targeted proteins there are a number of steps within the endocytic pathway that can be regulated. Proteins destined for membrane insertion can be retained in the Golgi complex (GC) or endoplasmic reticulum (ER). Early and late endosomes can provide feedback to the GC which may help the cell to decide their fate; recycled, degraded, or release of de novo trans-membrane proteins from the GC or ER.

transported from the plasma membrane to the nucleus where they can influence genomic activity. These are known as signalling endosomes, with tyrosine kinases receptors (Trk) and GPCRs being amongst the most extensively studied types of receptors involved in endosomal signalling.

Trk signalling is of interest to neuroscientists because activation of Trk receptors by neurotrophins such as nerve growth factor (NGF), brain derived neurotrophic factor (BDNF), neurotrophin-4 (NT4) or neurotrophin-3 (NT3) leads to expression of genes involved in cell survival. This is even though the distance between the activated receptor located at synapse can be over one meter away from the nuclear site of action. How activated Trk receptors cause nuclear activity is a matter of fierce debate. In the wave model, receptors are located at intervals along the axon so that once activated the signal is propagated down the axon in a 'domino' fashion until the signal eventually reaches the nucleus. Whilst the epidermal growth factor receptor (ErbB1) has been shown to utilise this method of signal propagation, there is no evidence of it happening with Trk signalling. Another method is called the signalling effector model. This model describes how activation of receptor causes a signalling molecule, such as cytosolic Ca^{2+} or a downstream kinase,

to be transported directly to either the nucleus or indirectly to a receptor located on the cell body followed by subsequent nuclear activation. However, Trk receptors appear to work independently of either model for two main reasons. Firstly, for Trk-mediated nuclear activity to occur activated Trk and bound ligand must be internalised. Secondly, this signalling endosome has to interact with the retrograde axonal transporter, dynein, and nuclear activity is only observed once it has been transported down the axon (Figure 11.24). Moreover, radio-labelling of the neurotrophin with ^{125}I has provided compelling evidence for the retrograde movement of Trk and bound neurotrophin from the synapse to the nucleus. Further studies have also shown that once in the nucleus this signalling endosome has the ability to phosphorylate intermediates involved in gene expression and subsequent gene induction (Sadowski et al., 2009).

Activation of Trk by neurotrophin binding causes the receptor to dimerise and auto-phosphorylate. The cytosolic domain of the receptor then interacts with a number of other proteins to form a signalling complex that can activate signalling cascades that include the mitogen-activated protein kinase (MAPK) pathway, the phosphoinositide 3-kinase (PI-3K) pathway and the phospholipase C-gamma (PLCγ) pathway. Once in the nucleus kinases such as

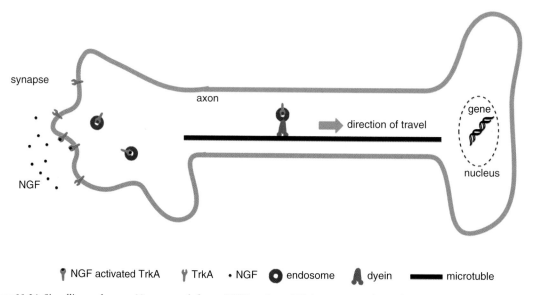

Figure 11.24 Signalling endosome. Nerve growth factor (NGF) activates TrkA receptors and is endocytosed into the cytosol to form a signalling endosome. The signalling endosome interacts with the retrograde axonal transport protein, dyein. Dyein and its cargo move down the axon to the nucleus. The activated tail of the TrkA receptor is free to interact with transcription factors to induce expression of genes involved in cell survival.

p90 RSK and ERK5 are thought to phosphorylate and activate transcription factors like cyclic AMP responsive element binding protein (CREB) which in turn induces gene expression. However, there is also evidence that CREB actually joins the signalling endosome in the axon and is transported to the nucleus.

Activity of this signalling complex can be ameliorated by its dephosphorylation, ubiquitination and disassociation of neurotrophin from the Trk. Translocation of the ligand bound receptor from its membrane compartment to another cellular compartment may also provide a different repertoire of signalling molecules with which it can interact and thereby have different cellular consequences. In addition, several splice variants of Trk exist which can interact with a different range of signalling complexes giving rise to another level of signalling complexity.

Trk receptors can be concentrated in membrane microdomains such as lipid-rafts, non-lipid rafts or calveolae, with internalisation being with or without the aid of scaffolding proteins such as clathrin, pincher or GPI-anchoring protein (Philippidou et al., 2011). Hence it is unclear as to whether specific micro-membrane domains and their associated proteins play a role in determining the receptor's fate. As Figure 11.25 shows, once inside the cell the Trk receptor/bound neurotrophin/signalling complex can become part of a macro-endosome or an early endosome. Receptors targeted for recycling or breakdown are directed from the early endosome towards recycling endosomes and lysosomes respectively. Otherwise the early endosomes can form either multi-vesicular bodies or late endosomes. Interestingly, the internalisation of receptors into multi-vesicular bodies prevents

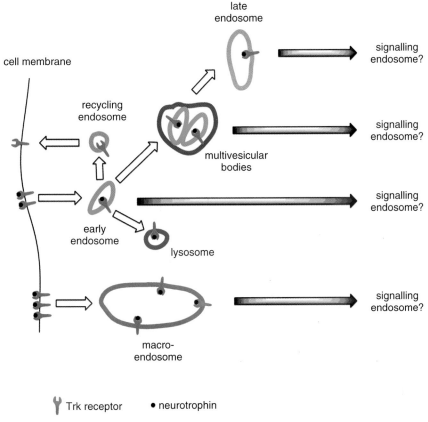

Figure 11.25 Showing possible candidates for signalling endosome. Trk receptor and bound neurotrophin are internalised and can become part of a macro-endosome or and early endosome. Early endosomes that are not targeted for recycling or degradation can coalesce to form a multi-vesicular body (MVB) where the activated tails are not exposed to the cytosol during axonal transport. Late endosomes have had this extra endosomal membrane (MVB) removed so that the tails of the Trk receptors are exposed to the cytosol. All four types of endosomes appear to participate in endosomal signalling.

them from interacting with their signalling molecules and hence suppressing signal activation. Labelling of the neurotrophin with ^{125}I or quantum dots, has shown that the Trk/neurotrophin complex is found in all types of endosomes raising the possibility that macro-, early-, multi-vesicular- and late-endosomes are all acting as signalling endosomes that are transported to the nucleus (Cosker et al., 2008; Miaczynska & Bar-Sagi, 2010). This may confer another level of complexity on endosomal signalling.

Disruption of axonal transport gives rise to a myriad of human pathologies with different ranges of severity. But many of these abnormalities are not solely attributed to deficits in endosomal signalling. However, a juvenile form of amyotrophic lateral sclerosis (ALS) has been associated with abnormal Trk endosomal signalling. Mutations within a gene associated with ALS (ALS2) results in the development of ALS as well as abnormal trafficking of neurotrophin signalling endosomes.

11.12 Summary

This chapter has explored the concept that many prominent signalling proteins (e.g. GPCRs, ion channels, tyrosine kinase linked receptors) exist as part of large multi-protein complexes often organised within specialised membrane domains such as lipid rafts. You should also appreciate some of the genetic and biochemical-based approaches that have been used to identify proteins associated with such complexes. However, a major task for the future is to understand the precise physiological role(s) of these complexes and how their dysfunction may contribute to disease progression. In the case of GPCRs, research to date indicates that signalling complexes regulate many functions of GPCR life including the targeting and trafficking of receptors to specific sites within the cell membrane, modulation of signal transduction, and receptor internalisation and recycling. The challenge for the future is to develop drugs that manipulate protein-protein interactions for therapeutic benefit.

References

Babuke T and Tikkanen R (2007) Dissecting the molecular function of reggie/flotillin proteins. European Journal of Cell Biology 86: 525–532.

Bernier V, Bichet DG and Bouvier M (2004) Pharmacological chaperone action on G-protein-coupled receptors. Current Opinion in Pharmacology 4: 528–533.

Bockaert J, Fagni L, Dumuis A, Marin P (2004) GPCR interacting proteins (GIP). Pharmacology and Therapeutics 103: 203–221.

Bockaert J, Perroy J, Bécamel C, Marin P and Fagni L (2010) GPCR interacting proteins (GIPs) in the nervous system: roles in physiology and pathologies. Annual Review of Pharmacology and Toxicology 50: 89–109.

Bouschet T, Martin S and Henley JM (2008) Regulation of calcium-sensing-receptor trafficking and cell surface expression by GPCRs and RAMPs. Trends in Pharmacological Sciences 29: 633–639.

Cosker KE, Courchesne SL and Segal RA (2008) Action in the axon: generation and transport signaling endosomes. Current Opinion in Neurobiology 18: 270–275.

Daulat AM, Pascal M and Jockers R (2008) Recent methodological advances in the discovery of GPCR-associated protein complexes. Trends in Pharmacological Sciences 30: 72–78.

DeWire SM and Violin JD (2011) Biased ligands for better cardiovascular drugs. Circulation Research 109: 205–216.

Fields S and Song O (1989) A novel genetic system to detect protein-protein interactions. Nature 340: 245–246.

Gavarini S, Bécamel C, Altier C, Lory P, Poncet J, Wijnholds J, Bockaert J and Marin P (2006) Opposite effects of PSD-95 and MPP3 PDZ proteins on serotonin 5-hydroxytryptamine$_{2C}$ receptor desensitization and membrane stability. Molecular Biology of the Cell 17: 4619–4631.

Hancock JF (2006) Lipid rafts: contentious only from simplistic standpoints. Nature Reviews: Molecular Cell Biology 7: 456–462.

Hay DL, Poyner DR and Sexton PM (2006) GPCR modulation by RAMPs. Pharmacology and Therapeutics 109: 173–197.

He X, Huang Y, Li B, Gong CX and Schuchman EH (2010) Deregulation of sphingolipid metabolism in Alzheimer's disease. Neurobiology of Aging 31: 398–408.

Husi H, Ward MA, Choudhary JS, Blackstock WP and Grant SGN (2000) Proteomic analysis of NMDA receptor-adhesion protein signaling complexes. Nature Neuroscience 3: 661–669.

Ji SP, Zhang, Y, Van Cleemput J, Jiang W, Liao M, Li L, Wan Q, Backstrom JR and Zhang X (2006) Disruption of PTEN coupling with 5-HT$_{2C}$ receptors suppresses behavioural responses induced by drugs of abuse. Nature Medicine 12: 324–329.

Kim M, Jiang LH, Wilson HL, North RA and Surprenant A (2001) Proteomic and functional evidence for a P2X7 receptor signalling complex. EMBO Journal 20: 6347–6358.

Leonoudakis D, Conti LR, Anderson S, Radeke CM, McGuire LM, Adams ME, Froehner SC, Yates JR 3rd, and Vandenberg CA (2004) Protein trafficking and anchoring complexes revealed by proteomic analysis inward rectifier potassium channel (Kir2.x)-associated proteins. Journal of Biological Chemistry 279: 22331–22346.

Lingwood D and Simons K (2010) Lipid rafts as a membrane-organizing principle. Science 327: 46–50.

Liu F, Pristupa ZB, Yu XM, Wang YT and Niznik HB (2000) Direct protein-protein coupling enables cross-talk between dopamine D5 and gamma-aminobutyric acid A receptors. Nature 403: 274–280.

Luttrell LM and Gesty-Palmer D (2010) Beyond desensitization: physiological relevance of arrestin-dependent signaling. Pharmacological Reviews 62: 305–330.

Magalhaes AC, Dunn H and Ferguson SSG (2012) Regulation of GPCR activity, trafficking and localization by GPCR-interacting proteins. British Journal of Pharmacology 165: 1717–1736.

McLatchie LM, Fraser NJ, Main MJ, Wise A, Brown J, Thompson N, Solari R, Lee MG and Foord SM (1998) RAMPs regulate the transport and ligand specificity of the calcitonin-receptor-like receptor. Nature 393: 333–339.

Miaczynska M and Bar-Sagi D (2010) Signaling endosomes: seeing is believing. Current Opinion in Cell Biology 22: 535–540.

Pascal M, Daulat AM, Broussards C, Mozo J, Clary G, Hotellier F, Chafey P, Guillaume J-L, Ferry G, Boutin JA, Delagrange P, Camoin L and Jockers R (2008) A generic approach for the purification of signaling complexes that specifically interact with the carboxyl-terminal domain of G protein-coupled receptors. Molecular and Cellular Proteomics 7: 1556–1569.

Parameswaran N and Spielman WS (2006) RAMPs: the past, present and future. Trends in Biochemical Sciences 31: 631–638.

Philippidou P, Valdez G, Akmentin W, Bowers WJ, Federoff HJ and Halegoua S (2011) Trk retrograde signaling requires persistent, Pincher-directed endosomes. Proceedings of the National Academy of Sciences (United States of America) 108: 852–857.

Pike LJ (2006) Rafts defined: a report on the keystone symposium on lipid rafts and cell function. Journal of Lipid Research 47: 1597–1598.

Ritter SL and Hall RA (2009) Fine-tuning of GPCR activity by receptor-interacting proteins. Nature Reviews Molecular Cell Biology 10: 819–830.

Sadowski L, Pilecka I and Miaczynska M (2009) Signaling from endosomes: location makes a difference. Experimental Cell Research 315: 1601–1609.

Saito T, Yokosuka T and Hashimoto-Tane A (2010) Dynamic regulation of T-cell activation and co-stimulation through TCR-microclusters. FEBS Letters 584: 4865–4871.

Salter MW (2003) D1 and NMDA receptors hook up: expanding on an emerging theme. Trends in Neurosciences 26: 235–237.

Sexton PM, Poyner DR, Simms J, Christopoulos A and Hay DL (2009) Modulating receptor function through RAMPs: can they represent drug targets in themselves? Drug Discovery Today 14: 413–419.

Sharma P, Varma R and Mayor S. (2006) The Biophysical Characterization of Lipid Rafts, in Lipid Rafts and Caveolae: From Membrane Biophysics to Cell Biology (ed CJ Fielding), Wiley-VCH Verlag GmbH & Co. KGaA, Weinheim, FRG.

Shenoy SK and Lefkowitz RJ (2011) β-arrestin-mediated receptor trafficking and signal transduction. Trends in Pharmacological Sciences 32: 521–533.

Simons K and Gerl MJ (2010) Revitalizing membrane rafts: new tools and insights. Nature Reviews: Molecular Cell Biology 11: 688–699.

Tse C, Shoemaker AR, Adickes J, Anderson MG et al (2008) ABT-263: a potent and orally bioactive Bcl-2 family inhibitor. Cancer Research 68: 3421–3428.

Vassilev LT, Vu BT, Graves B, Carajal D et al (2004) In vivo activation of the p53 pathway by small-molecule antagonists of MDM2. Science 303: 844–848.

Verma SP (2009) HIV: a raft-targeting approach for prevention and therapy using plant-derived compounds. Current Drug Targets 10: 51–59.

Violin JD, Dewire SM, Yamashita D, Rominger DH, Nguyen L, Schiller K, Whalen EJ, Gowen M and Lark MW (2010) Selectively engaging β-arrestins at the AT_1R reduces blood pressure and increase cardiac performance. Journal of Pharmacology and Experimental Therapeutics 335: 572–579.

Waheed AA and Freed EO (2009) Lipids and membrane microdomains in HIV replication. Virus Research 143: 162–176.

Wells JA and McClendon CL (2007) Reaching for high-hanging fruit in drug discovery at protein-protein interfaces. Nature 450: 1001–1009.

Yamada E (1955) The fine structure of the gall bladder epithelium of the mouse. The Journal of Biophysical and Biochemical Cytology 1: 445–458.

12 Recombinant Proteins and Immunotherapeutics

12.1 Introduction to immunotherapeutics

Site-specific delivery of therapeutic agents has been the major aim in pharmacology. However, traditional drugs were not able to attain 100% therapeutic success against metabolic and/or systemic diseases. This is mainly because most of these drugs act either via pharmacological receptors and enzymes or are dependant on successful delivery to their target sites. On the other hand, anti-microbial therapy is mainly dependant on manipulating the biochemical differences between the host and the invading organism. Therefore, they are subject to redundancy due to the development of 'resistance'. Also it is apparent that current therapies for major illnesses such as cancer, asthma, ischaemic heart disease (IHD), AIDS and inflammatory disorders, are not always effective. The understanding of gene expression has given rise to new molecules that can be targeted to manipulate normal and pathological processes. New and innovative methods in diagnostics, drug delivery and specific targeting are being attempted. This has led to new approaches in the design and development of novel therapies. The main focus of these novel therapeutic modalities is the site-specific delivery (many of which are achieved by using carrier technology) with maximum efficacy. Some of these techniques include:

- **early diagnostic tests** – quick and inexpensive diagnostic tests to identify pathogenic targets.
- **new classes of anti-infective agents** – these include combination therapies, serum therapy and so on.
- **exploitation of genomics** – mainly targeted for diseases affected by genetic polymorphisms (see chapter 7.0 for details) which is likely to yield new generations of fast acting drugs that are inexpensive to produce.
- **vaccine development** – very powerful but indirect, cost-effective way to reduce the need for antibiotics; and
- **immunotherapeutics** – represent the largest group of molecules that are currently being developed (and used) from monoclonal antibodies.

This chapter will briefly discuss the promise, the use and the future of these modalities, mainly focusing on immunotherapeutics.

Molecular Pharmacology: From DNA to Drug Discovery, First Edition. John Dickenson, Fiona Freeman, Chris Lloyd Mills, Shiva Sivasubramaniam and Christian Thode.
© 2013 John Wiley & Sons, Ltd. Published 2013 by John Wiley & Sons, Ltd.

12.2 Historical background of immunotherapeutics

Although the term 'immunotherapeutics' is relatively new, the concept of activating the body's immune system against illness started in the early 1890s when William Coley tried to use live bacteria as anti-cancer vaccines (Kim et al., 2002). Similarly during this period, immune serum-based therapies were used to treat a variety of bacterial infections including *Corynebacterium diphtheriae*, *Streptococcus pneumoniae*, *Neisseria meningitides*, *Haemophilus influenzae*, and *Clostridium Tetani* (Casadevall and Scharff, 1994; 1995). Building on this theory, in 1900, Paul Erlich suggested that molecules within the body ('*magic bullets*') might have the ability to fight tumours (Waldmann, 2003). The first major breakthrough in immunotherapeutics happened in 1975 when George Köhler and César Milstein developed the technology for generating monoclonal antibodies (Mabs). Following this, in 1986, the FDA approved the first monoclonal antibody Muromonab-CD3 [orthoclone (OKT3)®] to be used against organ graft rejection (Clark, 2000). The major drawback of early Mabs is the fact that they were initially produced in the mouse, and therefore in the human body they were recognised as foreign molecules by the human immune system (human anti-mouse antibody; HAMAs – see section 12.4) which destroyed the molecules. However, recent advances in hybridoma technology provide humanised monoclonal antibodies that are highly specific with reduced toxicity. In 1997, the first humanised Mab, rituximab (Rituxan® or MabThera®) was approved by the FDA to use as a single agent in non-Hodgkin's lymphoma (NHL). Thereafter different researchers tried to produce and use antibodies, mainly against cancer, asthma, ischaemic heart disease (IHD), infection and other inflammation related disorders. Before looking at their therapeutic values, it is important to understand the basis of their use in clinical practice.

12.3 Basis of immunotherapeutics

Most animals including humans, have a functional immune system to protect against invading organisms and grafts. This is achieved mainly by immunoglobulins (Igs) or antibodies. The true physiologic function of antibodies is producing humoral immunity. However, by manipulating their specific binding abilities, one can use these antibodies against disease processes. Conventional drug therapy targets the invading organism, tumour cells or other inflammatory mediators by disabling (or inactivating) these disease causative agents; thereby the body's immune system can effectively and easily destroy them. On the other hand, immunotherapeutics aims to activate the body's own defence mechanisms by triggering and/or 'mimicking' immune responses. Natural antibodies in humans, as well as other animals, protect their host by different mechanisms.

They would either bind to and neutralise protein toxins, block the attachment of viruses to the cells, activate complement or activate natural killer (NK) cells. The basic structure of a typical human immunoglobulin (antibody) is given in Figure 12.1. Antibodies consist of four polypeptide chains. Two long heavy chains and two short light chains organised as globular domains. These chains are not only linked between each other by disulphide bridges, but also pose intra-chain disulphide bonds to maintain stability. Each heavy chain has (i) **a variable** (V) and a diversity (D) region in which the amino acid sequences are highly variable; a joining (J) segment with moderately variable amino acids; and (ii) **a constant** (C) segment where the sequence is constant. Likewise each light chain has a V, a J and a C segment. The V domains contain the antibody-binding sites (Fab portion – see Figure 12.1). On the other hand, the Fc portion of the molecule mediates the reactions initiated by the antibody (also known as the effector portion).

Antibodies play an important role in the recognition of foreign antigens (such as toxins, bacteria, viruses etc.) and activate an immune response to them. They are the key contributors to the adaptive immune response. Therefore, it is possible to use antibodies in many immunotherapeutic approaches. With the emergence of hybridoma/monoclonal antibody technologies, recombinant DNA technologies, and other molecular cloning methods, it is now possible to raise antibodies against specific antigens (such as unusual antigens expressed in tumours). As they are extremely specific, any artificially produced antibodies have the potential to specifically target bacteria, viruses or a group of cells with minimal unwanted side effects. By this way, they also have the potential to suppress the body's own immunity. In theory, antibody-based therapies could be developed against any proteins or substances. Different types of immunotherapeutics are explained below in section 12.3. However for this to be successful, it is important that these 'artificial' antibodies should not be recognised as foreign by the host's own immunity. Some of the technologies used to produce highly specific chimeric (Mouse-Human), humanised and human antibodies are discussed in section 12.4.

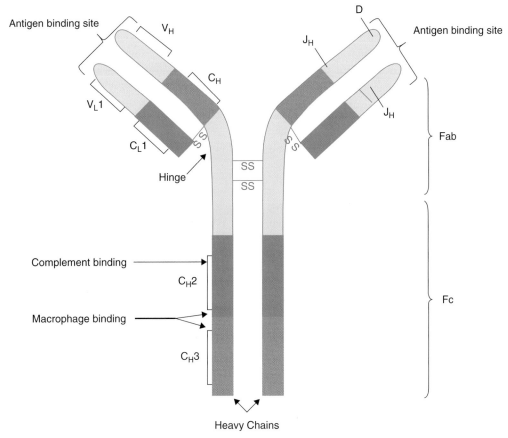

Figure 12.1 Schematic representation of a typical immunoglobulin (human antibody).
Fab and Fc are antigen binding and effector portions respectively. The constant regions are given in brown while variable regions are in light green. The constant regions of the heavy chains are subdivided into C_H1, C_H2, and C_H3 (and C_H4 in case of IgM and IgE). Each light chain has V, J and C segments.

12.4 Types of immunotherapeutics

This section describes different therapeutic applications of these novel antibodies. Clinically, immunotherapeutics has the potential to be used as i) non-specific immunotherapy, ii) naked monoclonal antibodies (those with no drug or radioactive material attached to them), iii) antibody conjugates (also known as immunoconjugates, or iv) antibody-directed enzyme pro-drug therapy (ADEPT).

Nonspecific immunotherapies
Non-specific immunotherapies utilise materials that have modulatory effects on the immune system [cytokines – such as interleukins (IL), interferons (IF) etc.]. These modulatory molecules are usually involved in stimulating macrophages, lymphocytes, and natural killer cells. They can either be used as single agents or in combination therapies (with another treatment) to improve the effectiveness of the primary treatment (as adjuvants). Some of the therapeutically significant cytokines include the ILs, IFs, tumour necrosis factors (TNFs), erythropoietin (EPO) and colony-stimulating factors (CSFs). Interleukins, such as IL-7, IL-12 and IL-21 have been studied in the treatment of cancer, both as single agents and as adjuvants. Currently, cytokines are being used to help to reduce the effects of traditional treatments such as chemotherapy. On the other hand, some genetically engineered cytokines are also being used to help boost the immune system and as adjuvant treatment with tumour vaccines. Cytokines are administered by injection, either into a vein or muscle, or under the skin.

Naked monoclonal antibodies

Naked monoclonal antibodies are the most widely used immunotherapeutic agent. At the beginning of this decade, they were used primarily after other therapies had failed. However due to their promise of successful reduction in tumour metastasis some of them are now being used as an earlier treatment option. These include Trastuzumab (Herceptin® – against breast cancer), Bevacizumab (Avastin® – against colorectal cancer), and Adalimumab (Humira® – against several autoimmune diseases). Monoclonal antibodies achieve their therapeutic effects through various mechanisms. They can have direct effects in producing apoptosis or (programmed cell death). On the other hand, they can block growth factor receptors and arrest proliferation of tumour cells. Their indirect effects are mainly brought about by recruiting cytotoxic cells, such as monocytes and macrophages. This is called antibody-dependent cell mediated cytotoxicity (ADCC). In ADCC the Fc gamma receptors (FcγR) on the surface of immune effector cells bind the Fc region of an antibody, which itself specifically bound to a target cell. The cells that can mediate ADCC are non-specific cytotoxic cells such as natural killer cells, macrophages, monocytes and eosinophils. Monoclonal antibodies can also bind complement, leading to direct cellular toxicity. This is known as complement-dependent cytotoxicity (CDC). In CDC, the C1q binds the antibody and this binding trigger the complement cascade which leads to the formation of the membrane attack complex (MAC). These mechanisms are summarised in Figure 12.2. Like most chemotherapies, these monoclonal antibodies are administered intravenously. Unlike traditional chemotherapies the side effects of naked Mabs are usually relatively mild. However not all the monoclonal antibodies are completely safe to use in any type of cancers. A good example is bevacizumab (Avastin®), a vascular endothelial growth factor (VEGF) inhibitor which, has been shown to produce side effects similar to traditional chemotherapies. It has been shown to produce severe bleeding, holes in the bowel and wound healing problems. Therefore the FDA has recently recommended withdrawing this drug from breast cancer treatment (see section 12.6 for details).

Antibody fragments

As explained in section 12.2, an active antibody fragment (Fv) composed of one variable domain in each of the heavy and the light chains. These domains shape the

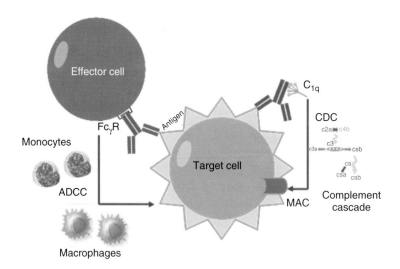

Figure 12.2 Schematic representation on monoclonal antibodies enhancing ADCC and CDC.
Schematic representation of the events produced by naked antibodies in enhancing cytotoxicity. In ADCC, the Fab portion of the monoclonal antibody can target the CD20 antigens expressed on the target (i.e. malignant cells). On the other hand, the Fc fragment binds the Fc receptors found on monocytes, macrophages, and/or natural killer cells. These cells in turn engulf the tumour cell and destroy them. In CDC, the monoclonal antibody binds to its receptor and initiates the complement cascade. The end result of this cascade is the formation of a 'membrane attack complex' (MAC) that literally makes a hole within the cell membrane, causing cell lysis and death.

- **Radio-immunoconjugates:**

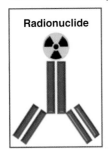

Using radio-immunoconjugates one can achieve targeted radiotherapy as a substitute for total body irradiation. It is a promising therapeutic approach for acute leukaemia. Monoclonal antibodies conjugated to the β-emitting isotopes are currently being used as standard treatment options for patients with CD20-expressing B-cell non-Hodgkin lymphoma (Dahle et al., 2007). They are also used as a diagnostic tool.

- **Immunotoxins:**

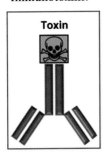

Immunotoxins are highly selective antibodies linked to toxic protein molecules that have been modified to remove their normal tissue-binding domains. Toxins used in the construction of immunotoxins are (a) bacterial toxins such as *Pseudomonas* exotoxin A, and diptheria toxin; or (b) plant derived toxin namely ricin, abrin, gelonin, and α-sarcin. These toxins inhibit the elongation step of protein synthesis.

- **Immunocytokines:**

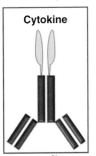

These are proteins that are genetically engineered by fusing cytokines into antibody sequences. They have the ability of specific targeting (antibody part) with the capability of stimulating immune destruction of target (mainly tumour) cells. Compared to systemic cytokine therapy these immunocytokines have minimal side effects. Immunocytokines containing IL-2 and IL10 have been shown to be efficacious against tumours and arthritis respectively (Pedretti et al., 2010; van de Loo and van der Berg, 2009).

- **Immunoliposomes:**

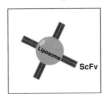

Liposomes are artificially made lipid molecules that are able to deliver therapeutic nucleotides. Selective toxicity can be achieved when liposomes are conjugated with ScFv domains of monoclonal antibodies (see section 12.3). Tissue specific delivery of tumour suppressor genes has been achieved in brain and breast cancers via immunoliposomes containing an antibody fragment (using ScFv) against the human transferrin receptor (Qian et al., 2002).

- **Antibody-directed enzyme prodrug therapy (ADEPT):**

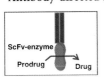

In this technology, ScFv domains of monoclonal antibodies are linked to a drug-activating enzyme. These ScFv domains are capable of selectively binding to the target cells. Thus subsequent to administration, a pro-drug (non-toxic) would be converted into a toxic drug only in malignant cells. This technology holds great promise in future oncology treatment (Bagshawe et al., 2004).

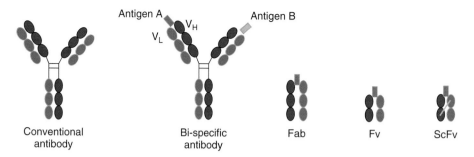

Figure 12.3 Structural differences between conventional.bi-specific antibodies and the antibody fragments. The antibody fragments Fab and Fv are generated by enzymatic cleavage of conventional antibodies (far left) whereas the ScFv fragment is created by molecular biology techniques. The yellow line on FcFv represents the linker between V_H and V_L domains. The fragments will differ from the full-size IgG molecule (far left) and bi-specific antibodies (middle) in characteristics such as affinity, immunogenicity, and circulating half-life.

antigen binding site (Fab) and determine the antibody specificity. It is now possible to artificially generate Fc and Fab domains by cleaving the Ig (antibody) molecule by the enzyme papain. Hence the variable regions of the heavy and light chains can also be fused together to form a single-chain variable fragment (ScFv), which is only half the size of the Fab fragment (Backovic et al., 2010). However it retains the original specificity of the parent immunoglobulin. Fab and ScFv fragments have an advantage over the larger mAb as they have faster clearance from circulation with high tissue penetration capabilities. For example, Fab fragments are used in the prophylaxis of snake bites and digoxin overdose (Hudson and Saurian, 2003). They are also useful in tissue imaging and diagnosis. Figure 12.3 compares the structural differences amongst conventional, bi-specific antibodies and antibody fragments (Backovic et al., 2010).

Although this technique is still in its infancy, significant success was made when ScFv against the human transferrin receptor were coupled with immunoliposomes (Flanagan and Jones, 2004.

Antibody conjugates

Antibodies conjugated with traditional therapeutic agents are more potent than naked monoclonal antibodies. Since antibodies are highly specific to their targets, it is believed that they can deliver the traditional drugs to specific cells and therefore produce selective toxicity. However since these traditional drugs are mostly radioactive substances or toxins, there is also a higher risk of side effects. This section summarises some examples of antibody conjugate technologies.

In addition to these modalities, techniques such as multi-step targeting have already been employed in cancer therapy to overcome the host response (HAMA) against antibody therapy. Bi-specific antibodies which have specificities to more than one antigen are usually used in this. In this technique, antibodies are first labelled with a tag (e.g. biotin) and injected into the host's body. This would allow some antibody molecules to attach/penetrate the tumour. The rest would be eliminated by the host response. After several days another non-active tag (e.g. strepavidin) which has high affinity to the first label (biotin) is injected and left for days. This would allow the second tag to either bind to the first tag-bound (e.g. biotynylated) antibody or be cleared from the circulation. Finally the radiolabelled form of the first tag (radiolabelled biotin) is injected which would have a higher chance of binding to the double labelled (strepavidin-biotynylated) complex; therefore minimising the chance of elimination by the host response. The sequence of events in multi-step targeting is summarised in Figure 12.4.

12.5 Humanisation of antibody therapy

Initially immunotherapeutics started with simple murine antibodies. These initial antibodies had several shortfalls which include i) a short half-life in vivo (due to host immune rejection); ii) limited penetration into target cells (such as tumour site), and iii) the inability to recruit host effector functions. The most important setback with murine antibodies is that being 100% murine proteins,

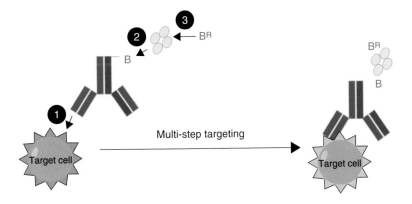

Figure 12.4 Sequences of events in multi-step tumour targeting.
The sequences of events is summarised on the left and the final effects are given on the right. ❶ Biotinylated antibody (B) is injected into the host. This allows the circulating biotynylated antibody to either bind to its target antigen or be cleared from the circulation by host reaction. ❷ Next strepavidin (light brown circles) which has a strong affinity for biotin, is injected. ❸ Again circulating strepavidin would either bind to antigen-bound biotinylated antibody or be cleared from the circulation. Finally, radiolabelled biotin (B^R) is injected which would either be rapidly cleared or bind to the tumour-bound strepavidin-biotinylated complex. By this specific targeting can be achieved.

and are recognised as 'foreign' by the human body and therefore they are rejected by an antibody-mediated immune response (human anti-murine antibodies – HAMA; produced by the host). To overcome these problems novel chimeric and humanised antibodies have been developed. To efficiently produce these antibodies, old techniques such as hybridoma technology have either been modified by using transgenic mice or replaced by recombinant DNA technology, and phage display. Figure 12.5 shows the structural differences between mouse, chimeric, and humanised in relation to human antibodies.

Currently, chimeric and humanised mouse monoclonal antibodies (that have therapeutic potential) are mainly produced by i) grafting complementarity-determining regions (CDRs) and ii) producing chimeric antibodies by splicing the mouse variable regions onto human constant regions. Fully human antibodies can also be generated by i) the selection of human antibody fragments from phage libraries, ii) transgenic mice and iii) through selection from human hybridomas (Rao and Schmader, 2007). These technologies are validated as commercially acceptable antibody drug discovery methods. Since the chimeric, humanised and human

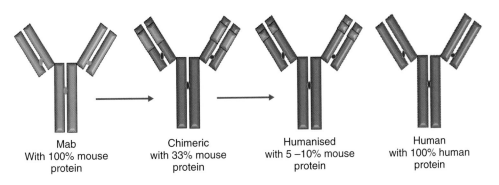

Mab
With 100% mouse protein

Chimeric
with 33% mouse protein

Humanised
with 5–10% mouse protein

Human
with 100% human protein

Figure 12.5 Evolution of immunotheraputics.
Chimeric Mab are usually produced from transgenic mice and/or hybridoma technology; humanised (zuMab) is produced by genetic engineering, CDR grafting, V gene cloning, and eukaryotic expression.

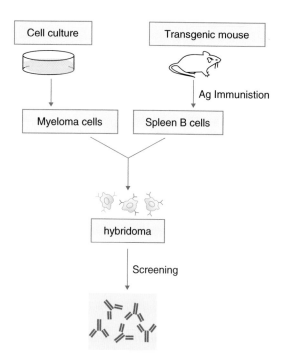

Figure 12.6 Schematic summary of steps involved in hybridoma technologies in producing chimeric antibodies. Hybridoma technology is similar to monoclonal antibody production except it starts with transgenic mouse. Cloning technology is mainly dependent on in vitro cell culture together with other molecular biological techniques.

antibodies have potential in future immunotherapeutic approaches, some technologies to produce these antibodies are briefly discussed in other sections.

Hybridoma technology using transgenic mouse

This technology is a slightly modified version of traditional hybridoma technology. Here, the hybridoma is produced from the spleen cells of transgenic mice in which the immunoglobulin genes are knockedout and replaced with human counterparts. This is followed by the antigen immunisation. The steps thereafter are similar to producing traditional monoclonal antibodies. The B cells from immunised transgenic mice are fused with myeloma cells derived from *in vitro* cell culture to produce immortalised hybridoma. These hybridomas are then screened for desired specificity. Once these specific hybridomas are produced, it is possible to generate hybrid-hybridomas. Figure 12.6 summarises the main steps involved in this method.

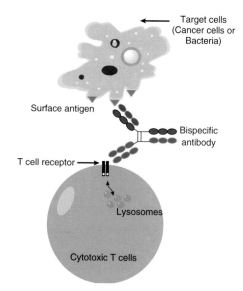

Figure 12.7 Model of action for effector cell retargeting by bi-specific antibodies.
One of the two arms in the variable domains of the bi-specific antibody is directed against an antigen of the target cell (either tumour or bacteria) and the other against a T-lymphocyte antigen such as CD3. Therefore the cytotoxic T cell gets activated and subsequently destroys the target cell.

These hybrid-hybridomas are obtained by fusion of two cells which contain the genetic information necessary for production of two different antibodies. In fact the formation of hybrid-hybridoma paved the first steps towards humanisation of mouse antibodies. They can also secrete chimeric antibodies made up of two non-identical halves. This new class of immunotherapeutic agents is also called bi-specific antibodies. This is beneficial in therapeutics as one arm of the bi-specific antibody binds to one antigen, the second arm binds to another. For example one arm of the antibody may bind to a marker molecule and the second to a target cell, creating an entirely new way of detecting and/or destroying tumour cells. This also has potentials in cancer immunotherapy as one arm of this chimeric antibody locks onto the tumour cells while the other may bind to a killer T cell to activate the destruction of tumour cells (see Figure 12.7; see also Figure 12.3).

Human antibody display

The human antibody library display technique uses phage, bacteria, yeast, mammalian cell and/or ribosomes to connect different antibody molecules. The most widely used

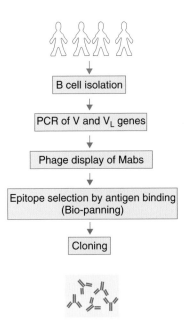

Figure 12.8 Overview of the Phage display system. cDNA encoding for VH, VL are amplified from human B cells by PCR and assembled. The assembled genes are inserted into a phage vector. Phage carrying specific-binding antibodies are then isolated using antigen and a series of cycles of binding, washing, elution, and amplification (i.e. bio-panning). Desired antibodies can be produced by cloning the gene from the selected phage into E.Coli.

library methodologies are based on the use of filamentous phage – a virus that infects *Escherichia coli*. By this way, antibodies can be synthesised and selected to acquire the desired affinity and specificity for immunotherapy. This technique involves three basic steps:

- **Antibody library construction and display onto the phage surface**
  Display libraries have high genetic diversity or repertoire size (commonly 10^9–10^{13}). The genetic diversity in these libraries is commonly created by cloning the Fv or Fab fragments from a large number of human donors. Figure 12.8 summarises the important steps in phage display technology. Firstly the gene segments responsible for variable region of human antibody (Fv and/or Fab) are amplified from human B cells to construct the antibody library. The library is then cloned for display on the surface of the phage (Marasco and Sui, 2007). In this way, the fusion product will be incorporated into the mature phage coat and its genetic material will reside within the phage particle. This connection

between ligand genotype and phenotype allows the enrichment of specific DNA (i.e. using selection on an immobilised antigen) (Dally et al., 2002).

- **Selecting the library against specific antigen targets ('*panning*')**
  Selection against the antigen is then performed using the phage display library. Desired antibodies are selected by successive rounds of bio-panning which involves several washes, during which the non-specific antibodies are washed away. Finally the phage with specific antibody from the display can be eluted and its DNA amplified by cloning into a vector (usually *Escherichia coli*).
- **Screening for desired specificity**
  After multiple selection rounds, the antibody with the desired specificity can be screened by using either ELISA or fluorescent-activated cell sorting (FACS). In cases where the target is a cell-membrane bound protein, genes of antibody variable regions can be cloned into whole human IgG expression vectors and transfected into cell lines to produce fully human Mabs.

Recombinant antibodies by cloning v-region genes

As explained before in section 12.1, the functional structure of the antigen-binding site is determined by genes of both heavy (H) and light (L) variable (V) domains. Therefore in this technology, the cDNA responsible for the V domain is extracted from mouse monoclonal cell lines and cloned into a mammalian expression vector. Then the vector is transfected into mammalian cells [usually Chinese hamster ovary (CHO) cells] which can generate the humanised/chimeric antibodies. Figure 12.9 summarises the steps in this technology. Cloning of mouse variable genes into human constant-region genes generates chimeric as well as humanised antibodies depending on the size of the clone.

Memory B-cell immortalisation

This technique involves isolation of human memory B cells from peripheral blood mononuclear cells (PBMCs) of infected patients. These B cells are then immortalised using Epstein Barr Virus (EBV) in the presence of a polyclonal B cell activator (mostly CpG oligodeoxynucleotide). These transformed cells are capable of producing a human monoclonal antibody with desired antigen specificity. Finally the culture supernatants are screened directly for specific antibodies. Positive cultures are further cloned and fully humanised. The main limitation of B-cell immortalisation is the antibody produced are only specific to the antigen from the infected organism

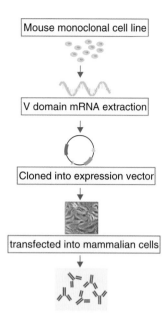

Figure 12.9 Steps involved in producing recombinant antibodies.
The mRNA responsible for the V domains is extracted and cloned into an expression vector. Then the vector is transfected into mammalian cells in order to generate humanised antibodies.

(as humans cannot be immunised to produce the desired antibodies). The sequence of events in B-cell immortalisation are summarised in Figure 12.10.

CDR grafting (antibody reshaping)

CDR grafting is the most advanced approach in which the CDR residues from the variable region of a mouse mAb are transferred to human constant and variable domain frameworks that have high sequence homology with the mouse counterparts. First of all, it is important to determine the variable region DNA in the mouse antibody to be amplified by RT-PCR. Then a human framework (FR) region should be selected to combine with mouse CDRs. Once the human FRs and mouse CDRs are selected, it is imperative to asses any conflicts between the two in order to eliminate mismatches.

Finally DNA and protein sequences of the CDR-grafted humanised antibody are designed incorporating any additional changes in the FR to maintain identical antigen specificity and to eliminate any rejection from HAMA. In this way, the final product would have high specificity with minimal rejection by HAMA. Figure 12.11 summarises the steps involved in CRR grafting.

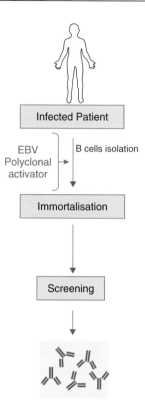

Figure 12.10 Schematic representation of Memory B-cell immortalisation.
Isolated human memory B lymphocyte subpopulation is transfected with EBV in the presence of a polyclonal B cell activator. This is followed by selecting a human B memory lymphocyte clone which has the capacity to produce specific human monoclonal antibody.

12.6 Immunotherapeutics in clinical practice

Research in immunotherapeutics started over 100 years ago. Now, this vision has become a reality in standard preclinical evaluation as well as in clinical practice. This is due to the rapid development of genetic and molecular biological techniques. The WHO appointed body for International Non-proprietary Names (INN) has given different post-fixes to these antibodies to identify their origins. According to INN, the official non-proprietary names given for monoclonal, chimeric humanised and fully human antibodies end with the postfix as *−oMabs, -xiMabs, -zuMab,* and *−muMbs* respectively. As explained in section 12.1, Muromonab (Orthoclone OKT3®),

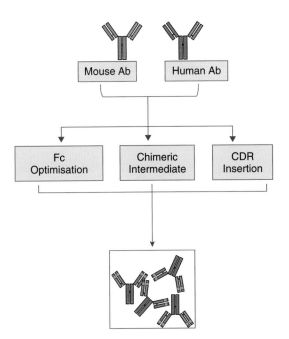

Figure 12.11 Schematic representation of flow chart involved in CRD grafting.
CDR grafting produces humanised antibodies with grafted amino acids from mouse (or rat) hypervariable regions. Therefore it retains around 90 to 95% of human identity.

the first FDA-approved therapeutic murine monoclonal antibody. Since then the therapeutic market for monoclonal antibodies has grown exponentially and there are now several FDA approved antibodies used in clinical practice.

Chimeric antibodies (postfix -xiMabs)

Chimeric antibodies (−*xiMabs*) are murine molecules that were engineered to remove their immunogenicity with improved immunological efficiency. As explained in section 12.3, chimeric antibodies contain around 33% mouse protein (mainly V regions). These are produced by fusing the antigen-binding variable domains of murine to human constant domains. That is mouse VL to human CL and mouse VH to human CH1–CH2–CH3 for light and heavy chains, respectively (see Figure 12.1). Some examples of chimeric antibodies that are currently used in clinical practice are given in Table 12.1.

Humanised antibodies (postfix -zuMabs)

Generation of high-affinity humanised antibodies requires the transfer of one (or more) additional residues from the framework regions (FRs) of the parent Mab. At present there are only a few examples of humanised antibodies in clinical practice. The first therapeutic CDR grafted antibody was developed against CAMPATH-1, an antigen expressed on the surface of human lymphocytes and monocytes (Riechmann et al., 1988). In this development, the heavy and light chain CDRs of rat anti-CAMPATH-1 antibody, YTH34/5HL

Table 12.1 Examples of Chimeric antibodies that are used in clinical practice.

Name	Clinical use	Clinical application
Infliximab (Remicade®)	Anti-inflammatory (against TNFα)	Rheumatoid arthritis, Crohn's disease, Ulcerative Colitis
Basiliximab (Simulect®)	Anti-inflammatory (against IL-2 receptor; CD25 subunit)	Against graft rejection In kidney transplants
Rituximab (Rituxan® and MabThera®)	Anti-cancer (against the protein CD20)	Non-Hodgkin's lymphoma
Cetuximab (Erbitux®)	Anti-cancer EGFR inhibitor	Colorectal cancer and Head and neck cancer
Abciximab (c7E3 Fab) (ReoPro®)	Anti-coagulant glycoprotein IIb/IIIa receptor antagonist	Prevent coagulation during coronary angioplasty; IHD and unstable angina

EGFR =Epidermal Growth Factor Receptor
IHD = Ischemic Heart Disease

Table 12.2 Examples of humanised antibodies that are used in clinical practice.

Name	Clinical use	Clinical application
Bevacizumab (Avastin®)	Angiogenesis inhibitor (against VEGF)	Colorectal cancer, Age related macular degeneration
Certolizumab pegol (Cimzia®)	TNF-α signalling inhibitor	Crohn's disease, rheumatoid arthritis
Daclizumab (Zenapax®)	Against IL-2Rα receptor	Currently in clinical trials to suppress graft rejection
Eculizumab (Soliris®)	Complement system protein C5	Paroxysmal nocturnal hemoglobinuria
Palivizumab (Synagis®)	Against F protein of respiratory syncytial virus	Respiratory syncytial viral infections
Trastuzumab (Herceptin®)	Against ErbB2 – HER2 (interferes with the HER2/neu receptor)	Breast cancer

VEGF = *vascular endothelial growth factor*
Erb2 = v-erb-b2 erythroblastic leukemia viral oncogene homolog 2
HER-2/neu = neuro/glioblastoma derived oncogene homolog (avian)

were spliced into the V regions of the human myeloma protein heavy chain and the Bence Jones protein light chain. The resultant CDR grafted antibody was found to be more efficient in cell-mediated lysis than rat antibody.

Anti-allergy antibody Omalizumab (Xolair®) is a successful example of humanised antibody in clinical practice. This antibody selectively binds to IgE forming an omalizumab-IgE complex. This prevents IgE binding to receptor sites on mast cells and basophils. In addition, the removal of circulating IgE by omalizumab would result in down-regulation of IgE receptors. This gives symptomatic relief from allergic asthma. Other examples that are currently used in clinical practice are given in Table 12.2.

Fully human antibodies (postfix -muMabs)

As already explained in section 12.5, human antibodies are usually obtained from single-chain variable fragments (ScFvs) or Fab phage display libraries. These antibodies have the highest specificity amongst most of the artificially produced antibodies. They can also be obtained from transgenic mice that are transfected with human immunoglobulin genes. Interestingly, these antibodies, which are produced from transgenic mice, have the advantage of not requiring humanisation prior to therapeutic use. In 2006, the first fully human antibody panitumumab (Vectibix®), an antibody directed against the epidermal growth factor receptor (EGFR) was approved by the FDA. Many cancer cells actually require signals medi-

ated by EGFR for their survival. Panitumumab binds to EGFR, preventing EGF and Transforming growth factor alpha (TGFα) from binding to the receptor. Both EGF and TGFα are known to promote carcinogenesis due to their mitogenic effects on tumour invasion. Thereby panitumumab interferes with the signals that would otherwise stimulate growth of the cancer cell and allow it to survive. Since it is a human antibody, it is expected to have the safety profiles such as, a low incidence of infusion reactions, antigenicity and allergic response. These are attributes currently being investigated in clinical trials. A few examples of fully human antibodies that are under development and/or undergoing clinical trails are summarised in Table 12.3.

12.7 Advantages and disadvantages of immunotherapy

Immunotherapeutic agents comprise an increasingly important class of compounds that have the ability to treat a variety of diseases ranging from cancer, neurodegenerative disorders, infectious, autoimmune and cardiac diseases. Currently over 25 antibodies have been approved for clinical use, and another 350 are in clinical trials (Casadevall et al., 2004). Compared to traditional therapeutic modalities (such as chemotherapy of cancer, subtype specific targeting for asthma, antibiotics against microbial diseases etc.), molecules used in

Table 12.3 Examples of fully human antibodies in development or undergoing clinical trails.

Name	Clinical use	Applications
Adalimumab (HUMIRA®)	Inhibition of TNF-α signalling	Rheumatoid arthritis (Auto-immune disorders) [CT]
Golimumab (Simponi)	Inhibition of TNF-α signalling	Spondylarthropathies and Psoriatic Arthritis (immuno-sppressive) [CT]
AIN457 (under research)	Inhibition of IL17	Psoriasis, Rheumatoid arthritis [UR]

CT = clinical Trials
UR = under research

immunotherapy have fewer side effects. Antibody-based therapies that use human or humanised antibodies have even lower toxicities and higher specificities. Therefore they offer improved quality of life for patients compared to some other cancer therapies. Due to their targeted delivery, they provide long-term benefit to a short-term therapy. This is particularly true in the field of antimicrobial immunotherapy. Due to their high specificity, at least in theory, they will not pave way for selecting resistant organisms. They also can be used as diagnostic tools; to test the responsiveness of cells before administering the drug or to identify the status of the disease (e.g. identification of cancer metastases using radiolabelled antibodies).

However, immunotherapeutics have disadvantages too. The major hurdle for antibody therapeutics has been the inherent immunogenicity (host response by HAMA). Since most of the Mabs are rodent derived, they would be considered as 'foreign' by the host and therefore be rejected. Although it is now possible to produce Mabs with reduced host rejection, these advanced technologies are expensive and time consuming. On the other hand, antibody-based therapies target only single cell types (or micro-organism). Therefore more than one antibody preparation might be required to target disease with high antigenic variation (involving different cell types). Moreover, some antibodies are found to produce severe adverse reactions similar to traditional chemotherapy. Other serious side effects include:

- Severe allergy-like reactions which in very few cases lead to death.
- Reduction of red blood cells, white blood cells and platelets.

- Heart problems including heart failure and a small risk of heart attack.
- Skin problems. Sores and rashes which can cause serious infections in some cases.
- Bleeding. Some of the monoclonal antibody drugs are designed to stop cancer from forming new blood vessels, for example, bevacizumab (Avastin®)].

12.8 The future

Due to the rapid development of genetic engineering and molecular cloning techniques, the future of cancer immunotherapy continues to be promising. Immunotherapeutics have the potential to overcome many problems that hindered traditional drug therapy. This includes, i) the increased prevalence of drug-resistant tumours/micro-organisms; ii) genetic polymorphisms of targeted receptors; iii) the emergence of new pathogens; iv) the re-emergence of old pathogens and v) the difficulties involved in treating infections in immuno-compromised patients. Also problems, such as the heterogenic nature of different tumours can be solved by antibody therapy as most of the antibody targets are proteins that can be mapped to detect the binding site (i.e. epitopes). Characterisation of these target epitopes will aid in the discovery and development of new therapeutics, vaccines and diagnostics. Therefore, there is a promise for immunotherapeutics as stand alone or in combinatory Therapeutic modalities. In the future, immunotherapies are expected to become the treatment of choice for cancer. It can also be used in combination with surgery, radiotherapy and chemotherapy.

In order to overcome current limitations, such as host rejection response, multi-step antibody targeting techniques can be employed. It is also possible to combine many variable gene elements to synthesise antibodies against large number of antigens, which would result in higher affinity antibodies with more diversity in specificity. Therefore in the future, it is possible for immunotherapeutics to become the main modality for treating currently incurable diseases.

12.9 Summary

Immunotherapeutics aims to activate the body's own defence mechanisms by triggering and/or 'mimicking' immune responses. Antibodies are the most widely used immunotherapeutic modalities. The development of molecular biological and gene cloning techniques have resulted in highly specific versatile antibodies that can be tolerated by the host. Several monoclonal, chimeric and humanised antibodies are already being used in clinical practice. New modalities for immunotherapeutics (such as fully humanised antibodies) are being either developed or undergoing clinical trails. Therefore, immunotherapeutics may become the treatment of choice for treating incurable diseases.

References

Backovic M, Johansson DM, Klupp BG, MettenleiterTC. Persson MAA and Rey FA (2010) Efficient method for production of high yields of Fab fragments in Drosophila S2 cells. Protein Engineering, Design & Selection 1–6.

Bagshawe KD, Sharma SK and Begent RHJ (2004) Antibody-directed enzyme prodrug therapy (ADEPT) for cancer, Expert opinion in Biological therapy 4(11):1777–1789.

Casadevall A, Dadachova E and Pirofski L (2004) Passive antibody therapy for infectious diseases. Nature Reviews Microbiology 2:695–703.

Cheson BD, Leonard JP (2008) Monoclonal Antibody Therapy for B-Cell Non-Hodgkin's Lymphoma. New England Journal of Medicine 359:613–626.

Clark M (2000) Antibody humanisation: a case of the 'Emperor's new clothes'? Immunology Today 21(8):377–388.

Dahle J, Borrebæk J, Jonasdottir TJ, Hjelmerud AK, Melhus KB , and Bruland S (2007) Targeted cancer therapy with a novel low-dose rate α-emitting Radio-immunoconjugate. Blood. 110(6):2049–2056.

Dally S, Dillon P, Manning B, Dunne L, Killard A, O'Kennedy (2002) Production and Characterization of murine Single Chain Fv Antibodies to Aflatoxin B1 Derived From a Pre-immunized Antibody Phage Display Library System. Food and Agricultural Immunology 14(4):255–274.

De Braud C, Catania C, Masini M, Maur S, Cascinu R, Berardi L, Giovannoni G, Spitaleri S, Boselli D, Emilia R (2010) Combinations of the immunocytokine F16-IL2 with doxorubicin or with paclitaxel investigated in phase Ib studies in patients with advanced solid tumours. Journal of Clinical Oncolology 28 (suppl; abstr e13017).

Flanagan RJ, Jones AL (2004) Fab antibody fragments: some applications in clinical toxicology. Drug Safety. 27(14):1115–1133.

Hudson PJ, Saurian C. (2003) Engineered antibodies. Nature Medicine 9: 129–134.

Kaminski MS, Tuck M, Estes J, Kolstad A, Ross CW, Zasadny K, Regan D, Kison P, Fisher S, Kroll, S, Wahl RL, (2005) ^{131}Tositumomab Therapy as Initial Treatment for Follicular Lymphoma New England Journal of Medicine. 352:441–449.

Kotzerke J, Bunjes D and Scheinberg DA (2005) Radio-immunoconjugates in acute leukemia treatment: the future is radiant. Bone Marrow Transplantation 36:1021–1026.

Marasco WA, and Sui J (2007) The growth and potential of human antiviral monoclonal antibody therapeutics. Nature Biotechnology 25:1421–1434.

Pedretti M, Verpelli C, Mårlind J, Bertani G, Sala C, Neri D and L Bello (2010) Combination of temozolomide with immunocytokine F16–IL2 for the treatment of glioblastoma. British Journal of Cancer 103:827–836.

Qian ZM, L, H, Sun, H, and Ho, K (2002) Targeted Drug Delivery via the Transferrin Receptor-Mediated Endocytosis Pathway. Pharmacological Reviews 5(4):561–587.

Rader C. (2009) Overview on concepts and applications of Fab antibody fragments. Current Protocols in Protein Science. Chapter 6:Unit 6.9.

Rao AV, Schmader K (2007) Monoclonal antibodies as targeted therapy in haematological malignancies in older adults. American Journal of Geriatric Pharmacotherapy. 2007 Sep;5(3):247–262.

Riechmann L, Clark MR, Waldmann H, Winter G (1988) Reshaping human antibodies for therapy. Nature 332:323–327.

van De Loo FA and van den Berg WF (2009) Immunocytokines: the long awaited therapeutic magic bullet in rheumatoid arthritis? Arthritis Research & Therapy 11:132.

Glossary

Acetylation

A post-translational modification and key regulatory mechanism that adds acetyl groups to proteins, for example to histones (see also *chromatin remodelling*).

Activated/inactivated receptor

When a receptor is activated by for example ligand binding it transduces an extracellular signal into a cellular response. However some receptors enter an inactivate phase where ligand is still bound but their transducing machinery (e.g. channel or G-protein) is inactive. This property is important because the receptor cannot be activated again until it returns to the non-activated state. Some drugs exploit this property and target the inactivated form.

Active transport

Movement of a substrate across a membrane that requires the input of energy.

Adenylyl cyclase

Enzyme which catalyses the formation of cyclic AMP using the substrate ATP.

Adjuvant

A pharmacological agent that modifies the effect of drugs or vaccine.

Affinity

A measure of how tightly a ligand binds to a GPCR.

Agarose

A polysaccharide with many hydroxyl groups.

Agarose gel electrophoresis

Technique widely used to separate DNA molecules using an electric field.

Agonist

A drug which binds to a receptor and activates it, producing a pharmacological response.

Allele

One of a set of alternative forms of a gene. In a diploid cell each gene will have two alleles, each occupying the same position (locus) on homologous chromosomes.

Allosteric modulator

Binds to a site other than the ligand binding site to modify a protein's (e.g. receptor or channel) activity.

Allosteric site

A ligand binding site on a receptor which is distinct from the orthosteric site. Some allosteric ligands are classed as non-competitive antagonists.

Alternative splicing

A process that creates different (alternative) transcripts from the same immature mRNA by either retaining or excising exons in different combinations; can vary from cell to cell.

Amnesia

A condition that is characterised by the loss of memory.

Molecular Pharmacology: From DNA to Drug Discovery, First Edition. John Dickenson, Fiona Freeman, Chris Lloyd Mills,
Shiva Sivasubramaniam and Christian Thode.
© 2013 John Wiley & Sons, Ltd. Published 2013 by John Wiley & Sons, Ltd.

Amphipathic molecules
A substance that has both hydrophilic and hydrophobic properties e.g. phospholipids.

Antagonist
A drug which blocks the effect on an agonist. Competitive antagonists reversibly bind to receptors at the same binding site as the endogenous ligand or agonist, but without activating the receptor. Most drugs classed as 'competitive antagonists' have been re-classified as inverse agonists.

Antibody-directed enzyme pro-drug therapy (ADEPT)
An artificially designed antibody which is linked to an enzyme designed for selective binding of a specific antigen and thereby capable of transforming the administrated pro-drug into an active drug

Antigen-binding fragment (FAb)
The region on an antibody that binds to antigens.

Antiporter
Transporter that moves substrate(s) using a co-transporter substrate which travels in the opposite direction across the membrane.

Antisense oligonucleotide
Single strands of DNA or RNA that are complementary to a selected sequence. Anti-sense RNA oligonucleotides can be used to inhibit RNA translation and thus prevent protein synthesis.

Anxiolytic
Referring to a drug that relieves anxiety.

Apical membrane
(luminal membrane) The part of the plasma membrane that borders the lumen.

Apoptosis
A form of programmed cell death.

Aptamers
Short single-stranded DNA or RNA-based oligonucleotides that selectively bind to intracellular proteins.

Aquaporin
A membrane protein that forms a highly selective channel allowing water molecules to cross the membrane.

Arrestins
A family of scaffolding proteins generally associated with the desensitisation of GPCRs.

Ataxia
Poor coordination leading to reduced movement.

Atrial/ventricular fibrillation
Irregular electrical activity in the atria or ventricles leading to cardiac arrhythmia.

Autoradiography
Technique in which a radioactive object produces an image of itself on a photographic film. The image is called an autoradiograph or autoradiogram.

Autosomal
An autosomal chromosome is any chromosome that is not a sex chromosome.

BAC library
A collection of bacterial artificial chromosomes (BACs), which contain clones of large DNA fragments, such as genomic DNA.

Bacteriophage
A virus that infects bacteria, such as the bacteriophages l and P1.

Basal transcription factors
Modulate/regulate constitutive gene expression.

Basolateral

The part of the plasma membrane that does not border the lumen. The basal membrane is furthest from the lumen, whist the lateral membrane is on the sides of the cell and is the site of contact between adjacent cells in a monolayer.

Biased agonist

A class of receptor agonist that promotes or inhibits only some of the signal transduction pathways associated with a specific receptor.

Bicistronic

Referring to a DNA fragment encoding two proteins.

Binary system

A system frequently used in genetic engineering to provide greater control over gene expression; it is based on the interaction of an effector molecule and a responder gene see conditional gene expression.

Binding element

DNA sequence where transcription factors can bind.

Bioelectrics

Movement of charge due to a biological system.

Bio-panning

A process of affinity selection to select the peptides that bind to a given target.

Bivalent ligand

An agonist possessing two functional pharmacophores linked by a chemical spacer.

Blastocyst

A stage during embryogenesis, when the embryo resembles a hollow sphere.

BRET

Bioluminescence Resonance Energy Transfer; the transfer of energy from a luminescent donor protein to a fluorescent acceptor protein.

Bronchiectasis

Pathological widening of part(s) of the bronchial tree with reductions in mucociliary secretions and airflow.

b-zips

Protein domains are formed when two proteins line up with moieties that intercalate to form a zipper like structure.

Cardiac arrhythmia

An irregular heartbeat.

Cardiac infarction

Blockage of a coronary blood vessel.

Caspase

A protease activated during the process of programmed cell death or apoptosis.

cDNA

Complementary DNA. DNA synthesised from a RNA template by reverse transcriptase to form an antisense 'copy' of the RNA.

cDNA library

A collection of cloned cDNA fragments, which can be synthesised enzymatically from mRNA.

CDR grafting

An attempt to minimize the mouse sequence by only cloning the mouse CDR sequence into a human variable domain.

Channel

A protein that forms pore and allows substrates to diffuse across membranes.

Channelopathy

A disorder caused by a dysfunctional ion channel.

Chaperone
A protein that aids the correct folding of other proteins.

Chemiluminescence
The emission of light as a result of a chemical reaction.

Chimeric antibodies
Genetically engineered antibodies that have the antigen binding fragment from one species fused with crystallisable fragment from another species.

Chimeric mouse
An animal consisting of two populations of cells with non-identical genotypes.

Chromatin remodelling
A heritable alteration of the chromatin structure, through changes in the methylation, ubiquitylation or acetylation status of histone proteins or DNA regions (not their sequence).

Chromatin
Tightly folded and packed DNA.

Chromatography
A method that separates mixtures of molecules based on their differential movement in a liquid or gaseous mobile phase through a stationary phase.

Cis-acting factors
DNA has two strands and cis factors interacting at sites in the stand that is to be transcribed, for example regulatory elements.

Classic genetics
see forward genetics.

Cloning of DNA
Creating multiple copies of a DNA fragment using molecular biological techniques commonly this involves inserting the DNA of interest into a vector (see recombinant vector).

Codon
See *genetic code*.

Comparative genomics
See *genomics*.

Concatemer
A DNA sequence consisting of multiple copies of the same DNA fragment arranged in a head-to-tail array.

Conditional gene expression
In genetics, the controllable expression of a gene, often achieved through exogenous inducers.

Conditional gene knockout
The tissue or organ specific deletion of a gene.

Confocal microscopy
Optical imaging technique that improves resolution and reduces out of focus information when compared to conventional light microscopy. It enables the production of three-dimensional images.

Conotoxins
Venoms produced by the cone sea snail.

Constitutive activity
GPCR-mediated activation of G-protein signalling which is independent of agonist-binding.

Constitutive gene expression
Expression of a continually active gene.

Crosstalk (signalling)

Where one cell signalling system affects another cell signalling system. For example the cAMP intracellular signalling pathway can result in the phosphorylation of Ca^{2+} channels, affecting their ability to conduct calcium ions.

Crystallography

See *X-ray crystallography*.

Cyclic AMP

Second messenger produced by the breakdown of ATP by the enzyme adenylyl cyclase.

Cyclodextrins

Cyclic sugar molecules widely used in food, pharmaceutical and chemical manufacture. In pharmaceutical applications they are used to help in the distribution of substances that are otherwise insoluble in water.

Cytochalasins

A family of fungal metabolites that bind to actin and interfere with the formation of microfilaments.

Cytochrome P450

A family of enzymes involved in drug metabolism.

Cytokines

A class of signalling molecule released by cells for intercellular communication.

DAG

Diacylglycerol; membrane-bound second messenger generated following the hydrolysis of phosphatidylinositol biphosphate (PIP_2) by phospholipase C. Responsible for the activation of protein kinase C.

Dalton (Da)

Unit of molecular mass approximately equal to the mass of a hydrogen atom (1.66×10^{-24} g).

Desensitisation

The reduction in the response to an agonist while it is continuously present at the receptor.

Diabetes

A metabolic disease that occurs due to abnormal glucose handing caused by a lack of, or inactivity of the hormone insulin.

Diploid

Having two sets of homologous chromosomes; thus each gene exists in two copies.

DNA

Deoxyribonucleic acid.

DNA ligase

An enzyme that forms phosphodiester bonds between two double-stranded DNA molecules.

DNA or RNA oligonucleotides

See antisense oligonucleotide

DNA recombinase

An enzyme with the ability to recognise corresponding DNA motifs and carry out site-specific recombination, namely excision, inversion, insertion, duplication and translocation.

Domain

The tertiary structure of a protein can be divided up into domains consisting of between 100 and 200 amino acids.

Down-regulation

The loss of total receptor number from a cell as a consequence of agonist-induced endocytosis followed by proteolytic degradation.

EC$_{50}$
The molar concentration of an agonist which produces 50% of the maximal response possible for that agonist.

ECG
Electrocardiogram; a test that records the electrical activity of the heart.

Ecto-nucleotidase
A class of plasma membrane bound enzymes that metabolise extracellular nucleotides.

Efficacy
The intrinsic ability of a drug-receptor complex to stimulate a functional response. Agonist efficacy refers to the variation in the size of response produced by different agonists even when occupying the same number of receptors. High-efficacy agonists trigger maximal responses whilst occupying a lower proportion of receptor sites compared to low efficacy agonists which cannot elicit the same maximal response even if occupying all available receptor sites. Compounds displaying low efficacy are referred to as partial agonists

Electrochemical gradient
The distribution of anions and cations across a membrane are dependent upon their concentration (chemical) and charge (electrostatic pull). Although there is a concentration gradient, repulsive/attractive forces due to charge may prevent ions from diffusing so that their concentration is equal on both sides of the membrane. This gives rise to a difference in potential across the membrane which is measured in volts.

Electrophoresis
Describes the movement of a molecule under the influence of an electrical field.

Electrophysiology
The measurement of bioelectrical activity. Extensively used to investigate ion movement across cell membranes.

Electroporation
The use of a large pulse of electricity to transiently permeabilise a cell, allowing the entry of foreign material (e.g. DNA or drugs).

Electroporation
The use of electric currents to permeablilise cell membranes and transfer molecules, such as vector constructs, into the cell.

E$_{max}$
The maximum possible effect for an agonist.

Embryonic stem cells
Undifferentiated pluripotent embryonic cells, which have the ability to develop into any cell type of the foetus.

Endocrine glands
Glands that secrete signalling molecules into the bloodstream.

Endocytosis
The removal of receptors from the plasma membrane into membrane-bound vesicles.

Endogenous ligand
The agonist(s) for a receptor that are produced by a particular organism.

Endogenous
Originating from within (e.g. endogenous gene).

Endomembrane
Membranes in the cytosol that form discrete structures such as the endoplasmic reticulum.

Endoplasmic reticulum
A specialised membranous organelle within eukaryotic cells responsible for synthesis of many membrane proteins.

Endosome
A membrane-bound organelle or vesicle involved in the process of endocytosis.

Enterotoxigenic

Produce enterotoxins.

Epigenetics

The study of mechanisms that an organism can employ to alter the phenotype of many genes without changing the genotype.

Epimodification

An alteration of the chromatin structure (see *chromatin remodelling*).

Epitope

The surface portion of an antigen capable of eliciting an immune response.

Epitope tag

See protein tag.

Excitotoxicity

Process where excessive excitatory neurotransmission leads to neuronal death.

Exogenous

Originating from outside (e.g. exogenous DNA or transgene).

Exocrine glands

Glands that secrete molecules into ducts that are external to the cell (e.g. salivary glands).

Exon

Coding region of a protein-coding gene.

Exporter

Transporter which moves substrate(s) in an outward direction.

Expression cassette

A DNA segment consisting of a promoter, a cDNA/gene and a polyadenylation signal.

Expression

Production of an observable phenotype by a gene – usually by the synthesis of a protein.

FISH

Fluorescence *in situ* hybridisation.

Fluorescence

The act of a molecule absorbing light at one wavelength and then emitting light of a longer wavelength.

Fluorochrome

See *fluorophore*.

Fluorophore

Functional group which absorbs energy at one wavelength and then emits energy at a different wavelength.

Forwards genetics

A traditional approach to identify genes, which are responsible for a particular gene product or phenotype.

Fragment crystallisable region (Fc)

The tail region of an antibody that interacts with cell surface receptors called Fc receptors.

Fragment-based screening

The screening of biological targets with small libraries of chemical fragments in order to identify important functional chemical groups.

FRET

Fluorescence Resonance Energy Transfer; the transfer of energy from a fluorescent donor protein/molecule to a fluorescent acceptor protein/molecule.

Gag region/protein

A structural protein of the human immunodeficiency virus (HIV).

Gain-of-function mutation

A new or altered function of a gene product as a consequence of a gene mutation.

Gene knockdown

Experimental reduction of a particular gene transcript, usually without the need of genetically modifying the gene itself.

Gene knockin

The insertion of mutated or altered genes into an organism.

Gene knockout

The deletion of a gene from an entire genome.

Gene silencing

See gene knockdown.

Gene targeting

Site-specific manipulation of a host genome through homologous recombination and a vector targeting the selected site.

General transcription factors

See basal transcription factors.

Genetic code

A set of rules that determines the translation of DNA or RNA sequences into protein sequences; it consists of triplets of nucleotides (codons) which specify amino acids or the termination of protein synthesis.

Genetics

The study of heredity and variations in living organisms.

Genome

The entire genetic information of a cell or an organism.

Genomics

The study of a genome, often involving the comparison of genomes from different species.

Genotype

The genetic constitution (i.e. alleles) of an organism.

Germ cells

The reproductive cells, that is, eggs (oocytes) and sperm (spermatozoa).

GFP

Green Fluorescent Protein; a protein originally isolated from the jellyfish *Aequorea victoria* which displays green fluorescence when exposed to blue light. Many mutations have been genetically engineered to produce a range of different colour variants such as yellow fluorescent protein (YFP) and cyan fluorescent protein (CFP).

Glycocalyx

The glycoprotein and glycolipid components on the outside face of the plasma membrane. It helps distinguish between "self" and foreign material or damaged cells.

Glycosylation

A post-translational modification that adds carbohydrates to proteins.

GPCRs
G-protein Coupled Receptors; a large family of transmembrane receptors which when activated couple to heterotrimeric G-proteins.

GRK
G-protein coupled receptor kinase; a family of enzymes which catalyse the agonist-induced phosphorylation of G-protein coupled receptors.

Haemolysins
Bacterial exotoxins if secreted into animal circulatory system cause lysis of red blood cells.

Haploid
Having just one set of chromosomes, such as in sperm and oocytes.

Haplotype
A set of single nucleotide polymorphisms found within a single gene.

Hemichannel
The smallest functional unit of a channel, usually found in gap junctions.

Heterochromatin
A genetically inactive part of the genome.

Heterodimer
A dimer composed of two different GPCR protomers.

Heterologous
Deriving from another species; for example, heterologous expression refers to the expression of a gene from one organism in another.

Heteromeric
Protein composed of different subunits.

Heterotrimeric G-protein
A class of guanine nucleotide protein composed of three different protein subunits.

Heterozygous
A diploid cell or organism carrying different alleles at the same genomic location on the two homologous chromosomes; for example, a transgene or other exogenous DNA may only be found at one site in a genetically engineering animal.

High-throughput screening
A method for screening large numbers of potential drug compounds using start-of-the-art robotics.

Homodimer
A dimer composed of two identical GPCR protomers.

Homologous DNA
A gene, chromosome or other DNA fragment, which is similar in sequence to another.

Homologous recombination
A naturally occurring process in living cells, whereby genetic material is reciprocally exchanged between homologous chromosomes; it is frequent during the generation of germ cells (meiosis), and experimentally used for gene targeting.

Homomeric
Protein composed of the same subunits.

Homozygous
A diploid cell or organism carrying identical alleles at the same genomic location on the two homologous chromosomes.

Housekeeping genes
Are usually involved in maintain a basic cellular function and constitutive expressed at similar levels in all cells of an organism.

Human genome project

The first project designed to sequence the complete human genome in order to identify and accurately map all its genes it was completed by an international consortium and a private corporation.

Humanised antibodies

Non-human species antibodies whose protein sequences have been modified to increase their similarity to antibody variants produced naturally in humans.

Hybridoma

A cell hybrid produced in vitro by the fusion of a lymphocyte that produces antibodies and a myeloma cells.

Hydropathy analysis

A method of predicting cytosolic (hydrophilic) and transmembrane (hydrophobic) regions of a protein based on amino acid sequence and their polarity; it is usually displayed as hydropathy plot.

Hydropathy plots

See *hydropathy analysis*.

Hydrophilic

A molecule with a strong affinity for water.

Hydrophobic

A molecule with a low or no affinity for water.

Hyperglycaemia

High blood glucose levels, pathologically usually characteristic of diabetes.

Hyperplasia

Increase in the rate of proliferation of cells above the normal range.

Hyperpolarise

The potential difference is more negative than normal.

Hypertension/hypotension

High/low blood pressure.

Hypertrophy

Increase in cell volume above the normal range.

Hypnotic

Referring to a sleep-inducing substance.

Hypoxia

Reduced oxygen levels in the blood.

Immunisation

A process of exposing a foreign material or antigen into an organism to promote the production of antibodies against that particular antigen.

Immunocytochemistry

Technique that detects specific antigens in cells using antibodies that are labelled with either fluorescent dyes or enzymes such as horseradish peroxidase.

Immunocytokines
A hybrid molecule formed by binding a cytokine to a monoclonal antibody.

Immunoglobulins
Antibody peptides that always folds into the same functional structure.

Immunohistochemistry
Technique that detects specific antigens in tissues using antibodies that are labelled with either fluorescent dyes or enzymes such as horseradish peroxidase.

Immunoliposomes
A hybrid molecule bearing a liposome chemically coupled monoclonal antibody.

Immunoprecipitation
A frequently used method to purify specific proteins from complex samples such as cell lysates or extracts using antibodies.

Immunotherapeutics
A field of medicine to enhancing the immunity of an individual by administrating natural or artificially produced antibodies and adjuvants.

Immunotoxins
A hybrid molecule formed by binding a toxin to a monoclonal antibody to achieve cell specific destruction.

Importer
Transporter which moves substrate(s) in the inward direction.

In silico
Performed using a computer.

Inotropic
A drug which increases the force of muscle contraction.

***In situ* hybridisation**
A molecular biology technique that uses labelled complementary antisense nucleic acids to detect transcripts of interest in the tissue (i.e. *in situ*).

Integrin
Transmembrane receptor proteins that are involved in cell-cell interactions and cell-matrix interactions. They function as receptors for fibronectin, laminin and other extracellular adhesive glycoproteins.

Intergenic
Referring to a DNA sequence located between genes.

Interlukin
A subset of signalling molecules of the cytokine family.

Internalization
The loss or removal of receptors from the plasma membrane.

Intrachromosomal recombination
The result from the crossing over between two linked homologous DNA regions.

Intron
Nucleotide sequence between exons in DNA which does not code for protein.

Inverse agonist
Binds to the same receptor as an agonist but induces a pharmacological response opposite to a full or partial agonist.

Ion channel
Pore-forming proteins involved in the movement of ions across membranes.

Ionophore

Lipid-soluble molecules that can facilitate transport ions across cell membranes. They are usually synthesised by microorganisms and act by either shielding the charge on an ion or forming a hydrophilic pore that allows the ion to diffuse across the membrane unhindered.

Ionotropic

A neurotransmitter or receptor which mediates its effects via the modulation of ion channels.

Iontophoresis

Using a small current to cause movement of a substance. Used in the cystic fibrosis sweat test to cause pilocarpine to penetrate the skin and stimulate the sweat glands.

IP$_3$

Inositol 1,4,5 trisphosphate; a water soluble second messenger generated following the hydrolysis of phosphatidylinositol biphosphate (PIP$_2$) by phospholipase C. Triggers the release of Ca^{2+} from intracellular stores.

Ischaemia

Reduced blood flow due to a blockage of a blood vessel.

Isoelectric point

The pH value at which a protein carries no net charge. The protein will not move when placed in an electrical field.

Isogenic DNA

A chromosomal fragment of identical sequence to another one.

Knockin mouse

The result of introducing a gene or other exogenous DNA into the genome of a mouse, using the gene targeting protocol.

Knockout mouse

The loss of gene function that is achieved through the gene targeting technique; also referred to as null allele.

Leucine zipper

An example of a b-zip where leucine moieties on opposing protein subunits dimerise via their intercalation.

Ligand

A molecule that binds to a specific site on a protein.

Ligand-based virtual screening

Computer-based (*in silico*) screening of chemical libraries for compounds that display similar chemical features.

Ligase

See *DNA ligase*.

Linkage disequilibrium

A measure of how often alleles are inherited together.

Lipid kinase

An enzyme that transfers the terminal phosphate group of ATP to a specific amino acid of a target lipid.

Lipid rafts

A specialised plasma membrane domain that is enriched in specific lipids, cholesterol and proteins.

Lipolysis

The enzymatic breakdown of fats by hydrolysis.

Lipoplexes

Plasmids coated in lipids that are traditionally used in gene therapy to get nucleic acids into cells. However, they can also be used to transfer other substance such as peptides and drugs. Basically the cargo (DNA, RNA, peptides, drugs etc.) is encased in the lipid covered plasmid and endocytosed by target cells.

Loss-of-function mutation
The partial or total loss of the function of a gene due to a gene mutation.

Luciferase
A generic term for a class of oxidative enzymes which catalyse the production of light from the substrate luciferin.

Lumen
The space inside a tubular structure (e.g. pancreatic duct).

Luminescence
The act of emission of light from a chemical that does not require heat. Fluorescence is thus strictly a form of luminescence (photoluminescence). In a biological context luminescene is used to describe emission of light in the absence of excitation light.

Lysosome
An organelle that contains many digestive hydrolases present in animal cells.

Magnetic resonance imaging (MRI)
An imaging method based on the behaviour of atomic nuclei (particularly H) within a strong magnetic field.

Magnetofection
Use of a magnetic field in association with DNA coupled to magnetic particles to introduce DNA into cells.

Mass spectrometry
A powerful analytical technique that can be used for identifying chemicals based upon their mass-to-charge ratio. Widely used for identifying proteins and sequencing peptides.

Meiosis
The production of reproductive cells; see germ cells.

Membrane potential
Difference in concentration and valencey of charged ions and proteins across a membrane. This can generate a chemical and electrostatic gradient which can be used as a driving force for movement of substrate(s) across a membrane.

Methylation
A post-translational modification that adds methyl groups to proteins (see also *chromatin remodelling*).

Micelle
An aggregate of amphipathic molecules in water, so that the non-polar portions of the molecules amass in the interior whilst the polar portions at the exterior surface and hence the water interface.

Micro-array
A collection of protein or DNA molecules which are attached to a solid surface.

Mimetic peptide
Pseudopeptides that contain no peptide bonds. Used in drug discovery/design.

Modifying transcription factors
Factors involved in inducing (or repressing) gene expression in response to the demands of the cell.

Molecular cloning
A process that introduces an isolated piece of DNA into a vector (recombination) and generates multiple copies (clones) of it.

Molecular genetics
See reverse genetics.

Molecular Pharmacology
An area of pharmacology concerned with the study of drugs and their targets at the molecular or chemical level.

Monoallelic
Referring to a single allele.

Monoclonal Antibody
Antibodies that are made by identical immune cells and have monovalent affinity.

Morula
A stage of the embryonic development after cleavage of the zygote and prior to the blastocyst stage.

Mosaic mouse
An animal consisting of two populations of genetically different cells, all of which developed from the same fertilised oocyte (zygote).

Mucociliary escalator
Mucus produced by the respiratory tract traps dust, bacteria etc. and cilia clear it from the airways. It is an important defence mechanism of the respiratory tract.

Multiphoton confocal microscope
A confocal microscope that uses more than one photon to excite a fluorescent molecule. The excitiation wavelength is longer, so the energy of an individual photon is less than a conventional confocal. It requires two or more photons arrive almost simultaneously to excite the fluorophore. Multiphoton confocals can penetrate deeper into samples, have better spatial resolution, and are less likely to cause photobleaching than conventional confocal microscopes.

Mutagenesis
A process of causing genetic mutations.

Myocarditis
Inflammation of the myocardium layer of the heart.

Myristoylation
A post-translational modification of a protein which involves the covalent addition of the 14-carbon saturated fatty acid myristate.

Naked antibody
A natural state antibody molecule without any other molecules attached to it.

Neonate
Newborn.

Nephrotoxic
A substance that is nephrotoxic can damage the kidneys.

Neutral antagonist
An antagonist which binds to a GPCR without discriminating between the inactive or the active state and hence does change the level of receptor activity.

N-glycosylation
The attachment of a sugar residue to the nitrogen of asparagine or arginine side chains.

NMR spectroscopy
Nuclear magnetic resonance (NMR) spectroscopy is an analytical chemistry technique used for determining structure.

Nociception
Pain perception.

Non-coding RNA
A transcript that is not translated into protein.

Non-genic
Referring to a DNA sequence that does not contain a gene.

Non-synonymous

A single nucleotide polymorphism that changes a codon coding for one amino acid to a codon coding for a different amino acid.

Northern blotting

A molecular biology technique used to detect RNA expression in a tissue or cell using a cDNA probe.

Nuclear receptor

A class of proteins that detect a diverse family of ligands including steroid hormones and function as transcription factors.

Nuclear transfer

A technique that is used to generate a genetically identical copy (clone) of a living animal.

Null allele

see knockout mouse.

Olfactory

Referring to the sense of smell.

Oligonucleotide

A short RNA or DNA strand up to 100 bases in length.

One-dimensional (1D) gel electrophoresis

The separation of proteins based on their mass using sodium-dodecyl sulphate polyacrylamide gel electrophoresis (SDS-PAGE).

Oocyte

A female germ cell (i.e. egg).

Open channel probability

A term used in electrophysiology in connection with ion channel activity. It refers to the probability that a channel is open.

Open-reading frame

A piece of DNA that contains a series of translatable codons, but no stop codon.

Optical probe

The use of light to report on some aspect of cell physiology.

Orphan GPCR

A GPCR whose endogenous ligand is not known.

Orthologue

A gene that exists in different species as a consequence of speciation events during evolution. It has a common ancestral gene.

Orthosteric site

The primary binding on a GPCR for the endogenous ligand(s).

Ototoxicity

A substance that is ototoxic can damage hearing and or the sense of balance/movement, which reside in the inner ear.

p53 protein

A tumour suppressor protein that is involved in the regulation of gene expression.

Palmitoylation

A post-translational modification of a protein which involves the covalent addition of the 16-carbon saturated fatty acid palmitate.

Pancreatic insufficiency

Refers to the inability of the exocrine pancreas to supply enough digestive enzymes to properly digest food.

Pancreatitis

Inflammation of the pancreas.

Paracellular

Paracellular transport refers to movement across an epithelia layer that occurs around the sides of cells, rather than directly through the interior of cells. Thus substances will not need to cross plasma membranes in order to traverse epithelia, though it does require that the tight junctions are sufficiently leaky to allow the substance to pass.

Partial agonist

An agonist that produces sub-maximal functional responses despite full receptor occupancy.

Patch clamp electrophysiology

A method of investigating cellular bioelectrics that involves attaching the tip of a micropipette to a cell. There are four possible configurations. Cell attached, where the pipette is attached to the outside face of the membrane, whole cell, where the patch pipette is still attached to the cell, but the plasma membrane directly underneath the pipette has been permeabilised, or two forms of excised patch, where the patch pipette is removed from the cell, taking with it a patch of plasma membrane.

Pathogenic

Ability to cause disease.

PCR Polymerase chain reaction

A method for detection of nucleic acids by amplifying the number of specific sequences of DNA.

PDZ domain

A widespread structural domain of 80-90 amino acids found in many signalling proteins that binds to short concensus amino acid sequences.

Pharmacogenetics

An area of pharmacology which investigates the influence of genetic variation within a single gene on drug response to pharmaceuticals.

Pharmacokinetics

The process by which a drug is absorbed, distributed, metabolised, and eliminated by the body.

Phase I

Clinical trial testing of a drug on a small number of healthy volunteers. The aim is to assess drug safety, tolerability, pharmacokinetics and pharmacodynamics.

Phase II

Clinical trial larger scale trials and often involving patients.

Phase III

Clinical trial large randomised multicentre trials involving large patient groups.

Phasic activity (neuronal)

Some neurones exhibit phasic (bursting) activity.

Phenotype

The observable physical or biochemical characteristics of an organism.

Phosphatase

Enzyme that removes a phosphate group by hydrolysis.

Phosphodiesterase

An enzyme that catalyses the breakdown of the second messenger cyclic AMP or cyclic GMP.

Phospholamban

A protein that plays a vital role in regulating the activity of the sarcoplasmic reticulum Ca^{2+}-ATPase and hence cardiac muscle contractility.

Phospholipase A$_2$

An enzyme that catalyses the release of fatty acids from the second carbon of glycerol within phospholipids.

Phospholipase C
An enzyme that cleaves phospholipids. Typically associated with the hydrolysis of phosphatidyl-inositol biphosphate (PIP_2) to generate IP3 and DAG.

Phosphorylation
The addition of a phosphate monoester to a protein or other macromolecule, catalysed by a specific enzyme (kinase). Proteins can be phosphorylated on the amino acid side chains of serine, threonine and tyrosine. Phosphorylation can alter the conformation of a protein, resulting in modulation of the protein's activity.

Phylogenetic
Referring to the evolutionary relationship between different species.

PI-3K
Phosphoinositide 3-kinase; a family of enzymes that catalyses the addition of a phosphate group to membrane inositol containing phospholipids e.g. phosphatidyl-inositol 4,5 biphosphate (PIP_2) is phosphorylated producing phosphatidyl-inositol 3,4,5 trisphosphate (PIP_3).

Plasmid
A self-replicating piece of circular DNA.

Pluripotent
see embryonic stem cells.

Point mutation
A mutation affecting a single or a few of nucleotides (e.g. substitution, insertion, deletion).

Polyadenylation
The addition of multiple copies of adenosine monophosphate to mRNA. This affects the stability of mRNA and its export from the nucleus.

Polyclonal antibody
Antibodies that are obtained from different immune cell resources and consist of a combination of immunoglobulin molecules secreted against a specific antigen, each identifying a different epitope.

Polymerase chain reaction
The polymerase chain reaction (PCR) is used to amplify a specific DNA.

Polymorphisms
Genetic variations among individuals.

Polyplexes
Plasmids coated in polymers that are traditionally used in gene therapy to get nucleic acids into cells. However, they can also be used to transfer other substance such as peptides and drugs. Basically the cargo (DNA, RNA, peptides, drugs etc.) is encased in the polymer covered plasmid and endocytosed by target cells.

Pores
Also known as a channels, allows small substances to transverse membranes.

Post-translational modification
Enzyme catalysed change to a protein made after it is synthesised. Examples are cleavage, glycosylation, methylation, phosphorylation, prenylation and ubiquitination.

Prenylation
A post-translational modification of a protein which involves the covalent addition of the 16-carbon saturated fatty acid palmitate.

Promoter
A region of DNA, usually upstream of a gene that is involved in regulating that gene's expression.

Pronuclear injection
A technique used for the genetic manipulation of an organism; it involves the injection of DNA into the male pronucleus in a fertilised oocyte.

Pronucleus
A haploid paternal nucleus, in a fertilised oocyte, deriving from either the female egg or the male sperm.

Proteases
Enzymes that degrade proteins by cleaving peptide bonds.

Proteasome
A large multi-protein complex involved in the proteolytic degradation of proteins targeted to the proteasome by ubiquitination. The most common form of the proteasome is known as the 26S proteasome.

Protein A
Protein obtained from *Staphylococcus aureus* that binds immunoglobulin molecules without interfering with their binding to antigen. Widely used in purification of immunoglobulins and in antigen detection, for example immunoprecipitation.

Protein G
Immunoglobulin binding protein isolated from Streptococcal bacteria. Widely used in purification of immunoglobulins and in antigen detection, for example immunoprecipitation.

Protein kinase A (PKA)
Enzyme that phosphorylates target proteins in response to a rise in intracellular cyclic AMP. First identified in skeletal muscle as part of the pathway of regulation of glycogen breakdown in response to adrenaline.

Protein kinase
An enzyme that transfers the terminal phosphate group of ATP to a specific amino acid of a target protein.

Protein kinase C (PKC)
Enzyme that phosphorylates target proteins in response to increases in intracellular diacylglycerol.

Protein Phosphatase
Enzyme that removes a phosphate group from a protein by hydrolysis.

Protein phosphorylation
The addition of a phosphate monoester to a protein or other macromolecule, catalysed by a specific enzyme (kinase). Proteins can be phosphorylated on the amino acid side chains of serine, threonine and tyrosine. Phosphorylation can alter the conformation of a protein, resulting in modulation of the protein's activity.

Protein tag
A short peptide that is fused onto a gene product of interest to facilitate the subsequent detection of the fusion product, with a tag-specific antibody.

Proteomics
The study of the complete set of proteins (proteome) encoded by the genome.

Protomer
The individual unit of an oligomeric protein complex.

Pseudogene
A gene that has lost its capacity to generate functional proteins.

Pseudo-pregnant mouse
A female mouse that has been mated with a vasectomised male; it is false pregnant but shows the signs associated with pregnancy.

Quantum dots
Are nano-molecules that emit light of characteristic colours when irradiated with light of specific wavelengths. They can be used to label probes that detect proteins or nucleic acids. Since they are so small the possibility of interfering with the normal function of proteins or hybridization of nucleic acids is minimised.

Radioimmunoconjugates
Combinations of therapeutic radionucleotide linked with specific antibodies used to specifically target certain cancers.

Ras

A monomeric guanine nucleotide binding protein.

Ratiometric optical probe

An optical probe that uses the ratio of fluorescence at two wavelengths to report on some aspect of cell physiology. In a calcium sensitive ratiometric probe, the fluorescence at one wavelength will refer to the probe that has calcium bound to it, whilst the other wavelength reports on the calcium free probe. Ratiometric probes are much less susceptible to artifacts than single wavelength optical probes.

Reading frame

See *open-reading frame.*

Receptor

Protein that binds a specific extracellular signalling molecule (ligand) and initiates a response in the cell.

Recombinant DNA

A DNA molecule that has been generated by joining (recombining) DNA molecules, which potentially derive from two different sources.

Recombinant vector

A vector with an inserted fragment of foreign or cloned DNA, which is also transcribed during the plasmid's own replication process.

Rectifying channels

Pores that allow the passage of ions and/or small molecules through its channel in one direction only.

Reporter gene

A gene encoding a product that is visually or biochemically easy detectable; frequently used to label individual molecules or cells.

Resensitization

The recovery of a functional response following desensitization.

Restriction endonuclease

An enzyme that cuts DNA at specific sequences to produce discrete DNA fragments.

Restriction enzyme

See restriction endonuclease

Reverse genetics

An approach in genetics whereby a selected gene is modified in order to characterise the function of the encoded product.

Reverse transcriptase

Enzyme that catalyses the synthesis of cDNA from a RNA template.

RFLP (Restriction fragment length polymorphism)

Variations in DNA fragment patterns obtained following restriction enzyme digestion and viewed using agarose gel electrophoresis. Caused by genetic variations (polymorphisms) that alter restriction enzyme cleavage sites.

Rhodopsin

A GPCR that is involved in sensing light.

RNA editing

A post-transcriptional and dsRNA-dependent event, in which nuclear ADAR (adenosine deaminase acting on RNA) enzymes hydrolyse adenosine to inosine, at selected nucleotide positions.

RNA interference

A mechanism by which double-stranded RNA molecules are processed into single-strand RNA molecules that base-pair with mRNA which inhibits translation and gene expression.

Salt bridge

A non-covalent interaction, usually electrostatic attraction and hydrogen bonds. In proteins these weak interactions between amino acids can help form secondary/tertiary structures.

SDS-PAGE
Polyacrylamide gel electrophoresis (PAGE) in which proteins are separated according to molecular weight in the presence of sodium dodecyl sulphate (SDS).

Second messenger
Small molecule that is formed in or released in the cytosol in response to an extracellular signal and helps to relay the signal to the interior of the cell. Examples include cyclic AMP, IP_3 and Ca^{2+}.

Serine/threonine kinase
An enzyme that catalyses the addition of a phosphate group to the amino acid side chain of serine or threonine.

Single-nucleotide polymorphism
A DNA sequence variation involving a change in a single nucleotide.

Site-directed mutagenesis
A technique for specifically altering (*in vitro*) the sequence of DNA at a defined point.

Somatic cells
Any cell of a developed organism except the germ line cells (i.e. eggs and sperm).

Southern blot
A technique for the separation of DNA fragments followed by detection of specific segments.

Spermatozoa
A male germ cell (i.e. sperm).

Spiking activity (neuronal)
Some neurones exhibit very high firing rates.

Spirometry
Lung function tests performed using a spirometer which measures air flow into and out of the lungs.

Spliceosome
Ribonucleoprotein complexes involved in splicing and ligation of exons.

Splice variant
A protein variant produced as a consequence of alternative splicing.

Split-ubiquitin yeast two-hybrid assay
A genetic approach for studying protein-protein interactions involving soluble and membrane proteins.

Stoichiometry of a receptor
The subunit composition of a multimeric receptor.

Stop codon
Nucleotide triplet sequence in messenger RNA which signifies the termination of translation.

Structural fold
A characteristic spatial assembly of secondary protein structures (e.g. α-helices and β-sheets) into a domain-like structure that is common to many different proteins. A particular structural fold is often related to a certain function.

Superovulation
Hormone-induced multiple ovulations.

Symporter
Transporter that moves substrate(s) using a co-transporter substrate which travels in the same direction across the membrane.

Synonymous
A single nucleotide polymorphism that does not alter the encoded amino acid.

Syntenic
Refers to genes which are located on the same chromosomal region; the existence of corresponding syntenic regions in the genomes of different organisms indicates evolutionary conservation of the arrangement of the genomes into chromosomes.

Targeting vector
A vector used in gene targeting for the modification of a predetermined chromosomal site.

Tonic activity (neuronal)
Some neurones are constantly active (firing).

Topology mapping
Method of predicting secondary and tertiary (folds) protein structure based on amino acid sequence.

Topology
The arrangement of protein sequences into hydrophobic and hydrophilic domains for the identification of membrane spanning domains. Especially useful in determining the two-dimensional structure of protein.

Trafficking
The intracellular movement of proteins or vesicles from one cellular compartment to another.

Trans-acting factors
DNA has two strands and trans factors interact across both strands for example transcription factors.

Transcription factor
A protein that regulates gene expression by binding to a specific DNA sequence.

Transcriptome
The entire collection of RNA transcripts generated by a genome.

Transfection
A process of deliberately introducing DNA or other nucleic acids into cells.

Transgene
The artificial transmission of a gene or exogenous DNA (e.g. a cDNA) into the genome of an animal a gene that may derive from a different species (heterologous gene).

Transgenic
See *transgene*.

Transporters
Membrane embedded protein(s) that facilitate the movement of ions, small molecules and peptides across the lipid bilayer.

Transposon
A small, mobile DNA element with the ability to replicate independently and insert itself into a new location of the genome.

Triplet
See *genetic code*.

Two-dimensional (2D) gel electrophoresis
The separation of proteins using two different properties of the protein. Usually begins with the separation of proteins based upon their isoelectric point using pH gradients (the first dimension) and followed by their separation based on mass (second dimension). This allows proteins with the same mass but different isoelectric point to be resolved.

Tyrosine kinase
Enzyme that catalyses the addition of a phosphate monoester to the amino acid side chain of tyrosine.

Ubiquitin
A small highly conserved protein of 76 amino acids that when covalently attached to other proteins functions as a signal for their degradation by the 26S proteasome.

Ubiquitination
The post-translational modification of proteins by the covalent addition of the protein ubiquitin.

Uniporter
Transporter that moves substrate(s) across the membrane without the using a co-transporter substrate to generate the energy for translocation.

Vasectomy
The sterilisation of a male through surgical interruption of the vas deferens.

Vasodilation/constriction
Occurs due to the lumen of a blood vessel either increasing or narrowing respectively. Important in determining blood pressure.

Walker domain
Characteristic domains found in ATP-binding proteins.

Western blot
Technique by which proteins are separated and immobilised on a paper sheet (membrane) and then analysed, usually by means of a labelled antibody.

Xenobiotic
A compound foreign to an organism.

X-ray crystallography
When a beam of electrons (X rays) strike a crystal they are diffracted. The angle and intensity of the diffraction depends upon the relative position of atoms as well as the chemical bonds employed. Extrapolation of the diffraction data enables the 3-D arrangement of structures such as nucleic acids and proteins to be determined.

Yeast two-hybrid assay
A genetic based approach for studying protein-protein interactions which is restricted to soluble proteins.

Zygote
The cell that results from the fusion of an oocyte and a sperm, and their pronuclei, after fertilisation.

α-helix
Secondary protein structure where amino acids interact to form a coiled structure (usually right-handed).

β-sheet
Secondary protein structure where chains of amino acids (peptides) interact with an adjacent parallel peptide chain to form a sheet like structure.

Index

References to figures are given in italic type. References to tables are given in bold type.

Molecular Pharmacology: From DNA to Drug Discovery, First Edition. John Dickenson, Fiona Freeman, Chris Lloyd Mills, Shiva Sivasubramaniam and Christian Thode.
© 2013 John Wiley & Sons, Ltd. Published 2013 by John Wiley & Sons, Ltd.